LOCAL FLAPS IN HEAD AND NECK RECONSTRUCTION

LOCAL FLAPS IN HEAD AND NECK RECONSTRUCTION

IAN T. JACKSON, M.D., F.R.C.S., F.A.C.S.

Head, Section of Plastic Surgery, The Mayo Clinics;
Professor of Plastic Surgery, Division of Plastic and Reconstructive Surgery,
Mayo Medical School, University of Minnesota,
Rochester, Minnesota

with 1090 illustrations

THE C. V. MOSBY COMPANY

ST. LOUIS · TORONTO · PRINCETON   1985

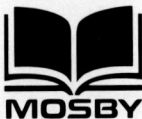

A TRADITION OF PUBLISHING EXCELLENCE

Editor: Karen Berger
Assistant editor: Sandra L. Gilfillan
Manuscript editor: Carlotta Seely
Designer: Jeanne Genz
Production: Mary G. Stueck, Suzanne C. Glazer

Copyright © 1985 by The C.V. Mosby Company

All rights reserved. No part of this publication may be reproduced, stored in a retrieval system, or transmitted, in any form or by any means, electronic, mechanical, photocopying, recording, or otherwise, without prior written permission from the publisher.

Printed in the United States of America

The C.V. Mosby Company
11830 Westline Industrial Drive, St. Louis, Missouri 63146

Library of Congress Cataloging in Publication Data

Jackson, Ian T.
  Local flaps in head and neck reconstruction.

  Includes bibliographies and index.
  1. Flaps (Surgery) 2. Head—Surgery. 3. Neck—Surgery. 4. Surgery, Plastic. I. Title. [DNLM:
1. Head—surgery. 2. Neck—surgery. 3. Surgical Flaps.
WE 705 J12f]
RD521.J285   1985   617'.510592   85-8844
ISBN 0-8016-2380-4

C/MV/MV 9 8 7 6 5 4 3 2 1   12/B/216

PREFACE

Facial reconstruction involves important choices for both patient and surgeon. The patient seeks the best possible reconstruction with the most natural-looking results. The surgeon, in an attempt to solve the patient's problem, often must decide whether to perform a quick reconstruction to cover a defect or carry out a carefully considered but more involved surgical procedure that combines an appreciation of form and function with an understanding of tumor biology. Complete tumor resection is always the first consideration and must never be compromised for reconstruction.

With each patient the surgeon must strive to attain the best possible result in facial reconstruction. This frequently presents a considerable challenge. Attention to detail is of critical importance, and each type of facial defect deserves the surgeon's complete skill and attention.

The ability to plan reconstructive surgery in the abstract comes only with experience. Thus in the early stages of one's practice the results of reconstructive facial surgery can be humbling. Competence and skill in these techniques can be achieved only through study, patience, and practice. Having lived through this painful process myself, I have attempted to translate my experience into the written word through this structured guide to learning the art of local facial flap surgery.

The book is organized according to the various regions of the face. The individual anatomic, aesthetic, and functional characteristics of each region are presented to ensure that these basic factors are not forgotten or ignored in the planning of reconstructive surgical procedures. Photographs of surgical series have been included where possible. These, together with Bill Westwood's superb drawings, provide step-by-step illustrations of each procedure presented in the text. I sincerely hope that this establishes a clear understanding of the fascinating array of available local facial flaps.

It is not the purpose of this book to present all the techniques for facial reconstruction that are used today; rather, it is to offer a detailed presentation of the approaches that I have found to be most successful for various facial defects. Viable alternatives are considered and examined, and their positive and negative aspects are discussed. An extensive bibliography is supplied for those who wish to delve deeply into the history and development of facial flaps.

It must be understood that the production of a book such as this would be impossible without assistance and cooperation from many quarters. I would be remiss in not mentioning several individuals who have worked with me on this undertaking.

I have greatly appreciated all the help, criticism, and encouragement given to me by Karen Berger, Editor-in-Chief, Clinical Medicine, of the C.V. Mosby Company. She and her Assistant Editor, Sandy Gilfillan, never hesitated to "go the extra mile" to ensure quality of production. Carlotta Seely, Senior Manuscript Editor, and Mary Stueck, Senior Production Assistant, cheerfully accepted text changes and extensive rearrangement of illustrations and by their skill and experience produced an end product beyond my initial expectations.

Bill Westwood was recommended to me as an excellent medical artist, and that he is. However, during the course of this project he became a good friend. What better spin-off could one have!

In an enterprise such as this, a good secretary is essential, and I wish to offer my heartfelt thanks to Jean Heiman. She has been the powerhouse of this whole project and, despite the undoubted stress that it has caused, remains my clinical secretary. The fact that she is still with me demonstrates her commitment to completing this book; there could have been no greater test to this relationship.

The other person who during this time has had added cause to leave me to my own devices is my wife, Marjorie. Fortunately, she has survived the ordeal and, as always, continues to be my constant encouragement in all my literary efforts.

Ian T. Jackson, M.D.

CONTENTS

1 General considerations, 1

2 Patient management, 35

3 Forehead reconstruction, 43

4 Nose reconstruction, 87

5 Cheek reconstruction, 189

6 Ear reconstruction, 251

7 Eyelid and canthal region reconstruction, 273

8 Lip reconstruction, 327

Bibliography, 413

Acknowledgments, 439

CHAPTER 1

GENERAL CONSIDERATIONS

*And ne'er did Grecian chisel trace
A Nymph, A Naiad or a Grace
of finer form or lovelier face!*

SIR WALTER SCOTT
The Lady of the Lake

*It is the common wonder of all men,
how among so many millions of faces,
there should be none alike.*

SIR THOMAS BROWNE
Religio Medici

The face and its features have been the subject of poetic and artistic endeavors throughout the ages. Because a person's face is highly visible and difficult to camouflage, any scars or imperfections are obvious to others and may be distressing to the affected individual. Particular skill is required of the surgeon reconstructing facial defects because the cosmetic result will have physical and psychologic implications for the patient. The surgeon's goal is to avoid unsightly scars while using the simplest, most effective reconstructive approach.

■ ADVANTAGES OF LOCAL FLAPS

Local flaps of donor tissue obtained from the area surrounding the defect provide an ideal solution for the problems encountered in facial reconstruction. With these flaps, skin used for reconstruction is likely to be similar in color and texture to the skin at the site of the defect. In addition, minor procedures can be performed as outpatient surgery under local anesthesia, and secondary defects can frequently be closed directly.

It can be argued that skin grafts are just as effective as local flaps and easier to perform. In fact, full-thickness skin grafts from the retroauricular area and the upper eyelids are satisfactory for use on the eyelids and the medial canthal areas. Nasolabial skin also has been used as a free full-thickness graft for the nose. Unfortunately, however, grafts do not have a 100% survival rate. Also, they often become paler or more pigmented than the surrounding skin. Occasionally the graft becomes pinker.

The theory that skin cancer is best treated by excision, skin grafting, and observation is fallacious because it ignores the possibility that excision of the tumor may be incomplete. There may be a limited resection in depth to maintain a vascular layer that will accommodate a skin graft. This is a frequent occurrence in the medial canthal area and has dire consequences for the patient. To ensure total resection, it is better for the surgeon to perform radical excision down to and including bone, if necessary, and then reconstruct with a local flap. In full-thickness defects of the nose, lips, eyelids, and ear, flap reconstruction is mandatory.

Functionally, flaps are much better than grafts because little or no scar contracture occurs. Thus ectropion and epiphora and loss of oral competence are prevented. A flap provides an additional blood supply, which is important in lower lip reconstruction where the tongue flap is used and in cases involving previous radiotherapy (see Chapter 8).

A surgeon who is experienced in the use of local flaps and plans the procedure carefully almost always succeeds with this type of surgery. Not only do local flaps provide better oncologic and functional results; they also offer the best aesthetic solution for the patient because the skin is the correct color and texture.

■ DISADVANTAGES OF SKIN FLAPS

The greatest drawback to the use of skin flaps is that they require planning and experience. If the flap is not planned properly, functional problems can occur; examples are ectropion and nasal obstruction. If functional complications occur, concurrent aesthetic complications frequently will result from scarring and distortion. In addition, skin of the wrong color and texture may be used, hairbearing skin may be moved into an area where hair is not normally present, or the flap may be too thick and bulky. When designing a flap, the surgeon should ensure that it is the same size and thickness as the defect to be reconstructed.

Local flaps are easy to use in the older patient but much less so in children because excess skin is not available. Scarring and distortion caused by rearrangement of local anatomy also is more of a problem with children.

For patients of all ages local anatomic landmarks, such as the temporal hairline and eyebrows, must be preserved because a poorly planned flap will alter the position of a mobile landmark and therefore cause obvious asymmetry.

When a flap fails, an area of tissue availability has been exhausted, and the surgeon must then use the less desirable skin graft. Since the graft is then a secondary reconstruction, more scarring and more functional and aesthetic deformity will result. This consequence further supports the need for close study of the design and use of skin flaps.

■ GENERAL PRINCIPLES

To use local flaps effectively, the plastic surgeon needs more than a simple understanding of the different techniques available for moving tissue. He must first understand some of the general principles governing the use of local flaps. Knowledge of geometry, skin biomechanics, and facial anatomy must be combined with a sense of aesthetics and an appreciation for shape, symmetry, and color. After identifying the areas of tissue availability and examining the defect, the surgeon needs information on the general and specific types of skin flaps, the principles by which these flaps are moved, and the advantages, disadvantages, and complications associated with these flaps. Finally, the surgeon must consider all this information and carefully plan the appropriate approach for each individual patient in order to achieve the best aesthetic result.

☐ Skin Biomechanics

Fundamental knowledge about the basic characteristics of skin is necessary in almost every surgical maneuver involving closure of a skin defect or tightening of skin.[7] Extension of skin is a mechanical property that is time dependent; continuing tension produces ongoing lengthening to a point. As skin stretches, because of increased load or force, a contraction occurs at right angles to the line of extension. Many materials, such as elastic, become narrower as they are stretched. In vivo this further increases the vascular compromise that results from the original stretching. It has been noted in vitro that the volume of the skin decreases with stretching (i.e., it becomes thinner), probably because of fluid extruding from its undersurface.

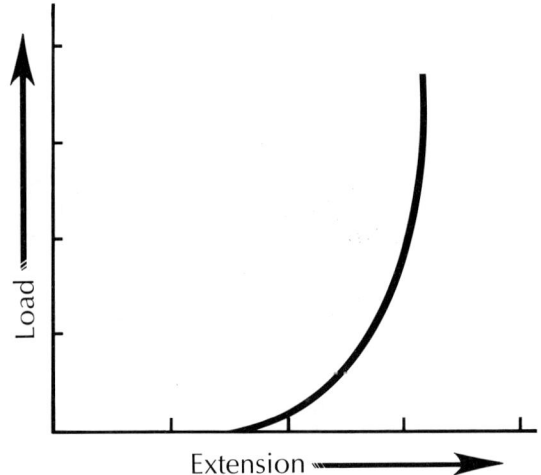

A graph of the in vitro extension curve shows great initial stretch with a small load. The upward sweep indicates that a small increase is obtained with rapidly increasing load, and the vertical part illustrates that after a certain amount of extension the skin will not stretch any further, no matter how much the load increases. In the clinical situation a balance between stretching and vascularity occurs. When the skin has been stretched beyond safe limits, there is likely to be a compromised circulation, with blanching and eventual distal necrosis of the flap tissue. Thus, to effectively plan surgery, the surgeon needs to understand two main characteristics of skin biomechanics: stress relaxation and creep.

STRESS RELAXATION AND CREEP

If a constant loading or stretching force is applied to any material, it will exhibit stress relaxation or creep. *Stress relaxation* occurs when a constant load applied to skin causes it to stretch. With time, the load required to maintain the skin in its stretched position decreases. *Creep* occurs when a sudden load applied to skin is kept constant. The amount of extension increases with the passage of time. Stress relaxation and creep are termed the *viscoelastic properties* of skin. The extent to which these phenomena occur depends on the size of the load applied and other factors, such as the extrusion of fluid from the skin framework, the stretching and subsequent compacting of the framework fibers, and the viscoelastic behavior of the collagen bundles.

What is the practical value of this phenomenon? In many situations it is necessary for the surgeon to use his knowledge of stress relaxation and creep; otherwise he would be unable to close many defects. Because the skin stretches, skin flaps can be taken and placed into larger defects without a resulting skin shortage or tightness. For example, in the case of a scalp flap that is too tight, if one pulls on the flap as hard and as steadily as possible for 5 to 10 minutes, stress relaxation and creep come into play, and the skin stretches and produces a closure under normal tension. The intrinsic viscoelastic qualities of skin may be the saving grace for many flaps, allowing the flap to fill a defect that is larger than the actual flap area. The tight suture line actually causes the flap to lengthen, and so the flap changes from white to pink, a positive sign.

An obvious antagonistic relationship exists between tension and vascularity, and the surgeon must judge the appropriate amount of extension the skin will permit before its blood supply is compromised. No measurements or theories can substitute for sound clinical judgment. For some surgeons, such judgment is second nature; for others, it comes by experience. However, this helpful aphorism should be imprinted indelibly in every plastic surgeon's mind: "On the face white flaps are safe flaps; they become pink."

Tissue expanders, which are used to supply local skin for large defects, rely primarily on the biomechanic phenomena outlined above.

■ PLANNING THE SURGICAL APPROACH
☐ Areas of Tissue Availability

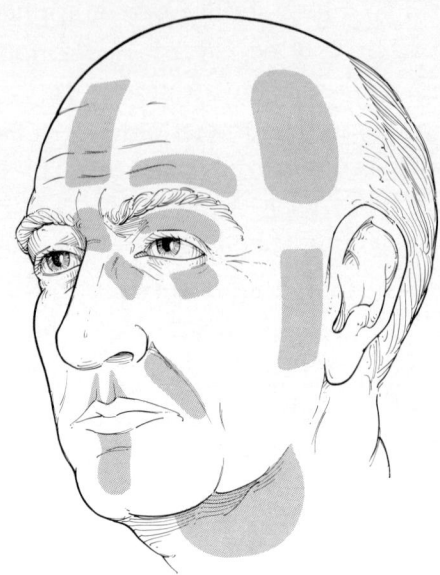

For effective use of local facial flaps, excess facial skin must be available. The regions containing this extra skin, called *areas of tissue availability*, need to be inspected carefully during the planning stages.

As a person ages, the amount of skin present in these areas (except for the lips) becomes more plentiful and aging lines or wrinkles appear. In biomechanics these are referred to as *lines of minimal relaxed tension*; that is, the skin tension is least at right angles to these lines and thus in this direction there is loose skin available for reconstruction.[3] Fortunately, skin cancer usually appears in older patients; since skin stretchability increases with age, more skin is available for reconstructing the defects left from tumor excision in these patients. Reconstruction of skin defects in the young is more challenging because of the reduced amount of donor tissue available.

☐ Examination of the Defect and Donor Area

The area of the proposed defect should be inspected to determine the best position for flap placement. Incision lines for the flap and donor area should fall into the lines of minimal relaxed tension. In this way the scars will heal effectively because they will have a minimal transverse force on them. In addition, if incisions are placed in this position, they will lie on the aging lines of the face and will be as inconspicuous as possible.

The skin surrounding the area to be reconstructed is also carefully examined. In the early planning stage the requirements for skin type and quantity are determined. Donor skin, which should be approximate the color and texture of the recipient area, must be of sufficient quantity to reconstruct the total surface contour.

☐ **Methods of Skin Movement**

GENERAL PRINCIPLES

Rotation

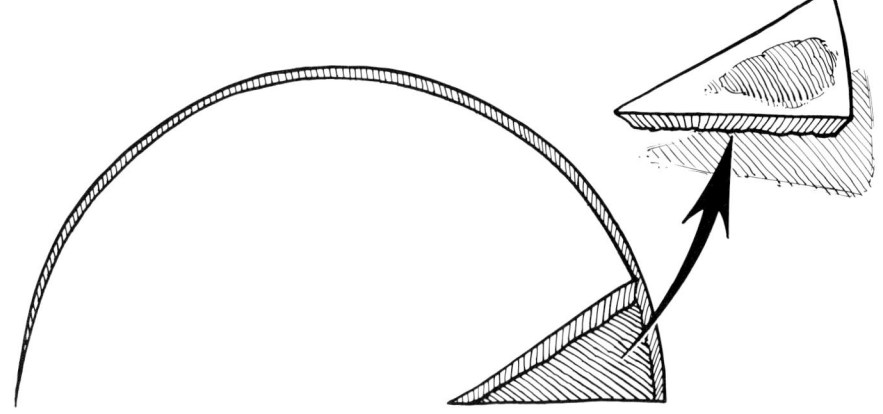

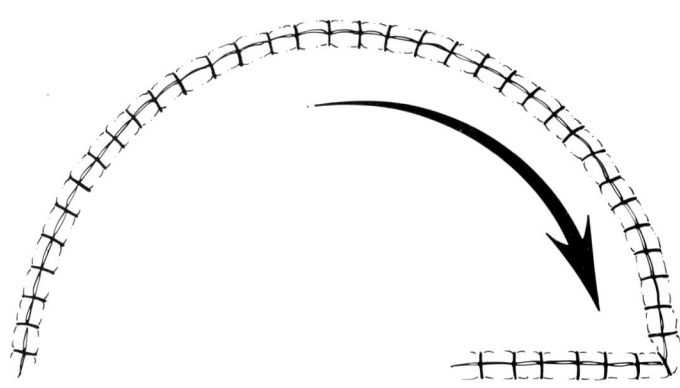

In this classic rotation method[9,10] the surgeon triangulates the defect, making the shortest side the base of the triangle. The base then forms a portion of the circumference of a circle, and a flap is constructed so that its leading tip will rotate around the circumference of the circle on which the triangular defect lies. In effect, the base of the flap is the radius of the large circle. When the flap is elevated, it can be rotated to close the defect. In situations where sufficient flap rotation is not possible, because of local circumstances such as skin tension or contour problems, a *back cut* is necessary. With a back cut, an incision is made toward the center of the circle; this allows a defect to open and makes further rotation possible. Usually the back cut is closed directly.

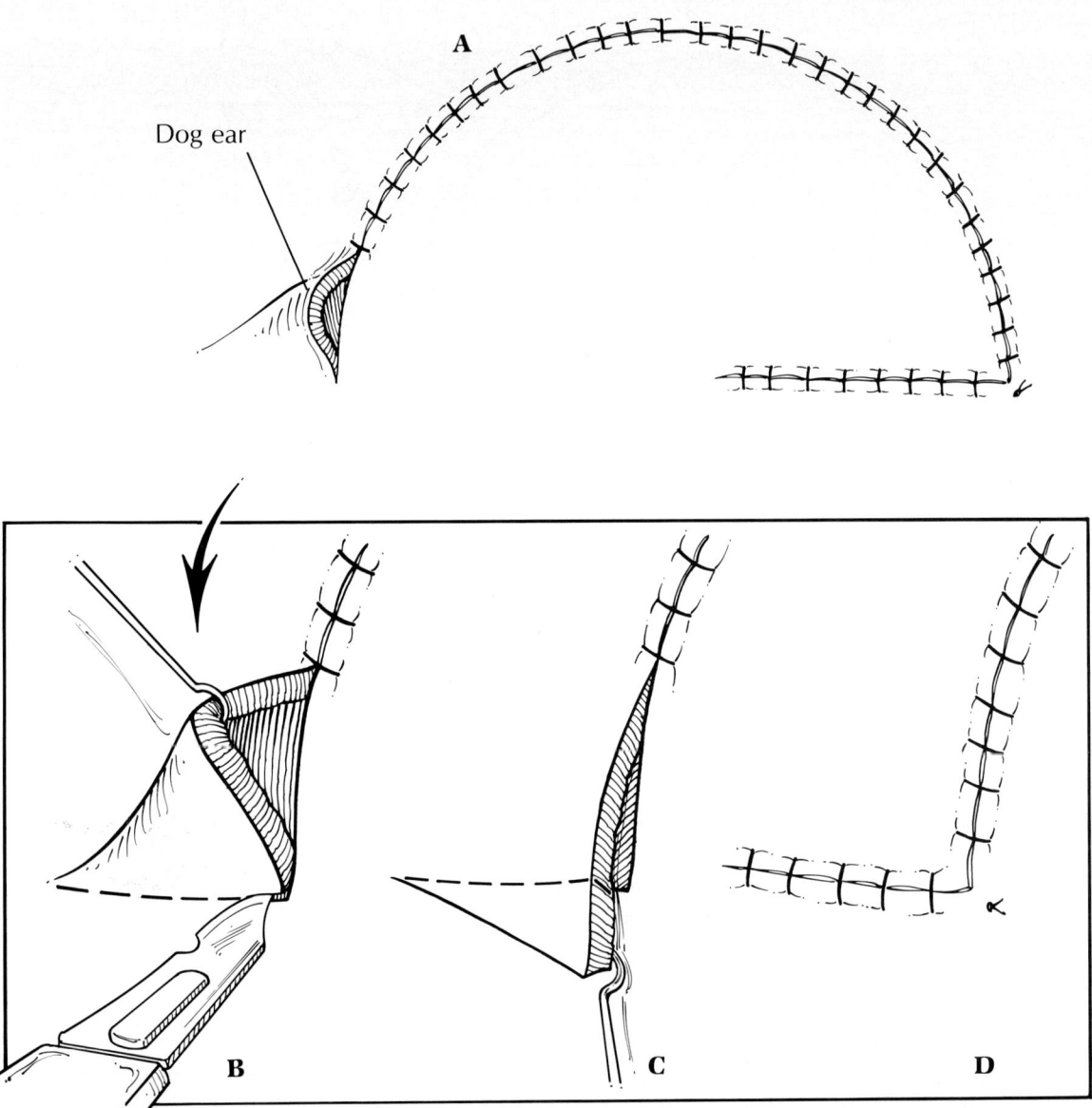

In cases where a rotation flap has been used without a back cut, the wound has a short inner edge and a longer outer edge. The excess of outer skin becomes a "dog ear" that is excised away from the flap. In this way there is no compromise of the flap base. The rotation flap works very well on convexities such as the malar area or the scalp.

A piece of gauze is used to assess whether a rotation flap will do what is required. The gauze is stabilized on the pivot point of the flap, and the rotation is checked.

CHAPTER 1
GENERAL CONSIDERATIONS

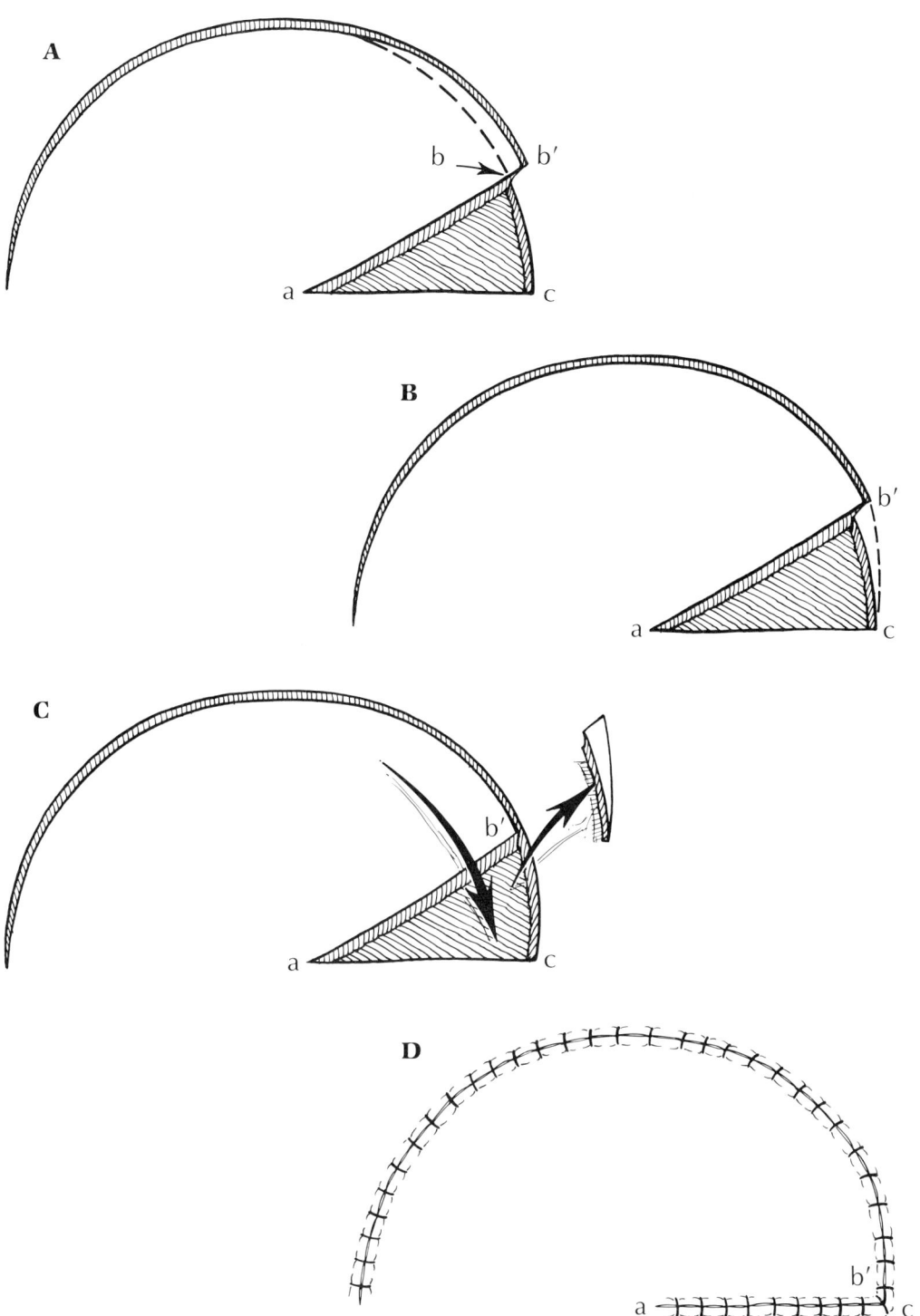

If the rotation flap is planned and a trial of rotation reveals that the flap will not close the defect without undue tension, the maneuver illustrated here should be used. The circumference of the rotation flap is moved out from b to b', thus lengthening the leading edge of the flap. On rotation, the defect is now closed comfortably. A small portion of skin may need to be excised from the outer edge of the defect to allow the flap to be inset in a more satisfactory fashion.

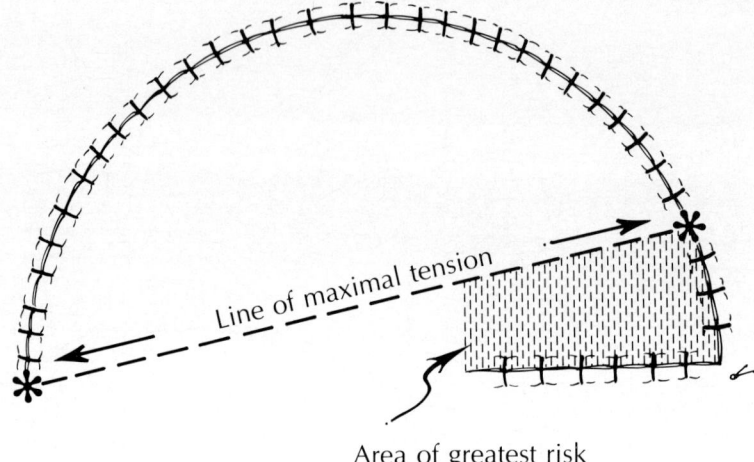

Area of greatest risk

In a rotation flap the line of greatest tension extends from the pivot point of the flap to where the edge of the defect nearest to the flap previously lay. If there is undue tension along this line, the area of the flap covering the defect will become ischemic and may not survive. Much of the movement of the rotation flap and of the transposition flap that follows is not consistent with mathematic analysis because of the biomechanic features of stretching skin described earlier.

Transposition

It is difficult to differentiate between rotation flaps and transposition flaps because they share certain characteristics of skin movement. The required flap movement may be small when the defect is immediately adjacent, or it may be taken farther around the circle of which the flap diagonal is the radius. The maximal possible transposition of the flap is 90 degrees from its original position.

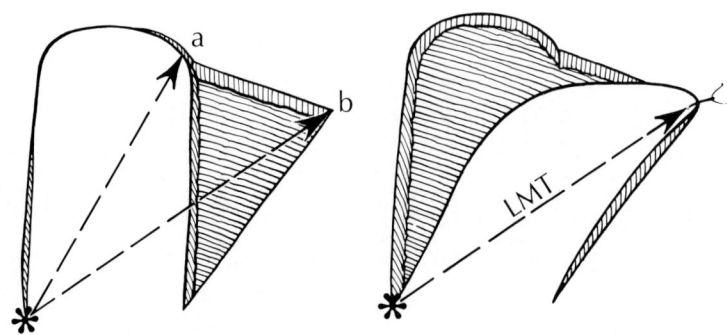

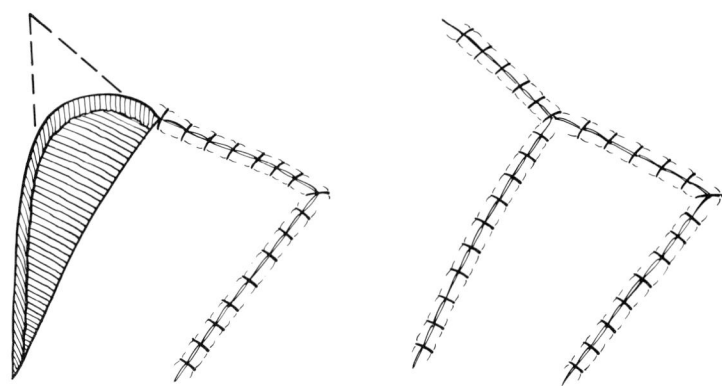

The transposition flap is rectangular and has rounded angles. When the defect is adjacent to the flap, it is triangulated. As with the rotation flap, the possible flap movement is assessed preoperatively with gauze. It is usually necessary to extend the flap beyond the defect because the flap becomes shorter as it rotates. If closure is difficult, a back cut may be used to give a little extra rotation. When a back cut is used, the pivot point changes and the circle of rotation is moved beyond the original circle of rotation; thus tension on the flap is reduced. The line of maximal tension (LMT) runs diagonally across the flap in such a direction that the most important portion of the flap will necrose if tension is excessive.

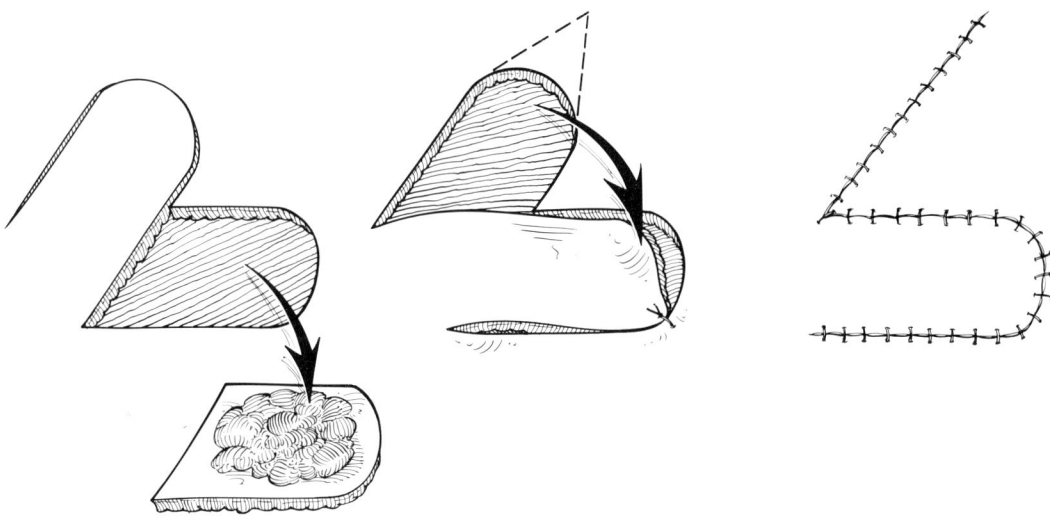

When the flap is transposed over a larger distance, for example, 90 degrees, there is an interpositional area of intact skin; it is usually possible to close all areas primarily. It may be necessary to trim the flap a little to obtain an exact fit into the defect. At the upper end of the donor site defect, a triangle of skin will be excised to facilitate direct closure.

Advancement

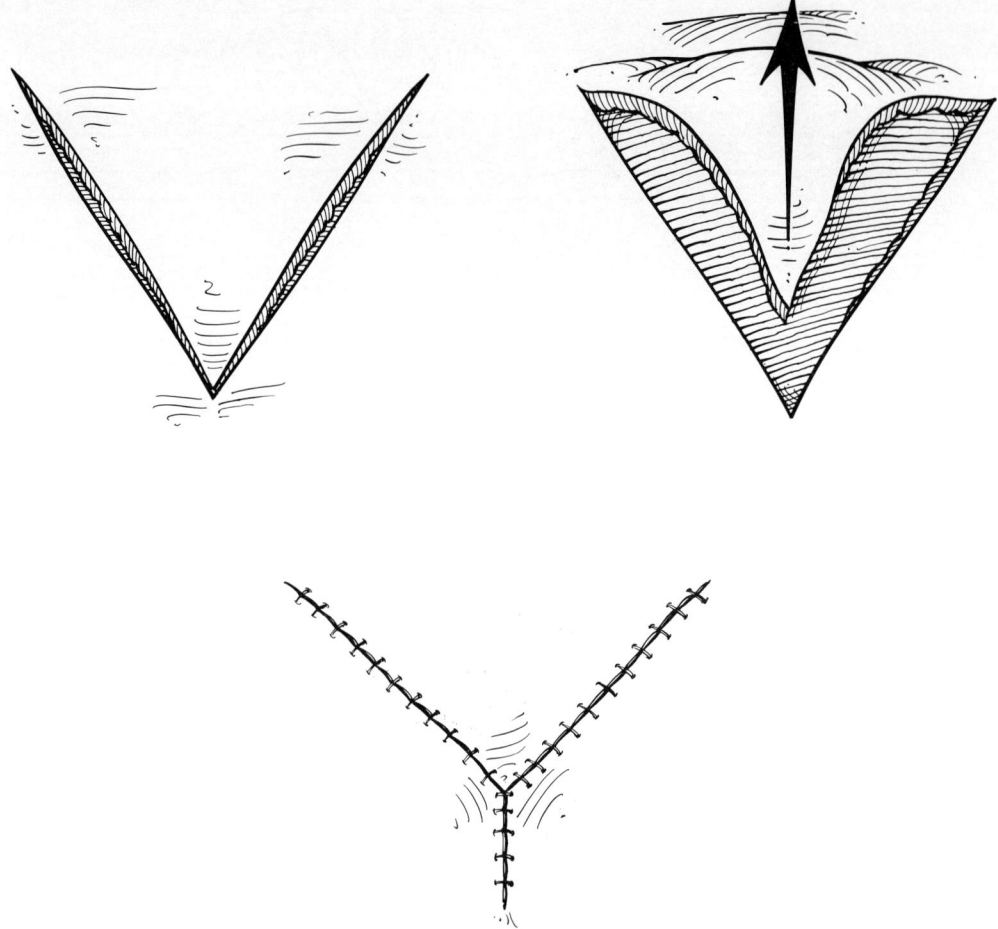

Although there are various types of advancement, the basic procedure is the same. As the name implies, this method of tissue movement involves sliding tissue forward for defect closure or for augmentation (e.g., to eliminate a notch in the lip margin after trauma or cleft repair). The simplest type of movement is the V-Y advancement. The skin is lifted as a V, moved forward, with direct closure of the posterior defect; thus a Y-shaped suture line is formed. The skin to be advanced can be converted into a triangular island flap that can be used to close a rectangular defect lying in front of the triangle. (For more information, see p. 235.) The extra movement is obtained as a result of the vertical subcutaneous pedicle lying below the island of skin.

CHAPTER 1
GENERAL CONSIDERATIONS

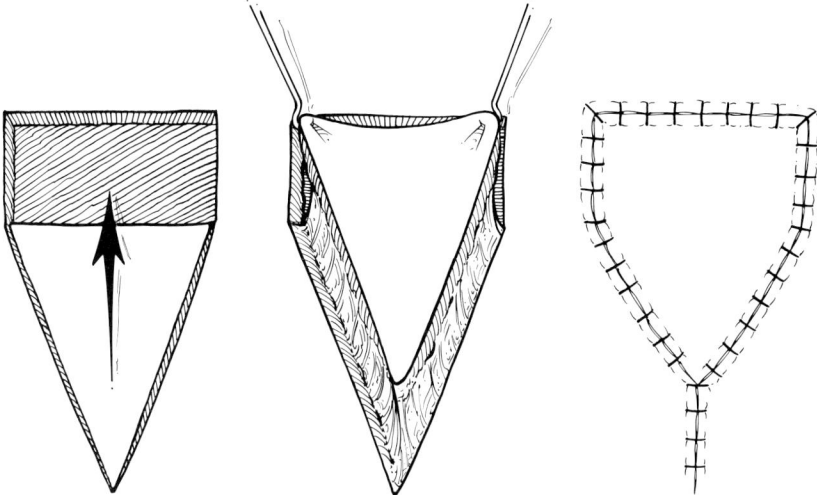

Another type of advancement flap is the direct type used for coverage of square defects. One of the sides of the square is chosen for donor tissue because of tissue availability, and a rectangular flap is drawn. This flap is elevated to its base and advanced. In some situations this is all that is necessary.

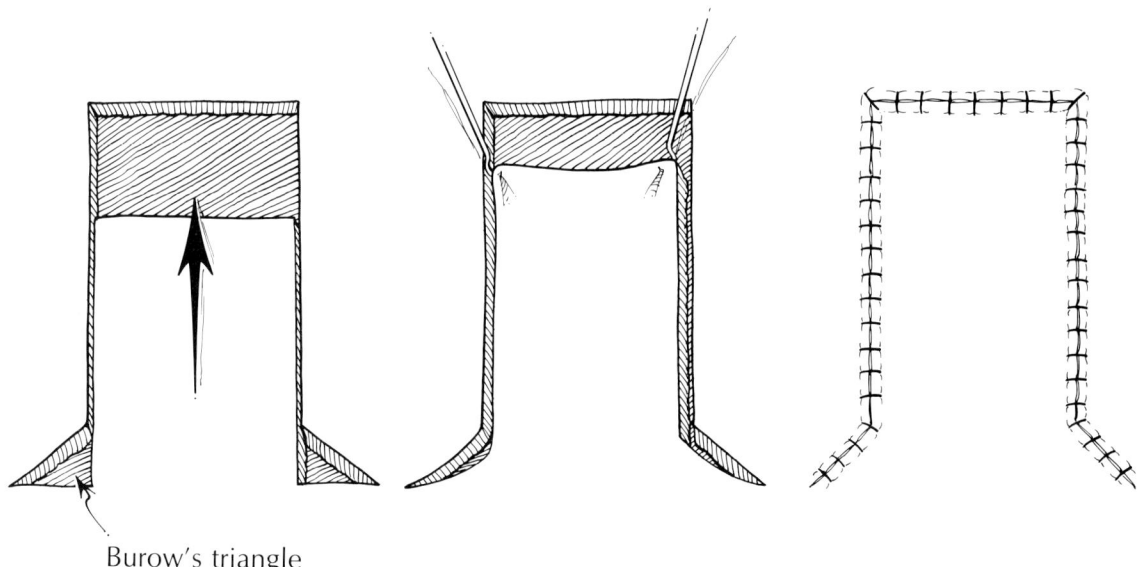

Burow's triangle

In others excess skin appears laterally as Burow's triangles. These triangles are excised lateral to the flap base.

Advancement flaps are very safe and probably underused.

Island Technique

Island flaps are of two types, depending on the flap blood supply. In one type the base is subcutaneous tissue without definite blood vessels. Of necessity, the flap pedicle is short and the arc of rotation is therefore limited. In the second type there is a definite vascular pedicle (e.g., temporal vessels); thus the pedicle can be longer and the arc of rotation more extensive.

The tumor is excised, and a defect is created. The surgeon then designs and marks the island, making sure that its arc of rotation allows it to move in such as way as to close the defect. If the flap has a subcutaneous pedicle, the pedicle is dissected out from under the skin and elevated from the underlying fascia.

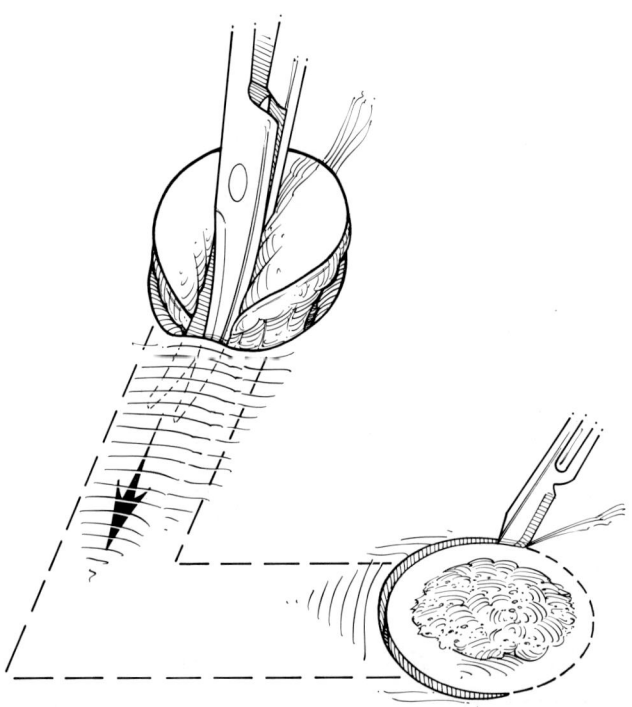

A tunnel is then made from the defect to the pedicle base.

CHAPTER 1
GENERAL CONSIDERATIONS

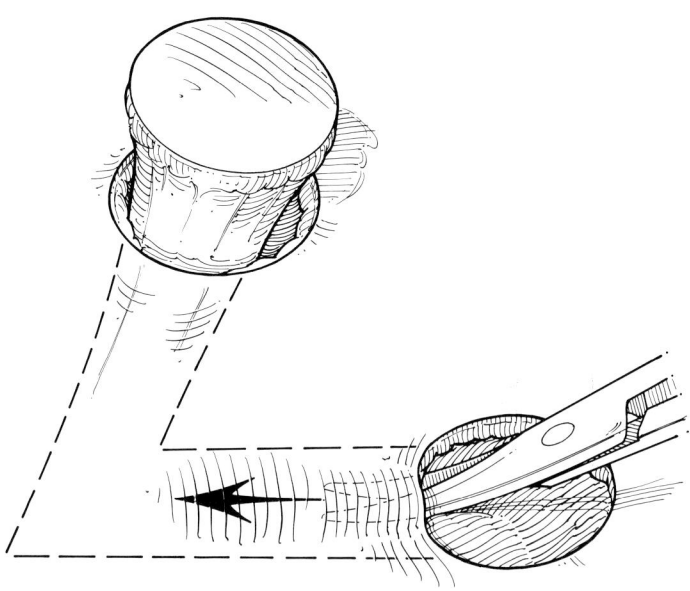

The island flap is transposed through the tunnel and into the defect.

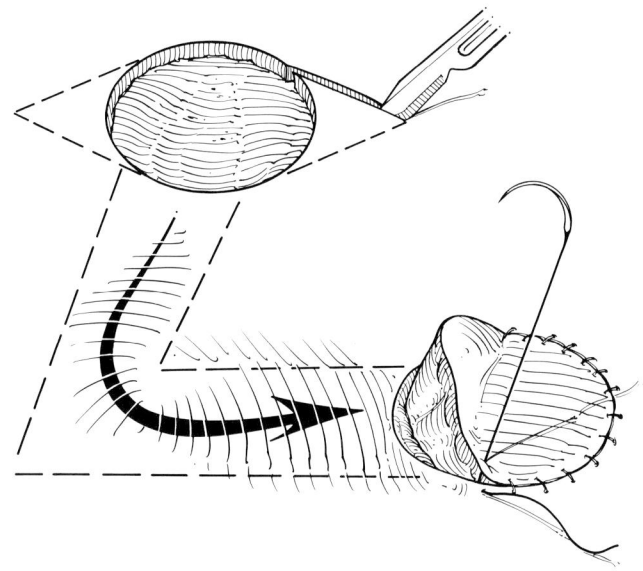

In a flap with a true vascular pedicle the vessels may be dissected out, allowing great facility of movement. The arc of rotation may be 180 degrees.

A particular variety of island flap, alluded to under advancement flaps, has a subcutaneous pedicle lying directly under the flap. It is extremely safe, but movement is limited to advancement. There is no arc of rotation (see p. 12).

In planning island flaps, the surgeon should not make the flap pedicle too long without a definite vessel because ischemia may occur. It is also important to create an adequately large tunnel to avoid constriction of the pedicle as a result of postoperative swelling. Such constriction may result in ischemia and necrosis of the flap.

☐ Specific Types of Local Flaps

Having discussed the various methods of skin movement, it is important to examine how these principles are incorporated into and modified in the commonly used local flaps.

RHOMBOID (LIMBERG) FLAP

Introduced by Limberg[11] in 1946 and further enlarged upon by him and others (see general bibliography), the rhomboid flap is an interesting procedure for skin movement in which a rhomboid defect is created and then closed with a rhomboid-shaped flap of a similar size.

The lesion is excised as a rhomboid. The orientation is such that the 120-degree angle of the rhomboid is placed where the excess of skin lies, the position of which is judged by pinching the skin between thumb and forefinger. This excess will form the rhomboid flap. An additional consideration is the position of the donor defect; it should lie, if possible, in the long axis of a line of minimal tension. Its closure should not distort local anatomic features such as hairline or eyebrow.

In designing a rhomboid flap, the surgeon draws a line from the outer point of the 120-degree angle; this line bisects the angle, with its length being equal to that of the side of the rhomboid. From the outer point of this line, another line is drawn at 60 degrees parallel to the side of the rhomboid defect. Its length again equals that of the side of the rhomboid. Before any incisions are made a further check of skin availability is made with thumb and forefinger. This checking procedure ensures that the donor defect will close. If it will not, the original rhomboid may be changed in position or another donor flap can be used.

CHAPTER 1
GENERAL CONSIDERATIONS

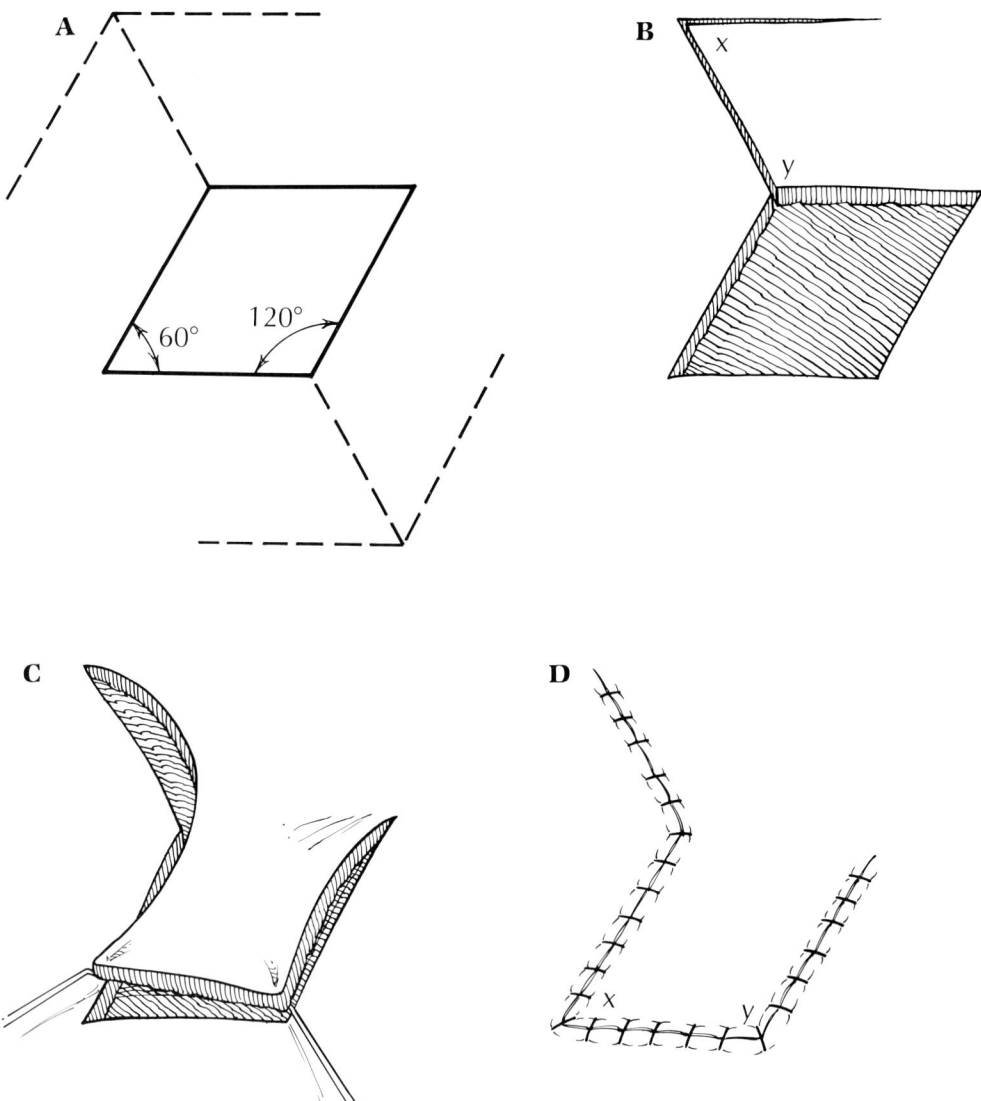

As depicted in **(A),** four potential flaps can be designed for each rhomboid. Using the principles outlined here, the surgeon chooses the most convenient one. The excision is completed and the donor flap is elevated **(B).** As with the Z-plasty, this elevation should extend slightly beyond the base of the flap **(C).** The excisional defect is usually closed without difficulty. The angles of the flap are fixed by three-point sutures. The donor site is closed directly **(D).** With good planning little or no trimming of the flap is necessary. If the facial contours are irregular, the flap may not fit exactly and more extensive modification will be required.

Double Rhomboid

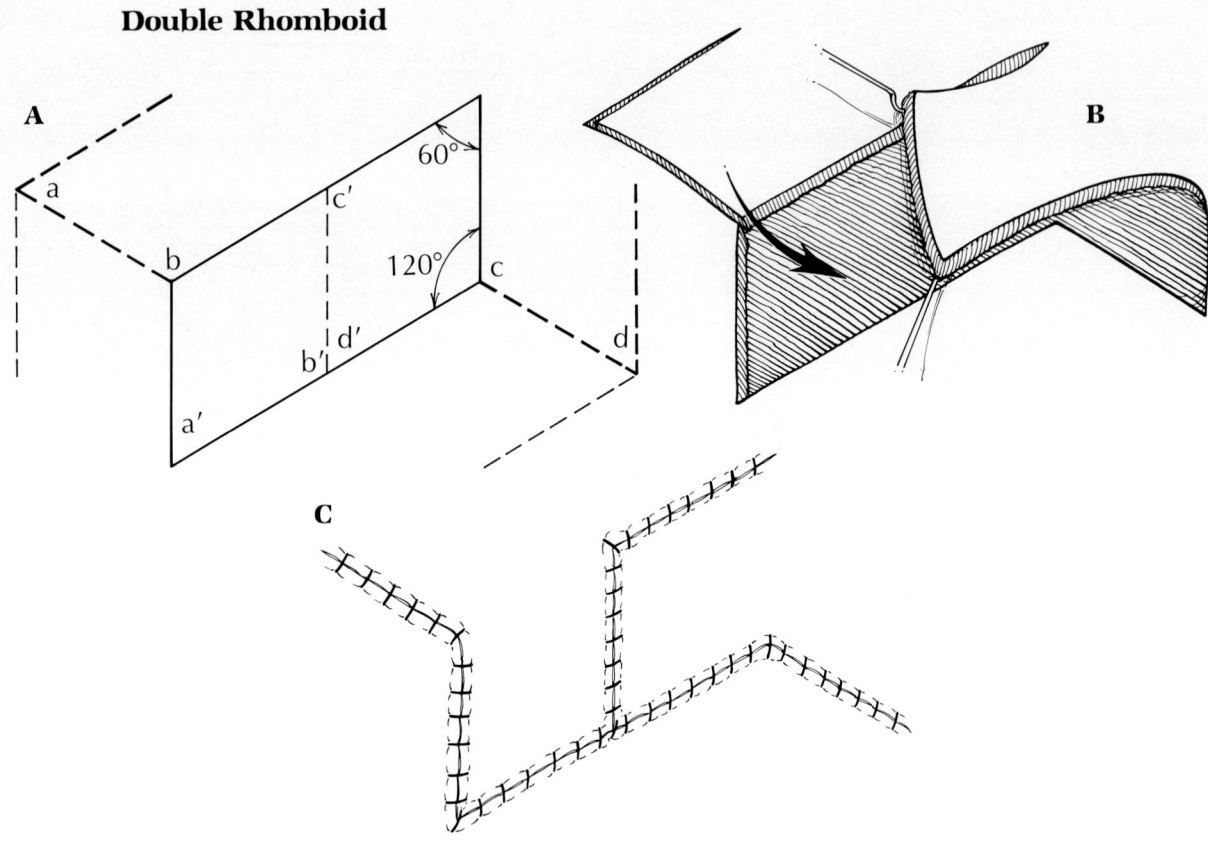

The rhomboid principle can be extended for closing long defects, which are made into parallelograms by placing two rhomboids end to end. It is possible to plan four available rhomboids on the 120-degree angles. The rhomboid flaps are chosen according to the requirements of the local situation.

In the arrangement shown at the top of the page, the use of the flaps is somewhat uncommon. The arrangement illustrated below is the one more frequently used. The rhomboid flaps are virtually diametrically opposed to one another. This seems most convenient in the majority of situations.

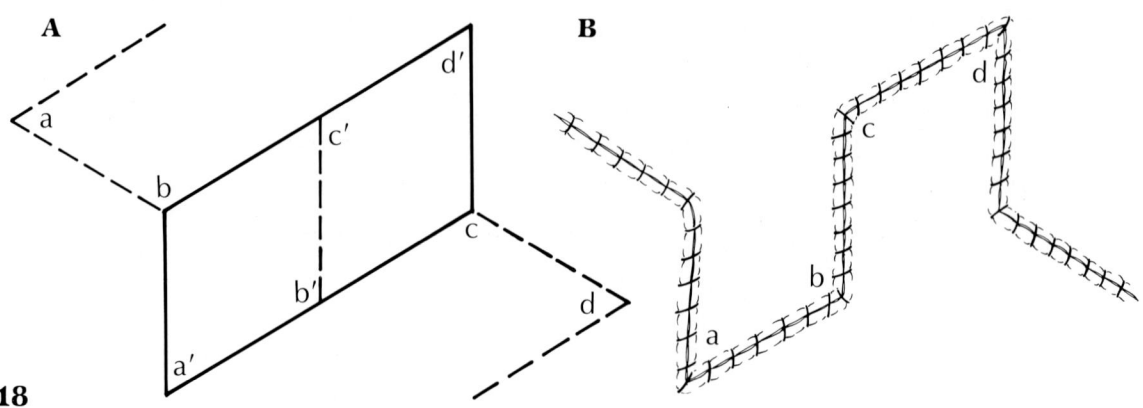

Triple Rhomboid

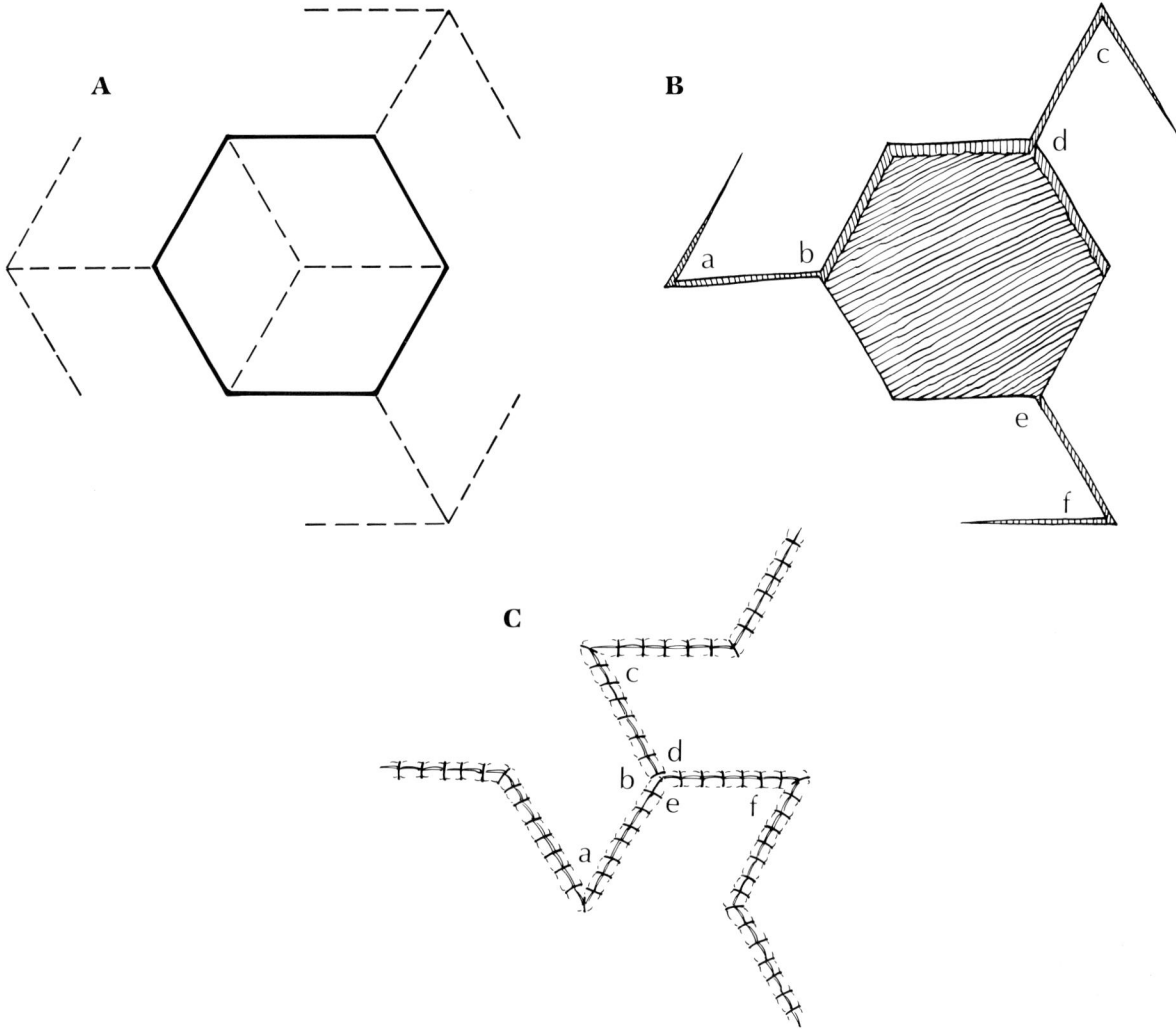

A large circular defect can be converted into a hexagon, and the hexagon in turn can be broken up into three rhomboids. Rhomboid flaps can be planned on the 120-degree angle, and thus six potential flaps are available. The three flaps are chosen as is convenient.

One interesting feature of the rhomboid flap is its lack of pincushioning or "trap-dooring," a common occurrence with circular flaps. The contraction of the circular scar line causes bunching of the flap tissue and a resulting contour defect. In contrast to the circular flap, the rhomboid flap possesses straight lines and angles. It is probably this combination that prevents scar contracture from having the same effect as in the circular type of flap. This fact should be taken into consideration in making the choice between one method or the other. Many other factors influence such a decision, including the excessive incision lines and consequent scars resulting from raising the rhomboid, and the area and amount of tissue availability.

DUFOURMENTEL FLAP
(LAMBEAU EN L POUR LOSANGE, "LLL" FLAP)

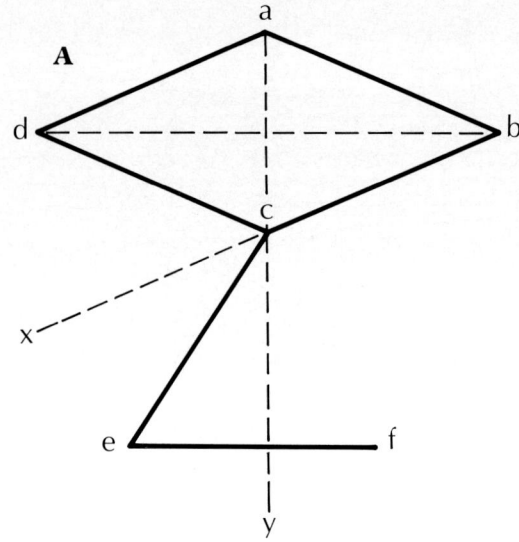

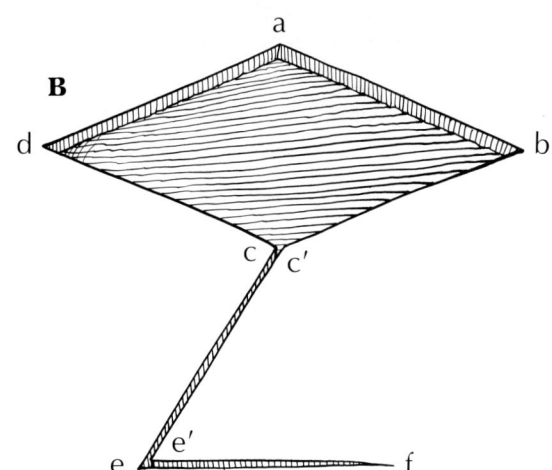

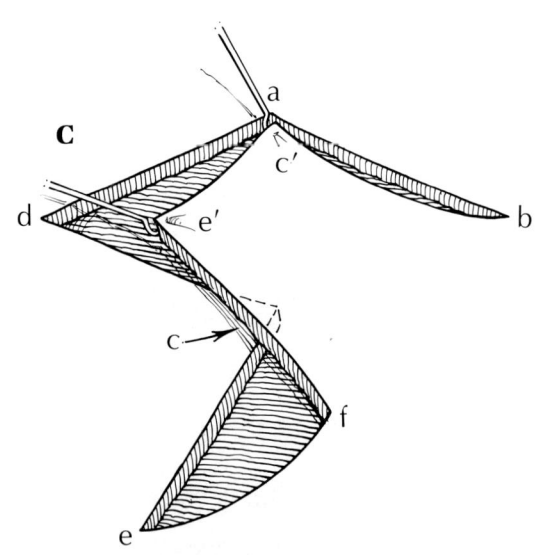

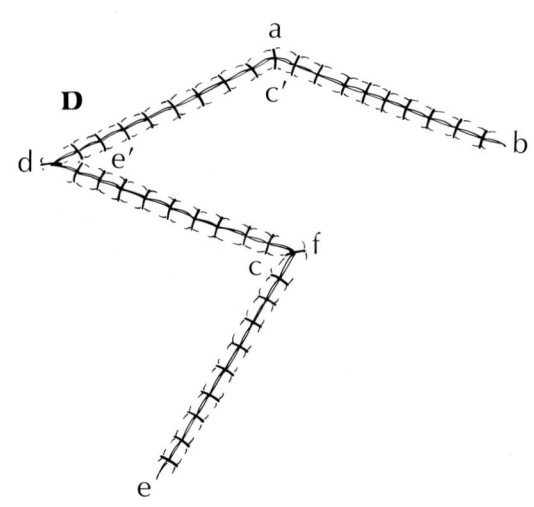

The Dufourmentel flap technique, described by Dufourmentel[5] in 1962, is a modification of the rhomboid flap. Although the originator has not given specific angle values, it is best to consider the narrow angle to be approximately 30 degrees and the wide angle to be approximately 150 degrees. The diagonals are drawn into the figure. On the wide angle, the short diagonal and one side are extended outward. The angle formed by these is bisected by a line that equals a side length. From the outer end of this line, to form an acute angle, the surgeon should draw another line of equal length parallel with the long diagonal. In this way the donor flap is fashioned.

This somewhat complex rhomboid type of flap undoubtedly provides more tissue to close the defect than is absolutely necessary; thus the closure of the donor defect may be slightly easier, facilitated by an actual mobilization of flap *dce*. Closure has then been achieved by means of an unequal Z-plasty. Thus in certain specific instances, when a rhomboid flap may give difficulty in donor site closure, and with proper experience, this technique may be chosen. As with the standard rhomboid flap, four potential donor flaps are available.

BILOBED FLAP

The bilobed flap was first described by Esser[6] in 1918 for use in nasal tip defect reconstruction. Zimany[15] described how the principles for this procedure could be applied to many areas of reconstruction. More recently McGregor and Soutar[13] have expanded the understanding of choosing the area in which to use the bilobed flap. They have explained the geometry in a clear fashion and have shown where this type of flap can be used to best advantage. In facial reconstruction the bilobed flap is most useful on the nose. This flap is basically a rotation flap that "spreads the load," masquerading as two transposition flaps. The planned defect is outlined, and two flaps are drawn, each slightly smaller than the other in transverse dimensions. The width of flap 1 is slightly less than the diameter of the defect, and that of flap 2 is correspondingly less than flap 1.

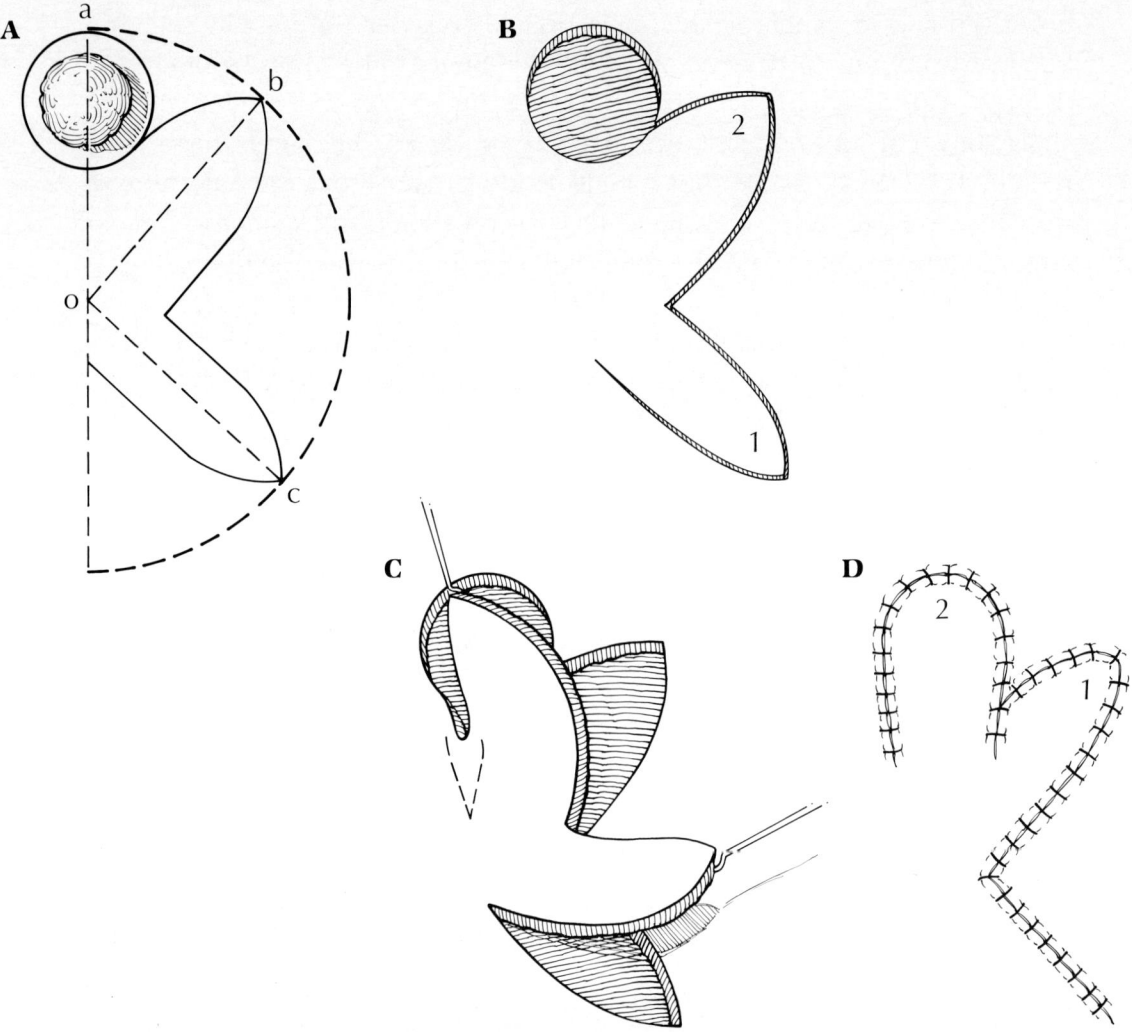

The flaps are fashioned so that they are in effect the radius of a circle on whose edge the outer rim of the defect lies **(A)**. Each flap may rotate 90 degrees or less **(B)**. The flaps must be elevated to their bases and beyond to achieve good movement **(C)**. The secondary defect of flap 2 should be capable of comfortable direct closure **(D)**. Trimming of the ends of the flaps and the dog ears resulting from the rotation may be necessary.

What has been achieved is a transfer of available tissue around the arc of the circle. To assess the feasibility of the flap, the surgeon must test tissue availability along the circumference of the circle of rotation to determine whether the tissue excess can be translated through 180 degrees or less. Since these are rounded flaps, there is a potential for pincushioning as the scars heal and contract. In addition, the area of scarring is extensive.

CRESCENTIC ADVANCEMENT FLAP

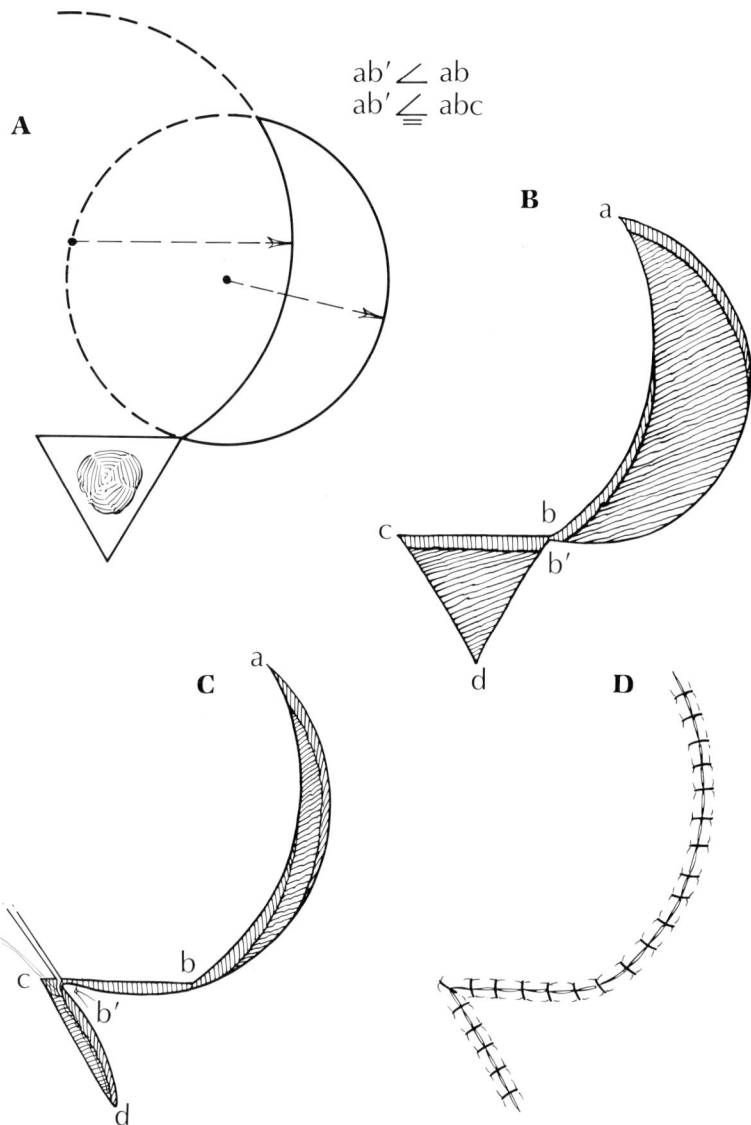

A crescentic advancement flap was first used for lip reconstruction by Webster.[14] It had been described by others in the past but in a less sophisticated way (see general bibliography). The principle involved in this type of flap is ideally suited to the perialar and upper lip regions of the face. The technique is ingenious and, like all good methods, intrinsically simple.

The tumor is resected, and a triangular defect is left **(A)**. An ellipse of skin is excised vertically above one end of the base of the triangle. This ellipse is fashioned so that its outer edge, *ab,'* is of a greater length than *ab*. It may equal or be slightly less than the combined length of the inner edge of the ellipse and the base of the triangle *cbd* **(B)**. The flap *ab'c* is undermined widely and advanced until complete closure is obtained without tension **(C** and **D)**.

☐ Procedures to Facilitate Flap Movement

Z-PLASTY

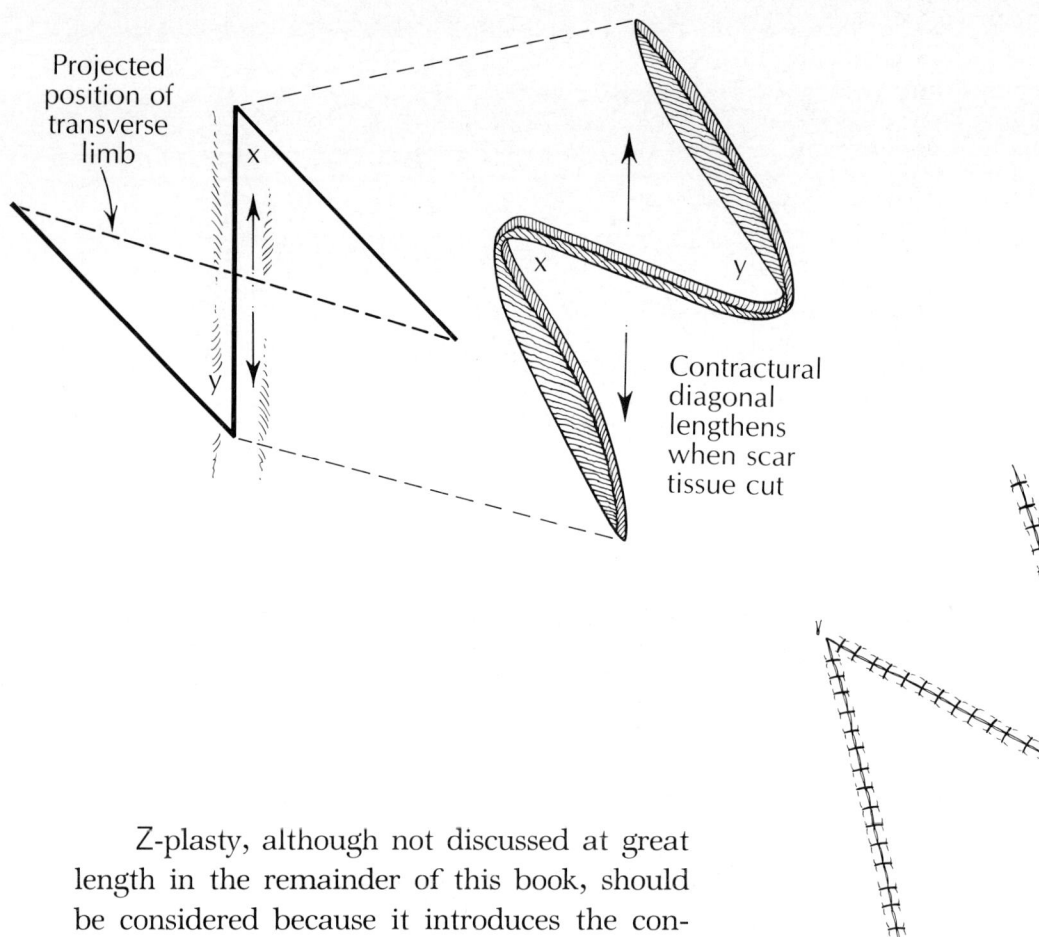

Z-plasty, although not discussed at great length in the remainder of this book, should be considered because it introduces the concept of a strict mathematic approach to a skin problem. It can be used in conjunction with some flaps to improve cosmesis or flap movement. The basic principle of the Z-plasty, initially described by Horner[8] in 1837, is to transfer a lateral skin excess transversely to lengthen the area along the line of the wound or a tight scar. This increase in length will prevent contracture and resulting contour deformities. It will also allow the subsequent scar to conform to surface irregularities such as convexities and concavities. The method of achieving this result is what makes the procedure fascinating.

CHAPTER 1
GENERAL CONSIDERATIONS

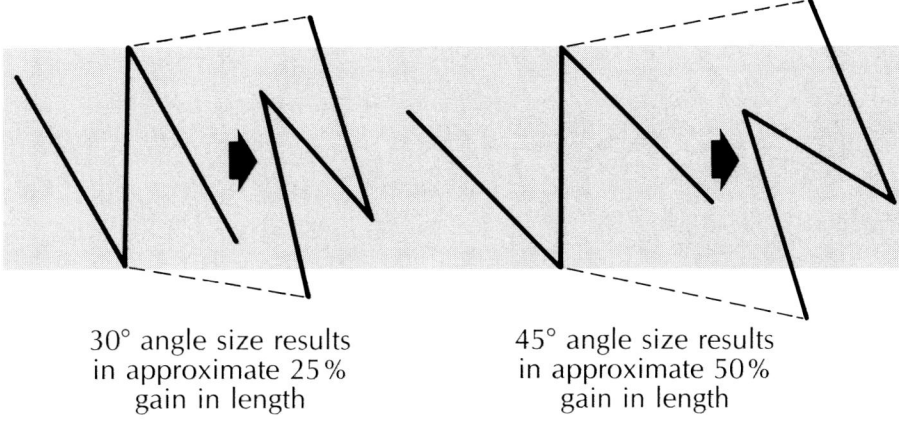

30° angle size results in approximate 25% gain in length

45° angle size results in approximate 50% gain in length

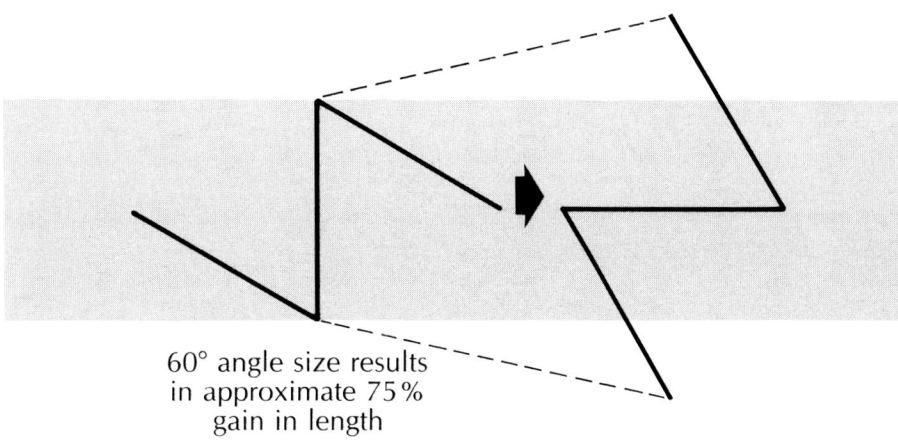

60° angle size results in approximate 75% gain in length

When planning flaps, the surgeon should consider where the transverse limb of the new Z-plasty will lie. According to the trigonometric studies of McGregor,[12] as the angle of the Z opens up, the amount of lengthening increases. In theory, an increase in length occurs as the Z-plasty angle increases up to 130 degrees; however, angles much greater than 60 degrees are not a practical proposition; thus this value is chosen in relation to the clinical situation. In some situations multiple Z-plasties will be used for long contractures; in these a series of 60-degree angles is most convenient. Sometimes unequal Z-plasties may be employed.

25

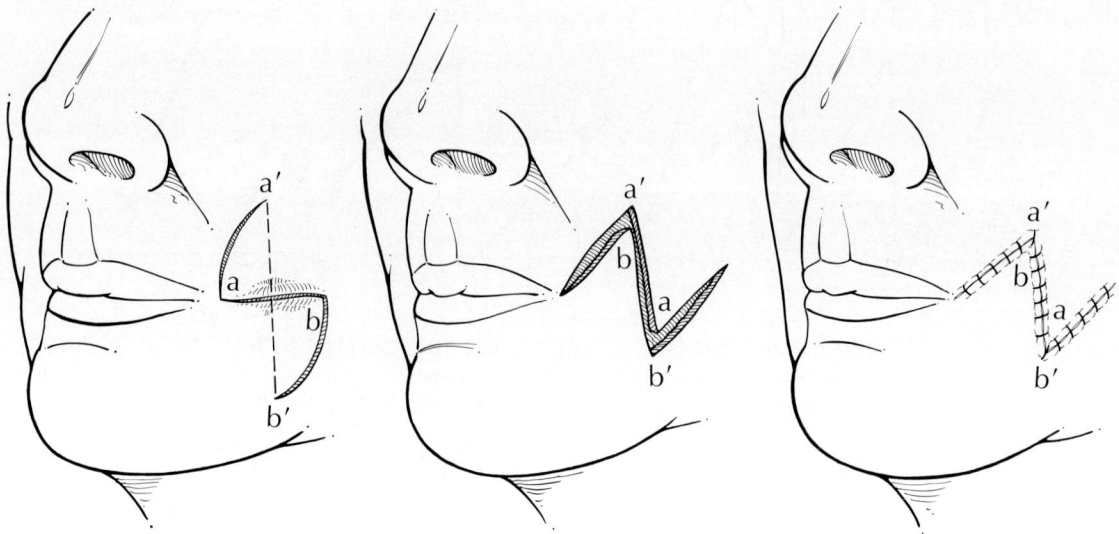

A few technical tips can make the performance of the Z-plasty somewhat easier. Forecasting where the transverse limb will lie is done by drawing its projected position across the scar to be revised and then outlining the flaps to establish their position.

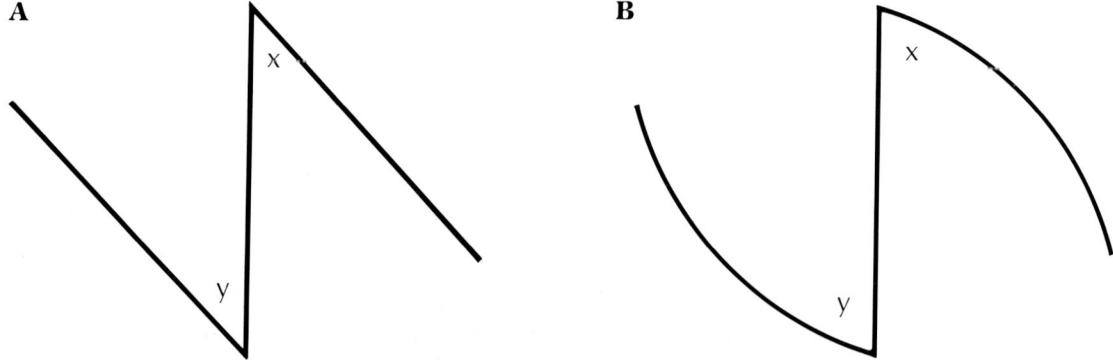

By curving the Z flaps, the surgeon can include extra tissue in the flap base and may augment flap vascularity, which can be important in heavily scarred or irradiated areas. The extra tissue may lead to a standing cone midway along the transverse limb. On the face this excess of skin should be trimmed. The flaps should be fully elevated, probably to slightly beyond their bases, allowing for ease of rotation. The tip of the Z-plasty should be stabilized initially with the Gillies three-point suture. If planning has been accurate, little or no trimming will be required.

CHAPTER 1
GENERAL CONSIDERATIONS

FOUR-FLAP Z-PLASTY

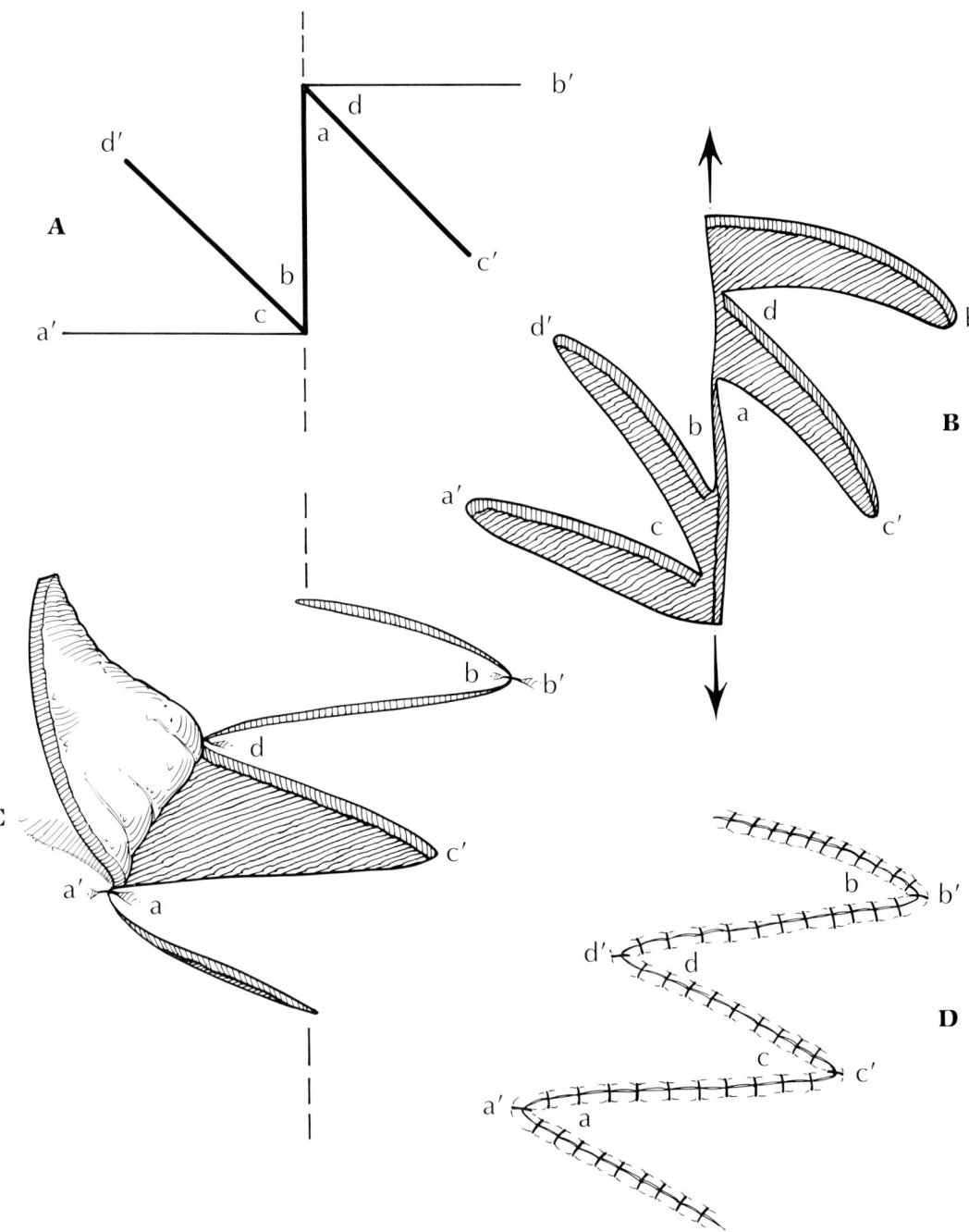

To obtain maximal lengthening a four-flap Z-plasty, first described by Berger[1] in 1904, may be used. In significantly scarred contracted areas this technique will bring unscarred skin into the central Z area. This is helpful in preventing further heavy scarring and contracture.

W-PLASTY

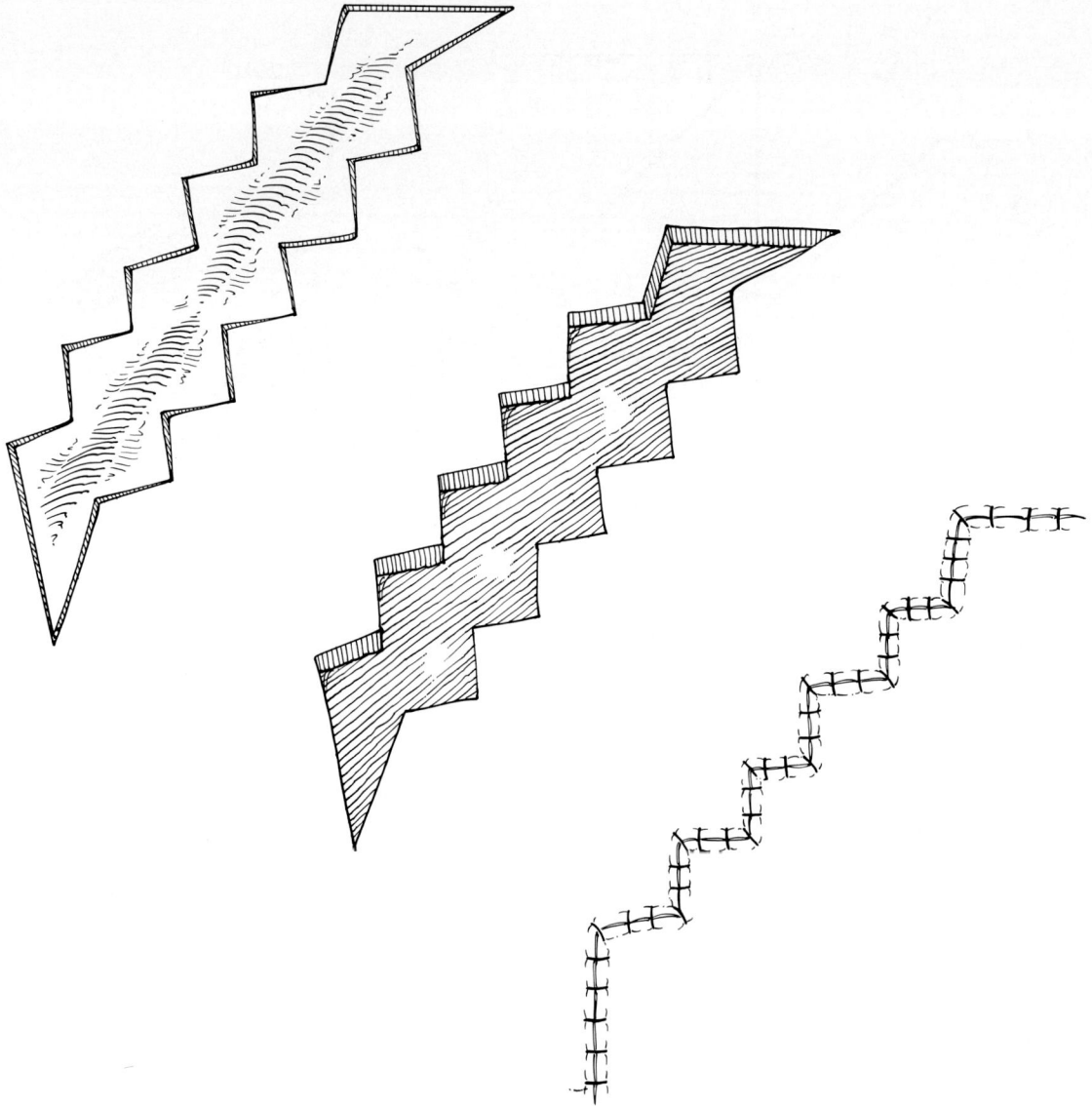

For the sake of completeness, the W-plasty technique is included here. The concept, introduced by Borges[2] in 1959, produces a zigzag scar in a simpler way than using a multiple Z-plasty. The main function of the W-plasty is in scar revision, and it is particularly useful in the forehead and cheek. There is probably a slight lengthening potential with this technique. Undoubtedly W flaps are also used to some degree in preventing scar contracture.

BACK CUT

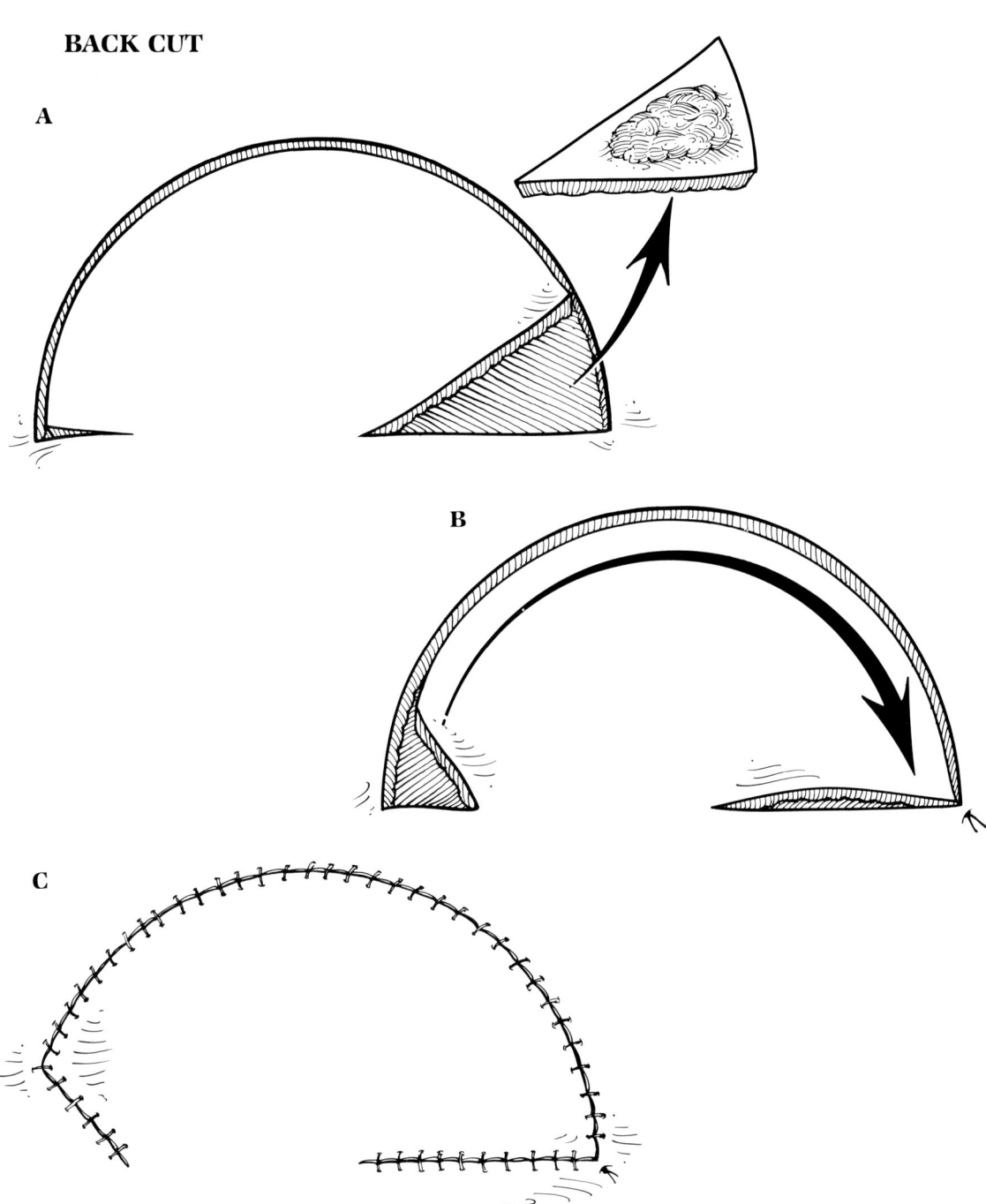

By using the back cut, the surgeon extends flap movement in rotation and transposition flaps. The cut is made gradually until the length required to produce adequate movement at the end of the flap is obtained. Failure to use a back cut can lead to a diagonal tension line across the flap, with ischemia distal to this tension line; this is a bad situation because it can mean loss of the most essential part of the flap. In making this back cut, a frequent maneuver in a scalp flap, vascularity may be prejudiced by reduction in the width of the base of the flap. The back cut in the donor area can usually be closed directly, but occasionally a skin graft may be required.

"DOG EARS"

As skin is moved around, "dog ears," or excess skin folds (the "standing and lying cones" of Limberg), are formed. With some preplanning, this excess skin can be incorporated into the reconstruction.

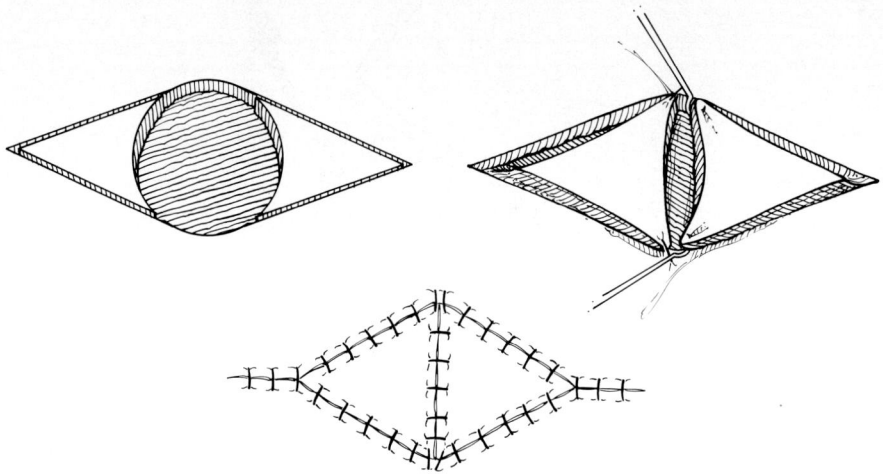

An attempt to close a circular defect results in skin excess lateral to the closure. Any existing tension may be released by making the skin excess into triangular island flaps based on a subcutaneous pedicle. These can then be moved medially, as advancement flaps, to close the main defect, with the V-Y principle applied for closure of the secondary defect.

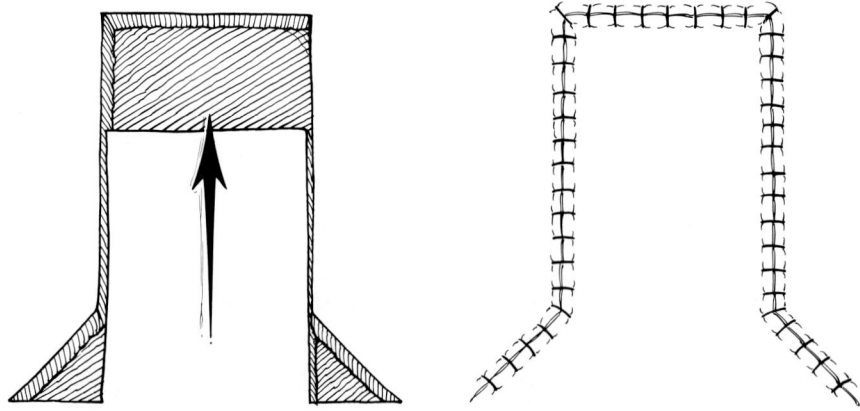

In a straight advancement flap, as the defect at the leading edge of the flap is closed, folds of skin appear bilaterally just lateral to the flap base. These can be excised as Burow's triangles[4] with a twofold effect: the contour problem is dealt with, and, as the skin is pulled toward the flap base, the tension is shared between the skin of the defect and the skin of the flap—an admirable compromise.

CHAPTER 1
GENERAL CONSIDERATIONS

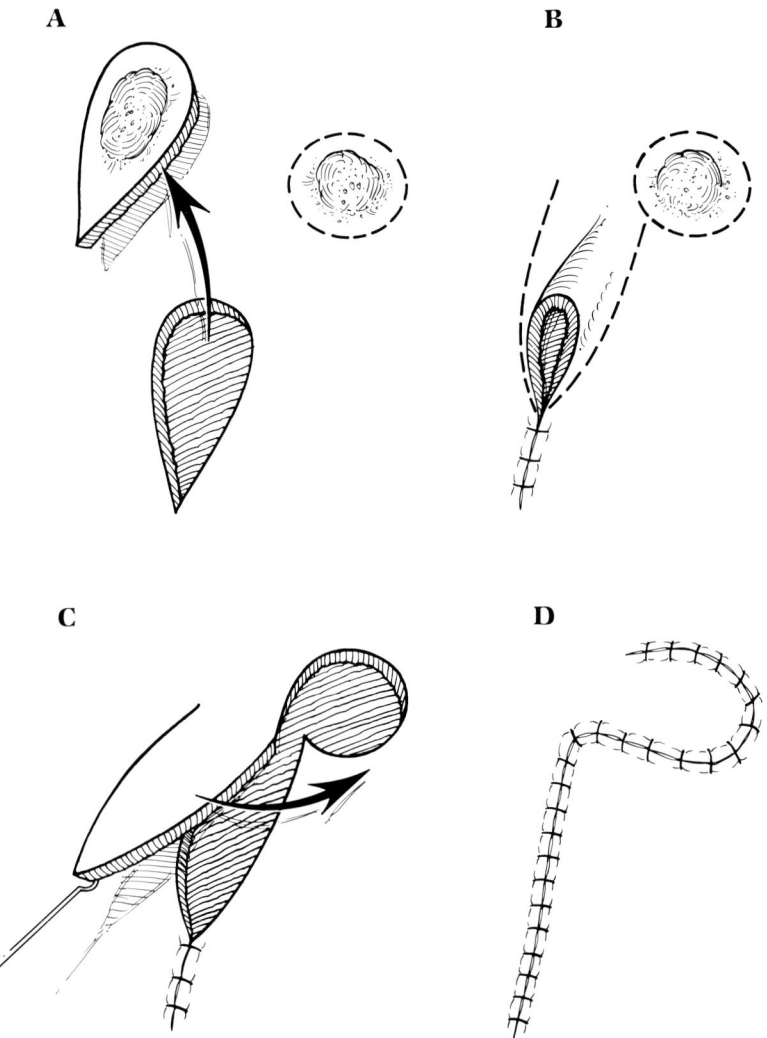

Occasionally, when circumstances are right, the dog ear can be used to form a flap to reconstruct another neighboring defect. In closing the primary defect and leaving a dog ear, the surgeon may elevate the dog ear as a long finger type of transposition flap, which can then be used to deal with a skin lesion within a 90-degree radius of it.

Although considerable emphasis has been placed on the mathematics of flaps, accepted mathematic theory relates to a plane surface and assumes that the size of the flap will not alter. This theory is faulty, however, because it does not take into consideration the viscoelastic properties of skin, which are additional aids to the surgeon. If the planning is not accurate, skin stretching will make up for geometric and trigonometric deficiences.

■ COMPLICATIONS OF LOCAL FLAPS

Almost all complications of local flaps result from errors in judgment, planning, and execution. The worst complication is tumor recurrence, which results from a failure to think in biologic terms and a desire to make the defect fit the flap. The lesion should always be widely excised. Even a basal cell carcinoma should be given 0.5 cm margins, except when it occurs directly under the eyelid. (Rarely do eyelid skin basal cell carcinomas extend into and over the lid margin). Only *after* the tumor has been completely excised and the defect has been created should the surgeon select a method of flap reconstruction. The defect *then* can be modified to fit the chosen flap reconstruction. With this technique local tumor recurrence is rare.

Flap loss is a serious complication that almost always results from a design or technical error. Reasons for flap failure include the following:
1. Using a small flap to fill a big hole (design fault)
2. Hematoma (technical error)
3. Damaging the blood supply (technical error)
4. Making the flap extend outside its blood supply (design fault)
5. Suturing the wound under tension, failing to use a back cut, or making a pedicle too short (all technical errors).

With experience and care, all these errors are preventable.

If radiation therapy has been used in the region previously, this presents a problem. Skin and subcutaneous tissue become less vascular, and if flaps are to be used, they should be based on a vascular pedicle that is absolutely secure. No tension should be present on the suture lines. If these conditions can be met, the results will be superior to those achieved with skin grafts. Failure to provide sufficient vascular support to the flap frequently results in flap necrosis.

Care must be taken to respect normal anatomy and visible landmarks such as the eyebrows. The branches of the facial nerve must also be protected, especially in the temporal and submandibular areas. An excellent reconstruction with a distal paralysis is a poor trade-off. A good working rule is to raise facial flaps in the face-lift plane. The medial canthus and the lacrimal apparatus must be preserved; they should be resected only if this is necessary for tumor clearance.

Pincushioning is another complication that can occur with local flaps. The frustrating aspect of this complication is its inconsistency. This deformity cannot be corrected until the scars are mature, approximately 12 to 18 months after surgery.

CHAPTER 1
GENERAL CONSIDERATIONS

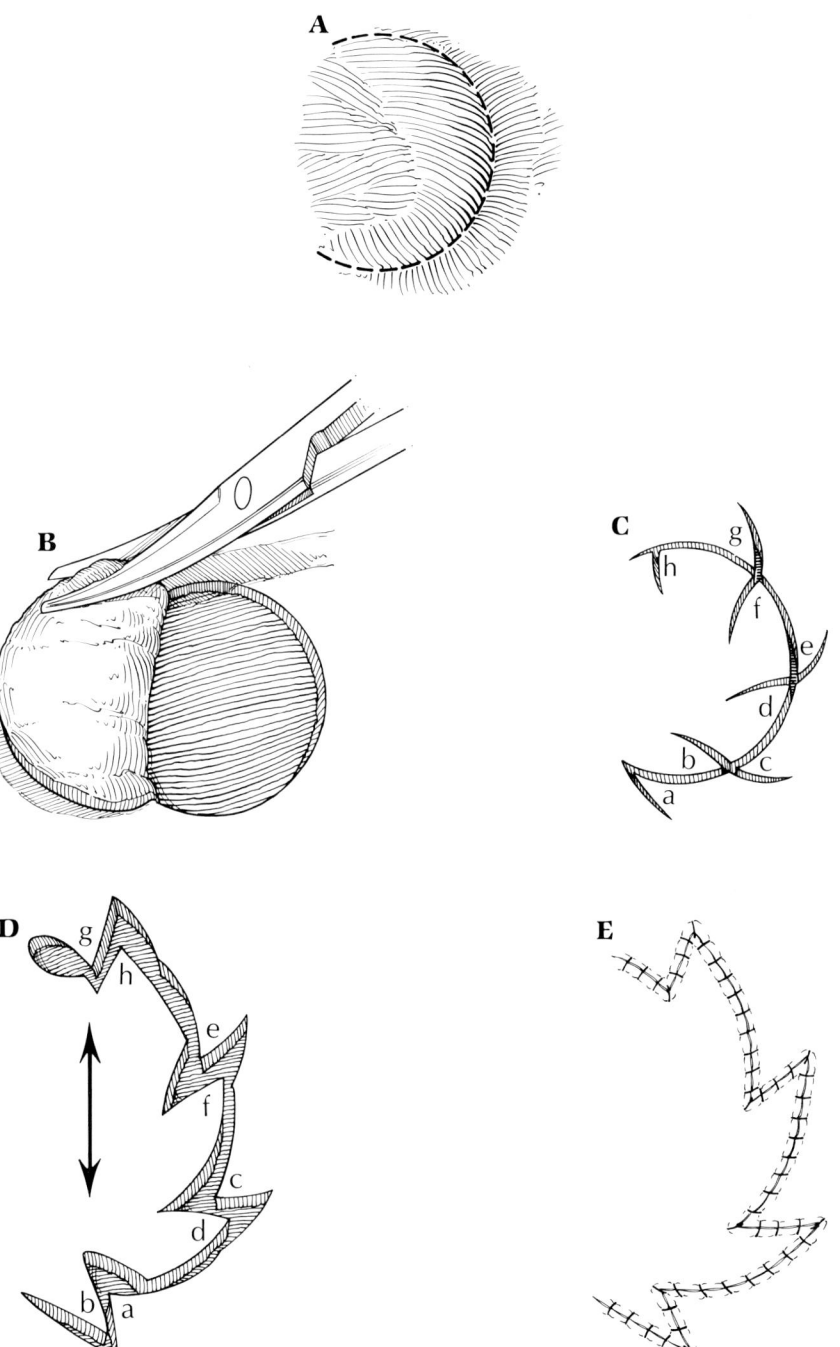

Correction is difficult. The old flap is elevated by excision of the previous scar. The undersurface of the flap is thinned by defatting. A series of multiple Z-plasties, the number and size of which depend on the particular situation, are performed. The Z flaps are widely elevated and sutured into position. This technique will frequently correct the contour problem. Unfortunately, further pincushioning may occur within the scars of the Z-plasty flaps.

☐ Conclusions

Success in using local flaps is directly related to knowledge of such flaps, careful planning, good technique, and experience. Wide excision in skin cancer is a valuable rule. The creation of the defect is of primary importance; closure is a secondary event. When the defect has been created, the surgeon should choose a flap of adequate size and shape, for wound closure without tension. Hemostasis should be meticulous. In large flaps suction drainage is used. Even in smaller flaps this method is becoming more popular because of availability of mini suction drains.

When a flap looks as though it is in circulatory distress (cyanosed with a sluggish or absent capillary refill), action must be taken. If a hematoma is present, sutures should be removed, hemostasis established, and resuturing performed. If suturing is too tight in one area, a few sutures can be removed. If these measures are unsuccessful, then all sutures should be removed and the flap returned to its original area. With what amounts to a "delay" the flap will probably recover and can be used another day, a situation that is preferable to total flap loss.

REFERENCES

1. Berger, P.: Autoplastie par dédoublement de la palmure, et échange de lambeaux. In Berger, P., and Banzet, S.: Chirurgie orthopedique, Paris, 1904, Steinheil.
2. Borges, A.F.: Improvement of antitension lines scar by the "W-plastic" operation, Br. J. Plast. Surg. **12:**29, 1959.
3. Borges, A.F., and Alexander, S.E.: Relaxed skin tension lines, Z-plasties on scars and fusiform excision of lesions, Br. J. Plast. Surg. **15:**242, 1962.
4. Burow, C.A.: Beschreibung einer neuen Transplantationsmethode (Methode der Seitlichen Dreiecke)—zum Wiederersatz verlorengegangener, Theile des Gesichts, Berlin, 1855, Nauck.
5. Dufourmentel, C.: Le fermeture des pertes de substance cutanée limitées "Le lambeau de rotation en L pour losange" dit "L.L.L.," Ann. Chir. Plast. **7:**61, 1962.
6. Esser, J.F.S.: Gestielte Lokale Nasenplastik mit Zweizipfligem Lappen. Deckung des Sekundaren Defektes vom ersten Zipfel durch den Zweitzen, Dtsch. Z. Chirurg. **143:**385, 1918.
7. Gibson, T., and Kenedi, R.M.: Biomechanical properties of skin, Surg. Clin. North Am. **47:**279, 1967.
8. Horner, W.: Clinical report on the surgical department of the Philadelphia Hospital, Blockley, for the months of May, June, July, 1837, Am. J. Med. Sci. **21:**105, 1837.
9. Imre, J.: Lidplastik—und Plastiche operationen, An. Den Weichteile des Gesichts, Budapest, 1928, Studium, Verlag.
10. Imre, J.: Operationen an den Liden, in Thiel. Ophthalmologische Operations, Hamburg, 1942, Lehre.
11. Limberg, A.A.: Mathematical principles of local plastic procedures on the surface of the human body, Leningrad, 1946, Government Publishing House for medical literature (Medgiz).
12. McGregor, I.A.: The theoretical basis of the Z-plasty, Br. J. Plast. Surg. **9:**256, 1957.
13. McGregor, J.C., and Soutar, D.S.: A critical assessment of the bilobed flap, Br. J. Plast. Surg., **34:**197, 1981.
14. Webster, J.P.: Crescentic peri-alar cheek excision for upper lip flap advancement with a short history of upper lip repair, Plast. Reconstr. Surg. **16:**434, 1955.
15. Zimany, A.: The bilobed flap, Plast. Reconstr. Surg. **11:**424, 1953.

CHAPTER 2

PATIENT MANAGEMENT

Ne'er saw I, never felt, a calm so deep
WILLIAM WORDSWORTH
View from Westminster Bridge

Great events make me quiet and calm; it is only trifles that irritate my nerves.
QUEEN VICTORIA
In a Letter to King Leopold of Belgium

For the patient relatively minor facial surgery can be a major emotional experience. Fear of hospitals, worries about possible skin cancer, uncertainty about the quality of the surgical result, and dread of local anesthesia may cause considerable anxiety.

■ PATIENT EXAMINATION AND EVALUATION

Good patient management begins with a frank and informative office consultation as the plastic surgeon reassures the patient about the chances of successful removal of the lesion and the expectations of a good result. The patient should understand the proposed method of reconstruction and the technique of anesthesia to be used, since local flap reconstruction on the face is often performed with the aid of local anesthesia, usually on an outpatient basis. By expressing a sincere desire to make this experience as comfortable as possible, the surgeon can do much to allay the patient's apprehension.

A complete medical history should be taken. Because aspirin or aspirin-containing compounds may cause undue bleeding, the patient is asked to discontinue using these from 10 to 14 days before surgery. Allergy to epinephrine or other drugs should be established and noted. If a patient is excessively worried immediately before surgery, or if a history of hypertension or myocardial ischemia is a factor, a mild sedative such as Valium may be prescribed.

■ PREOPERATIVE CARE

The surgeon should be available in the operating room as soon as the patient is on the table and should again introduce himself to establish that the person in whom the patient has placed his trust is actually present and will perform the surgery. Gentle reassurance at this time will probably brings its reward in a calm patient with reduced systolic blood pressure during the procedure. The patient's allergies are checked against the preoperative record.

Careful, unhurried preparation by the resident or nurse, again with a full explanation of all movements, can further calm the patient. Particular care is taken to avoid irritation to the patient's eyes or spillage of cleansing solutions into the nose or mouth. The operating table is placed in the reverse Trendelenburg position to initiate some postural head and neck hypotension.

At this point the proposed excision and projected reconstruction are designed. Since this planning is done on the patient's face with a marking pen, the procedure must be explained beforehand, with particular emphasis on the fact that the patient will feel the pen as it traces the surgical plan. The patient should also understand that local, anesthetic infiltration will follow flap planning, with resulting deadening of the involved area. If a resident or colleague is present in the operating room, discussion about alternative methods of reconstruction may take place while the patient is being prepared for surgery. Reasons for this conversation should be mentioned to the patient and inquiries made as to whether this talking causes any concern. Many patients enjoy such a discussion because it is evidence that the surgeons are interested in and concerned with their medical problem.

At this time some patients will ask for tactile reassurance and may wish to hold a nurse's hand. This request should be granted quickly and pleasantly. The patient may ask to have music or, if music is being played, he or she may wish to have it turned off. These are reasonable requests and should be granted.

ADMINISTRATION OF ANESTHETICS

Local Anesthetic Infiltration

The local anesthetic agents used almost universally are lidocaine hydrochloride (Xylocaine) and epinephrine. The concentration varies; for small areas, 1% lidocaine and 1:200,000 epinephrine is used; for large areas and for children, 0.5% lidocaine and 1:400,000 epinephrine is advised. If a patient is sensitive to epinephrine, only lidocaine should be used. An additional drug that may be useful is hyaluronidase (Wydase*). One ampule is added to 20 ml of local anesthetic solution. This agent appears to aid the diffusion of the lidocaine, resulting in a less painful injection and more rapid and extensive anesthesia. It also allows nerve blocks to be executed more efficiently because of the spreading effect.

Unless the area to be anesthetized is limited, a 20 ml syringe should be used, thus obviating the necessity for refilling. The needle need not be unduly fine, but it should be sharp. Introducing the needle through the skin should be done with thoughtfulness and care. The surgeon should explain the procedure to the patient and again give reassurance. The skin is pinched in the area of the injection site; then, with the index finger and the thumb, it is stretched tightly, which produces skin blanching and enables the needle to be pushed rapidly and vertically through the skin with minimal pain. If the local anesthetic is injected *very* slowly, with concomitant explanation or conversation on the surgeon's part, this can be a virtually painless procedure. It is important to observe the patient's reaction; if there is any sign of pain, the surgeon should stop injecting the anesthetic and wait a few minutes before continuing.

Regional Nerve Block[1,2]

If possible, anesthesia should be produced by regional nerve block. This technique affords rapid regional anesthesia with *less* pain than would result from injection around the surgical site. Painless local infiltration of lidocaine and epinephrine to obtain vasoconstriction is then possible.

---

*Wyeth Laboratories, Division of Home Products, Box 8299, Philadelphia, Pa. 19101.

TECHNIQUE
Supraorbital Nerve

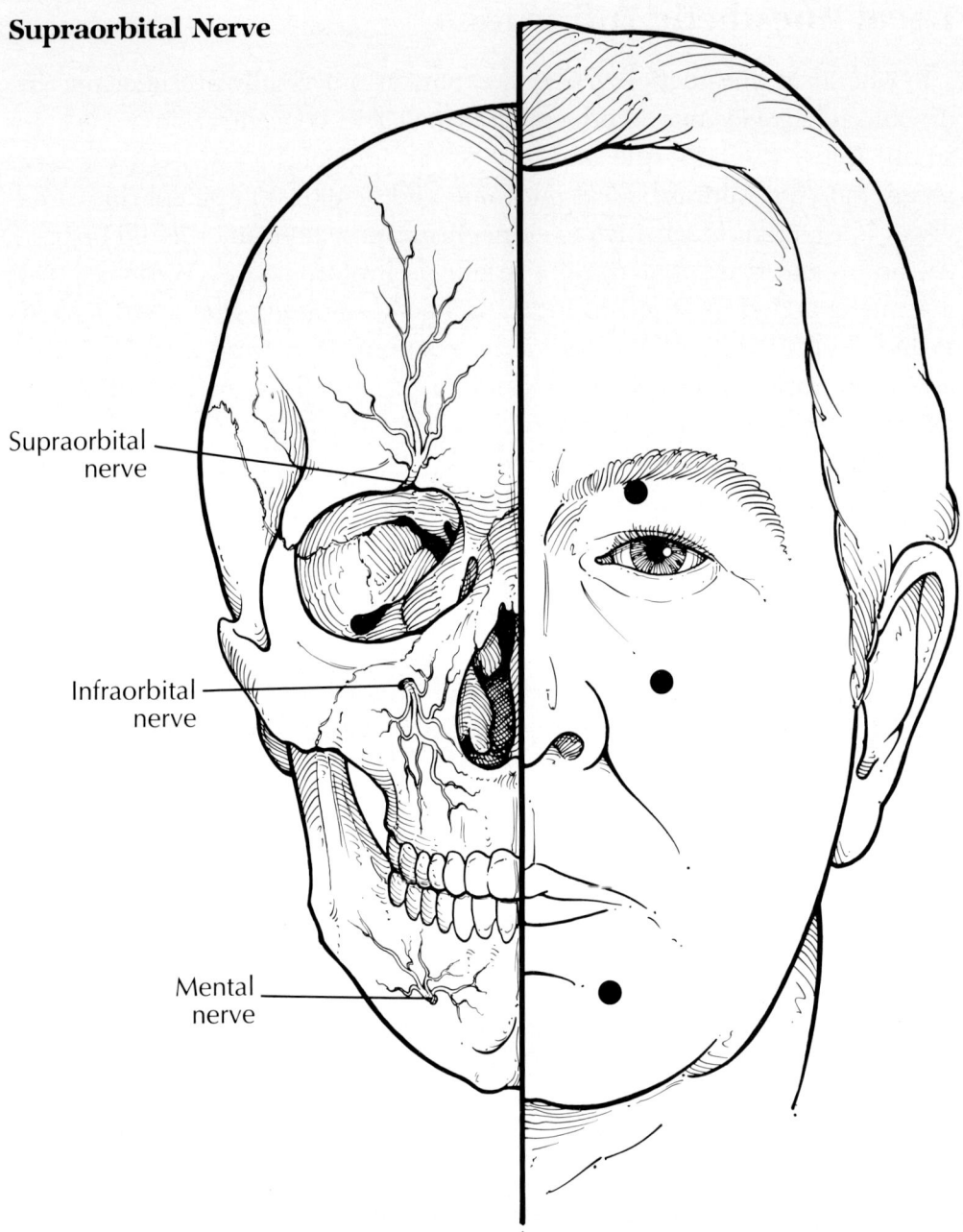

Much of the forehead can be anesthetized by infiltration of the supraorbital nerves. These nerves are located at the junction of the central and medial thirds of the supraorbital rim. The needle should be introduced just below the eyebrow, with the aim being the edge of the supraorbital rim. If hyaluronidase is used, accurate location of the nerve is not necessary; the lidocaine will spread rapidly and block the nerve.

Infraorbital Nerve

The infraorbital foramen is located at the junction of the central and medial thirds of the infraorbital rim. The infraorbital nerve exits from the foramen at a point 0.5 to 1 cm below the rim; here there is a concavity lying under the overhang of the rim. The needle should be placed directly into the area and the anesthetic infiltrated as described earlier. It is a mistake to move the needle around in this area; this increases discomfort without a corresponding increase in effectiveness. Satisfactory anesthesia is produced after administration of 0.5 to 1 ml of the anesthetic solution (probably the hyaluronidase helps in this respect). An alarming local phenomenon may occasionally be observed at this point: sudden and intense blanching over the area of distribution of the infraorbital nerve. Instant anesthesia is associated with this loss of color. Presumably it results from a "direct hit" on the nerve, causing profound vasospasm in all the vessels it controls.

With this block, anesthesia is obtained in the cheek, the ipsilateral half of the upper lip, a variable amount of the side and tip of the nose, and the upper alveolus and teeth on the injected side. Under normal circumstances, deadening will occur within 5 minutes. It is possible to perform the same block through the upper buccal sulcus. Perhaps because of previous dental procedures, most patients find the latter approach more frightening.

Mental Nerve

The mental nerve exits from its foramen in the mandible 1 to 1.5 cm above the lower rim in the region of the canine premolar teeth. The foramen lies approximately on a vertical line drawn through the supraorbital and infraorbital foramina. An injection through the skin to block this nerve can be painful. In contrast, an intraoral approach can be almost painless. The method to be used is carefully explained to the patient before the injection.

The surgeon stands behind the patient's head, and the index finger is placed down into the lower buccal sulcus just medial to the oral commissure. The lip is pulled downward and outward to stretch the lower buccal sulcus to the blanching point if possible. The needle is pushed quickly through the mucosa and the slow injection begins. Again, anesthesia is rapid. This block will anesthetize the corresponding half of the lower lip, alveolus, and teeth, as well as a varying portion of the cheek.

☐ Direct Local Infiltration

As can be appreciated from the previous description, much of the face can be comfortably anesthetized with nerve blocks. In some areas, however, direct infiltration is necessary. This may be done beginning in an area anesthetized by a nerve block. The secret to this approach is *very slow* infiltration; in addition, a large volume of anesthetic agent should be used. The latter will dissipate rapidly because of the hyaluronidase but will ensure adequate anesthesia and good vasoconstriction. Another essential ingredient for patient comfort is time. The lidocaine and epinephrine must be given time to work to maximal effect. A minimum of 5 minutes for injection and at least 5 minutes of waiting can convert an unpleasant experience into a surprisingly comfortable event. The surgeon may even want to mark the proposed excision and reconstruction, inject the area, and go for a cup of coffee or dictate for 10 to 15 minutes. The reward for this approach is a maximal level of anesthesia and vasoconstriction, an ideal operative field. This time allows the surgeon to further converse with the patient and set his or her mind at ease. Only when anesthesia is tried and tested should the surgery begin.

☐ Eye Anesthesia

Surface anesthesia can be obtained on the eye by means of a topical agent such as proparcaine, 0.5%, (Opthaine*). The procedure is explained to the patient, who should be told that there may be a stinging sensation. The patient looks to the side, holding the eyes open, and two or three drops are introduced onto the sclera. These drops must not be delivered from a height because this can cause an unpleasant sensation; the dropper should be placed close to the sclera. Effects of the anesthetic are evident in a few minutes.

☐ Intranasal Anesthesia

After infraorbital nerve block, intranasal anesthesia is produced by a combination of local anesthetic injection and packing with cocaine-soaked gauze (the latter procedure ensures anesthesia and mucosal vasoconstriction). The packing is prepared by placing 5 ml of a 10% solution of cocaine in a container into which is placed ribbon gauze or cotton-tipped applicators. An attempt is made to introduce the solution into all areas of the mucosa. A wait of 10 to 15 minutes is advised to obtain the optimal effect. Correct head-up posturing of the patient is very important to ensure a bloodless operative field.

---

*Squibb Pharmaceuticals, Box 4000, Princeton, N.J. 08540.

■ INTRAOPERATIVE CARE

If the patient becomes nauseated or light-headed during surgery and shows signs of fainting, the head of the table should be lowered and adequate time allowed for recovery from this condition before surgery is continued. The surgeon must be careful not to press on or traumatize the eyes during the procedure; this can be very disturbing. The patient's mood should be gauged during the procedure. If he or she wants to talk, this should be encouraged; if not, the surgeon should be prepared to operate in silence. At the completion of the procedure, all blood should be cleaned away. Special care needs to be taken to clean the patient's hair and ear canal; if the latter is forgotten, the patient may complain of reduction in hearing. A neat, tidy dressing is applied to allow the patient to appear in public with minimal embarrassment.

■ POSTOPERATIVE CARE

At the completion of the procedure, clear (preferably written) instructions should be issued to the patient. A prescription for analgesia is given with an explanation of the specific amount and how often it needs to be taken. The patient should be cautioned against taking aspirin-containing compounds, and the reason for this should be explained, with emphasis on the fact that they may cause bleeding and hematoma. An appointment for the first postoperative visit is given with a note of an emergency telephone number. Special emphasis is placed on explaining the extent and duration of the anesthesia and the consequent danger of burning the lips with hot liquids such as coffee or tea. If any oozing of blood occurs, the patient is detained for observation until it stops.

REFERENCES
1. Doberl, A.: Illustrated handbook in local anaesthesia, Copenhagen, 1969, Munksgaard.
2. Jenkner, F.L.: Peripheral nerve block, Berlin, 1975, Springer-Verlag.

CHAPTER 3

FOREHEAD RECONSTRUCTION

And freedom rear'd in that August sunrise her beautiful bold brow
>ALFRED LORD TENNYSON
>*The Poet*

The rapt one of the godlike forehead
The heather-eyed creature sleeps in earth
>WILLIAM WORDSWORTH
>*Extempore Effusion upon the Death of James Hogg*

Literary descriptions of the forehead emphasize that "the noble brow" is not an area to be taken lightly but one that merits careful study and consideration. The visible area of the forehead varies from individual to individual according to hairstyle; the actual area depends on the position of the hairline. The boundaries are the hairline above and lateral to the forehead and, inferiorly, the eyebrows, supraorbital rims, and glabellar region. The inferolateral extent is determined arbitrarily at the level of the lateral end of the eyebrow. To reconstruct this area a surgeon must be knowledgeable about the nerve, blood supply, and musculature, but more important he needs an appreciation of what can be referred to as "fixed aesethetic structures," such as eyebrows and lateral hairline. The position of these must be respected at all times to achieve optimal results.

■ ANATOMY
☐ Skin

APPEARANCE

The forehead skin of the young person is usually smooth, although some individuals have an overactive frontalis muscle that causes transverse wrinkles to form. Similarly, corrugator and procerus muscle overactivity will produce vertical frown lines in the glabellar area. With age these lines become more pronounced and may well influence the choice of reconstructive procedures for the forehead.

COLOR

The color of the forehead skin is often slightly paler than the nose and considerably paler than the malar region. This coloring may be altered by sun exposure.

TEXTURE

The skin texture of the forehead is smooth and often shiny, although it varies from person to person. The skin thickness is fairly uniform; the glabellar skin is somewhat thinner and certainly more pliable than that covering the rest of the forehead.

The full thickness of the main forehead area supplies a stiff, fairly thick layer for reconstruction. These textural characteristics are of importance when the forehead is being used for distant reconstructive procedures. For example, with the nose it is an *advantage* because it gives support; with the eyelid it is a *disadvantage* because it is too thick.

☐ Musculature

This region includes the frontalis, procerus, and corrugator muscles. These muscles usually provide symmetric movement to the forehead, but they are also capable of producing an asymmetric appearance, as in the quizzical raising of one eyebrow that is second nature to many individuals. Asymmetry of the vertical frown lines may also exist in the glabellar area.

CHAPTER 3
FOREHEAD RECONSTRUCTION

☐ Nerve Supply

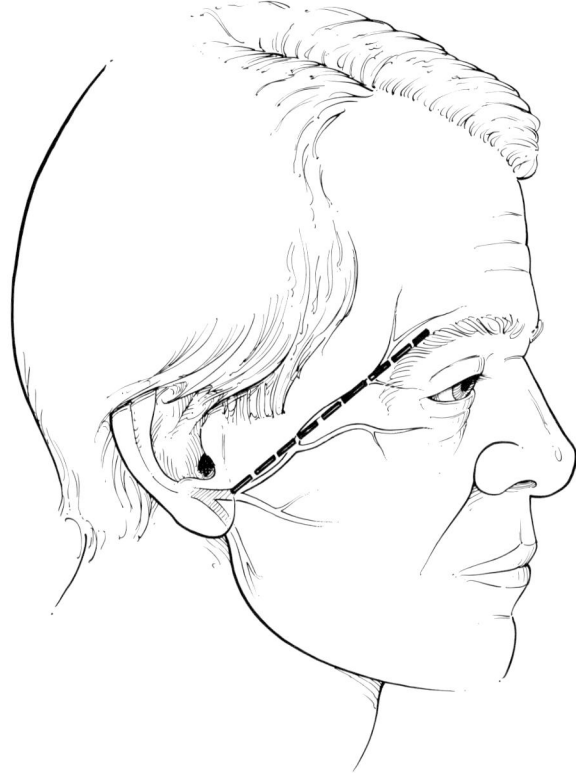

Sensory nerves are the supraorbital and trochlear from the trigeminal nerve (CN V). The motor supply is from the frontal branch of the facial nerve (CN VII). It is important to know the approximate position of the facial nerve. It lies on a line between the lobule of the ear and a point just lateral to the lateral end of the eyebrow. If this line is not kept in mind, the nerve will be injured during procedures done in the temporal and facial area.

☐ Blood Supply

The anterior branches of the temporal, supraorbital, and trochlear vessels provide the blood supply to the forehead.

☐ Lymphatics

The area just above the root of the nose drains into the submandibular group of lymph nodes. The remainder of the forehead and temporal region drains into the superficial parotid lymph nodes. These nodes, which lie just anterior to the tragus, are located on or deep toward the parotid fascia.

■ AESTHETICS

This obvious area of the face can be covered by hairstyling in the female, but camouflaging is not usually possible to the same extent in the male, particularly if he has male pattern baldness. Thus serious consideration must be given to any transgression of this area for reconstruction. If a lesion is excised from the forehead, the method chosen to fill the resulting defect must be carefully planned. The hairline should not be altered except in the most minor way. The eyebrows should not be displaced, and the frontal branch of the facial nerve should be spared unless resection is necessary for complete tumor removal. Similarly, the sensory nerves should not be wantonly sacrificed, even though recovery of sensation is usually complete.

■ PLACEMENT OF FOREHEAD INCISIONS

Ideally, the lines of minimal relaxed tension are chosen for scar position.[2] In the forehead these lines are transverse; in the glabellar region, vertical. If scars are placed in a frown line, the aesthetic result is quite acceptable. It is not always possible to choose the ideal scar line, and often the scar may be at right angles to the minimal relaxed tension lines, that is, vertical. With careful suturing, however, the results with vertical scars are often good, particularly if revised at a later date with a W-plasty. Scars running diagonally on the forehead are often the least satisfactory and may defy adequate revision. Occasionally it may be necessary to resort to a Z-plasty. This, however, may introduce the problems of bunching up, such as "trap-dooring" and "pincushioning," within the scars of the Z flaps.

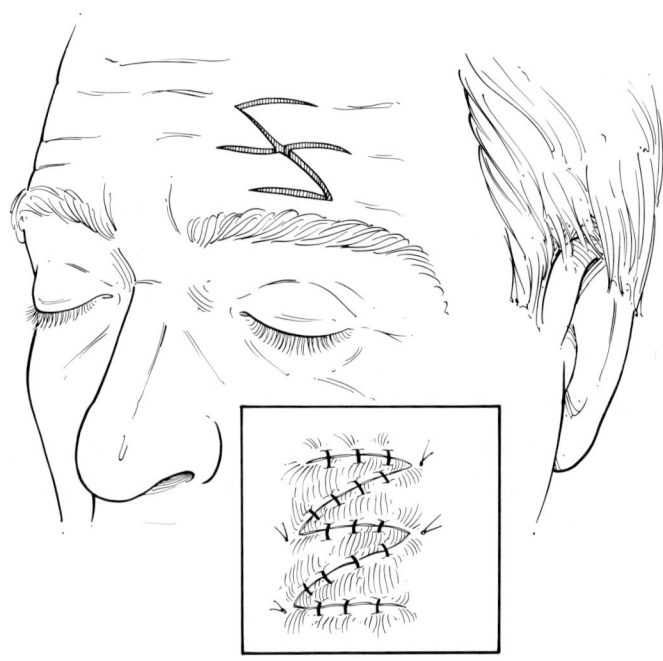

When raising flaps on the forehead, the surgeon should make all incisions vertically through the skin. We are all familiar with the pincushion effect of windshield injuries of the forehead in which the skin has been cut tangentially, raising small flaps. Even with careful incision placement, the pincushion effect may occur, particularly with round flaps; this may be caused by circumferential scar contracture. The introduction of angles into a flap (e.g., Limberg flap) prevents the pincushion effect from occurring (see p. 19), although the mechanism by which this happens is not known.

■ AREAS OF TISSUE AVAILABILITY

The natural mobility of the scalp allows the forehead to be rotated to close defects. Because the hairline and eyebrows form rigid boundaries on the forehead, care is taken in the planning of these flaps to prevent gross hairline irregularities. The skin for reconstruction lies within this demarcated area and must be moved around carefully to avoid disrupting these landmarks. The temporal region has loose skin; thus flaps can be moved within the constraints of its boundaries.

■ AREAS TO BE RECONSTRUCTED

The surgical options for forehead reconstruction are local flaps or skin grafts. Because of the color and texture of the transplanted skin, neither full-thickness nor split-thickness grafts provide satisfactory donor material, although reasonable results may still be obtained when these grafts are used for complete forehead resurfacing. Even in that situation, a thin, free vascularized flap is by far the best solution. The forehead can be divided into four areas: main forehead area, supraeyebrow area, temporal region, and glabellar region. It is convenient to consider the most suitable reconstruction in relation to these divisions because the flaps of choice are different for each region.

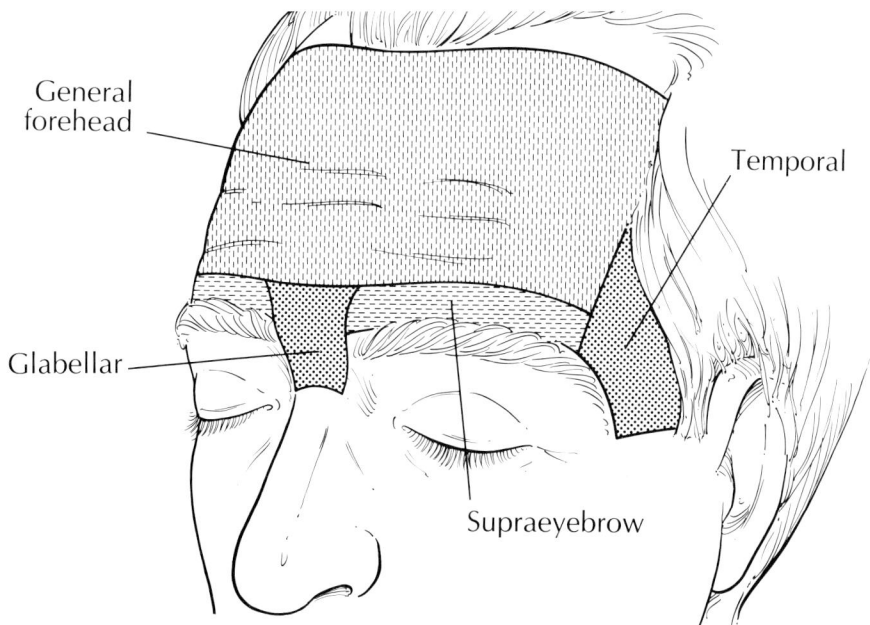

☐ Main Forehead Reconstruction

FACTORS TO CONSIDER

In the forehead region, scars, skin color, and texture are important considerations because the forehead is relatively flat, with few light and shade patterns; therefore any contour changes or alterations in skin color are quite obvious. Contour irregularities are highlighted in tangential light because room lighting is usually overhead or from the wall area. Flaps should be the same thickness as that of the skin excised in order to prevent pincushioning. Hairline and eyebrow symmetry should also be maintained. Scars should blend into natural skin lines. The frontalis muscle should not be damaged if possible, since a palsy or muscle dysfunction is easily noticed.

SCALP ROTATION

When possible, provided the hairline will not be significantly disturbed, rotation of the scalp is an ideal solution to many forehead defects. This reconstruction is particularly satisfactory when the scalp is moved from a posterior to an anterior direction in the bald male, since it reduces the bald area. The patient in the figure below illustrates this principle.

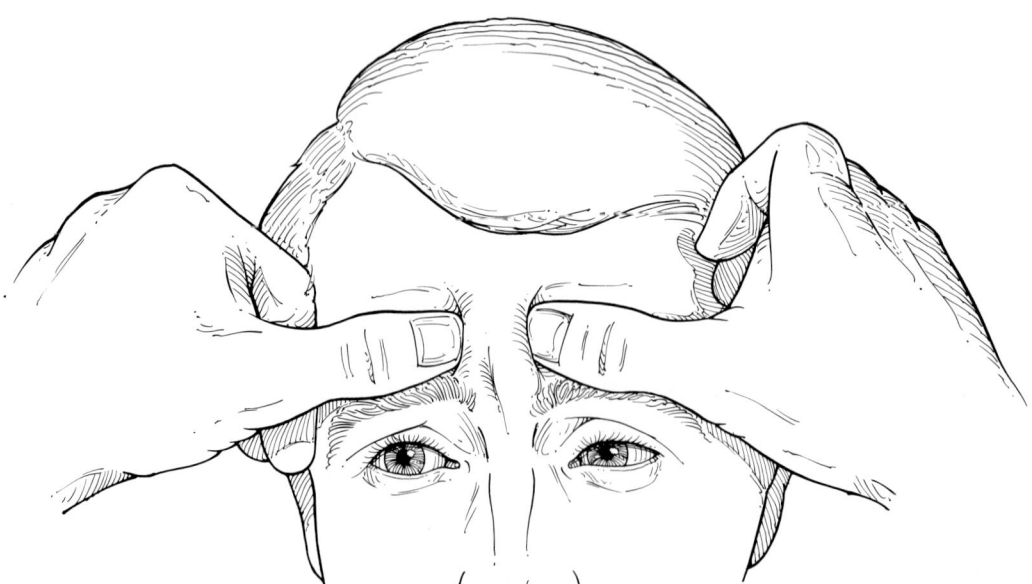

In most instances it is possible to assess the ability to perform a scalp rotation by estimating the looseness of the scalp. The scalp can be picked up by the fingers; if there is excess scalp, then reconstruction is simple. In addition, the overall rotational movement of the scalp on the periosteum assessed by the examining hand will give an idea of how much advancement may be obtained. This movement is judged by placing the fingertips on the scalp and pushing it in all directions. The amount of movement suggests how easy it will be to redistribute the scalp after the resection.

CHAPTER 3
FOREHEAD RECONSTRUCTION

UNILATERAL ROTATION FLAP

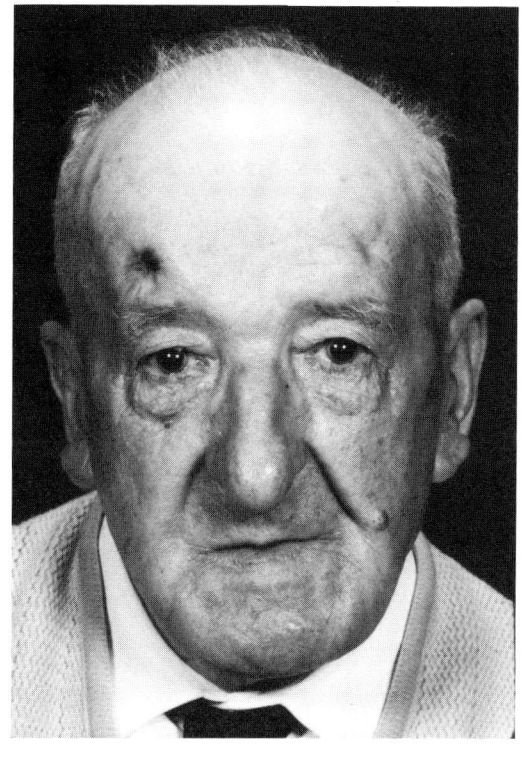

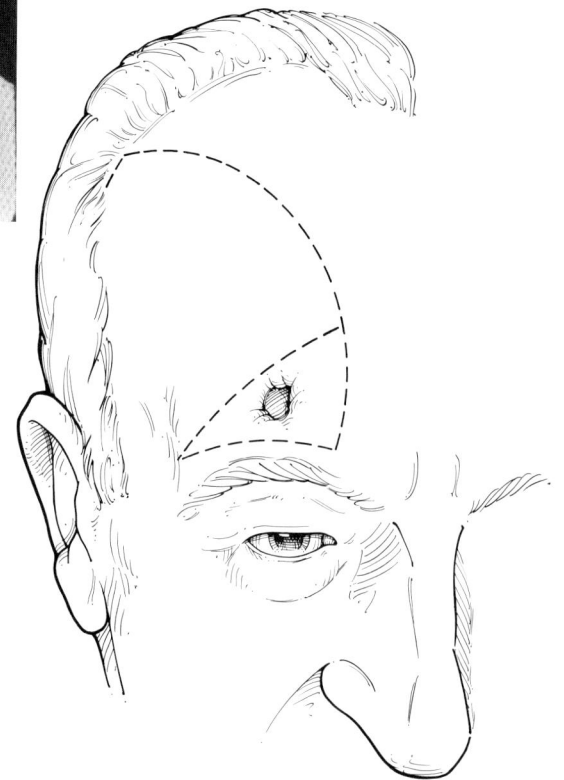

Resection of a lesion above the eyebrow makes forehead reconstruction difficult; any miscalculation in the reconstruction will elevate this natural landmark and cause facial asymmetry. The supraorbital basal cell carcinoma shown in the illustration above presents such a problem. The first move is to triangulate the excision with the base medially.

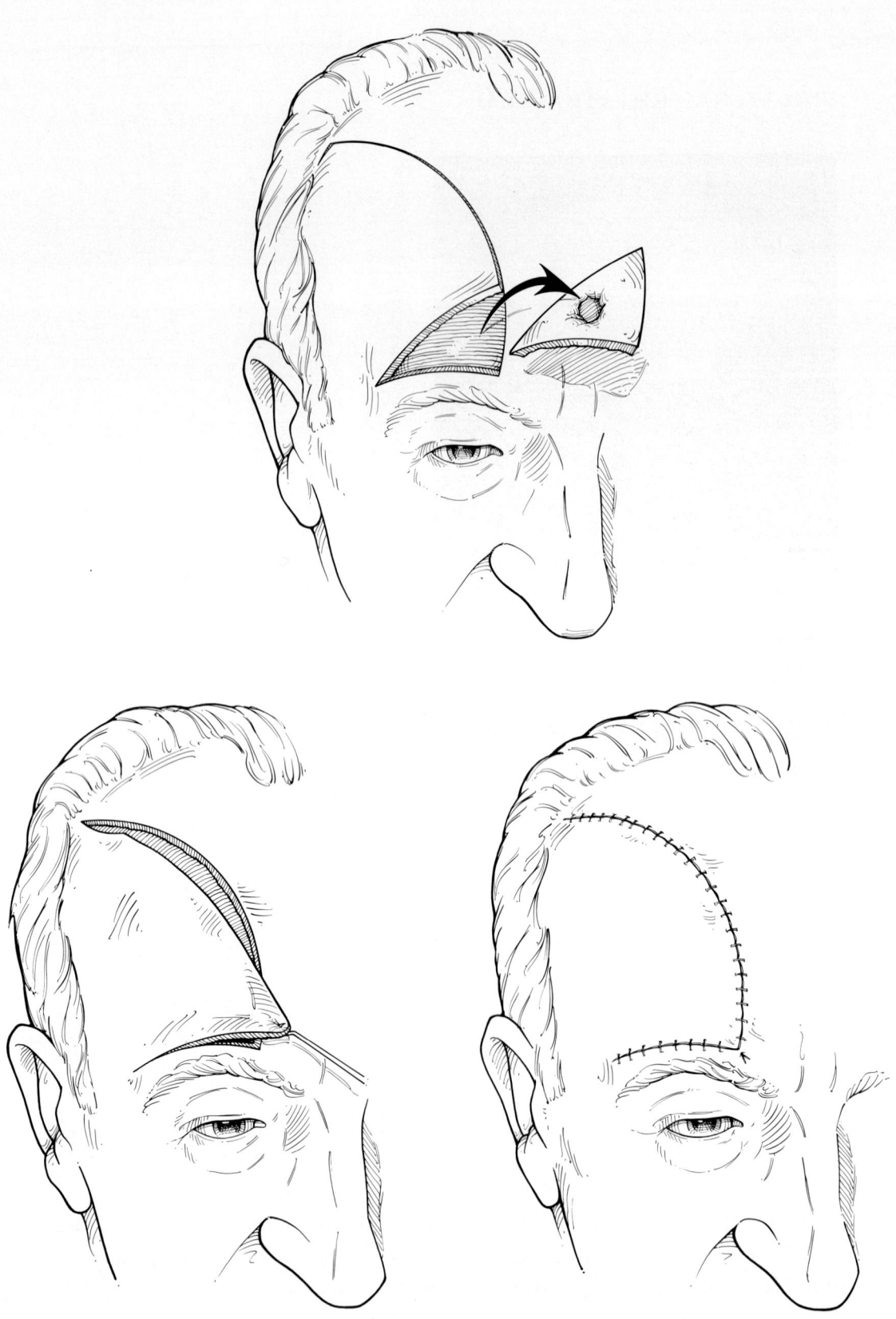

A triangular defect of this type can be closed with a rotation flap raised above the pericranium. This flap is based on temporal and some occipital vascular input and must be raised radically in the lateral area.

The rotation should be effortless and suturing should be without tension. Any tension will elevate the eyebrow and may compromise the blood supply of the tip of the flap. Should closure not be adequate, a back cut can be made at the most posterior extent of the flap. Such a cut allows greater ease of advancement, and in most cases this posterior secondary defect can be closed directly without difficulty.

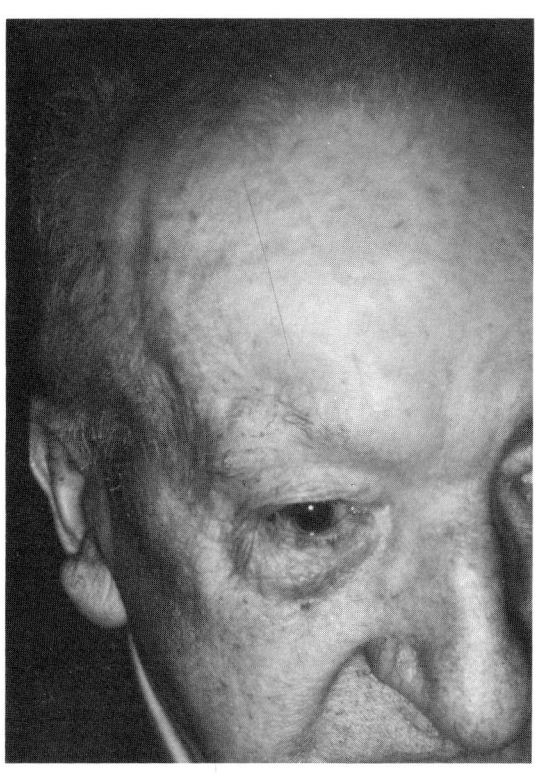

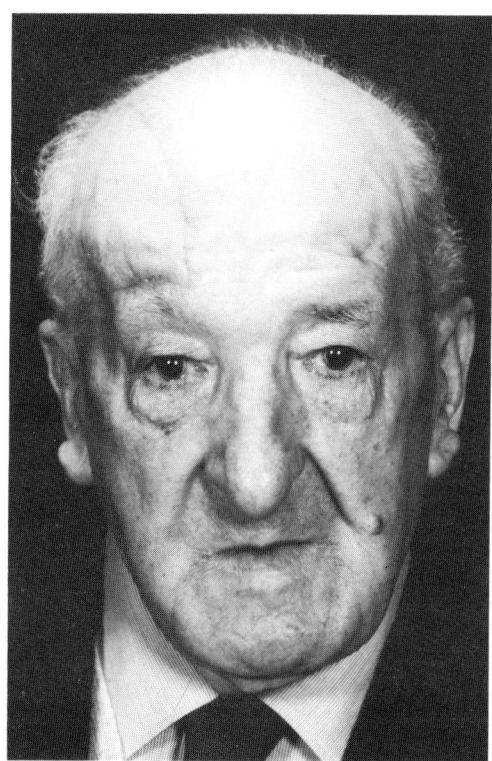

In the early postoperative phase an obvious scar and contour irregularity are present. With time this situation improves and a very acceptable result with maintenance of eyebrow position can be obtained.

PROBLEMS

Potential problems include hematoma under the flap and tightness and ischemia of the flap with eventual necrosis if flap tension persists. The hematoma must be released and, if necessary, a drain inserted. At the time of surgery the use of a drain is advised with a postoperative pressure dressing. If the flap has not been well planned and is tight, the circulation will be compromised. In this instance the sutures should be removed and the flap allowed to recover. A further attempt to remove the flap can be made in 1 to 2 days with a generous back cut to allow more mobility. Incisions within the hairline may not heal perfectly, with associated alopecia requiring later excision and resuture. Anesthesia or hypesthesia of the rotated portion of the forehead may occur; this condition will improve with time but may never be absolutely normal.

AIDING SCALP CLOSURE

GALEAL SCORING

Despite preoperative estimates, closure sometimes may be difficult, even with the use of a back cut. In this situation the technique of galeal incisions or scoring can be most useful. At 0.5 to 1 cm intervals, parallel to the leading edge of the flap, the galea is incised, with the underlying vessels preserved. If these cuts do not give enough movement, further galeal cuts at right angles to the previous ones are made to allow increased flap stretching.

SCALP STRETCHING

Occasionally, in large scalp defects, the phenomena of creep and stress relaxation may be used to achieve closure. These two principles are based on the viscoelastic properties of skin: when placed under a constant tension, skin stretches.

CHAPTER 3
FOREHEAD RECONSTRUCTION

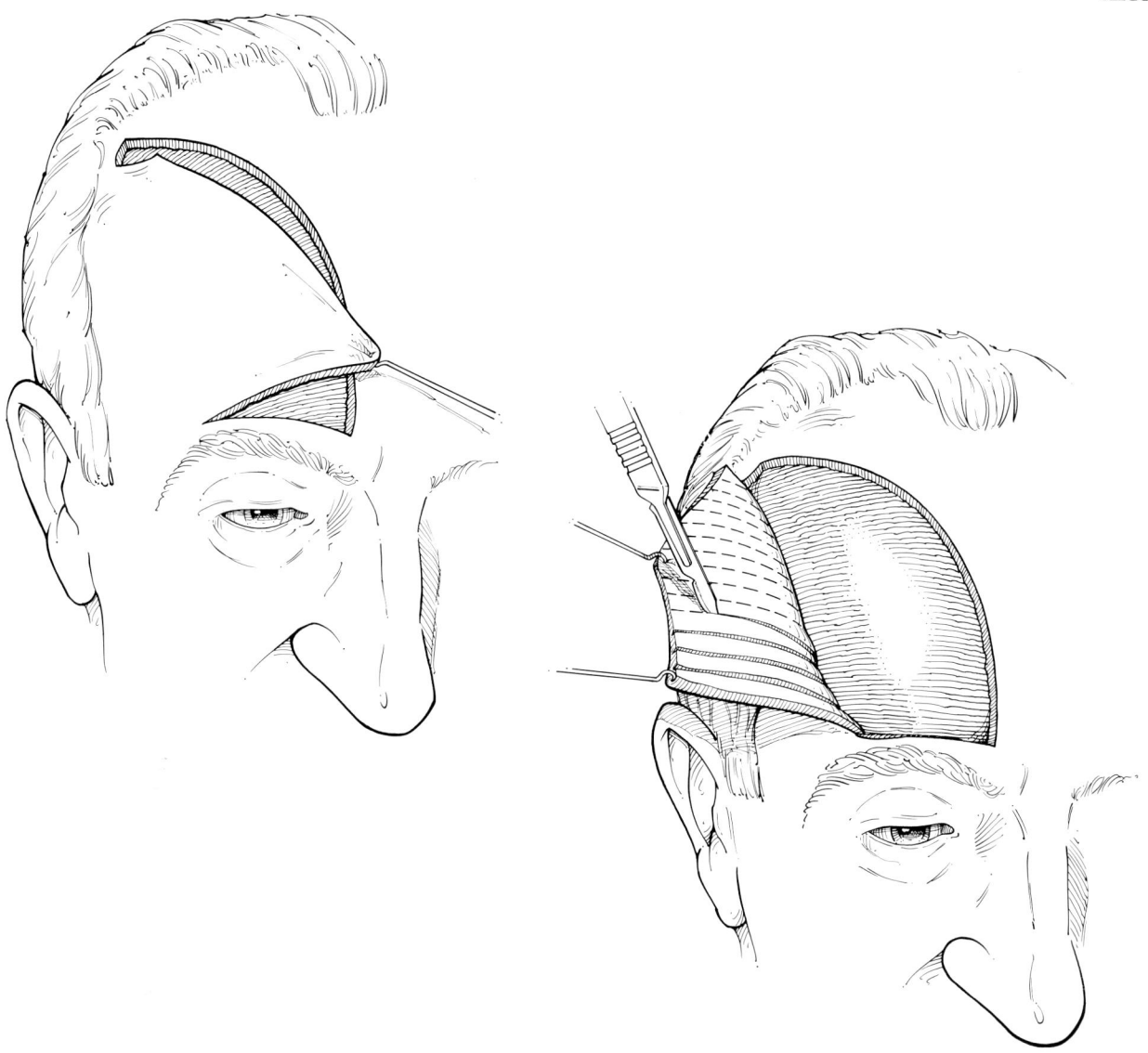

When the tension is discontinued, the skin does not return to its original length; it has become permanently stretched.[6,7,8] For closure of a large scalp defect, this stretching phenomenon is accomplished by placing two large hooks or rakes on the leading edge of the flap and pulling forcibly for at least 5 minutes.

SKIN GRAFTS

As a last resort for closure, a secondary defect may be accepted and a split-thickness skin graft applied. Grafting is possible only if the flap has been raised above the pericranium because skin grafts do not "take" on bare skull bone. This solution is not particularly desirable from an aesthetic point of view and, fortunately, is a rare eventuality.

WORTHEN ROTATION FLAP

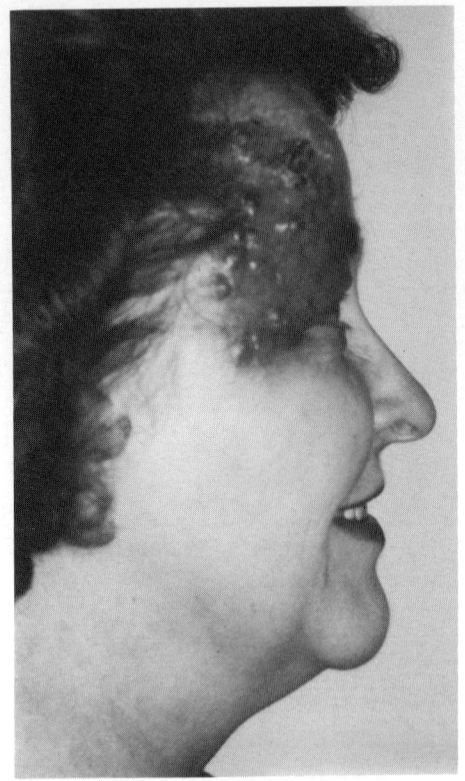

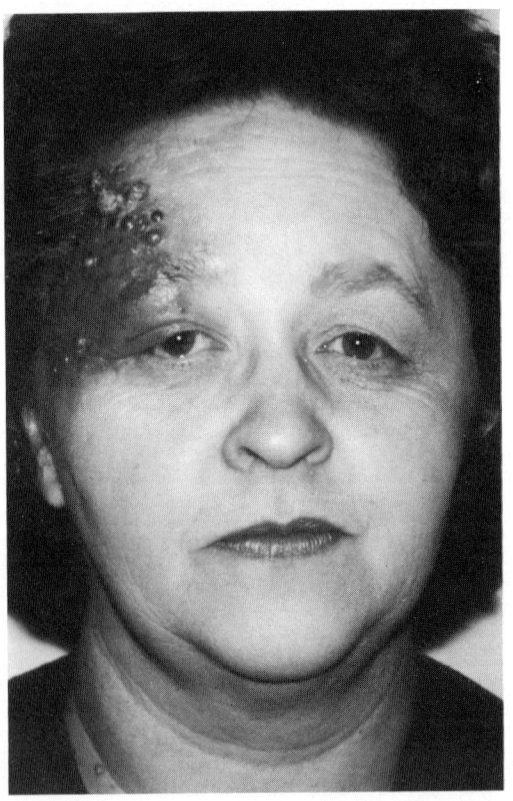

When large unilateral defects involving virtually the whole hemiforehead result from tumor resection, the concept advanced by Worthen[11] may be used. This technique has been applied to the right hemiforehead and upper eyelid nodular hemangioma, illustrated in the following patient.

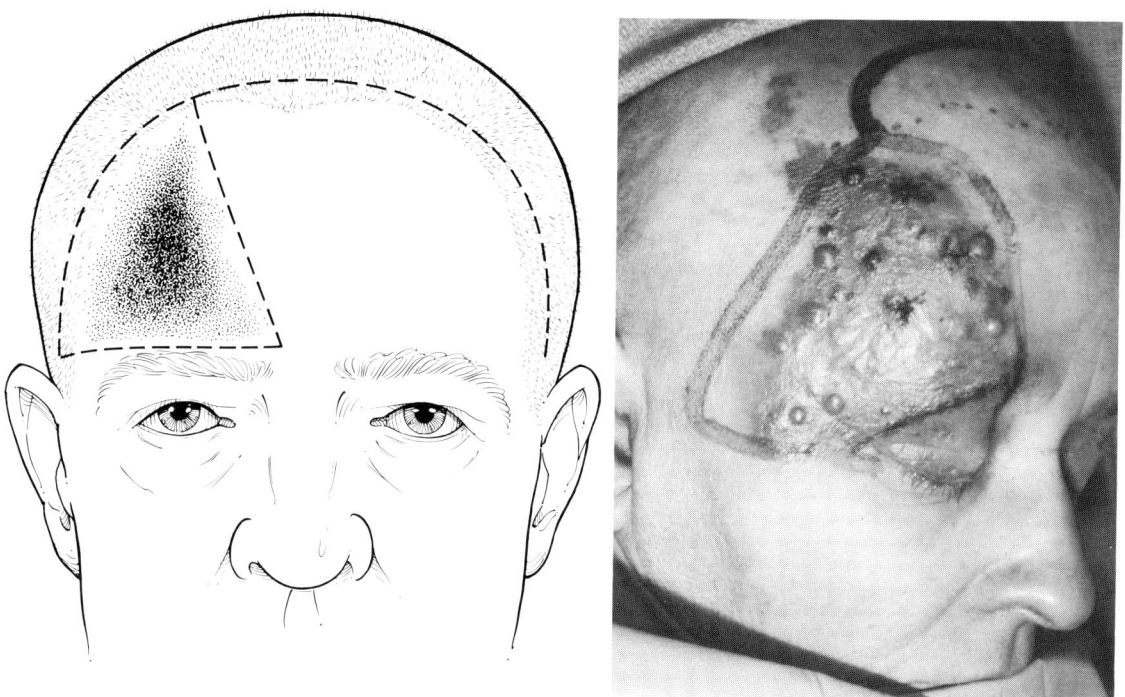

The vertical height of the forehead in the midline is approximately equal to the horizontal width of the hemiforehead just above the eyebrows.

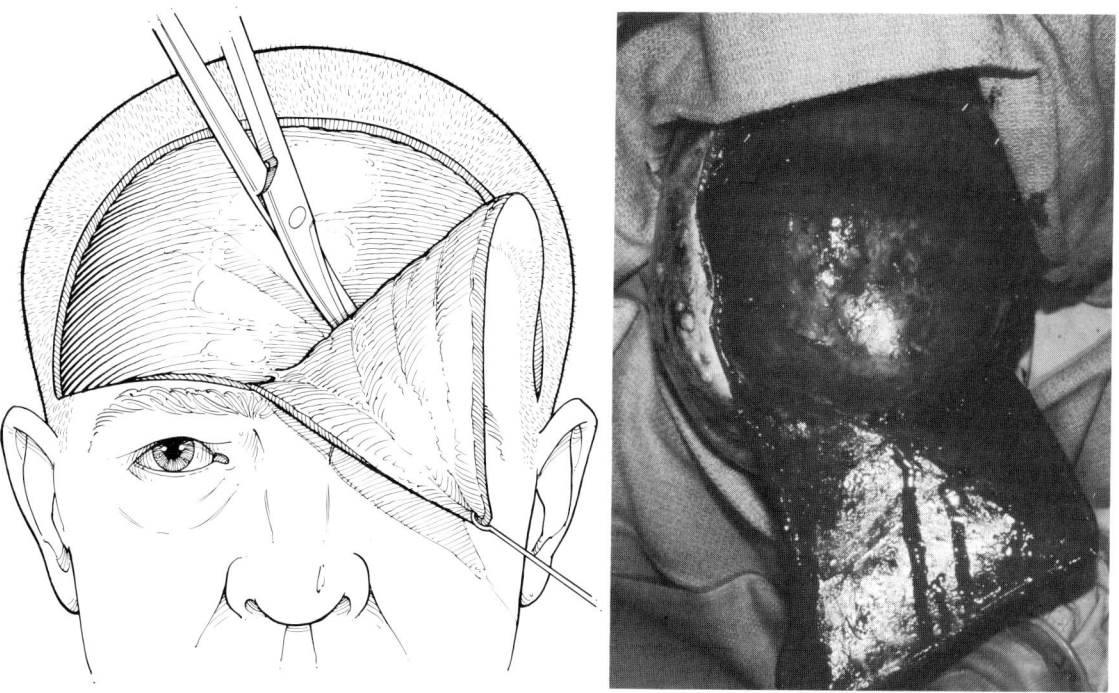

An incision completely within the hairline, or one initially in front of the hairline and then within the hairline down to the temporal region, will allow rotation of the whole remaining forehead.

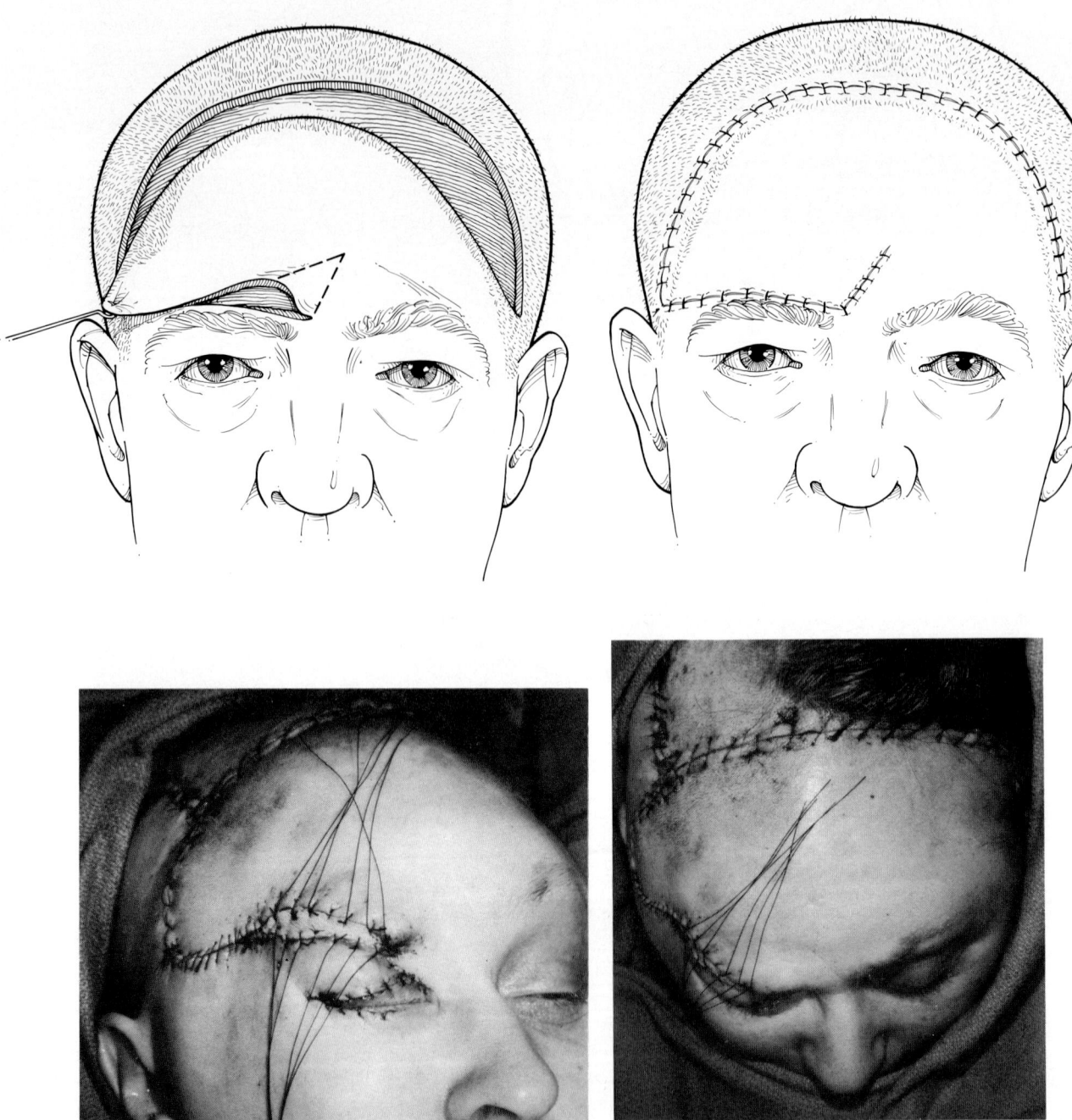

The vertical edge of the flap becomes the horizontal suture line. In this technique two rotational movements are being used: the loose scalp of the temporal area is being stretched, and the lateral scalp areas on both sides are being advanced.

CHAPTER 3
FOREHEAD RECONSTRUCTION

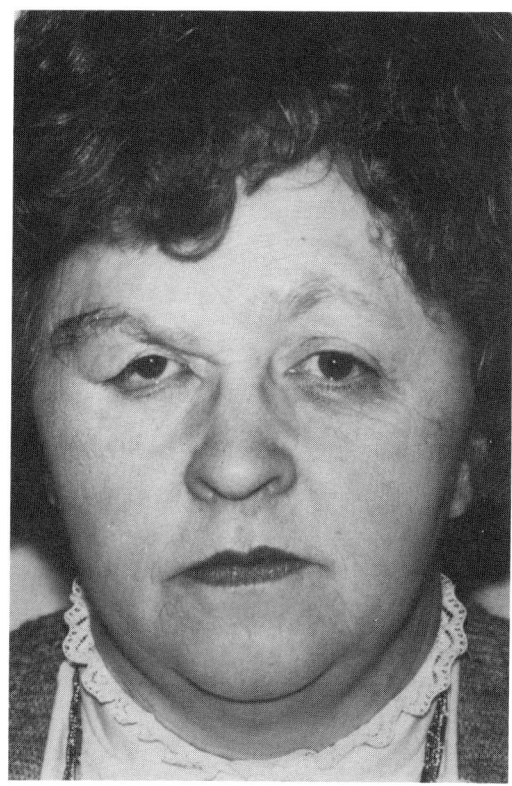

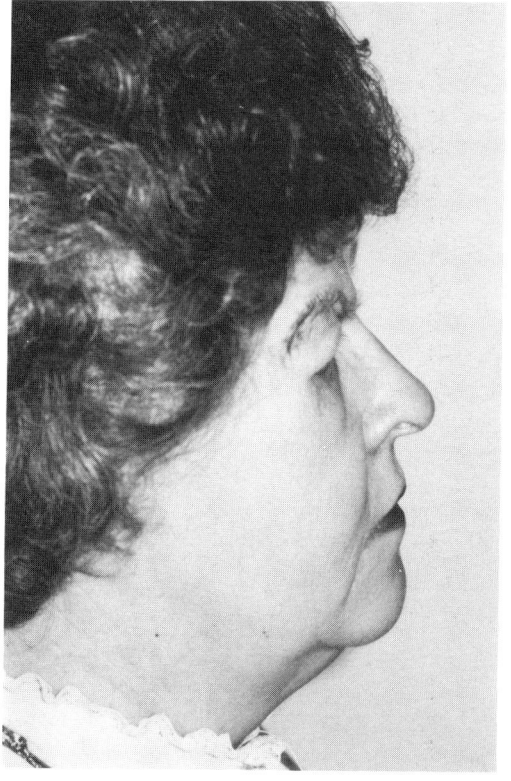

Some distortion of the eyebrows and the hairline may occur, but this is usually acceptable when compared to the original problem.

PROBLEMS

Careful preoperative assessment and planning is the secret to success for this procedure. If the hairline is low, the flap will not be large enough to close the defect. Wide undermining of adjacent scalp will be necessary for closure, but it will be under tension and necrosis of skin edges or parts of the flap may result. Even if healing occurs, the hairline and eyebrows may be distorted.

BILATERAL ROTATION FLAP

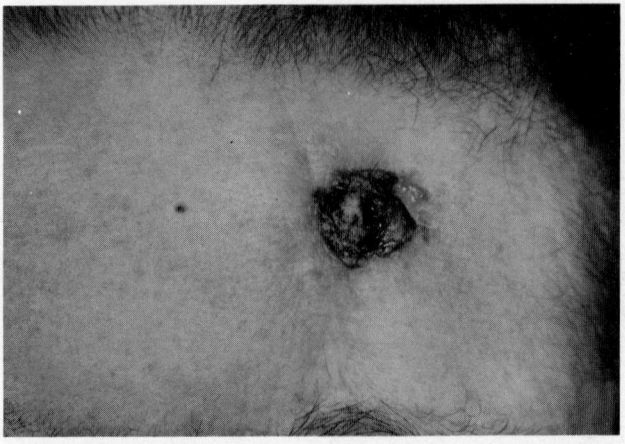

When scalp mobility is insufficient to obtain defect closure with one flap, bilateral rotation flaps may provide the solution. This method has been applied in a patient with recurrent forehead basal cell carcinoma after surgery and radiotherapy.

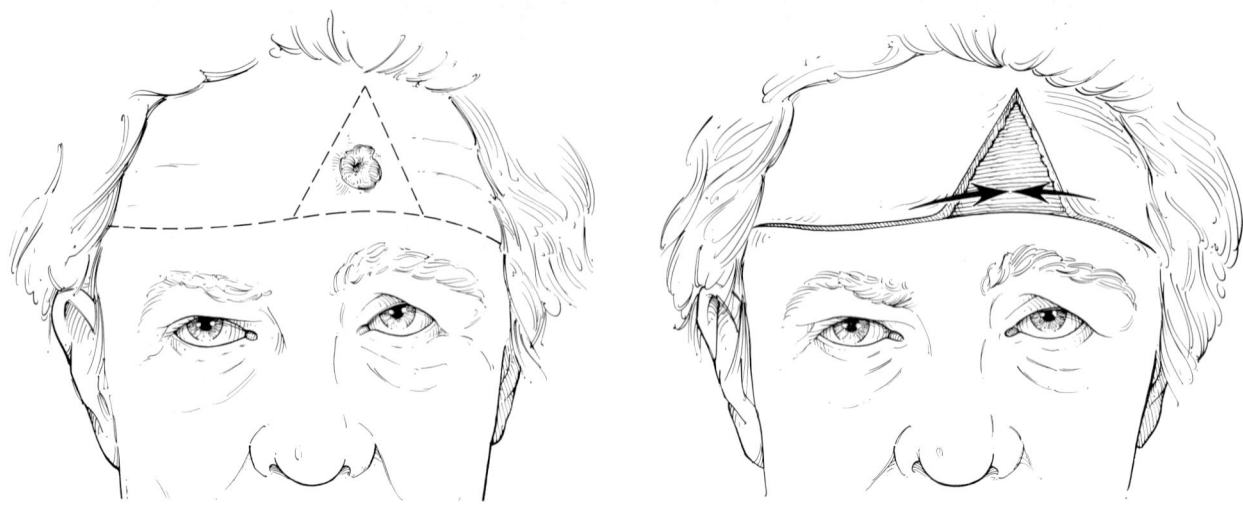

The defect is triangulated (the base being inferior) in a frown line, and the lesion is resected in this particular case with the underlying outer table of skull.

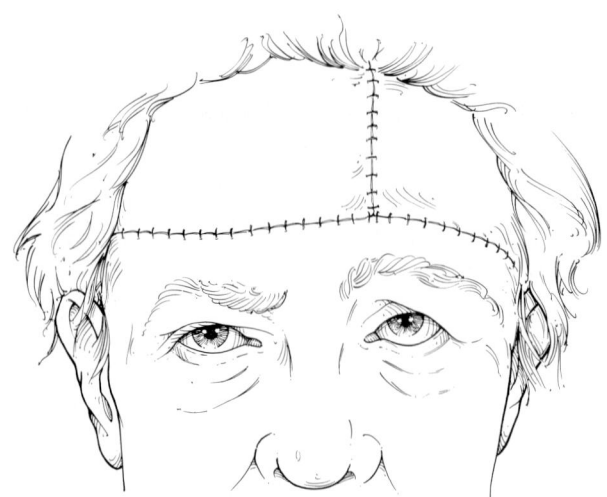

CHAPTER 3
FOREHEAD RECONSTRUCTION

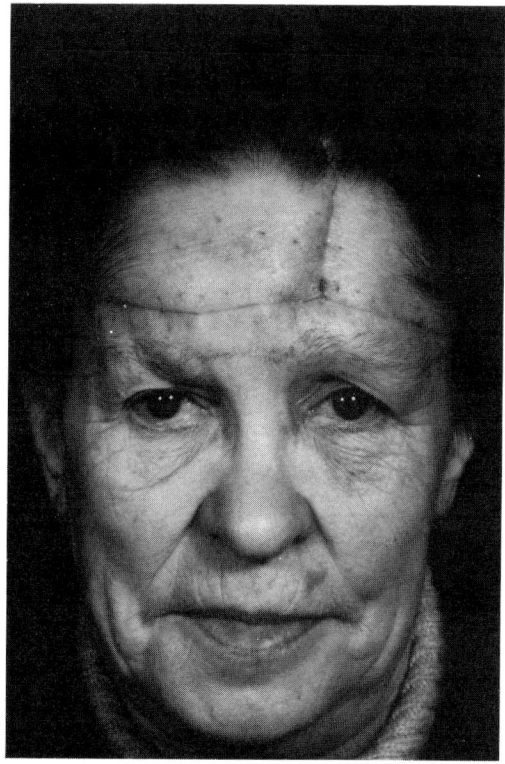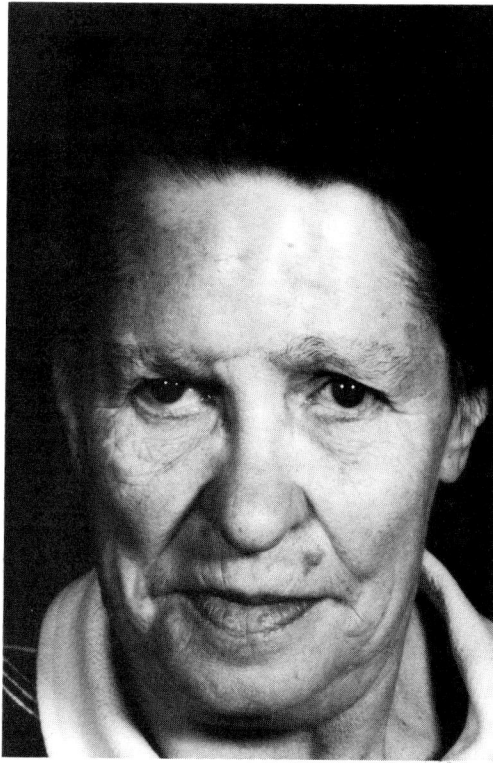

Posteriorly based bilateral scalp rotation flaps are raised above the pericranium and rotated anteriorly to close the defect. A dog ear will often appear at the superior angle of the triangle and needs to be trimmed to avoid a standing cone deformity. In rare instances bilateral back cuts may be necessary to facilitate closure. Again, these can usually be closed directly. The scars are in a fairly good position, but the forehead is denervated. Since these flaps are bilateral, symmetry is maintained, and the result is acceptable, especially after time has elapsed and the scars have matured.

PROBLEMS

Problems of bilateral flaps are similar to those encountered with unilateral flaps. If both flaps are unduly tight, bilateral necrosis may occur resulting in a bigger secondary defect.

Care must be taken in raising the flaps. It is possible to carry the lateral incisions too far posteriorly, thus depriving the scalp of circulation above these incisions. The surgeon must always stop before coming to the occipital vessels and perform a generous vertical back cut.

☐ Supraeyebrow Reconstruction

This is a difficult area to reconstruct, since the slightest error in judgement will lead to eyebrow displacement and noticeable asymmetry. A skin graft is not acceptable because of the obvious pale, mat skin patch appearance it creates. In the past a full-thickness forehead skin graft of half the dimension of the defect was taken from the same position on the other side with the thought that both eyebrows would be raised and symmetry maintained. Unfortunately, this skin also became pale, and the result was not satisfactory.

ISLAND FLAP

The island flap provides an ideal solution for reconstructing the supraeyebrow area and meets the requirements of flap selection: replacement of like tissue with like tissue and no distortion of normal anatomic landmarks.

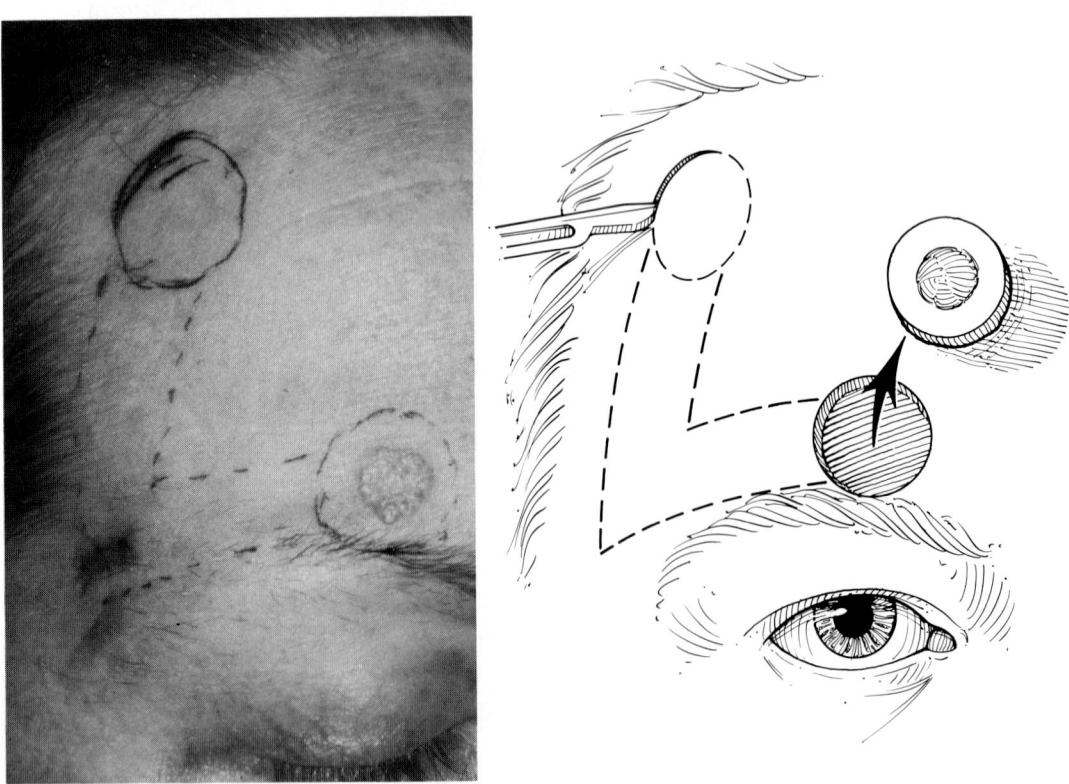

The patient shown above illustrates the effective use of these flaps in this area. This patient had a supraeyebrow basal cell carcinoma, and excision of this lesion left a significant defect. Direct closure of this defect would have caused unacceptable elevation of the patient's eyebrow.

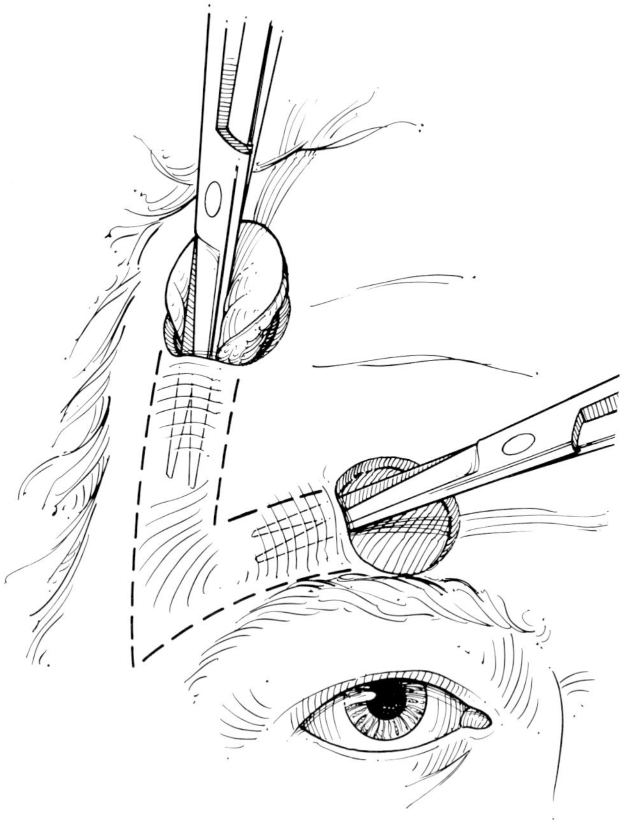

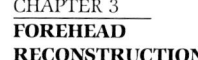
CHAPTER 3
FOREHEAD RECONSTRUCTION

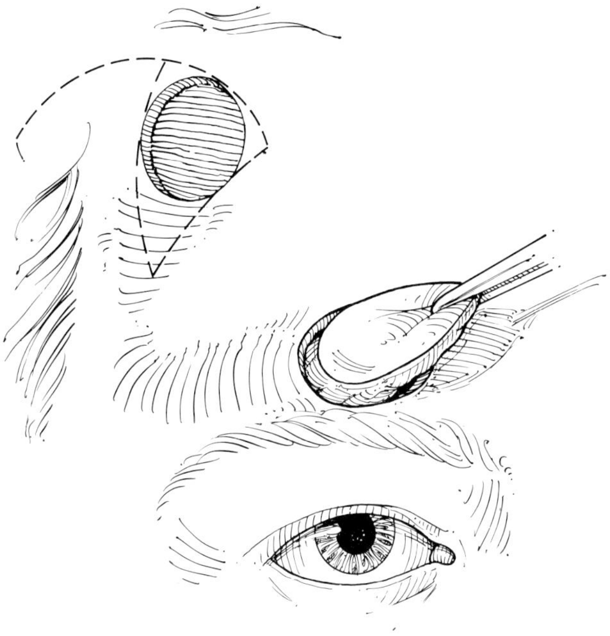

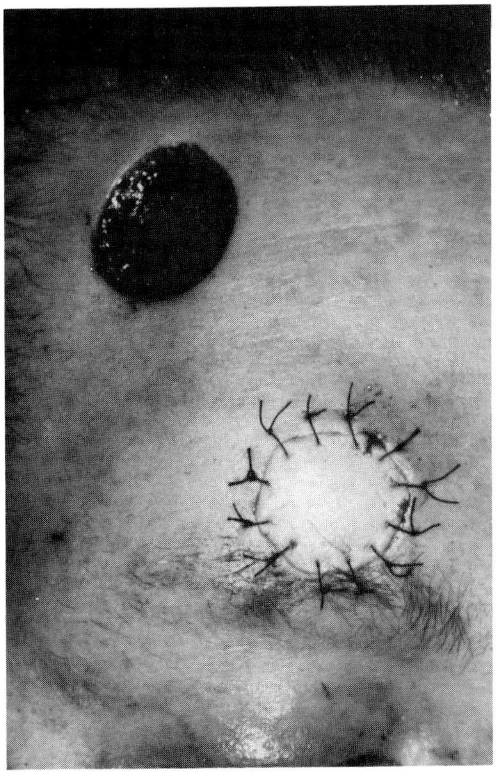

An island of skin with a subcutaneous pedicle taken to just above the periosteum and based on the superficial temporal vessels could be raised and tunneled under the forehead skin to close the raw area.

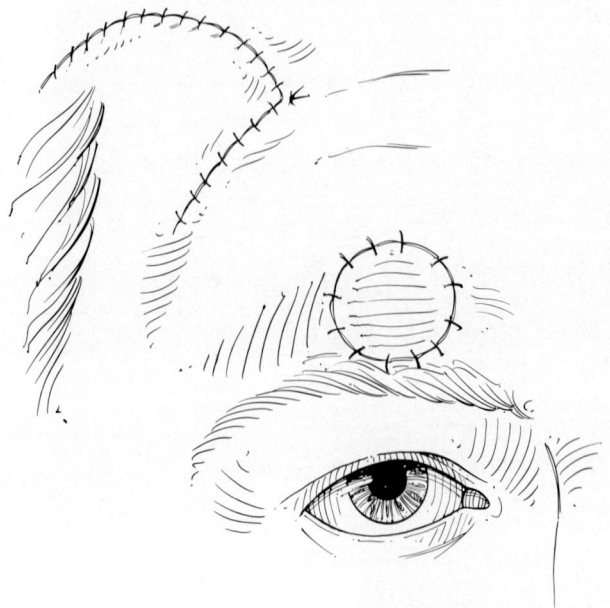

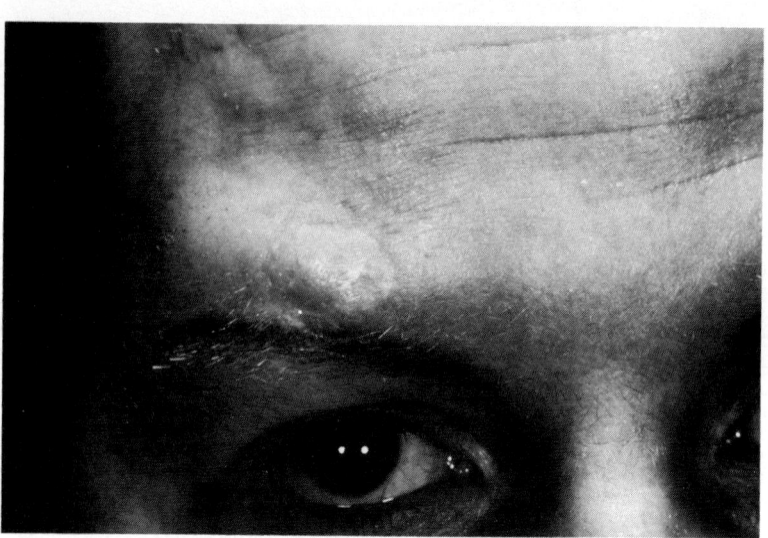

The donor site is closed with a small scalp rotation flap. This gives a good result without distortion of normal anatomic features.

This type of island flap need not always be raised on known vessels; it can be constructed on a subcutaneous pedicle based on a transposition flap design, which is known to work.[1] Absolutely no tension must be present on the pedicle, and the tunnel to the excisional defect must be generous in the extreme. It may be possible to close the secondary defect as an ellipse and end with a scar in a frown line.

PROBLEMS

The island is planned carefully on a known vascular pattern. Sometimes a definite vessel will be included in the pedicle. Ischemia will occur if the pedicle is too long, under tension, or constricted within its tunnel. As with any other flap, serious vascular impairment requires replacement of the flap back in its original position. Since the flap is circular, it may pincushion.

HATCHET FLAPS

The use of hatchet flaps, described by Emmett,[5] is shown above. When a lesion is excised in a circular fashion, the triangles of skin that would have to be excised laterally to convert the circle into an ellipse can be used in closure of the defect. It is from these that hatchet flaps are constructed. The hatchet flap is basically a V-Y advancement flap. The shaft of the hatchet provides a skin pedicle in addition to the subcutaneous pedicle. If the skin pedicle is sacrificed, the hatchet flap becomes a kite flap.[4]

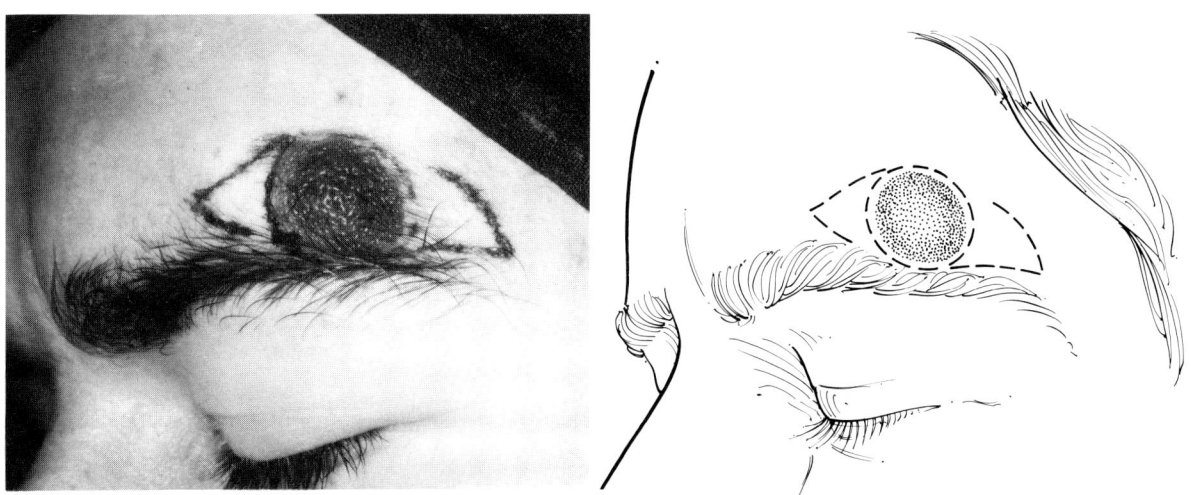

The patient shown here had a nevus above the left eyebrow; its excision created a small but significant defect. A small raw area in this region can be a considerable reconstructive problem, requiring the addition of tissue. Simple closure means deformity and asymmetry because of eyebrow displacement.

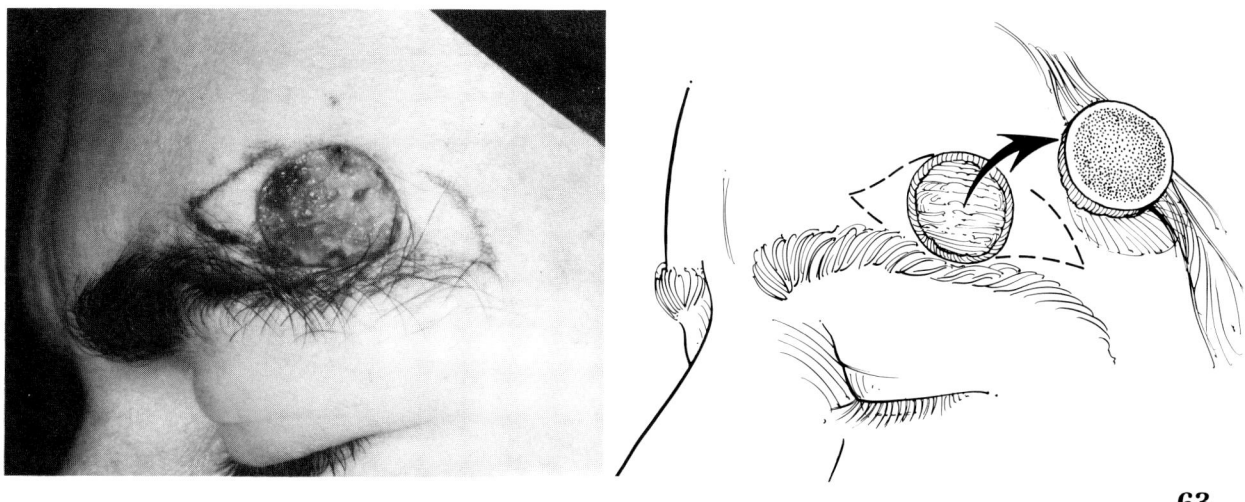

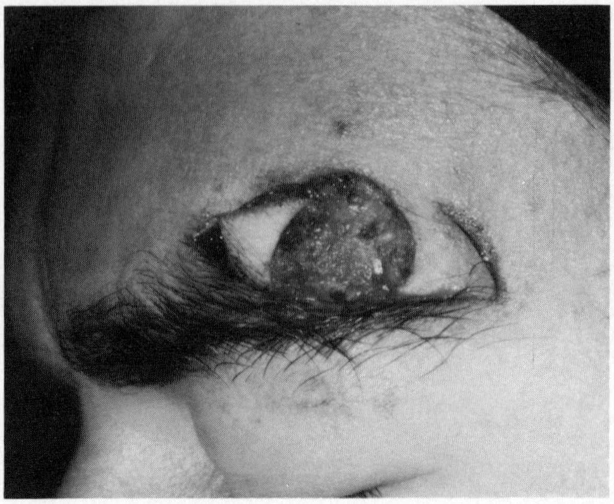

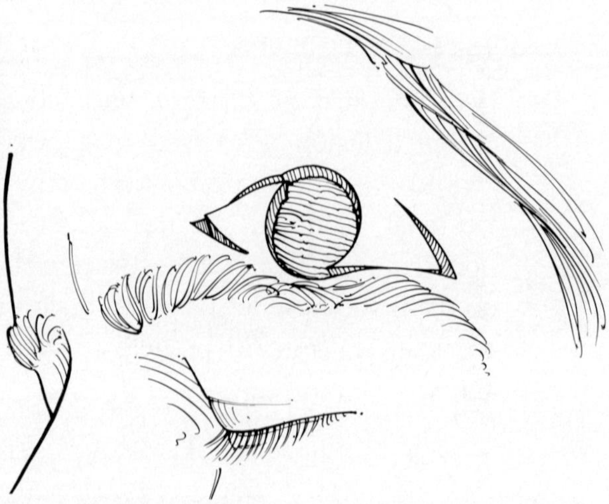

The flaps are raised as bilateral triangles on subcutaneous pedicles situated immediately under the flaps, but they also have small skin pedicles.

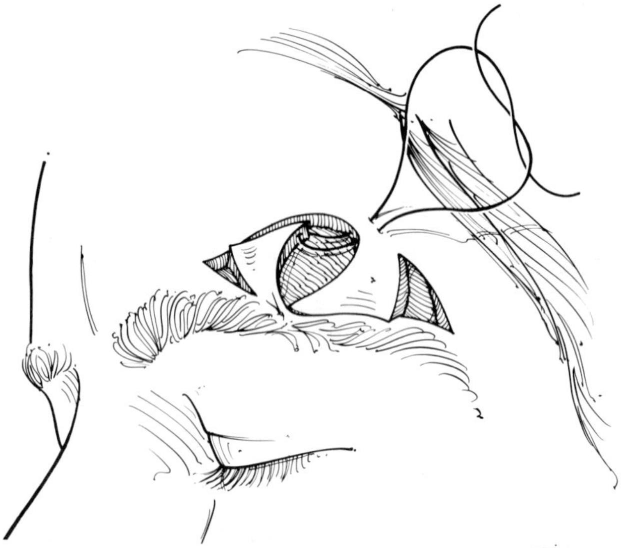

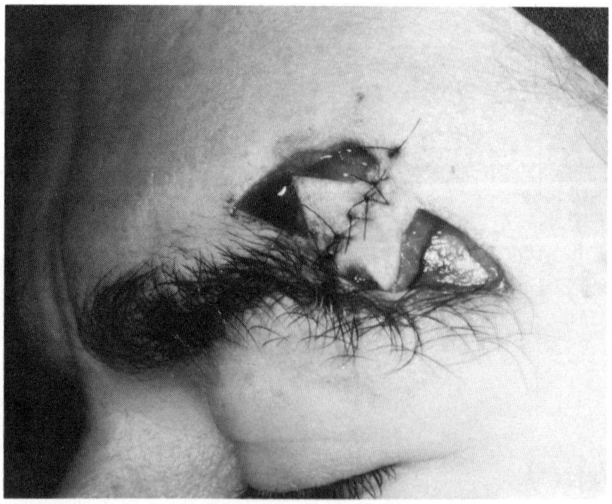

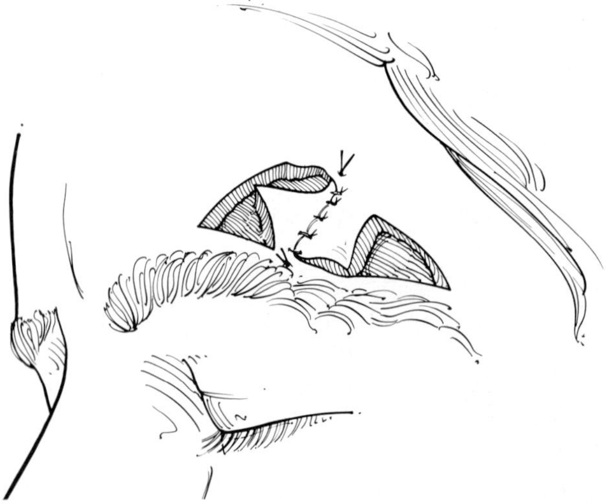

64 As dissection proceeds around the flaps, medial movement is facilitated, and closure is possible without tension.

CHAPTER 3
FOREHEAD RECONSTRUCTION

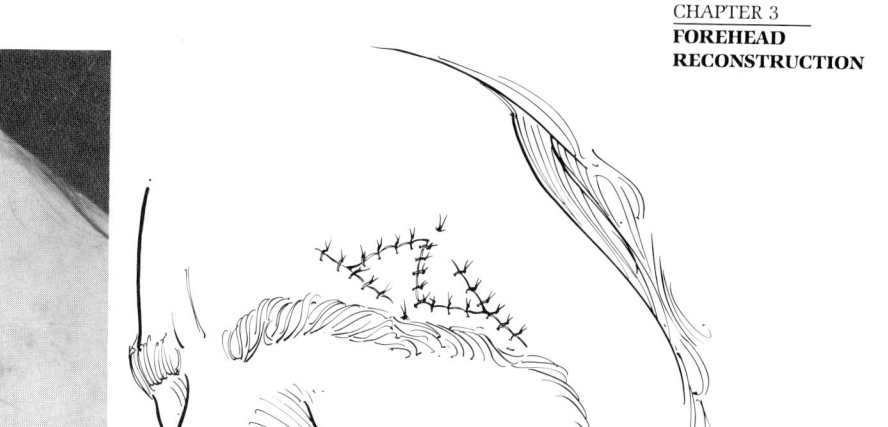

As the bases of the triangles are approximated, the resulting defect is closed directly. Closure is achieved in a V-Y fashion.

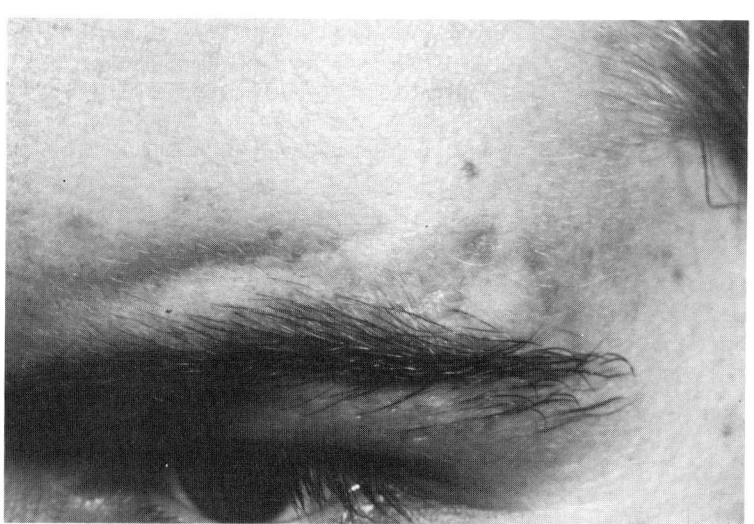
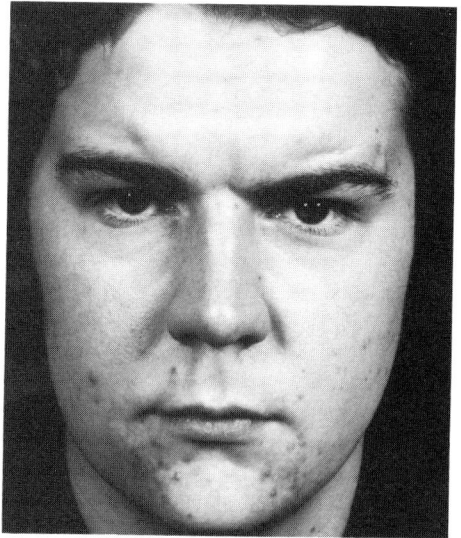

The position and contour of the eyebrow are maintained. Vascular insufficiency has not been encountered.

PROBLEMS

Hatchet flaps seldom become ischemic, but this possibility exists if they are sutured under tension and subsequent compromise of the pedicle circulation occurs.

Multiple scars are produced with this approach; if healing is not good, these may be obvious and require revision or dermabrasion.

RHOMBOID OR LIMBERG FLAP[9,10]

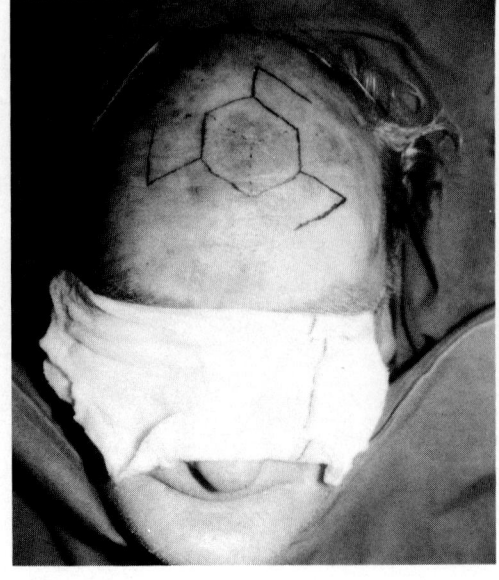

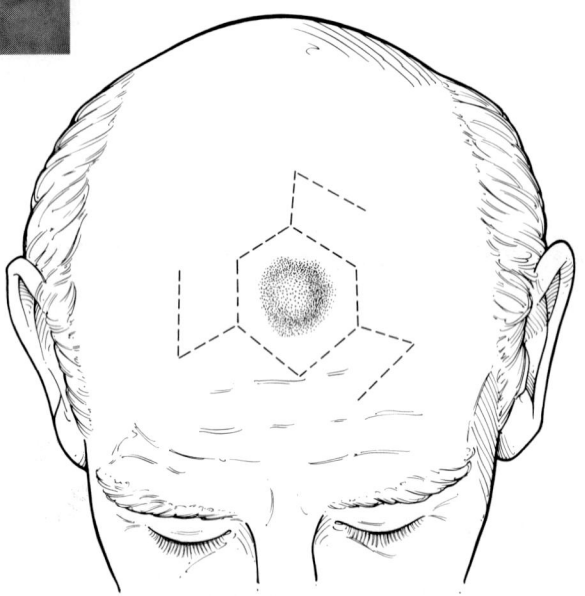

The rhomboid principle can be adapted to forehead and anterior scalp resections in bald males. It may be possible to reconstruct small defects with single rhomboid flaps, but this is not usually the case. From the viewpoint of tension and vascularity it is much better to spread the load. In the upper forehead superficial squamous cell carcinoma, a triple rhomboid (hexagonal) excision is planned. The three projected rhomboid defects can then be reconstructed with three rhomboid flaps. As illustrated on p. 48, the feasibility of success is determined by pinching the skin in the area of the projected rhomboid. If the fingertips can be brought together comfortably with the intervening skin, the reconstruction is possible.

CHAPTER 3
FOREHEAD RECONSTRUCTION

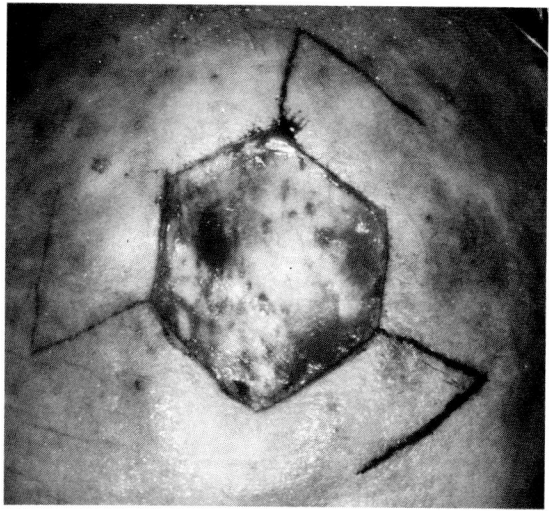
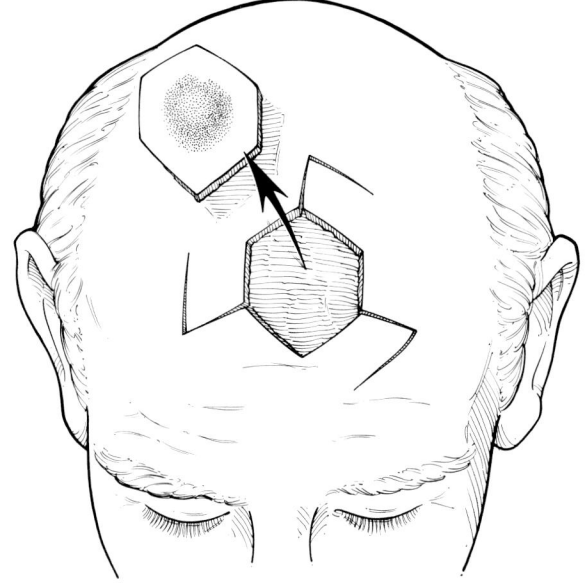

Following hexagonal excision of the lesion, the three rhomboid flaps based on the component rhomboids of the hexagon are planned.

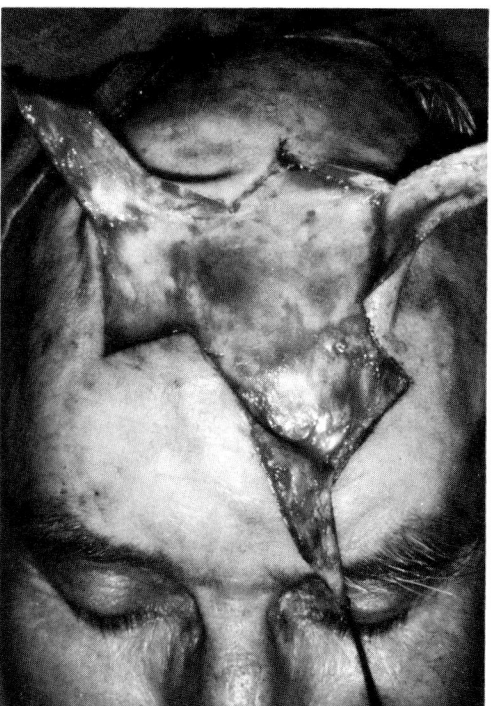
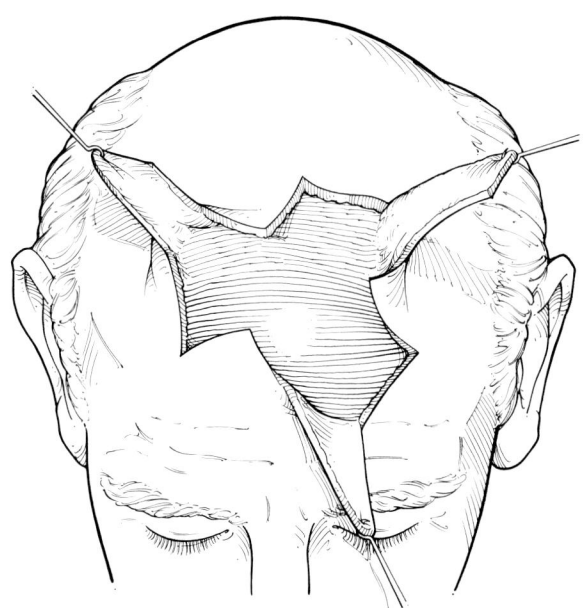

The rhomboid flaps are incised and then elevated. The elevation should be complete; to achieve adequate transposition, undermining should be taken beyond the bases of the flaps.

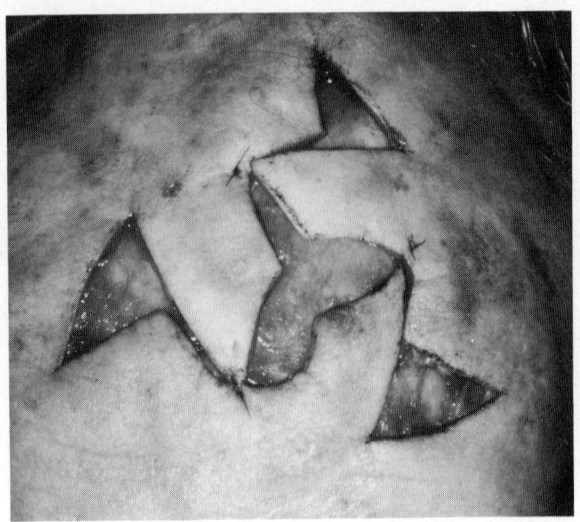 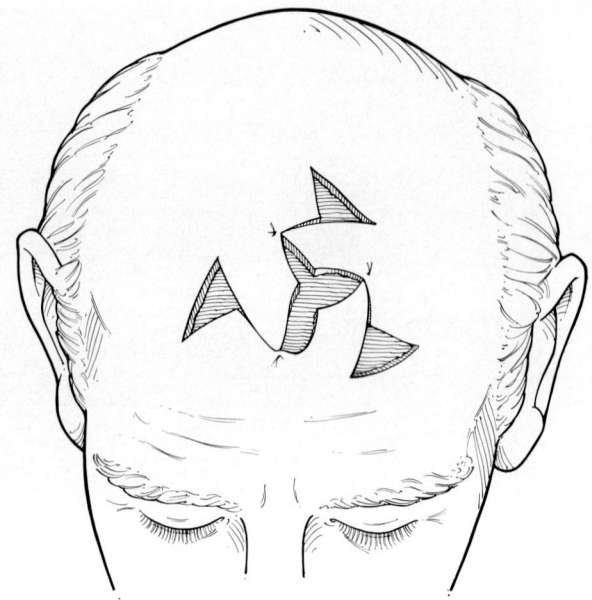

When the flaps are transposed, there should be minimal tension on them. Should tension occur, further dissection under the bases of the flaps is necessary.

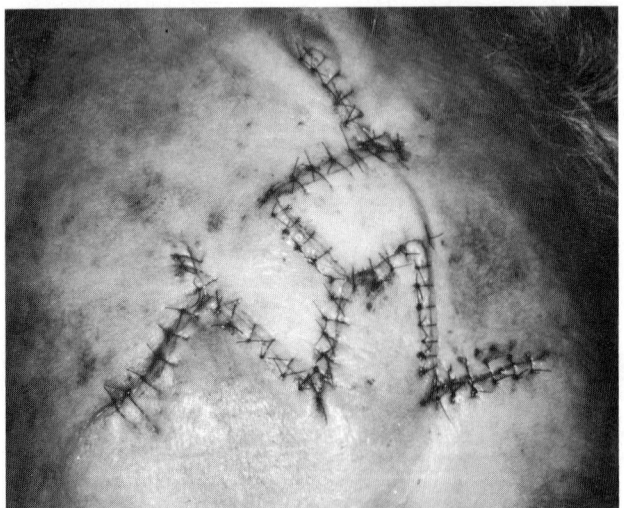 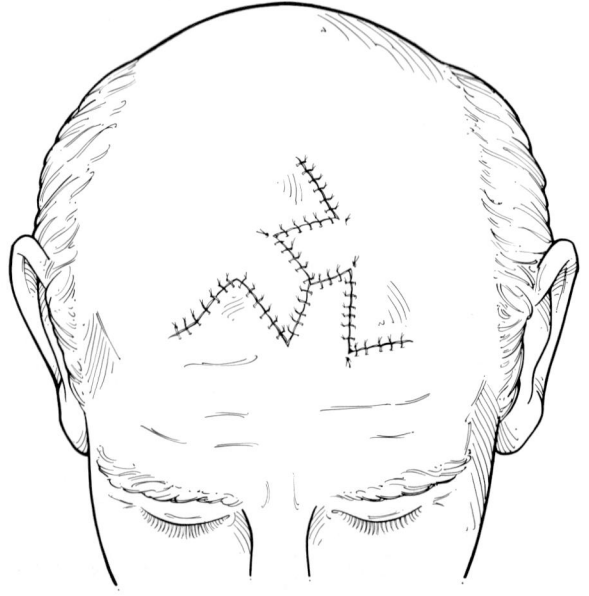

Closure of the secondary defects is often difficult; again, this may require some scalp undermining to prevent undue tension in the closure.

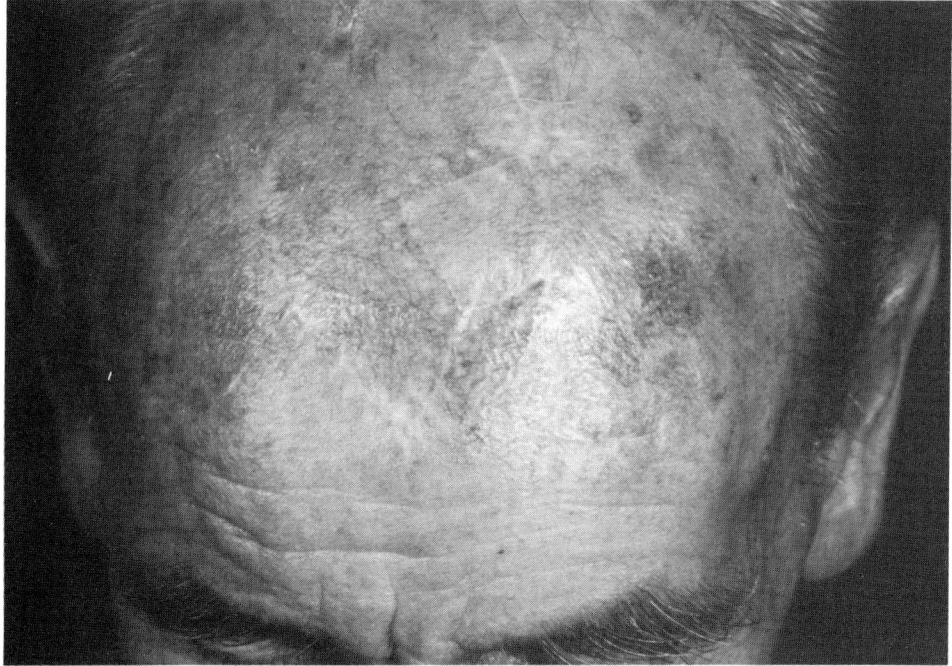

The result in this exposed area is very acceptable.

PROBLEMS

The disadvantage of this use of the Limberg technique is the multiplicity of scars. There is no possibility of placing these in ideal lines. The lack of pincushioning (trap-dooring) is a feature to be noted. If any type of circular flap is used, this would most certainly occur.

This procedure should be attempted only by those experienced in the use of rhomboid flaps. There is a delicate and narrow line between outstanding success and disastrous failure, particularly if the pericranium has been sacrificed. The all-too-familiar sequence of tension, ischemia, necrosis, exposed bone, and "where do we find another flap?" results from a failed flap procedure in the forehead.

The most significant problem resulting from this technique is the multiple scars it produces. These scars are aesthetically and oncologically undesirable. In cancer excision it is best to produce the simplest scars possible. Nonetheless, as in the case illustrated, this procedure can yield acceptable results.

☐ Reconstruction of Temporal Skin Defects

The margin for reconstructive error in the temporal area is small because it has well-defined, obvious anterior and posterior boundaries, the lateral end of the eyebrow and the temporal hairline. Any distortion of these natural landmarks is obvious and unacceptable. In addition, the lateral canthal area can be distorted by ill-planned reconstructive ventures that cause obvious asymmetry.

RHOMBOID OR LLL FLAP

The rhomboid flap, or the LLL flap of Dufourmentel,[3] can provide an ideal solution for reconstructing the temporal area, provided care is taken with the position of the hairline and the lateral end of the eyebrow.

LLL Flap

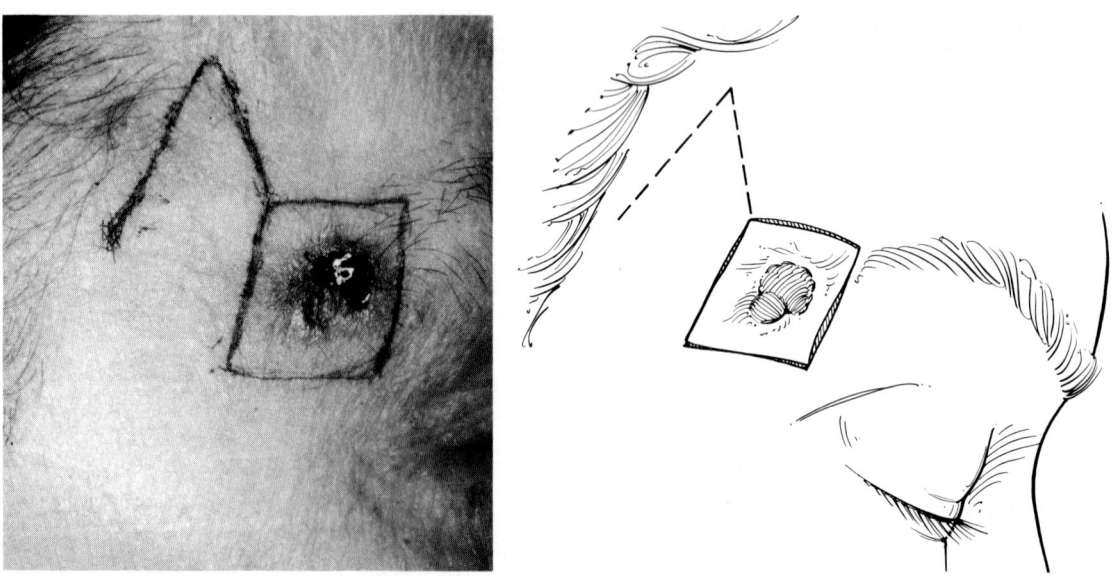

In the basal cell carcinoma shown here, an LLL flap reconstruction was performed. This patient had a basal cell carcinoma involving the lateral eyebrow and temporal area. Primary closure of the defect in any direction would cause deformity of the eyelid or the eyebrow. To obviate this problem an LLL reconstruction was planned.

CHAPTER 3
FOREHEAD RECONSTRUCTION

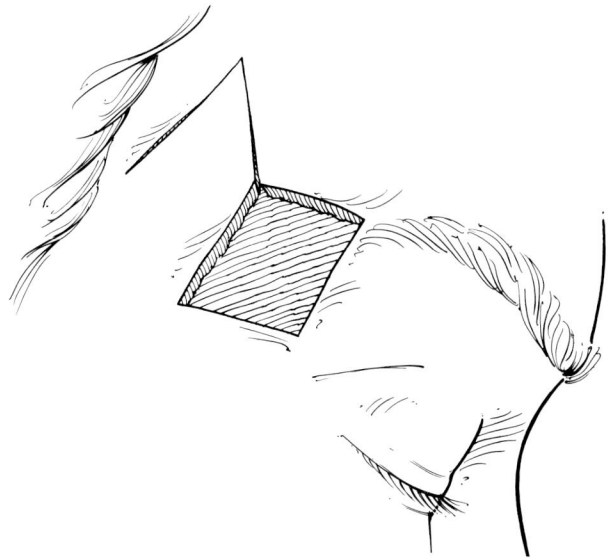

The planned rhomboid excision is completed and the LLL flap incised.

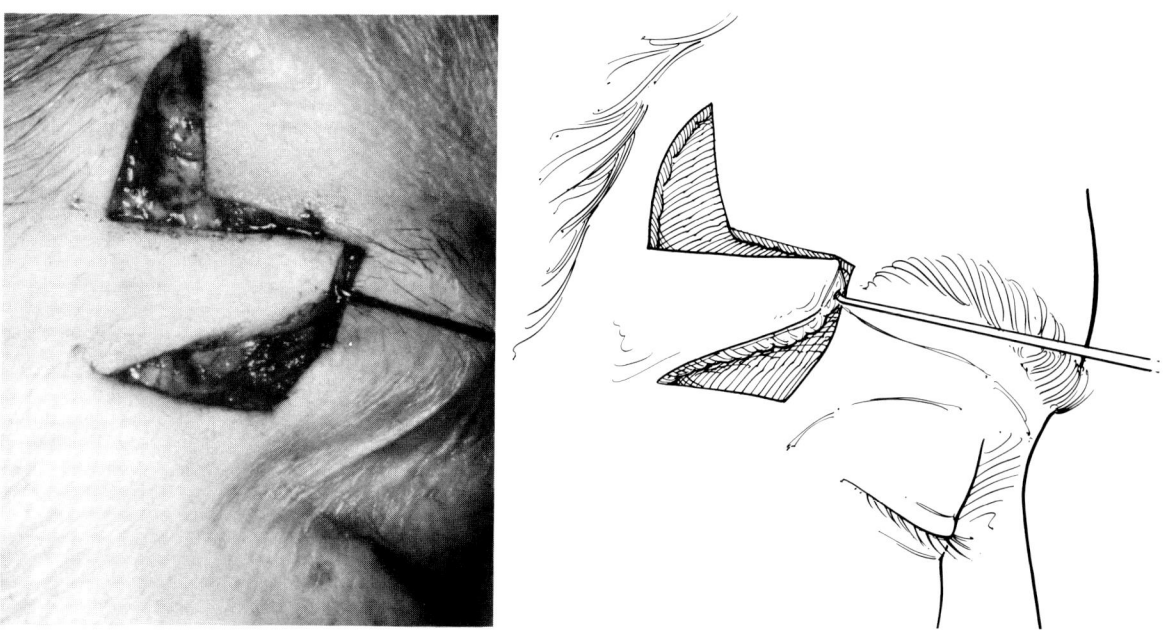

The flap is transposed without difficulty into the rhomboid defect. Again, undermining beyond the base of the flap has been performed.

71

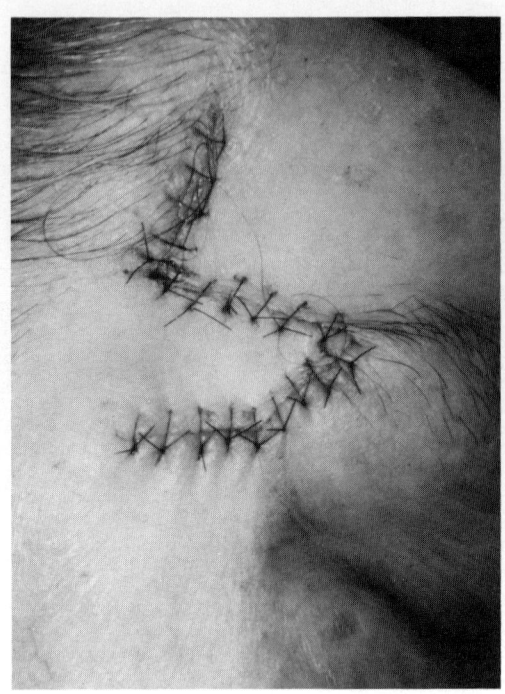
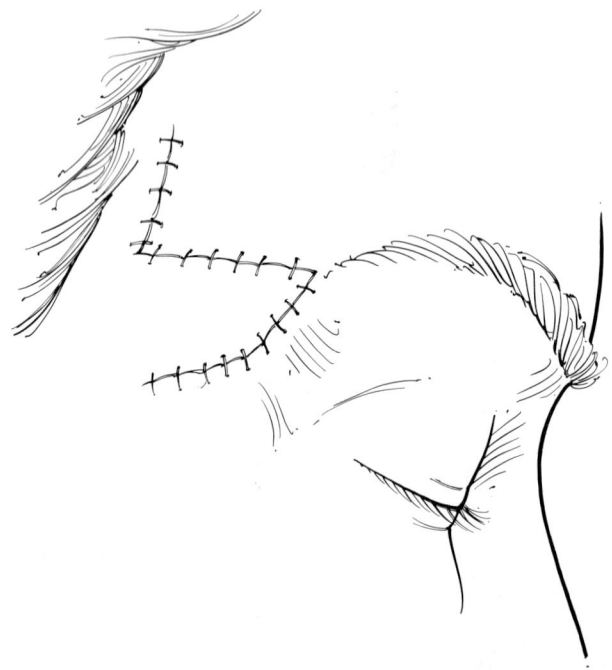

The defect is closed without tension and undue distortion of natural anatomic landmarks.

DOUBLE RHOMBOID FLAP

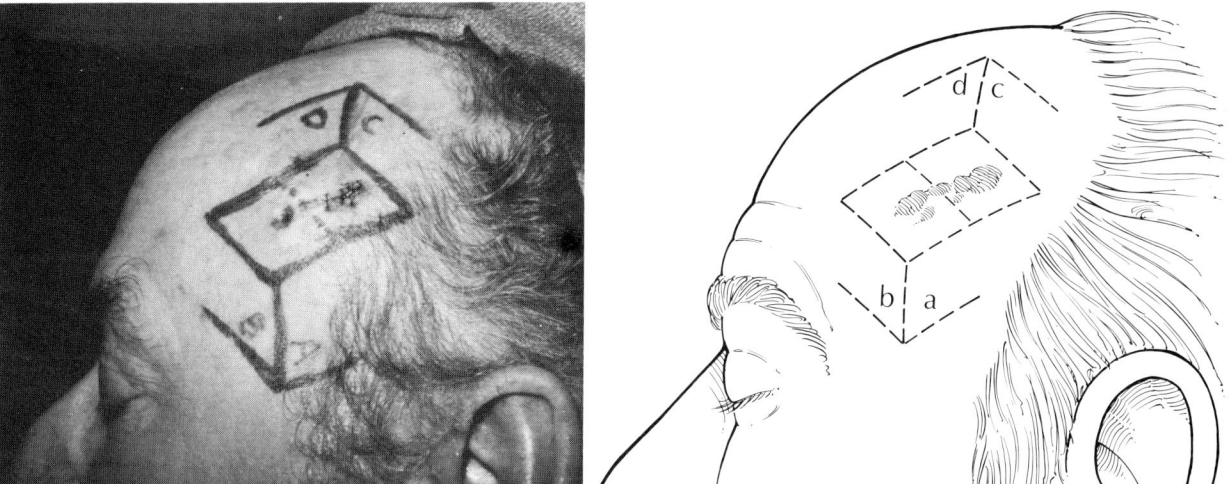

If the lesion is large, it is convenient to establish a long defect composed of two rhomboids, one on top of the other. This defect is oriented in such a way that a forehead and a cheek rhomboid can be constructed. The defect can then be closed without disturbing the anterior and posterior boundaries of the area. The various possible permutations of rhomboids are shown here. The defect may be closed with flaps *d* and *a* or flaps *c* and *b*.

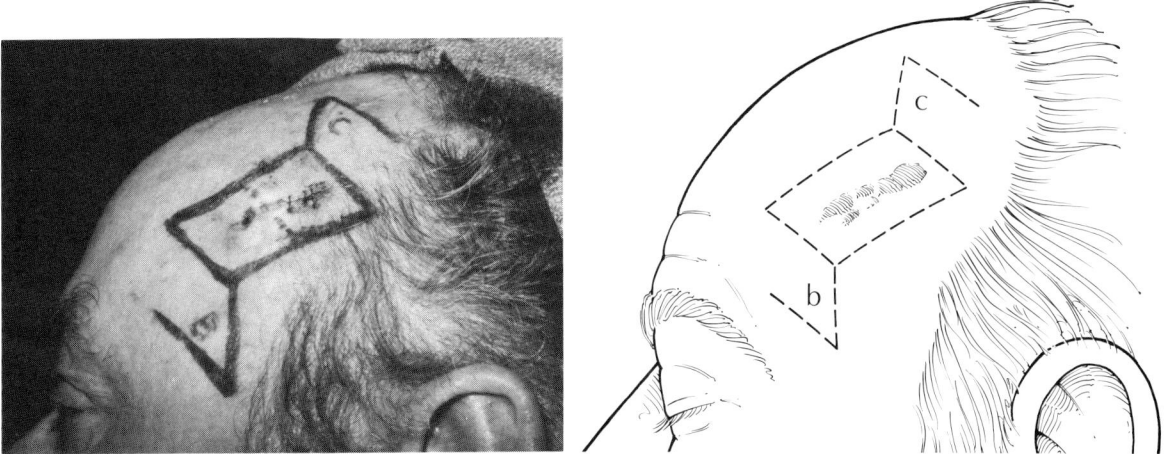

In choosing, the plastic surgeon should be aware of tissue availability (see Chapter 1) and should use the flaps that will cause the least disturbance of anatomic landmarks. The thicker upper skin is replaced with forehead skin, and the lower area receives the upper cheek skin.

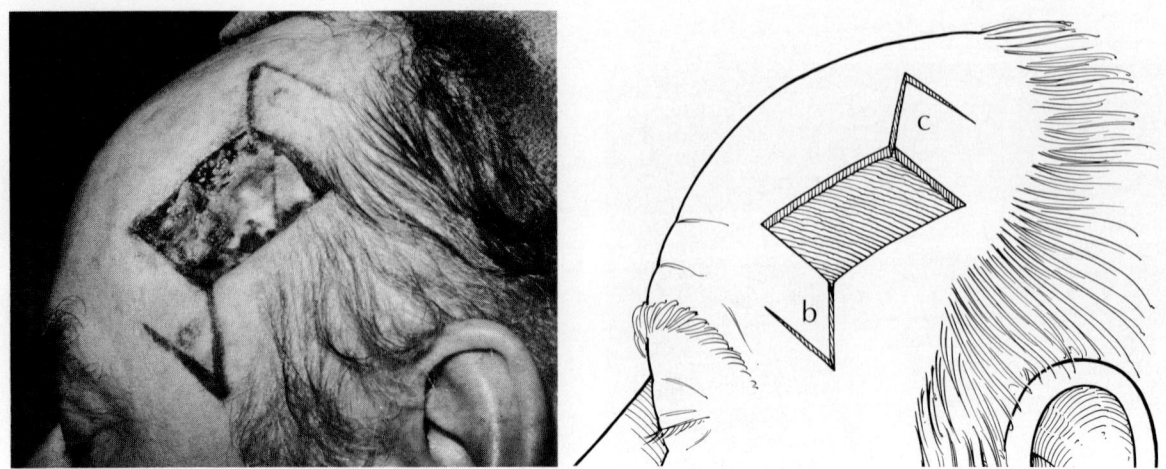

After excision of the basal cell carcinoma the plan for this patient is to close the postexcisional defect with two rhomboid flaps: one of thick upper forehead skin and one of thinner skin from the upper temporal area.

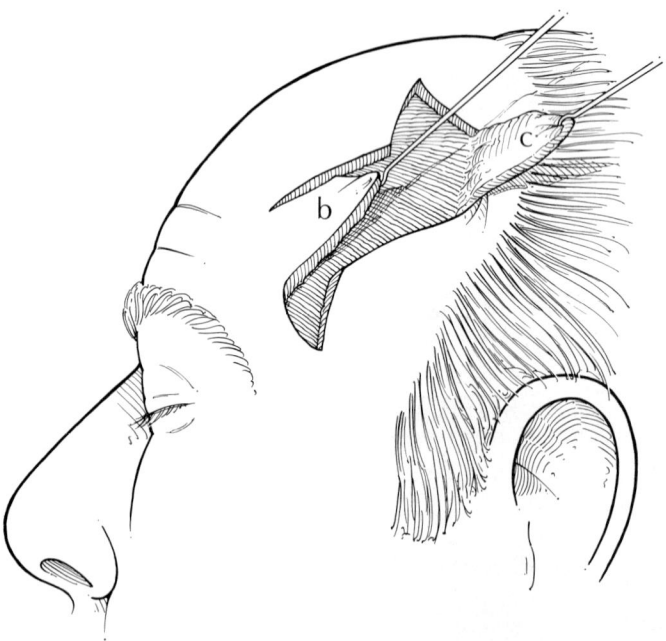

These flaps are widely undermined until they can be transposed in an effortless fashion.

CHAPTER 3
FOREHEAD RECONSTRUCTION

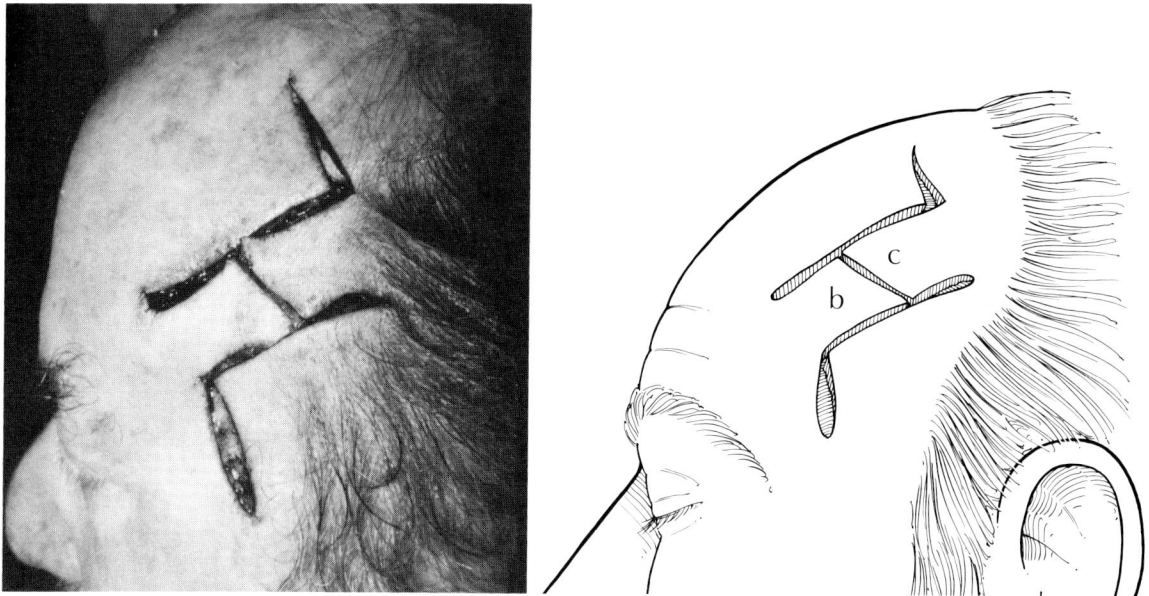

If the undermining has been sufficient, the flaps should lie comfortably, without tension, and the donor defects close almost automatically.

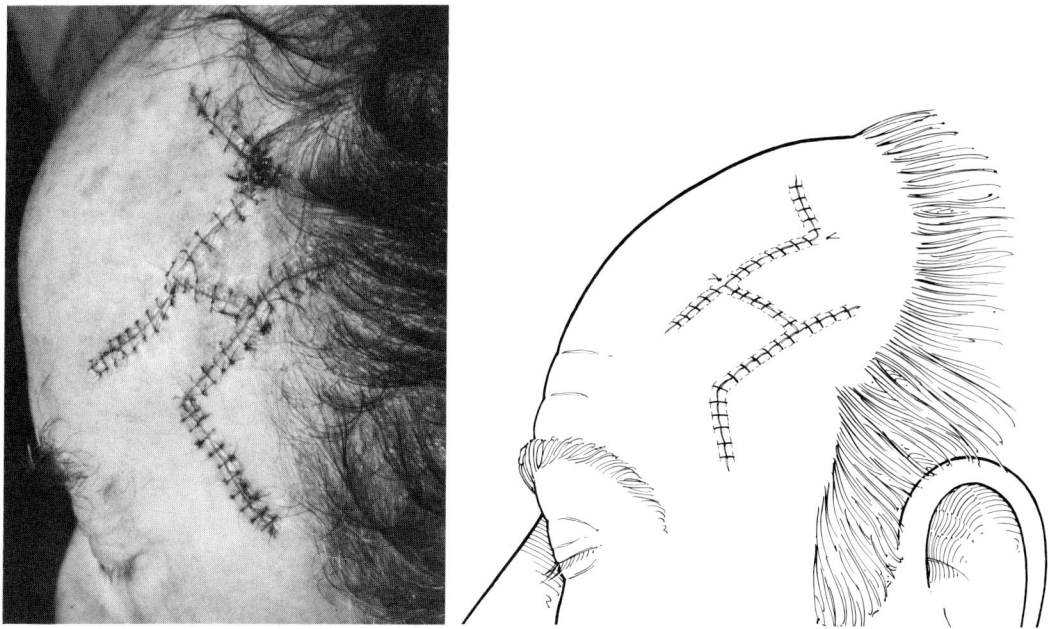

The flaps have been sutured in position and the donor defects closed with minimal trimming and adjustment of skin.

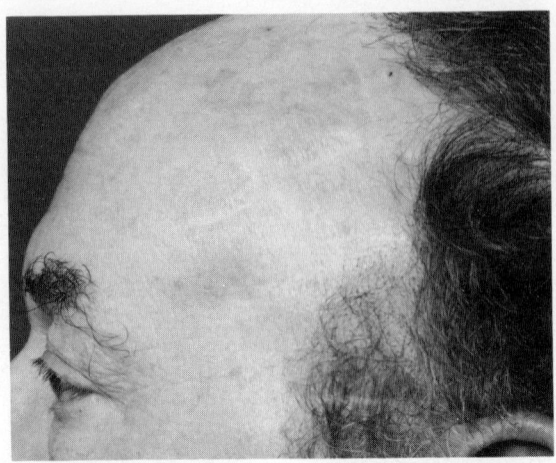

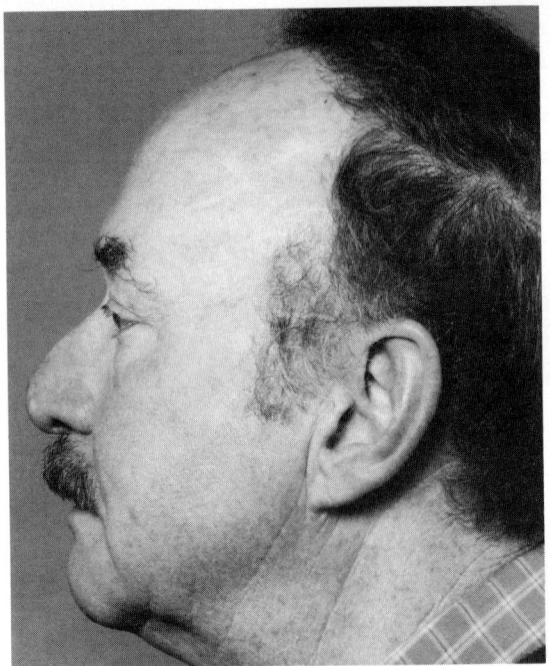

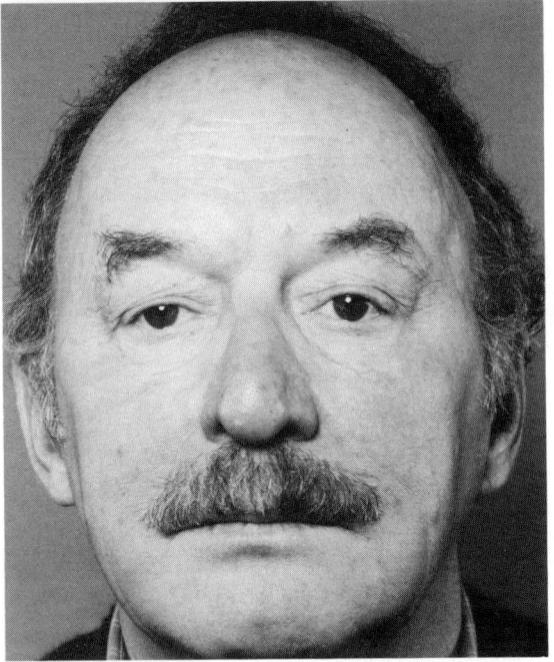

The aesthetic result is usually satisfactory with no displacement of normal features.

PROBLEMS

The Dufourmentel flap is complex to design and rarely chosen over the much simpler rhomboid flap. Both have the advantage of being predictable and geometrically conceived. Unfortunately, both flaps have the disadvantage of producing many scars. If any error of planning is made, there may be difficulty in rotating the flap into the defect or in closing the donor site. Usually this problem can be overcome by wider undermining or modification of the flap.

CHAPTER 3
FOREHEAD RECONSTRUCTION

☐ Glabellar Reconstruction

Since the skin in the glabellar region is mobile, relatively large defects may be closed directly, especially in a vertical direction running with the lines of minimal relaxed tension. If a defect stretches to the medial end of the eyebrows, however, direct closure will cause approximation of the eyebrows. In addition, removal of excess skin above and below this area would necessitate a long scar running up onto the forehead and down onto the nose. The reconstruction must maintain the medial ends of the eyebrows in a good position and also not interfere with upper lid function. Closure of a defect in this area is challenging and necessitates the use of a single transposition flap in case of small defects or several if the defect is of significant size.

RHOMBOID FLAPS

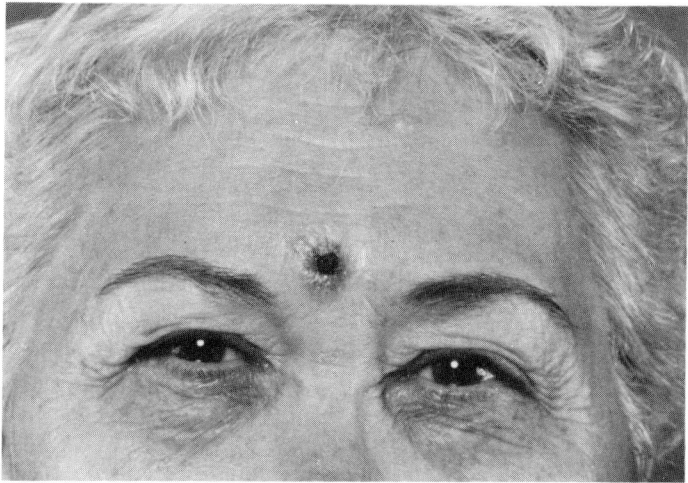

The defect created by excision of this moderately large basal cell carcinoma of the glabellar area is such that direct closure would result in unacceptable medial movement of the eyebrows.

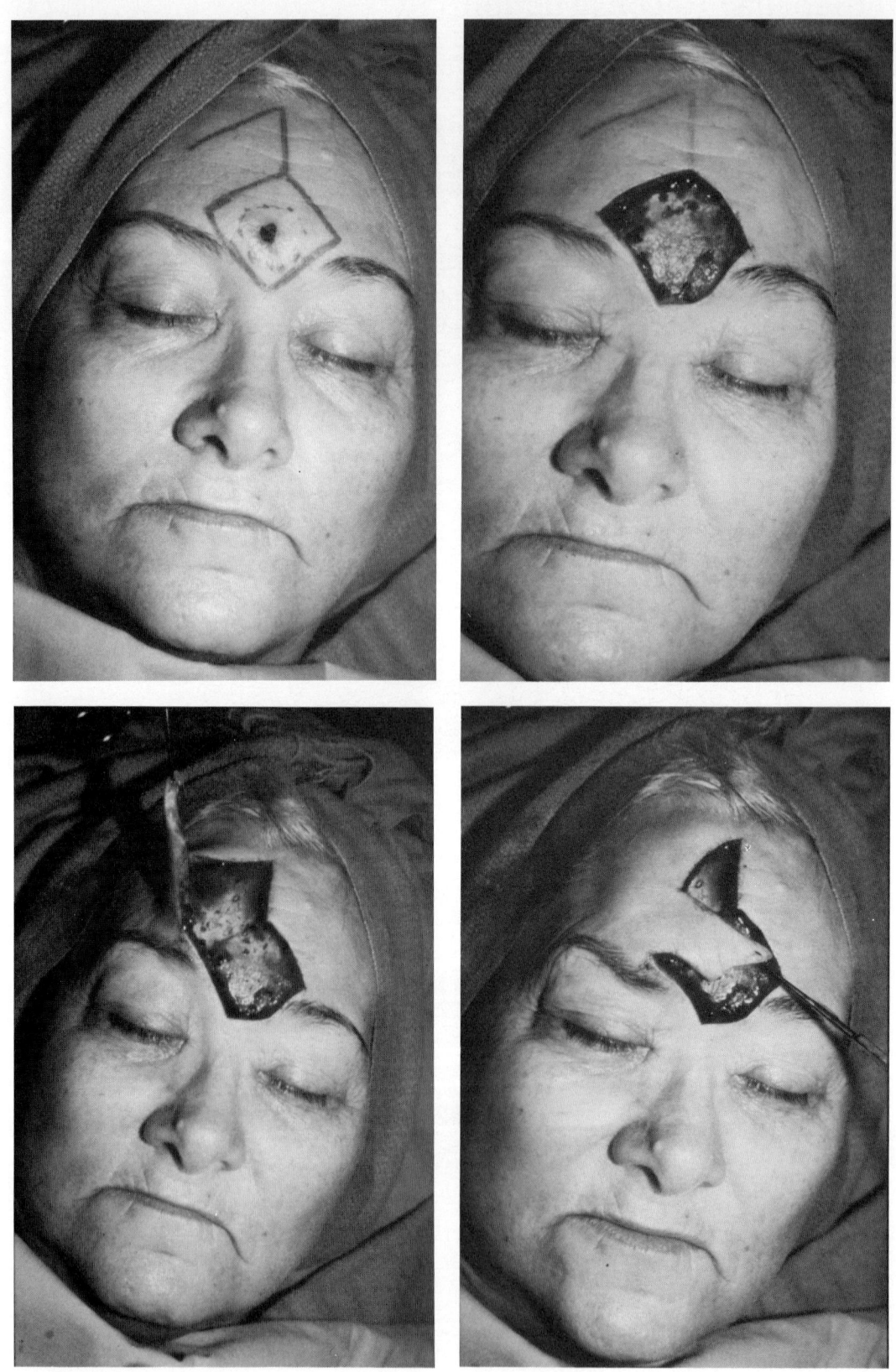

78 Is it therefore excised as a rhomboid and a superior rhomboid flap is used to close this defect.

CHAPTER 3
FOREHEAD RECONSTRUCTION

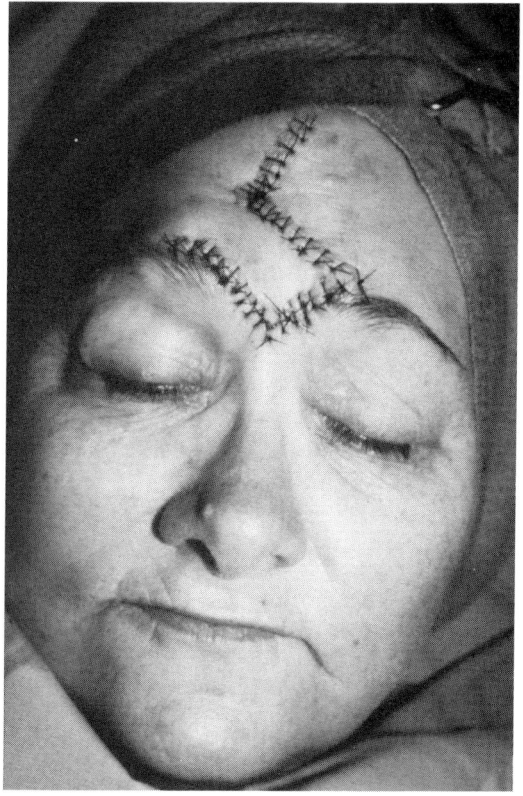

The flap donor site closes directly because of the transverse laxity of the forehead.

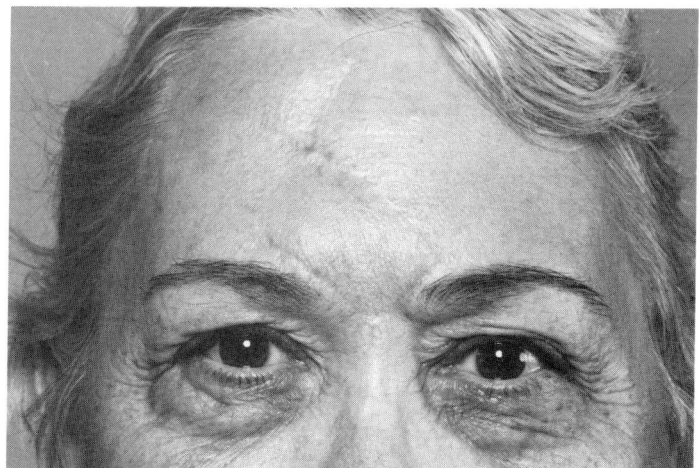

The postoperative result after 6 months shows good scar resolution and a satisfactory reconstruction without disturbance of local anatomic features.

79

MULTIPLE TRANSPOSITION FLAPS

Rhomboid transposition flaps are satisfactory on the forehead provided that the skin is available and the donor scar is in a good position. Tissue steal is shared by using bilateral flaps in large defects. The principle fundamental to all midline reconstructions requires that eyebrows always be moved in a symmetric fashion to preserve facial harmony.

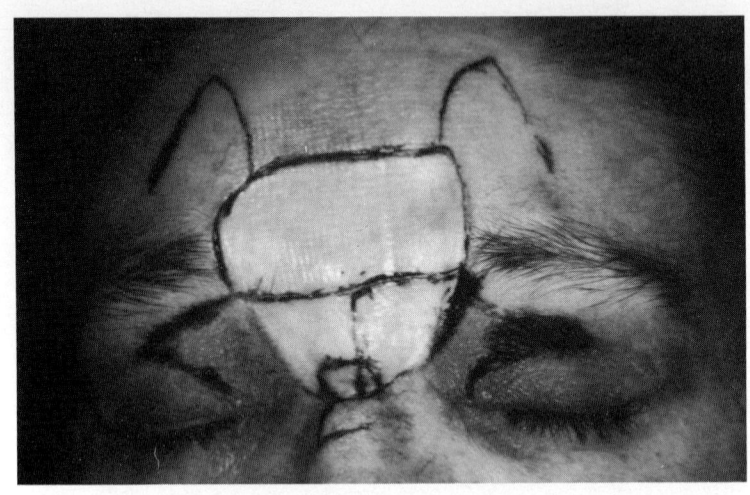

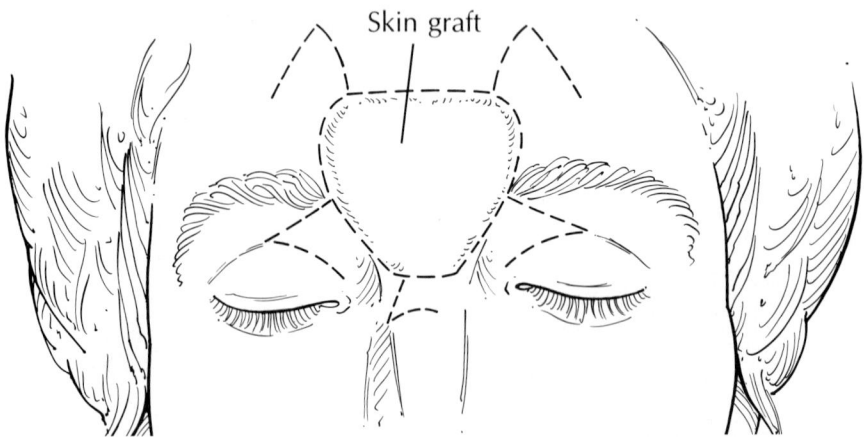

This patient had a malignant melanoma that was excised several years previously. The resulting large raw area was covered with a split-thickness skin graft. The patient wished reconstruction, and thus the imagination was significantly taxed. Five rhomboid flaps were used: two from the forehead laterally, two from the upper eyelids, and one from the central region of the nose.

CHAPTER 3
FOREHEAD RECONSTRUCTION

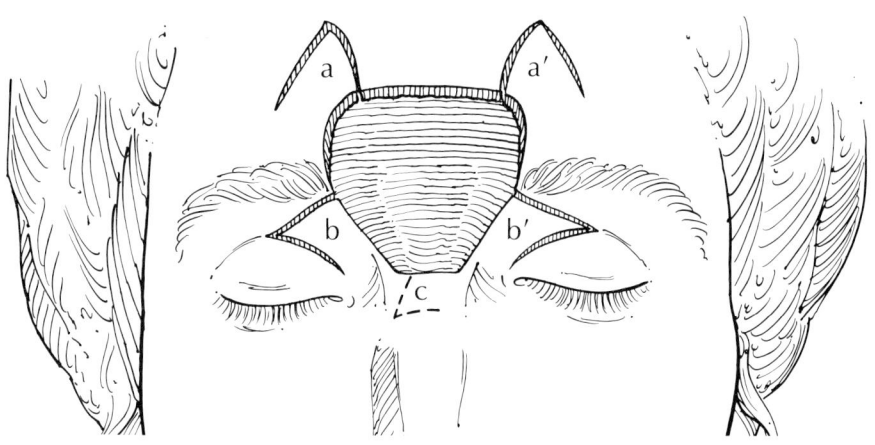

The shield-shaped defect has been created by excision of the old skin graft. The five rhomboid flaps—a, a', b, b', and c—are incised.

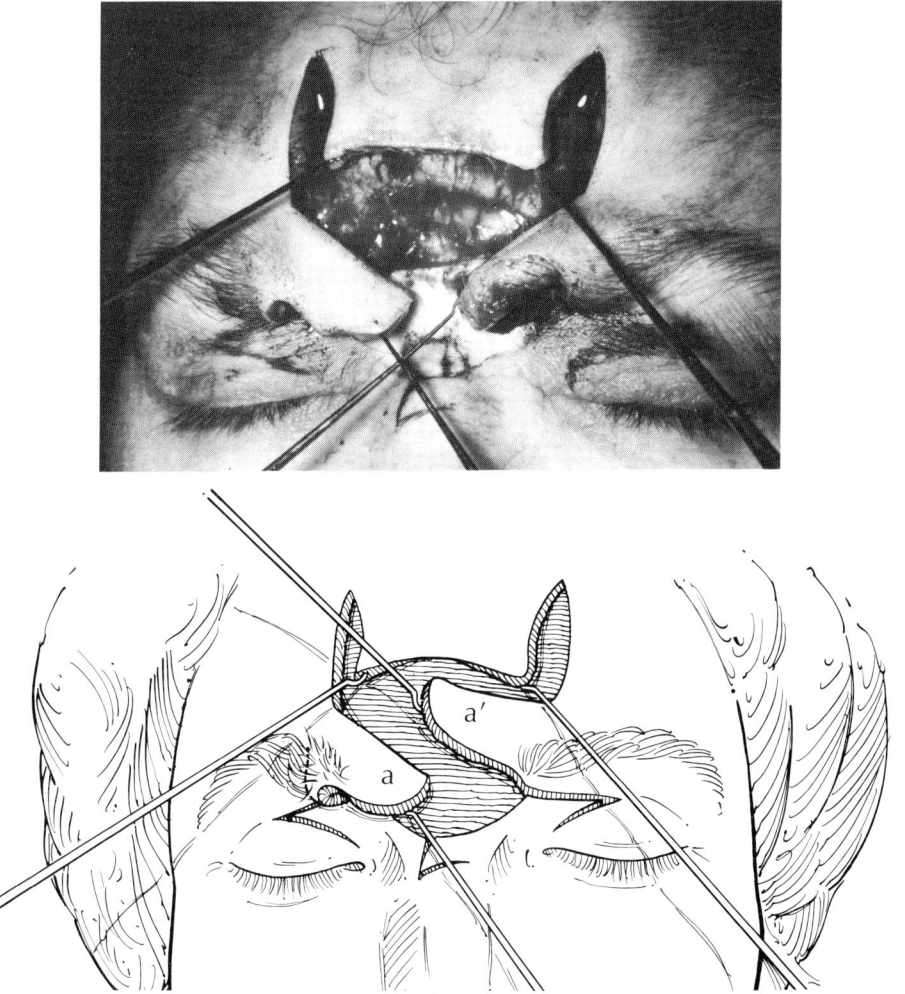

The forehead rhomboids are elevated, their bases are undermined, and their rotation is assessed. The ease of closure of the donor defects is also evaluated.

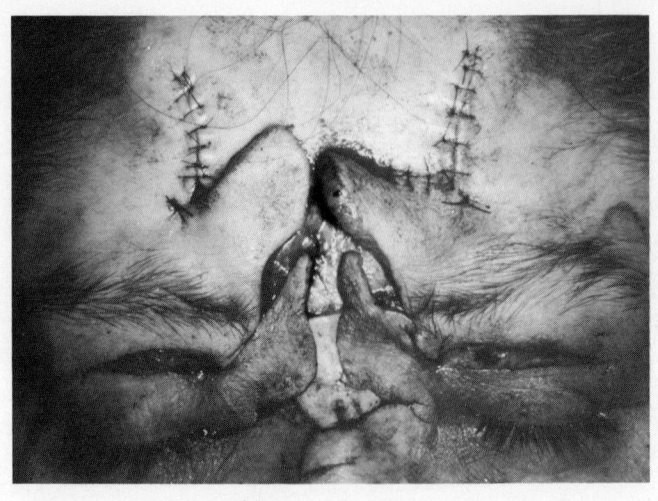

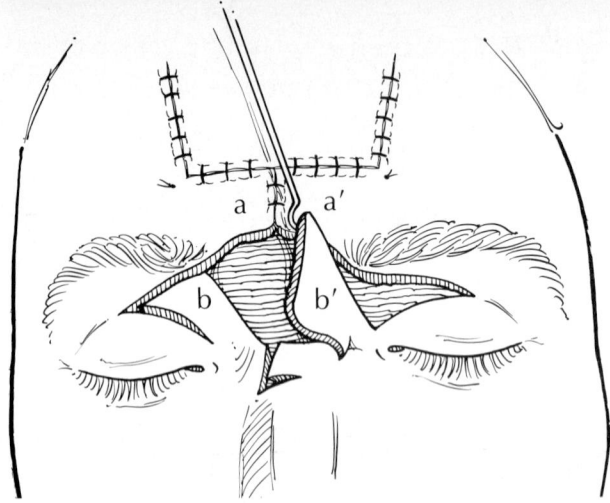

The forehead donor site defects are closed directly, and the forehead rhomboid flaps are rotated down medially and sutured into position. The upper eyelid rhomboid flaps based inferiorly are incised.

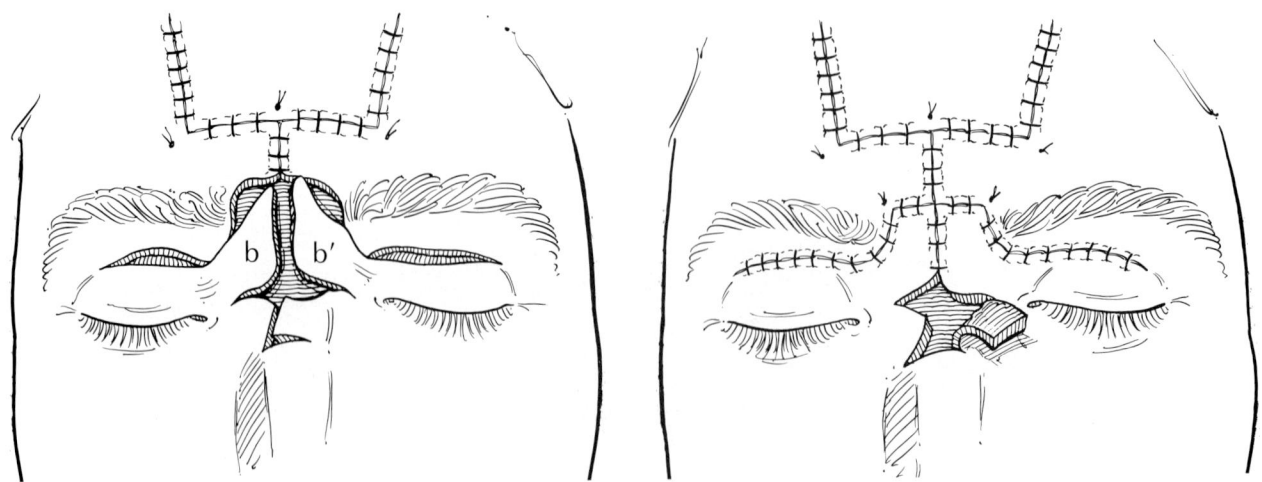

These thin upper eyelid flaps are transposed to close most of the lower portion of the glabellar defect. The donor sites on the upper eyelids are closed directly as in a blepharoplasty. The nasal bridge rhomboid is incised and elevated.

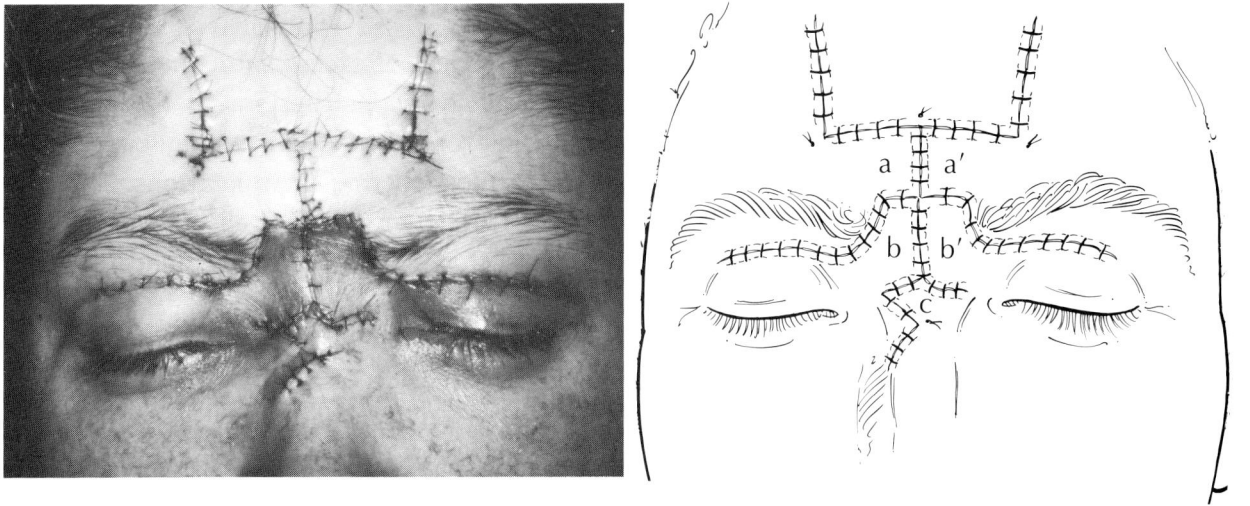

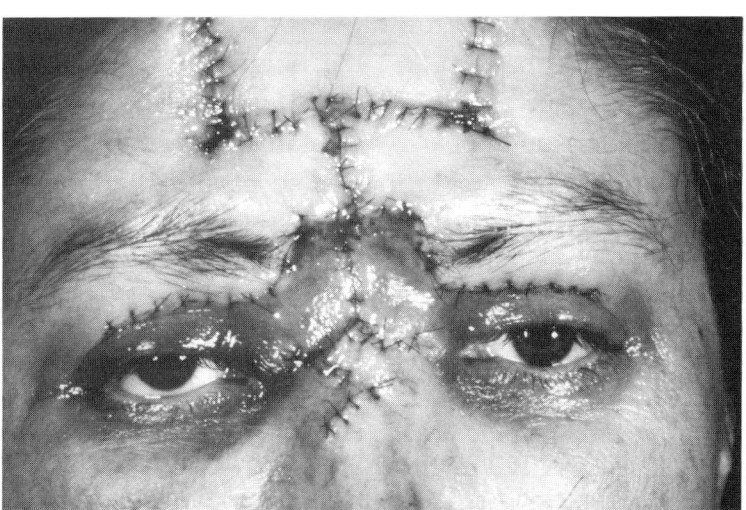

The nasal bridge rhomboid is sutured into position without tension, and the defect is closed directly. It can be seen in the early postoperative phase that even with maximal swelling there has been little or no distortion of the eyebrows or eyelids and that the flaps lie comfortably to close this large defect.

PROBLEMS

Poor flap design may cause distortion of natural anatomic features such as the eyebrows, canthi, and eyelids. Multiplicity of scars is a disadvantage, and the mixture of various types of skin can also result in a poor aesthetic result. However, as in the last case illustrated, there may be no other reasonable alternative.

CHAPTER 4

NOSE RECONSTRUCTION

> Lightly was her slender nose
> Tip tilted like the petal of a flower
>
> ALFRED LORD TENNYSON
> *The Idylls of the King, Gareth and Lynette*

> A nose as strange as a nose could be!
> Of vast proportions and painted red
>
> EDWARD LEAR
> *The Dong with the Luminous Nose*

> Thine has a great hook nose like thine
> Mine has a snub nose like to mine
>
> WILLIAM BLAKE
> *The Everlasting Gospel*

The nose, most prominent of all facial features, presents a challenging reconstructive problem for the surgeon. This hollow organ has a complex surface contour and a skin covering that lacks uniformity in texture, color, and appearance.

The contour of the nose varies from area to area. The lines of minimal relaxed tension are vertical in the glabellar area (frown lines) and transverse over the remainder of the nose. Transversely across the bridgeline, the nose is convex. A vertical cross section through the midline may be concave or convex, or it may even alternate along its line from one to the other. The sides of the nose are concave but tend to be convex toward the rims. If the alar rim is considered in an anteroposterior plane, it is convex. Junction areas such as the nose-cheek, nasolabial, alar-lip, and columellar-lip regions have their own characteristic form that must be preserved in any reconstructive endeavor. Noses vary in size and shape and in ability to function. Some noses allow for clear breathing, whereas others are almost totally obstructed. The cause for nasal obstruction may also vary; it may be truly mechanical, as in posttraumatic airway obstruction, or it may be the result of an allergic rhinitis.

ANATOMY

Skin

The nasal skin varies in texture, color, and appearance in different areas of the nose. In the glabellar area the skin is thin, pale, and pliable and may contain a significant element of eyebrow skin, depending on the position of the medial ends of the eyebrows.

The skin covering the bony skeleton and the sides of the nose is usually pale, thin, and of mat texture.

The skin in the nasal tip area exhibits considerable variation. It is always thick, but for some individuals, particularly males, this skin is much thicker; it is soft and oily, with a shiny surface. Frequently the pores are wide and obvious, and the color may appear pink, deep red, or even slightly purple. The skin color changes with age; in older patients it is often more lightly colored. Telangiectasia and the presence of hair may be evident in varying degrees. Slight rhinophyma frequently occurs, as do comedones. In the black patient the skin is shiny, and hairs and pores are less obvious; the color is slightly darker than that of the remainder of the face.

The alar rims may be thickened and rather spongy or, in the female, sharply etched and refined. The form of the columella is variable; it may hang low, exposing the vibrissae, or it may be retruded and not visible on profile.

The nose is lined with hairbearing squamous epithelium.

Musculature

The muscles of the nose are the procerus, compressor naris, and depressor septi. The procerus muscle arises from the nasal bone and inserts into the glabellar skin. It produces the transverse wrinkles at the nasal bridge. Extending from the maxilla lateral to the incisor teeth to the nasal bridgeline, the compressor naris muscle compresses the nasal aperture. The depressor septi muscle arises from the maxilla above the incisors and is inserted into the septum. It helps to widen the nasal aperture.

Nerve Supply

All muscles are supplied by the upper buccal branches of the facial nerve. Skin sensation is provided from the ophthalmic nerve through the infratrochlear and the external nasal branches, and the infraorbital branch from the maxillary nerve.

☐ Blood Supply

The alar region and the lower part of the septum are supplied by the alar and septal branches of the facial artery. The dorsum and the lateral areas are supplied by the dorsal nasal branch of the ophthalmic artery and the infraorbital branch of the maxillary artery. Venous drainage is provided by the anterior facial and the ophthalmic veins.

☐ Lymphatic Drainage

The external nose drains to the facial lymph nodes lying in relation to the anterior facial vein. The anterior part of the nasal cavity drains to the submandibular glands. The remaining portion of the intranasal area drains to the upper deep cervical nodes. The posterior part of the nasal floor is drained to the parotid lymph nodes.

■ AESTHETICS

The nose is a very positive facial feature, and any change in its shape, color, or skin cover is obvious. Therefore no effort must be spared to maintain its normal appearance. The surgeon must carefully choose a method of reconstruction, bearing in mind skin color, texture, and nasal topography.

■ PLACEMENT OF INCISIONS

The incisions should follow natural lines if possible; they should be vertical in the glabellar area and vertical in the main nose area or along the junction of the lateral nose and the cheek. It is important that no incisions be placed across concavities. Bridling caused by scar contracture will occur and will require later revision.

■ AREAS OF TISSUE AVAILABILITY

To reconstruct nasal defects, the surgeon can use local flap tissue available in six facial areas: (1) nose, (2) forehead, (3) glabellar region, (4) retroauricular region, (5) cheeks, and (6) neck.

Many ingenious methods have been devised to transport skin to the nose from the areas of availability. The method selected should produce the best nasal form and contour and provide the closest match in skin color and texture. It should not deform the area from which it is taken.

■ AREAS TO BE RECONSTRUCTED

In considering nasal reconstructive options, it is convenient to divide the nose into several distinct areas: the medial canthal region, the side of the nose, the nasal tip, and the columella. Partial and total composite nose reconstruction should be considered separately. The nasal contours are of such complexity that each site presents a unique challenge. Many options exist for reconstructing each of these regions. An unwise choice of procedure, however, can pose significant problems later.

☐ Medial Canthus

Nonhairbearing skin is essential for reconstructing the medial canthal area. This skin must be contoured into the biconcave form of the canthal region. Any flap must be extensive in case the medial ends of the eyelids also need to be reconstructed.

Although full-thickness skin grafting can give reasonably good results in this area, it cannot be used if the full thickness of skin must be sacrificed down to and including the periosteum to effect resection of the tumor. A skin graft will not take it if is applied directly to bone. In such a situation a glabellar skin flap is the treatment of choice.

GLABELLAR FLAPS

The glabellar donor area contains an abundant source of skin for resurfacing nasal defects. Because the skin in this area is thin, it provides a good color and texture match for the upper nasal area. The glabellar flap can be transferred in three ways: as a rotation flap, as a midline transposition flap, and as an island flap. The last two types are more flexible and can be enlarged and contoured as required.

CHAPTER 4
NOSE RECONSTRUCTION

Classic Glabellar Flap

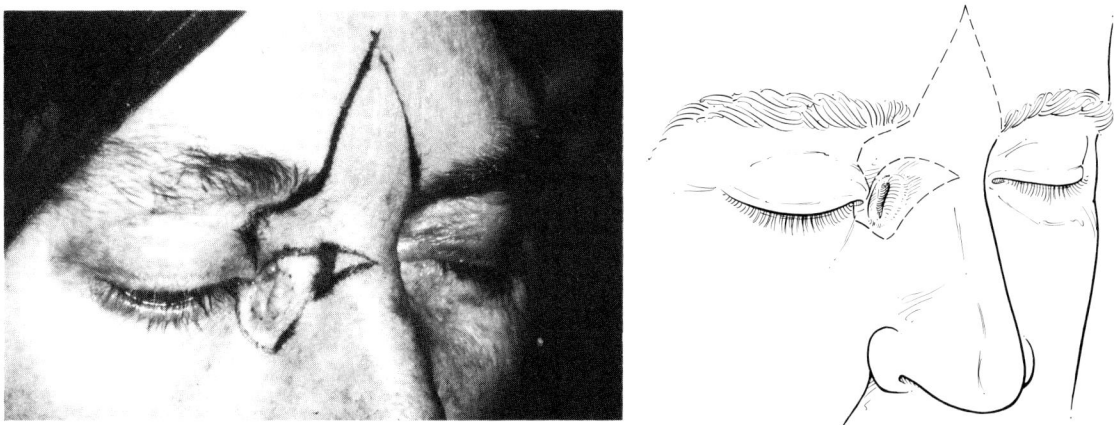

The classic glabellar flap is a rotation flap that incorporates a V-Y advancement in the glabellar region. The use of this technique can be seen in the illustration above, which shows a patient with a basal cell carcinoma of the medial canthus and a glabellar flap outlined for closure.

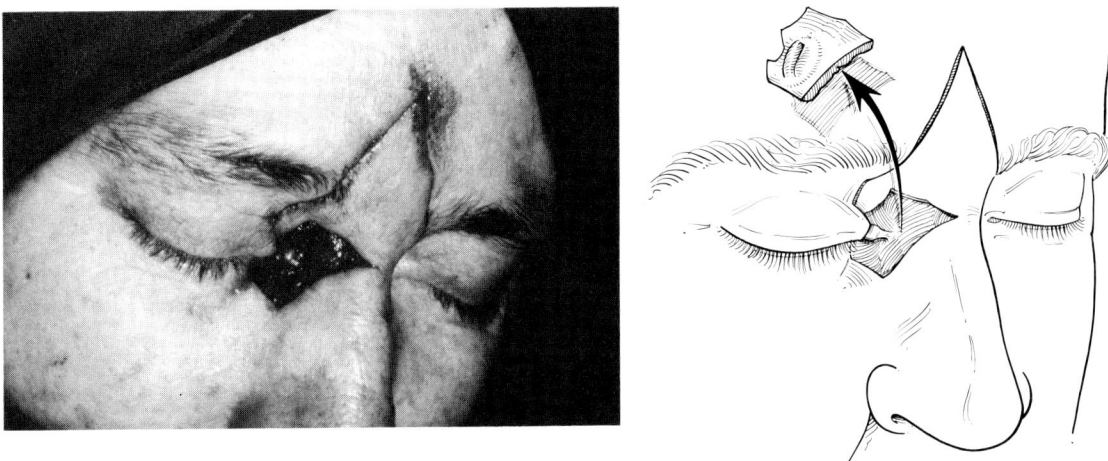

The lesion is resected in a triangular fashion. The flap is designed and raised at the level just above the glabellar musculature.

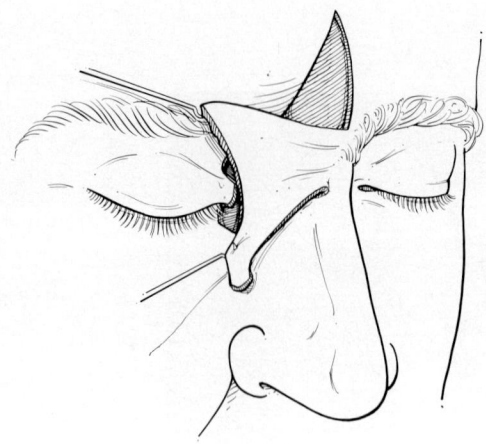

The movement of the flap is part rotational, part transpositional.

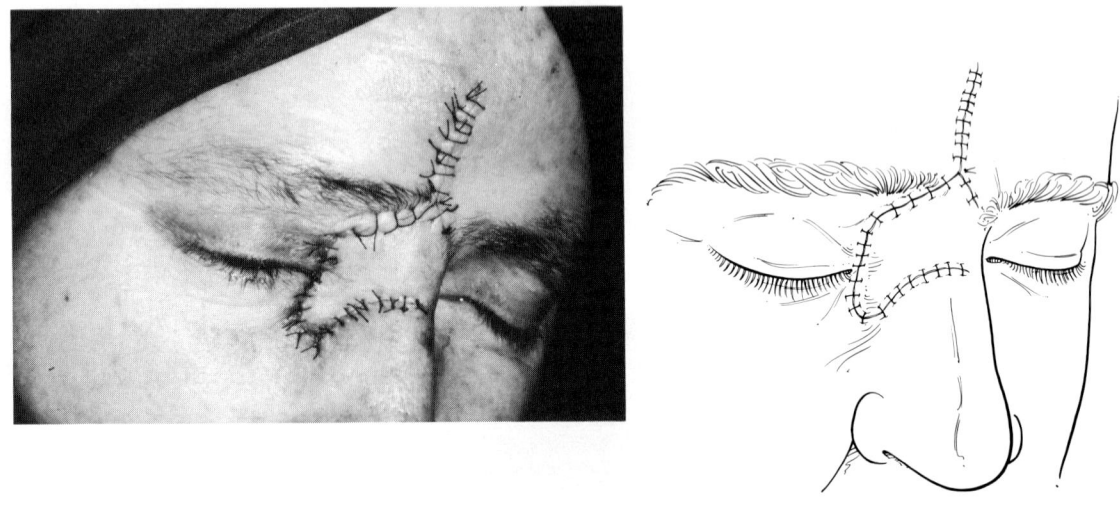

The donor defect is closed without difficulty and with only slight distortion of the medial end of the right eyebrow.

CHAPTER 4
NOSE RECONSTRUCTION

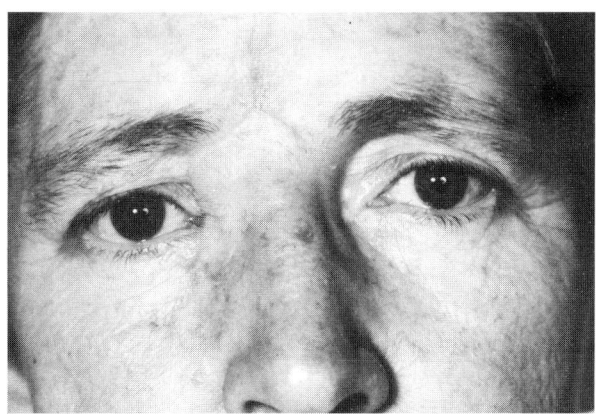

Although the classic glabellar flap is the time-honored method of reconstruction in this area, it has some defects and is *not* the method of choice. In this patient the result looks fairly good, but close examination reveals some eyebrow hair in the medial canthal area.

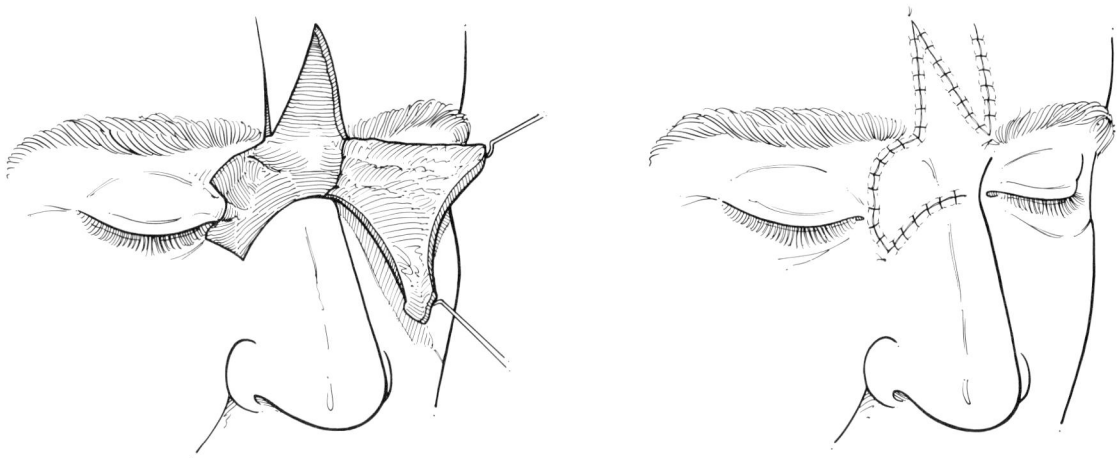

For cases in which larger flaps are used, a superior Z-plasty is planned. This approach has the advantage of increased movement of the flap toward the involved canthus as the secondary defect is closed by transposition of the Z flaps. The scars are usually acceptable, but there is always a risk of increased deformity when scar complexity is increased.

PROBLEMS

In many patients eyebrow hair is present in the glabellar region area, and the rotation of this skin moves the hair bearing area down into the medial canthus. This is unacceptable. Unfortunately, the thickness of the glabellar skin is greater than that of the skin removed from the medial canthal area, and this causes some convexity in this region (rather than the natural concavity). This can be a bonus if nasal bones need to be removed; the resulting defect is neatly filled by the flap bulk.

When the medial ends of the upper and/or lower lids require reconstruction, the design of the glabellar flap does not allow the required lid reconstruction to be accomplished satisfactorily. The reason is that the flap dimensions are fixed; the flap is not readily extensile.

Finger Flap

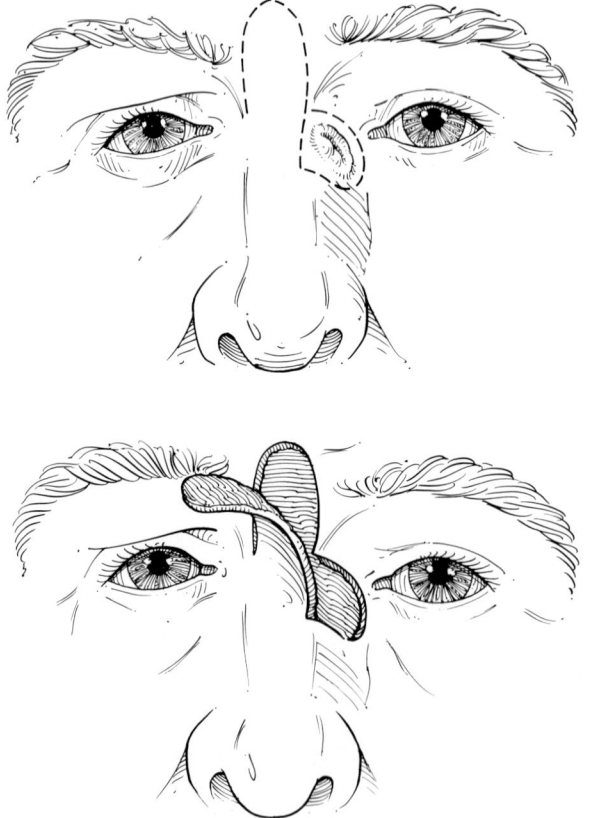

A midline transposition flap, or finger flap, is probably the most versatile approach to reconstructing the glabellar region and is the method of choice. This flap can be used in the reconstruction of a defect after excision of a medial canthal basal cell carcinoma.

CHAPTER 4
NOSE RECONSTRUCTION

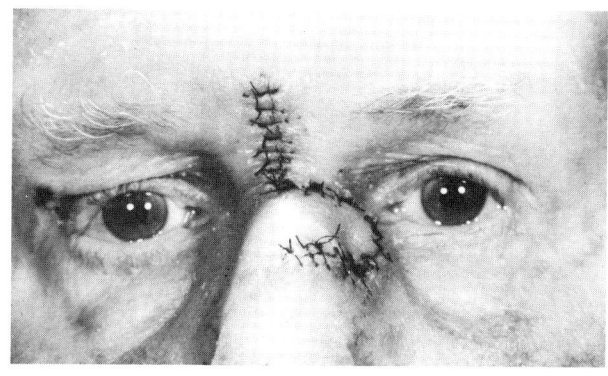
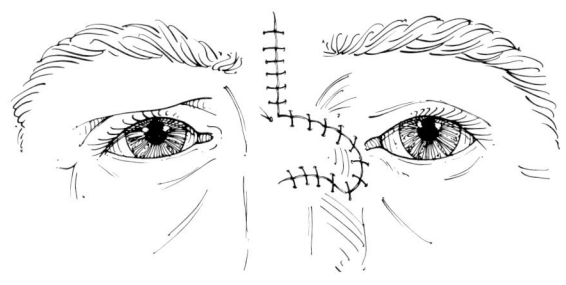

The finger flap has a simple design and allows transfer of nonhairbearing, thin skin by suitable transposition. The secondary defect is closed directly with ease.

If the flap has any skin excess, it will be exhibited as a standing cone in the inferior rotation area. The excess can be trimmed without difficulty and without compromising the blood supply of the flap.

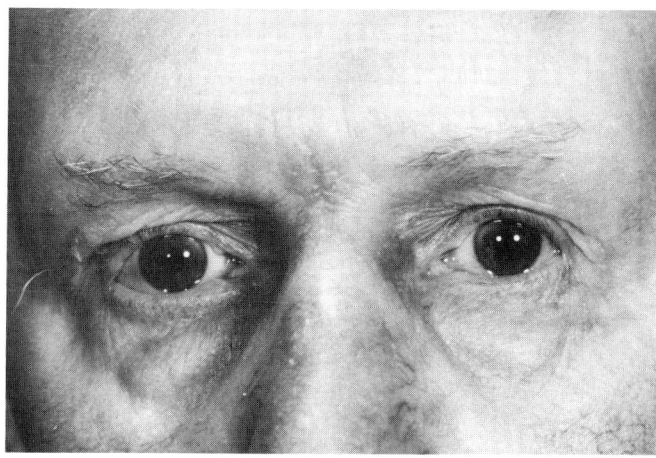

The result of any reconstruction involving this method is usually excellent.

If the medial portions of the upper and lower lids require reconstruction, a longer and perhaps slightly wider flap can be raised and incised to create a fork. The limbs of the fork are then set into the lid defects.

PROBLEMS

Although the midline transposition flap allows for ease of reconstruction, the skin is often somewhat thick for use with eyelid skin and may be noticeable on close inspection. In some cases a straight-line scar in the glabellar-nasal bridge concavity may result in a bridle deformity because of contracture along its length. Should this deformity occur, it will require later Z-plasty to ensure satisfactory contouring.

Glabellar Island Flap

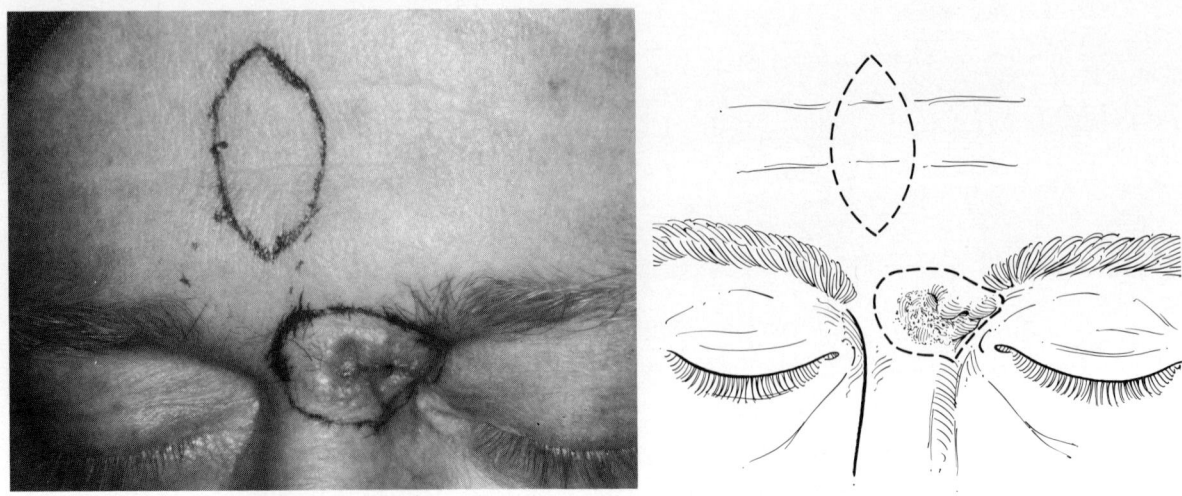

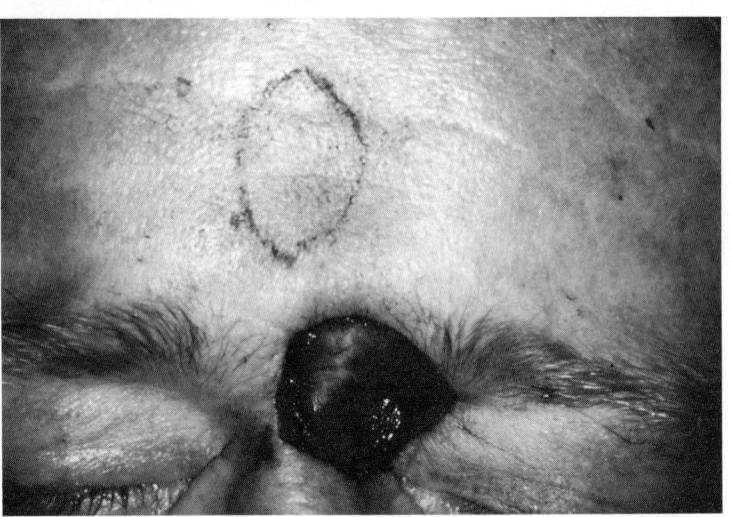

The glabellar island flap can be used instead of a transposition flap, with the same indications for its use. Although the procedure is interesting and elegant to perform, it takes longer and has little to recommend it over direct transposition. In addition, it cannot be used for eyelid reconstruction. The only advantage of this flap is its lack of skin deformity (e.g., a standing cone). Again, a medial canthal defect has been created by excision of a basal cell carcinoma. The principle for design of this flap is the

CHAPTER 4
NOSE RECONSTRUCTION

same as that of the Barron-Emmett flap[1]; the flap has a random subcutaneous pedicle extending from the undersurface of the flap down to the point of rotation.

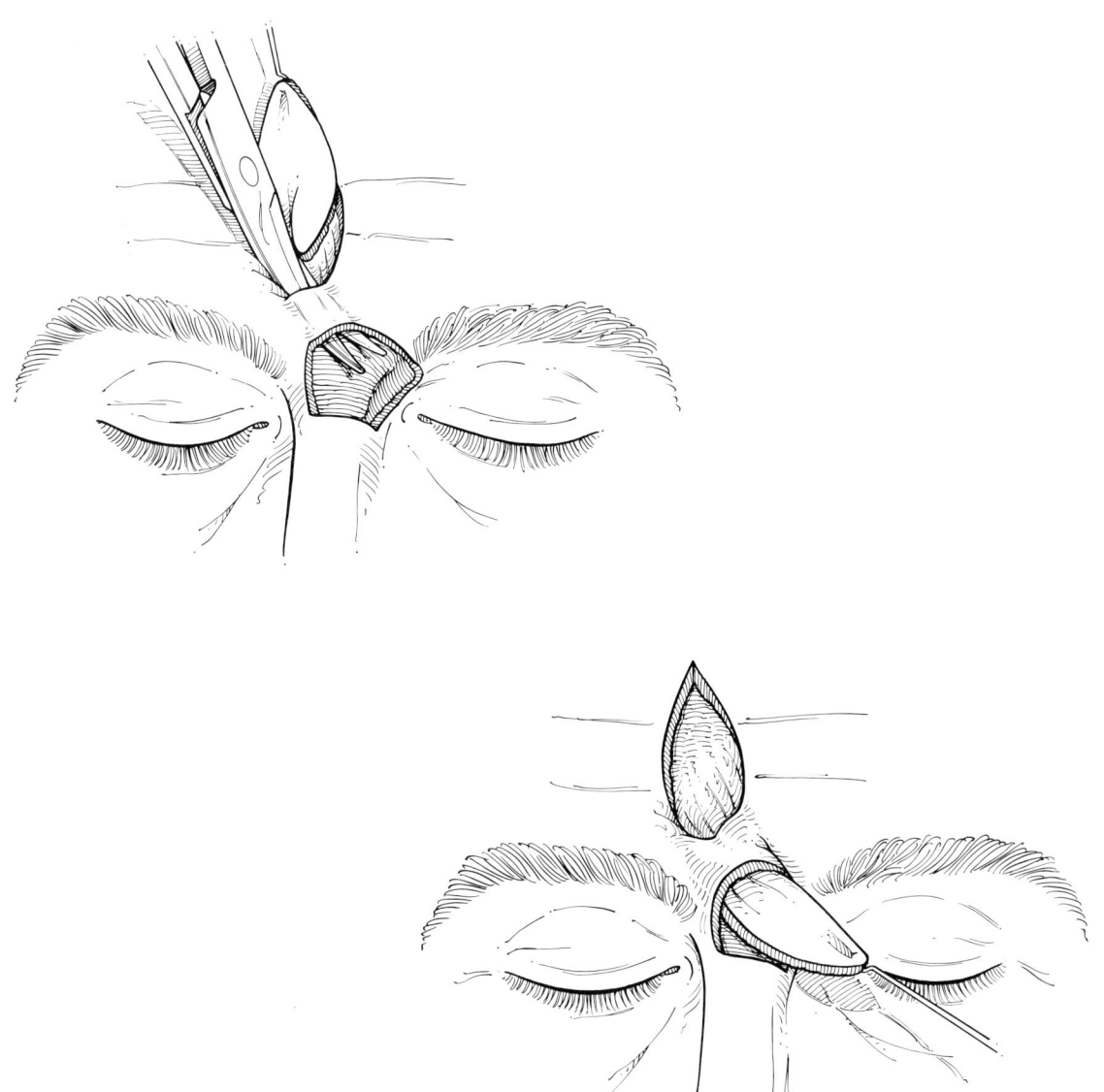

For extensive and long flaps it is probably wise to include some of the supratrochlear vessels in the pedicle if possible. A tunnel is created in the glabellar area to allow the flap to be drawn down and transposed into the defect. This tunnel should be spacious in order to prevent compression of the pedicle.

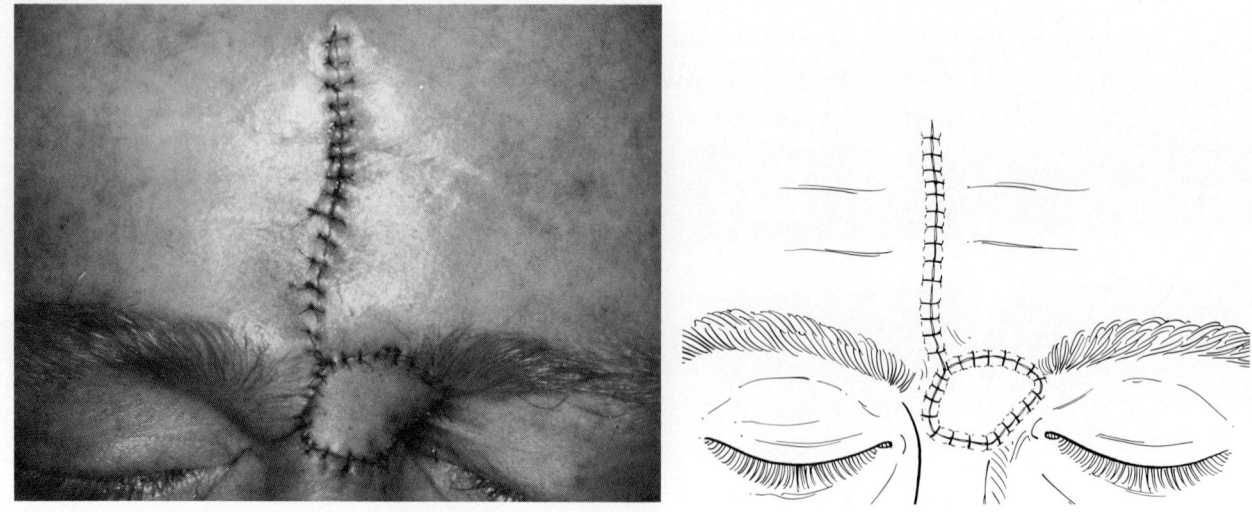

The donor defect is closed directly with excision of triangles of skin superiorly and inferiorly.

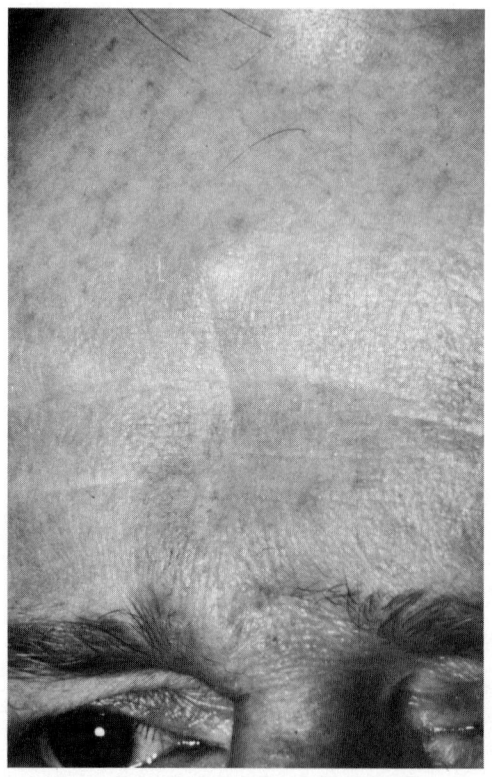

The result shows that the flap has contoured well to the concavity of the medial canthal area. Skin color and texture match are good, and the vertical forehead scar is aesthetically acceptable. There is no distortion of local anatomy.

PROBLEMS

The pedicle forms an obvious swelling in the nasal bridgeline area. Fortunately, in most cases this swelling will subside with time. The procedure is slightly complicated, and there is an element of risk because of vascular insufficiency not present in the direct transposition flap. As the flap is turned through 90 degrees and taken through the subcutaneous tunnel, the pedicle may be compressed and occluded, a problem that may become compounded by postoperative swelling. There may be more of a tendency for the island flap to "trapdoor" because of its circular design. Most significant is the fact that the procedure takes a long time to perform, always an important consideration.

SURGICAL TECHNIQUE OF CHOICE

The most versatile flap is undoubtedly the finger flap. It is reliable and extensile, and the skin color and texture provide a good match for the medial canthal area. The finger flap can be well contoured to the complex curvature of this region. Trimming, shaping, and splitting do not compromise its robust blood supply. Although in some instances the thickness of the flap may be a disadvantage, occasionally it may be a blessing. For example, when a radical resection of deep basal cell or squamous cell carcinomas is required, the underlying nasal bone and mucosa may be sacrificed. In this situation a thick flap with underlying subcutaneous tissue totally fills the resulting deep defect and obviates a contour deformity. In addition, there is no need to be concerned about nasal lining. It would appear that the intranasal defect, that is, the undersurface of the flap, becomes covered with mucosa, and this healing process has no effect on the external contours of the flap.

☐ Lateral Aspect of the Nose

This region is flat or slightly concave, but it is bounded by a convexity anteriorly and a concavity posteriorly. Its inferior margin is the alar rim, which is mobile, convex, and can be easily distorted. These natural boundaries should be respected; transgression with alteration of their distinct topographic features is unpardonable, since nasal asymmetry will inevitably result.

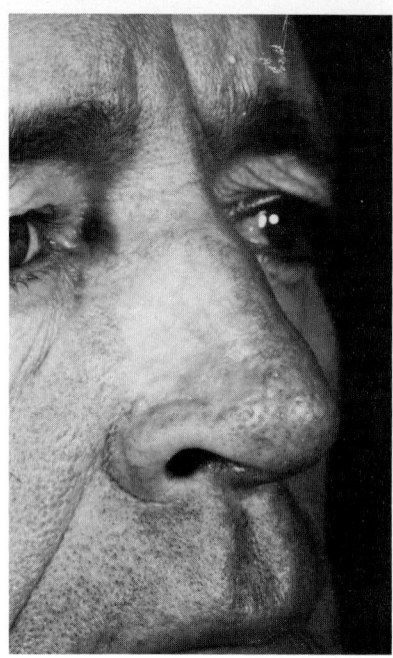
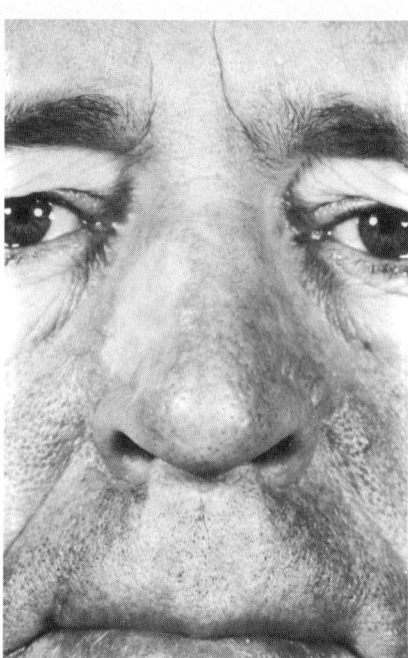
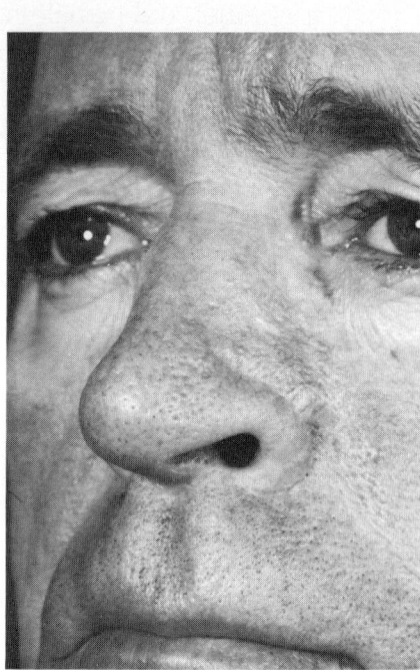

The lateral aspect of the nose is sometimes viewed as a cosmetic unit. As such, it can be reconstructed with a full-thickness graft, which sometimes gives an excellent result. The illustration shows such a reconstruction with postauricular skin, from the recommended donor site. The result is unacceptable, particularly when the ipsilateral side of the nose is considered; this area had a similar defect reconstructed with a local bilobed flap. Nose skin, especially in the male, usually defines a good match with a skin graft; the nasolabial area has been recommended as a good nasal skin donor site, but in practice it has not proved satisfactory.

BANNER FLAP

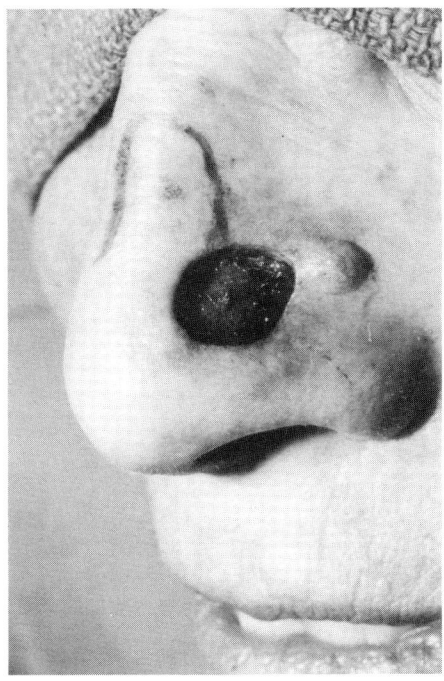
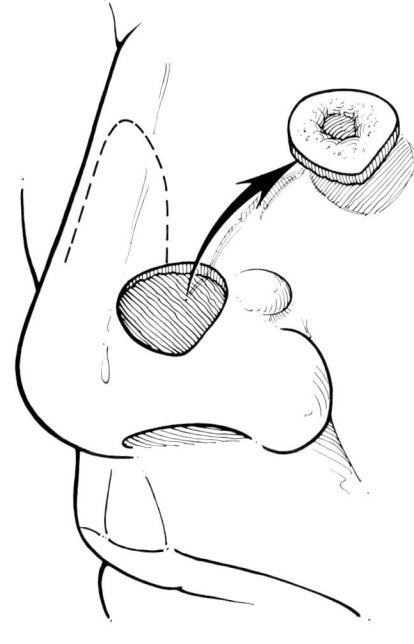

In small defects the transverse skin laxity can be used with the method shown here to reconstruct a lateral nasal defect resulting from excision of a basal cell carcinoma. The Banner flap, first described by Masson and Mendelson,[11] is virtually a small finger flap. The amount of skin available is judged by transversely pinching the skin between index finger and thumb. Skin availability decreases as the nasal tip is approached. A trial run of the transposition can be effected by using a strip of gauze in place of the skin flap; this will indicate the necessary width and length of the flap. The flap is designed by continuing the medial excision edge vertically. It is made a little longer than necessary and is pointed to allow later comfortable closure of the inevitable dog ear of the donor site. The lateral incision is taken vertically down to the superior resection edge.

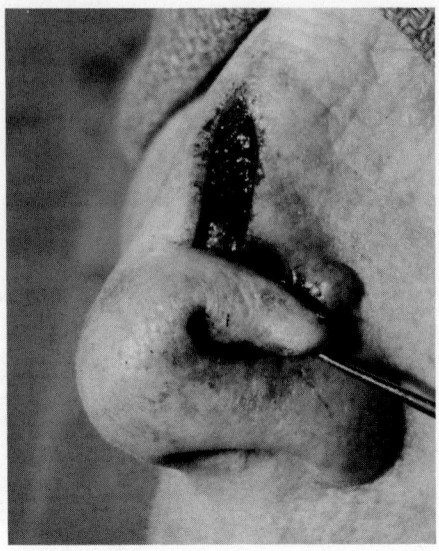 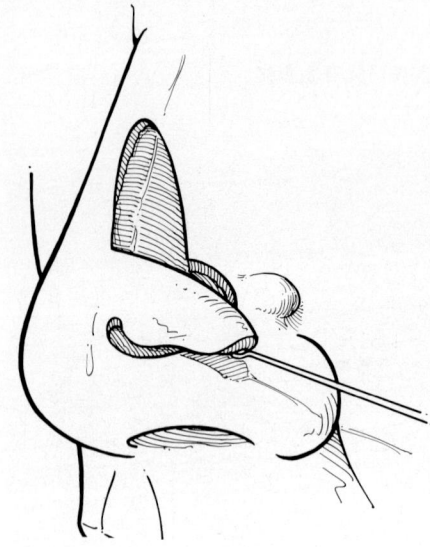

The flap is elevated just above the nasal musculature. The transposition is checked, and the vertical defect is closed directly. After it has been trimmed, the flap is sutured into place.

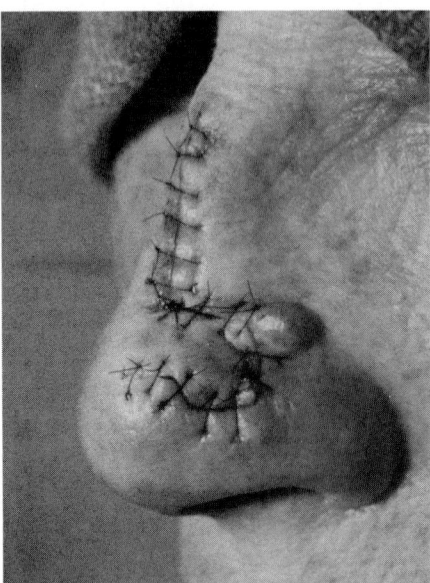 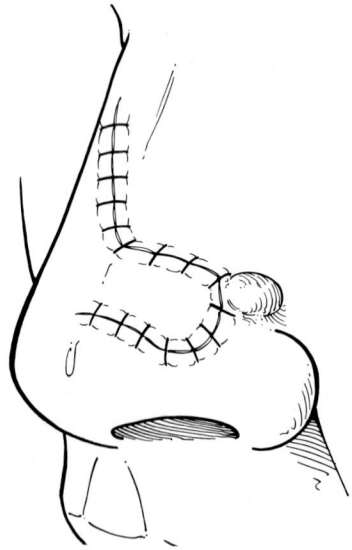

This results in an inferior standing cone, which must be removed in such a way that the base, and thus the blood supply, of the flap is not compromised.

PROBLEMS

Although the Banner flap is basically simple to design, some surgeons seem to find difficulty in removing the dog ears without compromising the pedicle base. As with all rounded flaps, there may be a tendency toward pincushioning. As the lower third of the nose is approached, less tissue is available and only small defects can be closed.

CHAPTER 4
NOSE RECONSTRUCTION

RHOMBOID FLAP

On initial consideration it may seem that there is not enough loose skin available on the nose to construct a rhomboid flap.

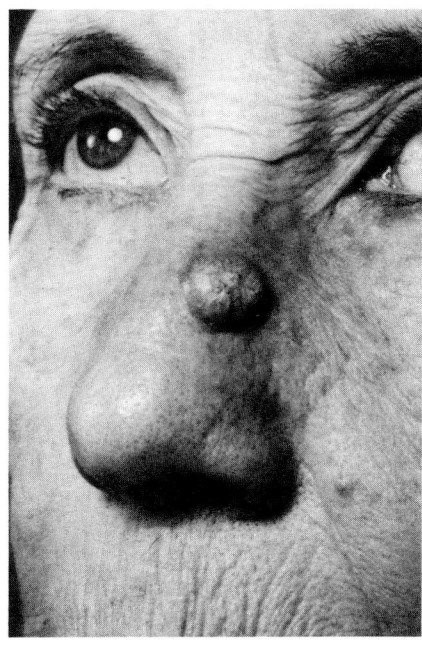
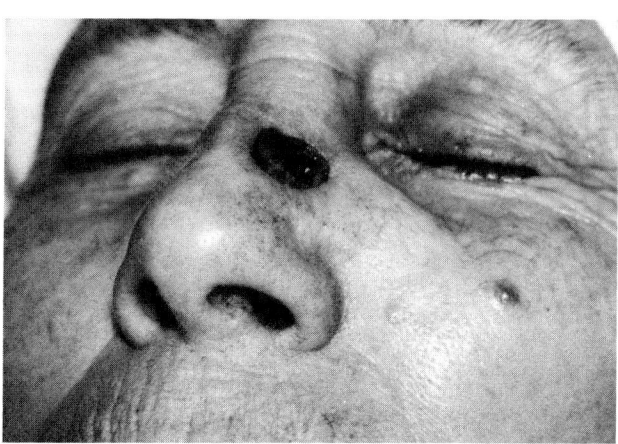
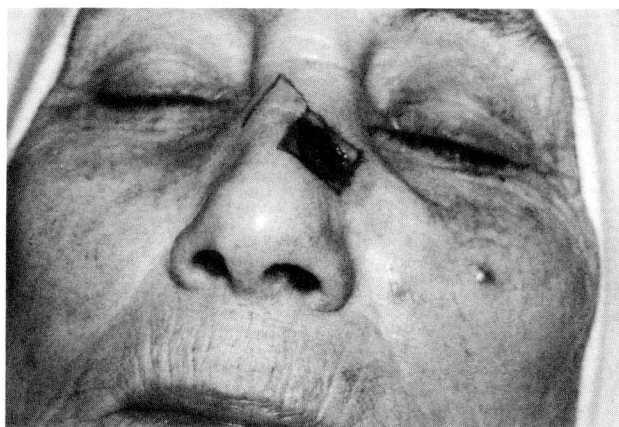
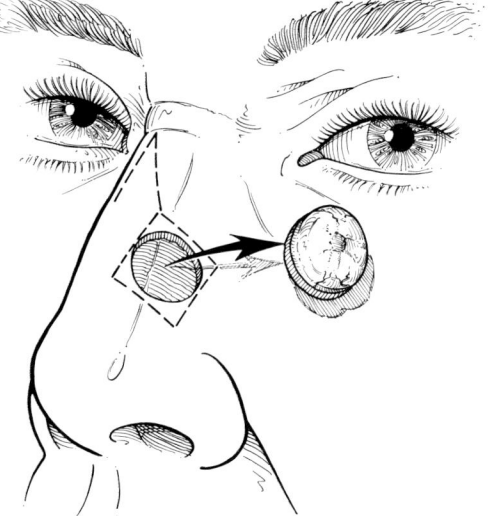

In the case of this patient with a basal cell carcinoma on the upper part of the lateral side of the nose, the excisional defect can be converted into a rhomboid.

103

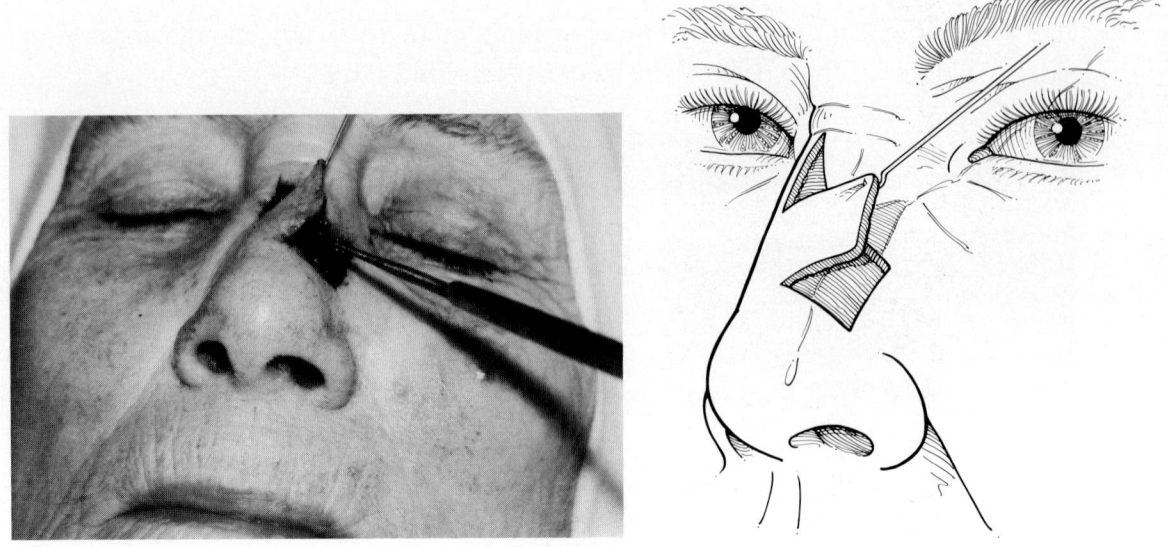

With the excess of skin transversely on the root of the nose, a rhomboid flap is constructed.

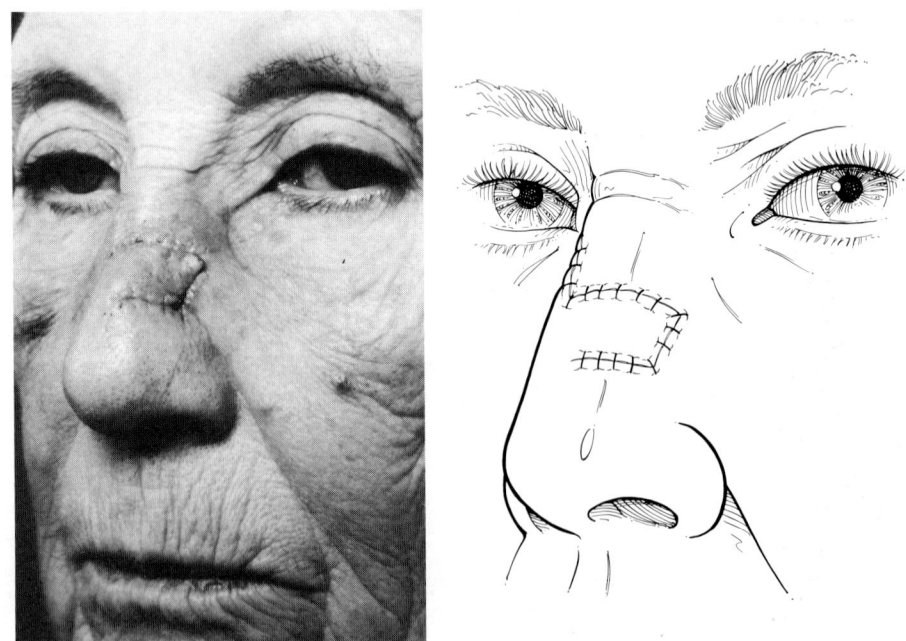

This is comfortably transposed to close the postexcisional defect, and the donor site is closed directly.

CHAPTER 4
NOSE
RECONSTRUCTION

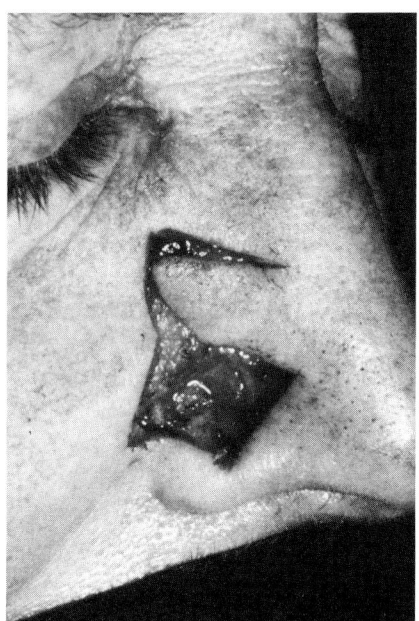

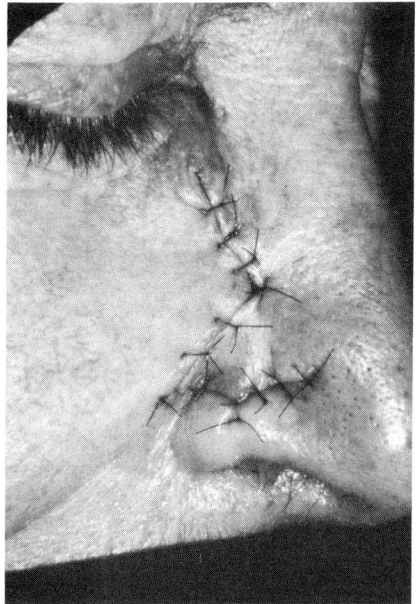

On the upper portion of the side of the nose vertically, skin is again available. In this case a rhomboid flap is used to reconstruct the extremely complicated area of the nasolabial, supraalar base, and alar rim. The flap can contour effectively into this complex surface anatomy.

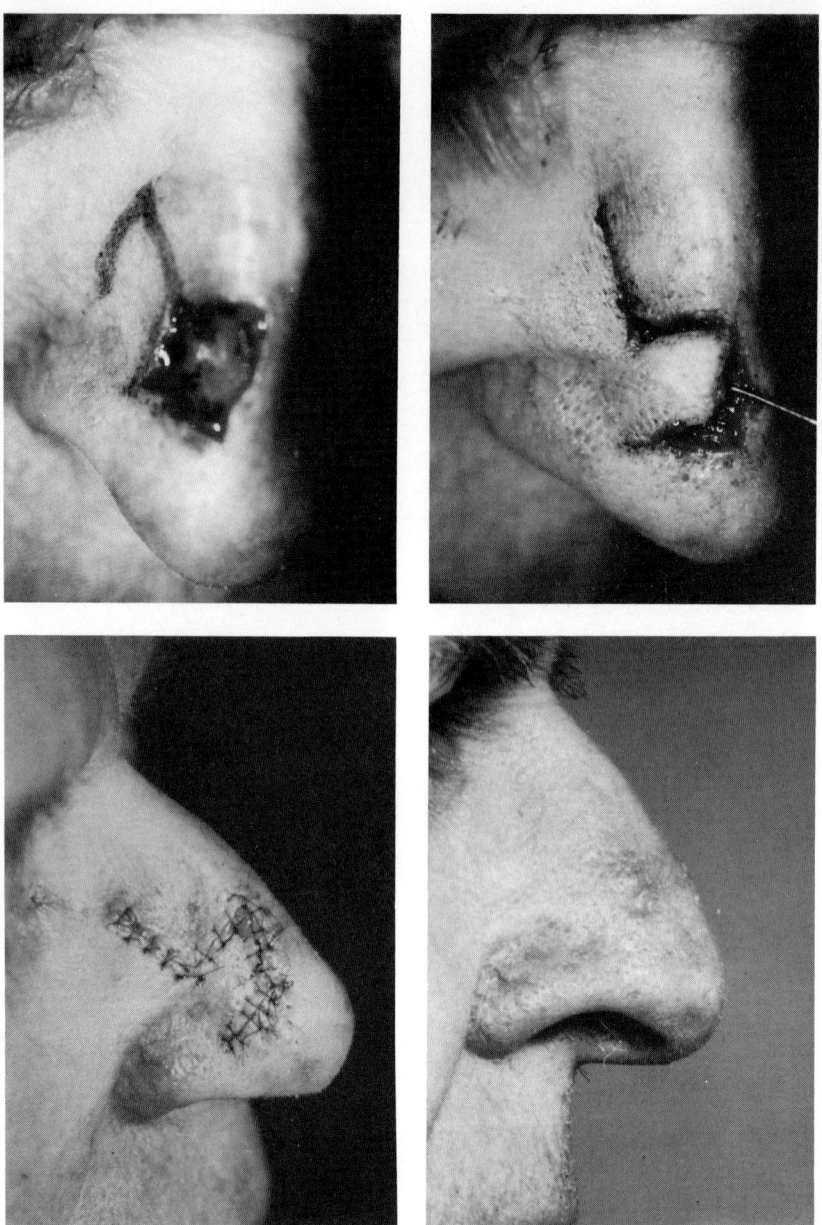

In some elderly patients there may be enough skin laterally, almost in the bridgeline area, to close postexcisional defects inferiorly and medially without skin tightness. In all of the patients presented in this section, there has been no distortion of the normal nasal anatomy.

PROBLEMS

The rhomboid flap is limited by the amount of skin available on the nose. The Banner flap is less complex to design. On the other hand, there is probably less pincushioning with the rhomboid flap.

CHAPTER 4
NOSE
RECONSTRUCTION

EXTENDED GLABELLAR FLAP

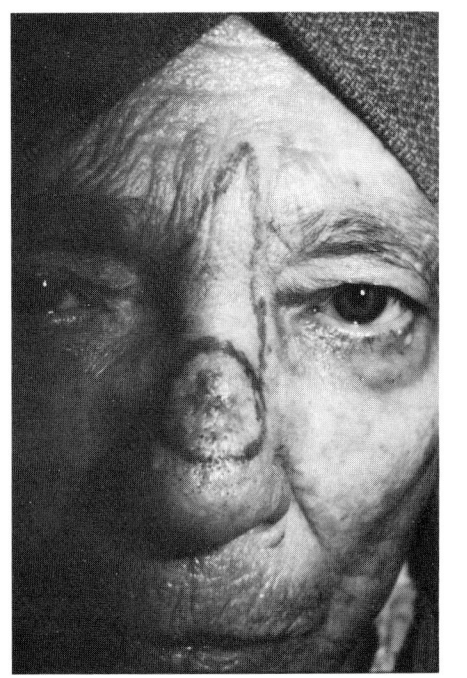
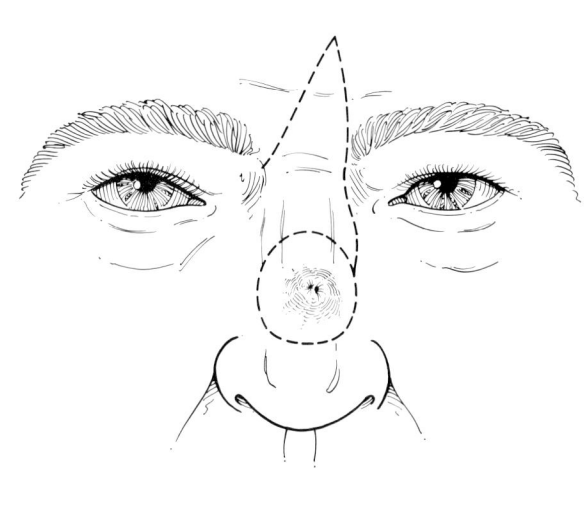

The extended glabellar flap, initially described by Gillies[3] and subsequently modified by Reiger,[14] could more accurately be called the hemi-nose flap. It has been used to reconstruct the defect left from excision of this patient's basal cell carcinoma of the nose.

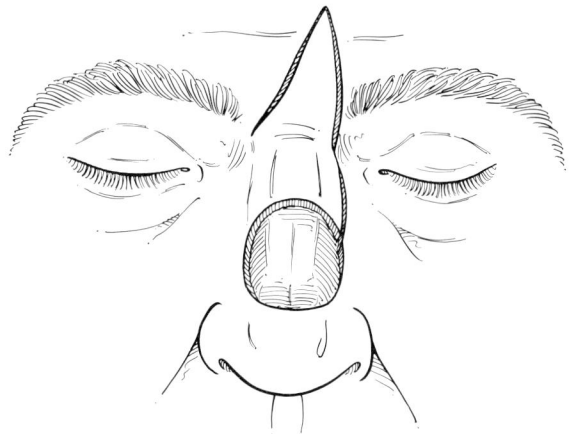

The lesion is excised as a triangle based laterally. The flap is designed rather like an extended glabellar flap; the skin is incised from the base of the triangular defect and taken up into the glabellar area. From here the incision is continued down to the other side of the nose.

107

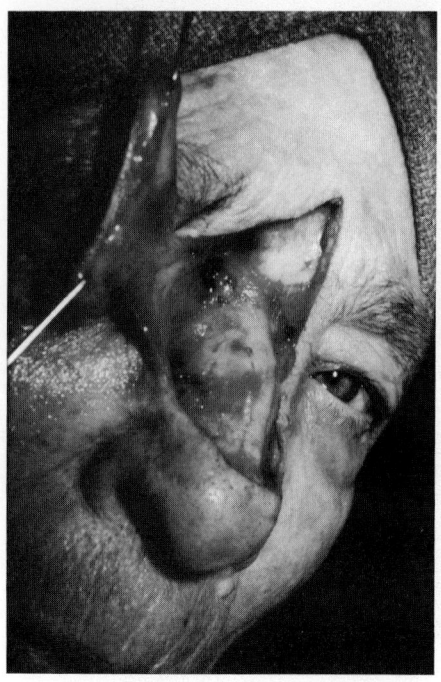
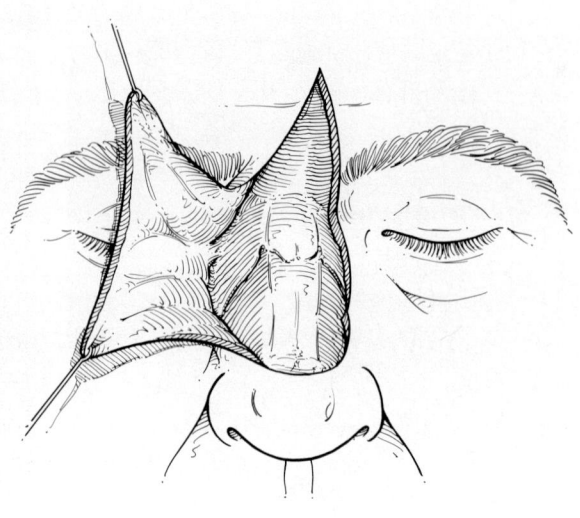

The skin of the nose superior to the defect is elevated completely down to and beyond its pedicle. Failure to do this will prevent adequate transposition to close the defect.

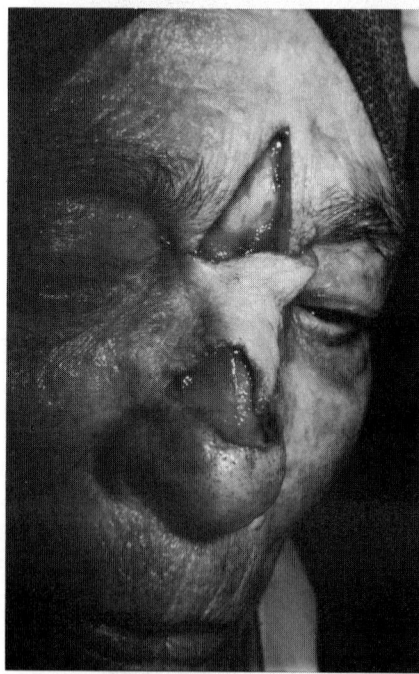
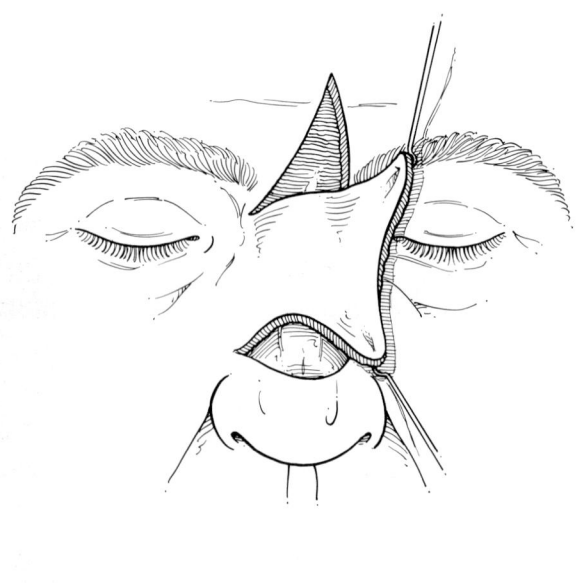

The flap is then swung down to close the defect and trimming of the inferior standing cone is performed.

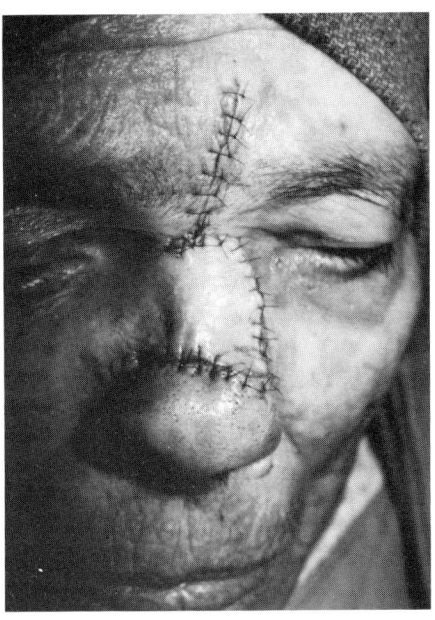
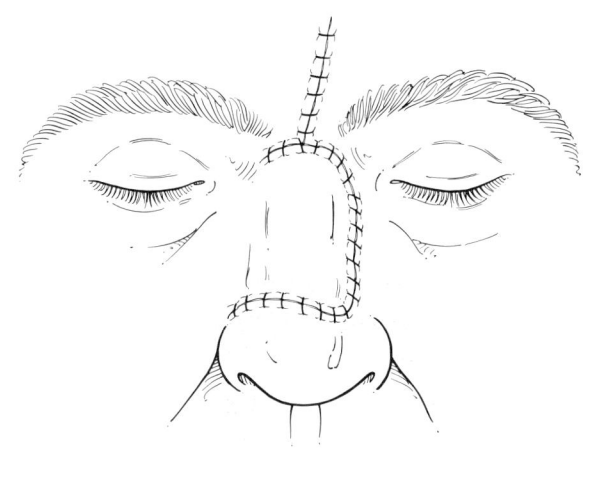

A glabellar Z-plasty is incorporated if this is considered necessary.

PROBLEMS

The disadvantage of the extended glabellar flap is the somewhat limited rotation obtained. If rotation is not sufficient, then the alar rim will be pulled up and nasal asymmetry will result. As the illustration shows, this asymmetry is not very noticeable when the defect is toward the midline. There is also the conceptual problem of raising such a large area of skin to close a relatively small defect. In spite of these objections, this type of flap is safe and certainly should be considered for lateral nasal resurfacing.

BILOBED FLAP

The bilobed flap, an old and ingenious type[2] can be used for reconstruction virtually anywhere, but it is best suited to the lateral aspect of the nose and the sole of the foot.[12] It is basically a method of transferring tissue through 90 to 180 degrees with a minimum of rotation, dissection, and disturbance of regional anatomy. The flap must be designed with extreme care or the results will be unsatisfactory.

An excess of nasal skin is present high in the middle of the nose or high on the lateral aspect of the nose. This skin can be used for lower nasal reconstruction. Defects toward the midline of the nose may be reconstructed with laterally based flaps. Unless small and situated toward the midline, lateral defects must *never* be closed with laterally based flaps. Flaps constructed in this way would lie across the cheek-to-nose concavity and would obliterate this normal anatomic contour, thus creating a deformity that would defy satisfactory correction later.

Flap Design

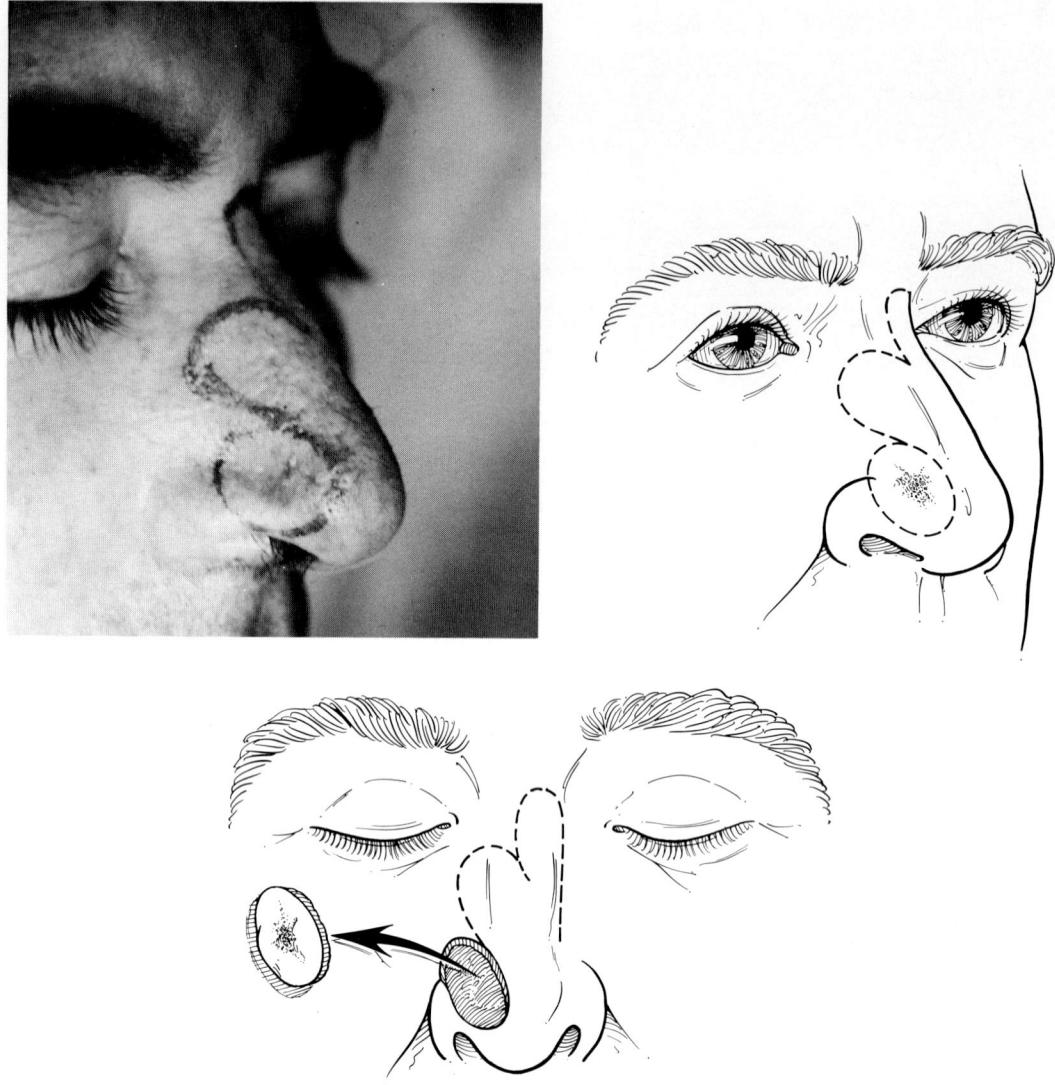

The defect is created and, depending on its position, the situation of the flap base is chosen. The flap for reconstructing the defect usually lies with its midaxis at 45 degrees to that of the defect; the flap is slightly smaller than the defect. To close the secondary defect, a flap is taken from the loose skin donor site (bridge of nose midline or lateral); its axis lies at 45 degrees to flap 1 and 90 degrees to the defect axis, and the flap is somewhat smaller than the secondary defect. This is well illustrated in this basal cell carcinoma lying just above the right alar rim.

CHAPTER 4
NOSE RECONSTRUCTION

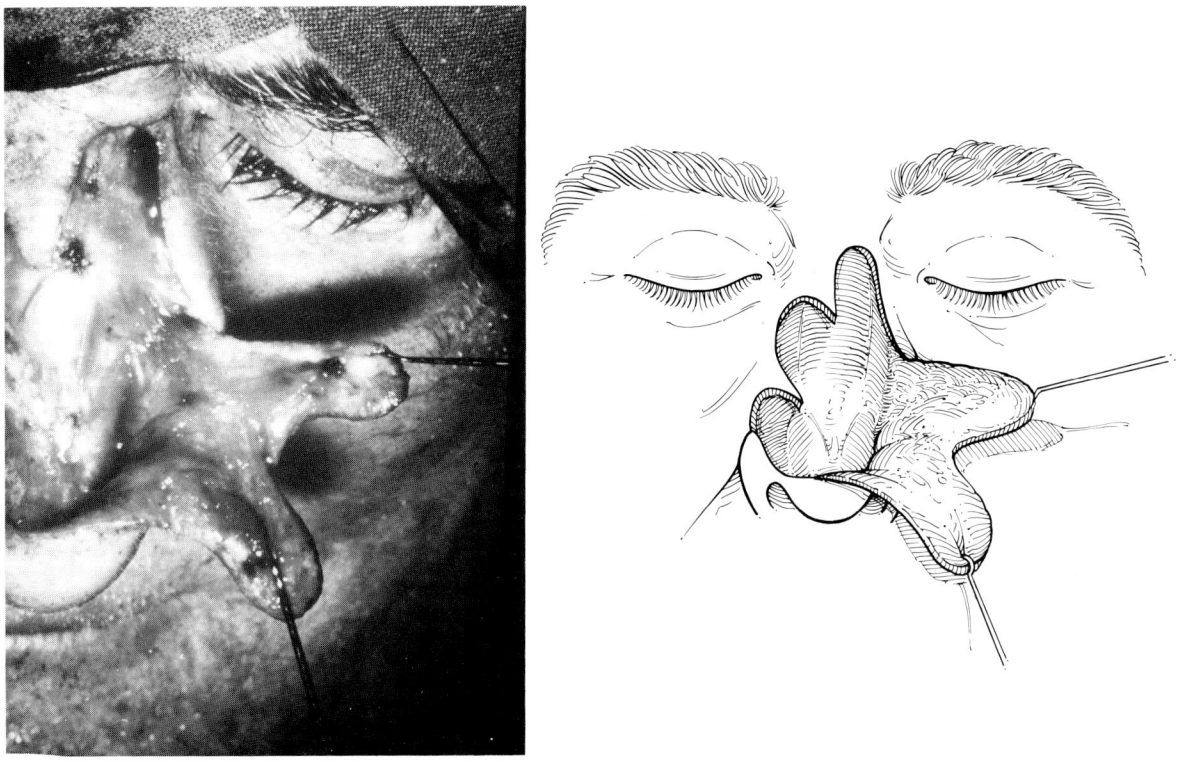

The flap is widely undermined to its base and beyond.

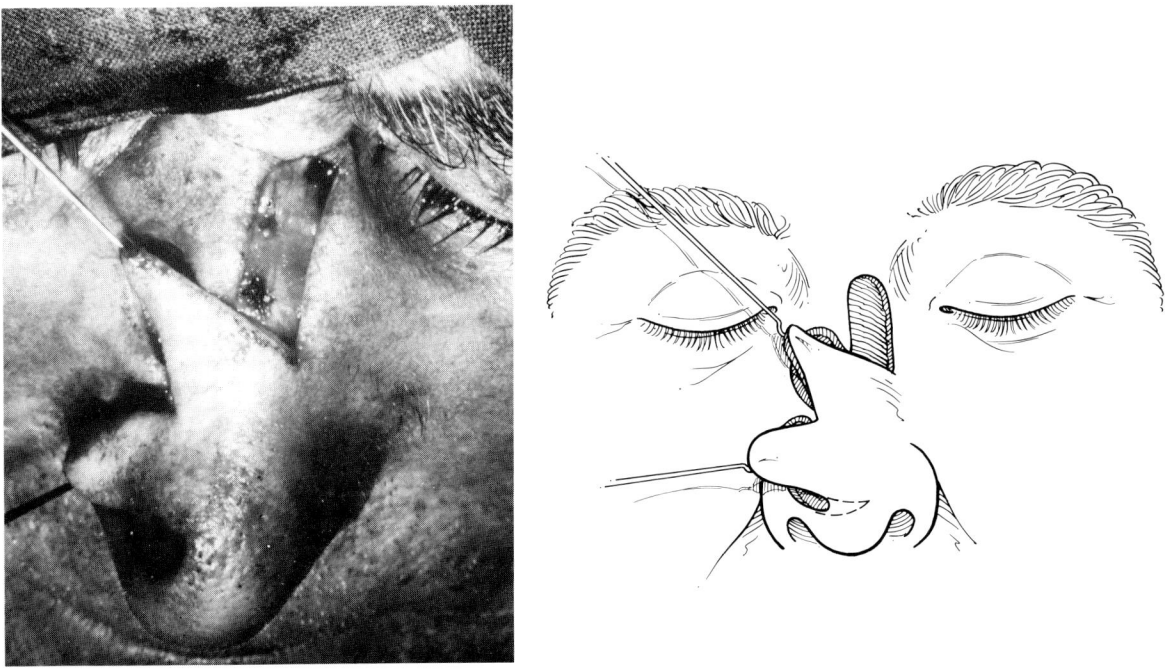

Flaps 1 and 2 are transposed to close the defects; this transposition should be possible with little effort.

111

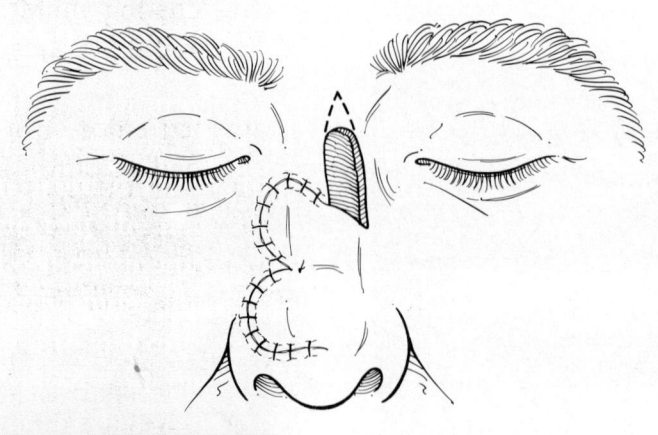

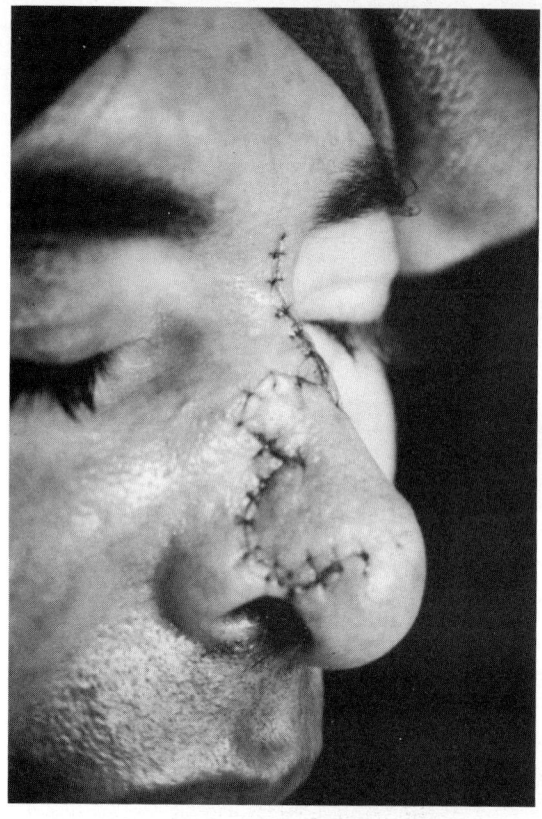

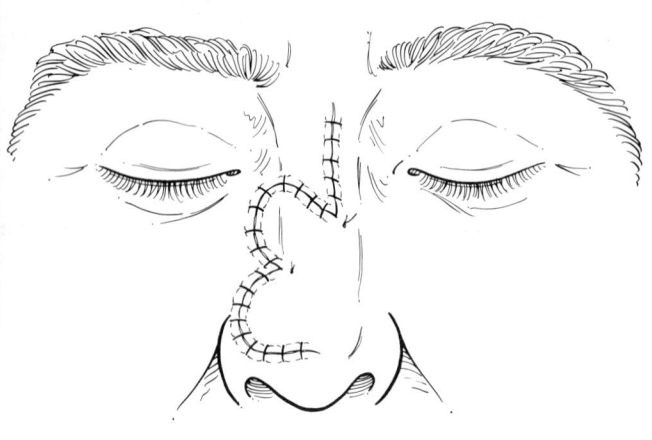

The donor site of flap 2 is closed directly. It is frequently necessary to trim the flaps as they are inserted into the defects. Any dog ears are carefully trimmed, with care taken to avoid the flap base, thereby avoiding interference with the blood supply.

Large defects can be closed in this way without distortion of anatomy. Poor flap design will cause tenting across the nasal cheek line, sometimes with pincushioning of the flap pedicle, a situation that cannot be corrected. It is possible to rotate each flap 90 degrees and in effect rotate tissue through 180 degrees. Such a maneuver becomes necessary when the defect is situated closer to the midline.

CHAPTER 4
**NOSE
RECONSTRUCTION**

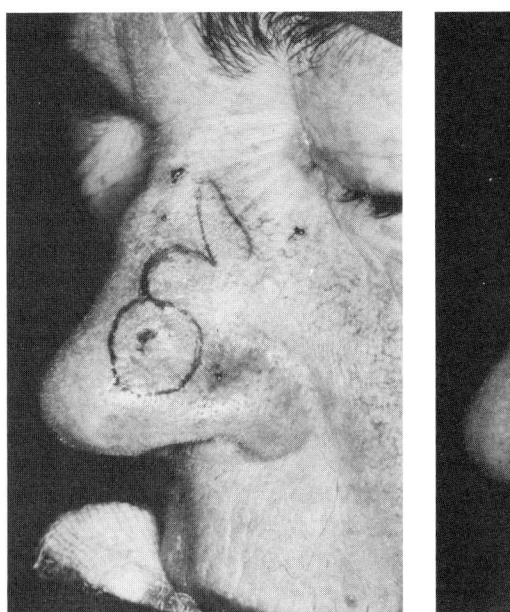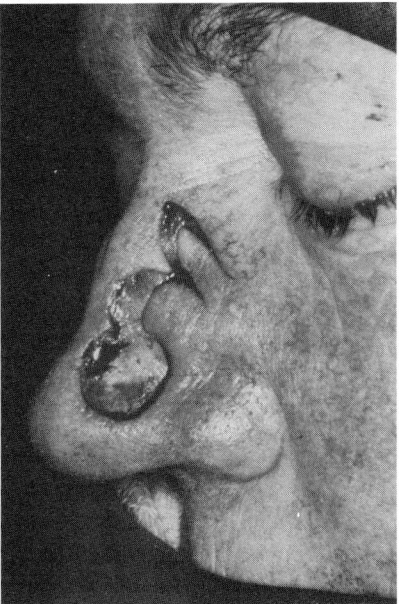

The patient shown here had a basal cell carcinoma present on the side of the nasal tip area. Care must be taken in planning a laterally based bilobed flap. The flap base is retained on the side of the nose itself.

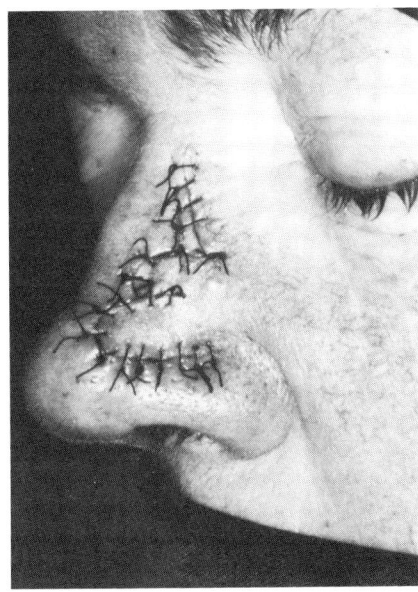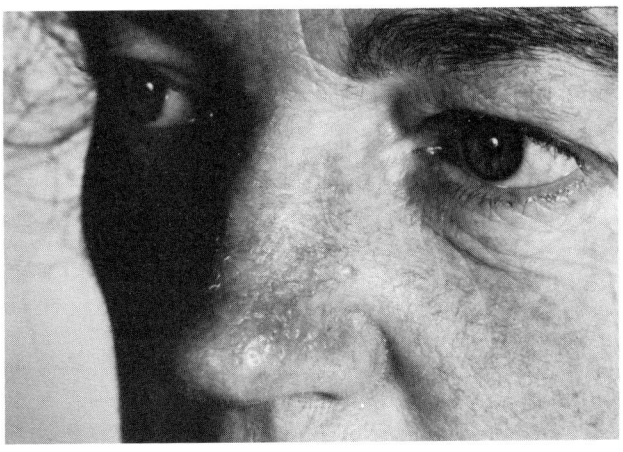

The remainder of the procedure is as described on p. 21. The result is most pleasing.

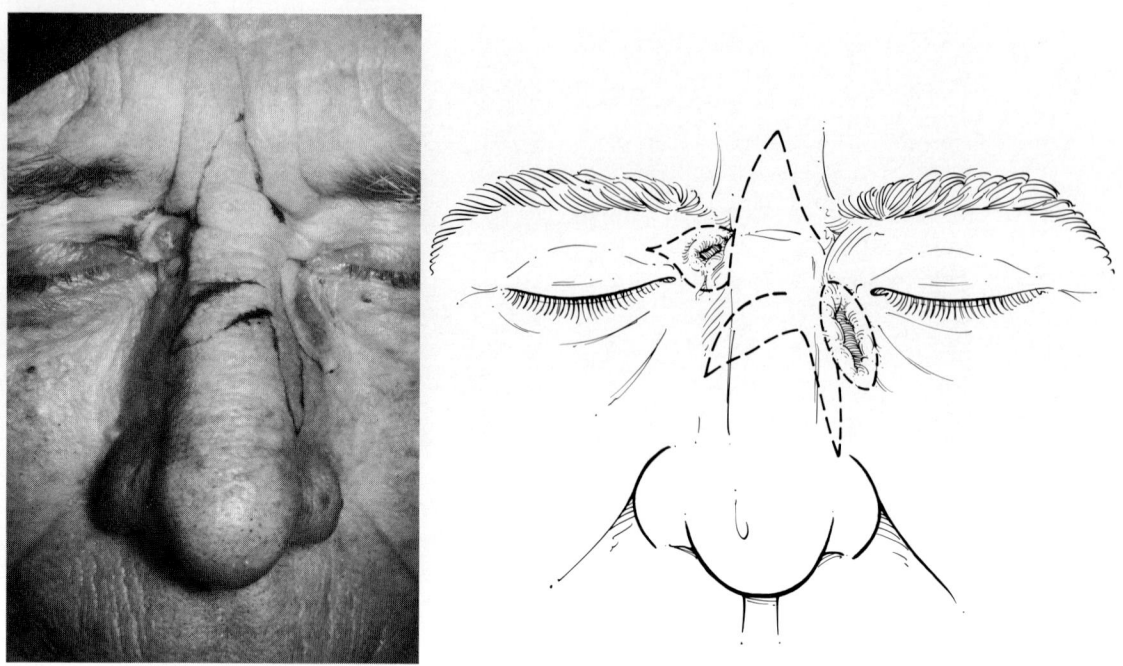

A bilobed flap may be conveniently used with other flaps to reconstruct complex contour defects. A case in point is a patient with basal cell carcinomas in both medial canthal areas.

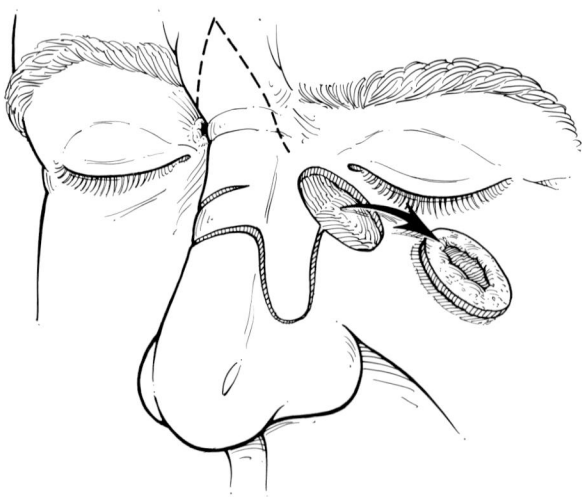

Reconstruction is planned to close the left side with a bilobed flap from the nasal bridgeline and the right side with a glabellar finger flap.

CHAPTER 4
**NOSE
RECONSTRUCTION**

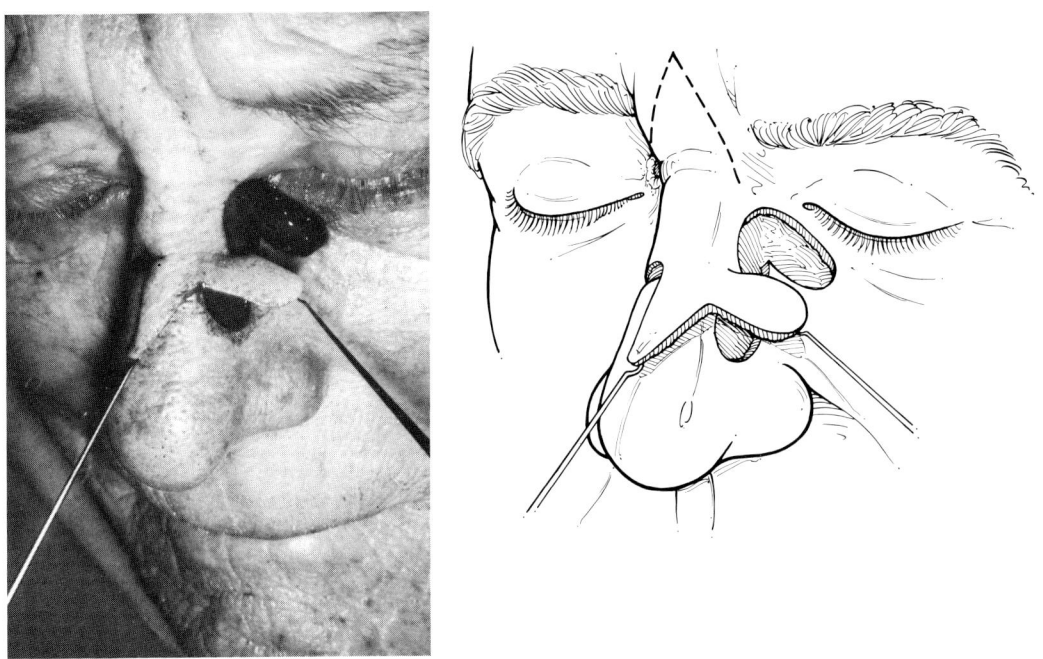

The lesion of the left medial canthus is excised, and the bilobed flap is widely elevated.

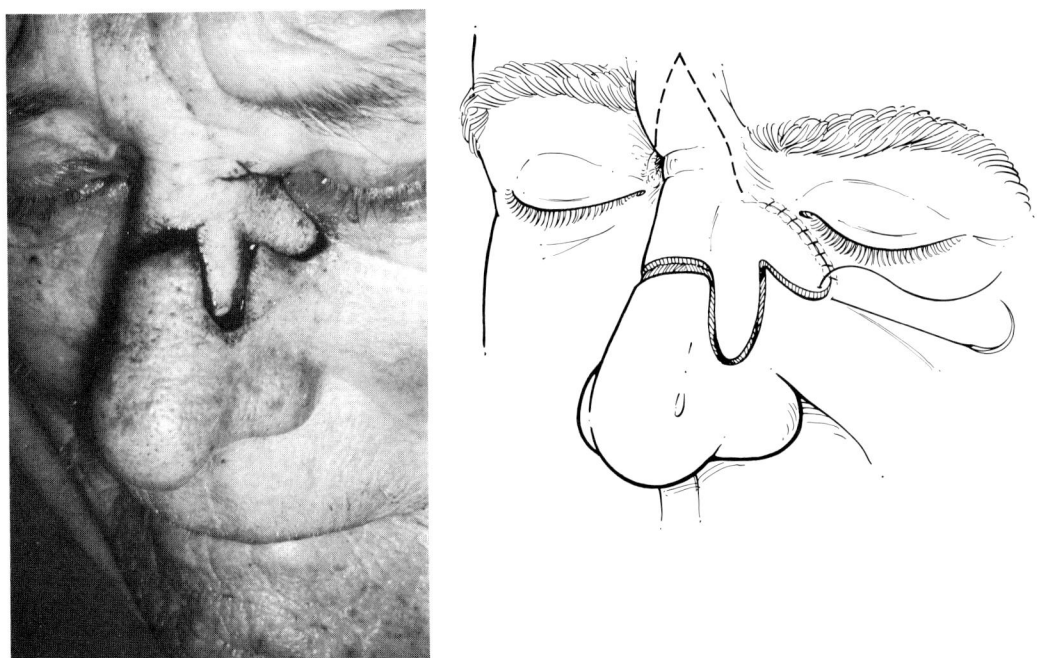

With the loose skin now available, the flap virtually falls into place.

115

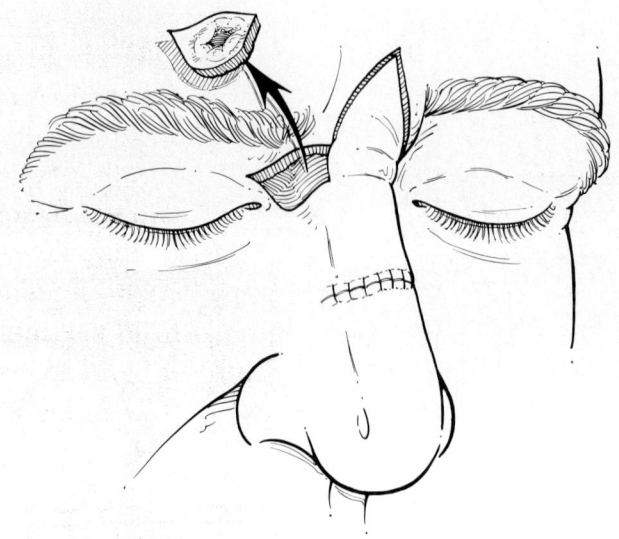

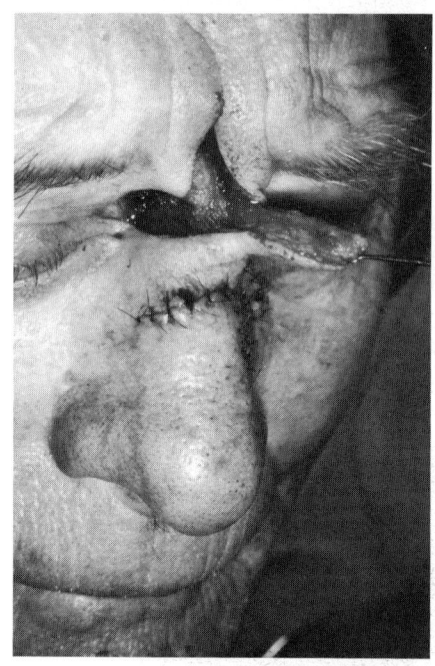

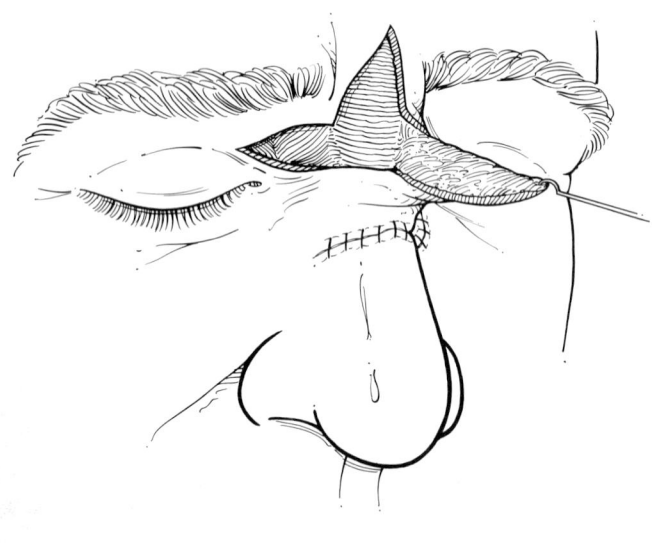

The lesion on the right side of the nasal bridgeline is resected, and the finger flap is elevated.

CHAPTER 4
NOSE RECONSTRUCTION

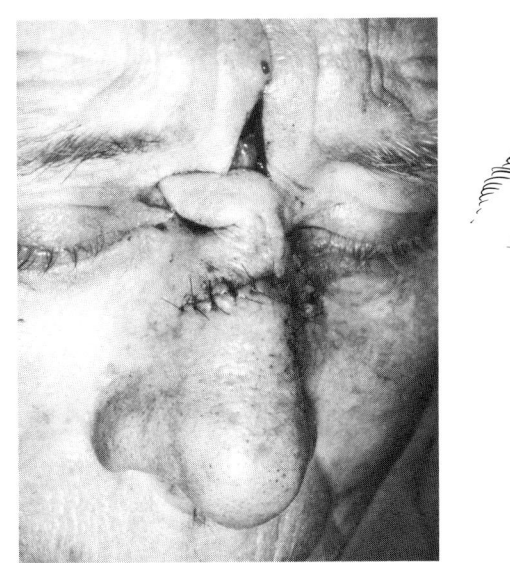
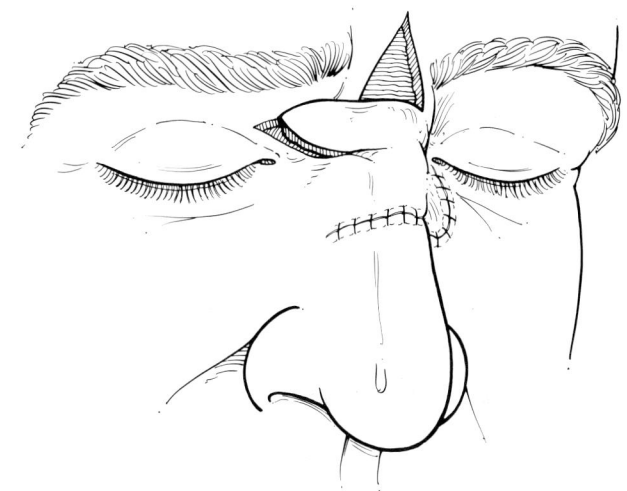

The flap can be rotated easily into position.

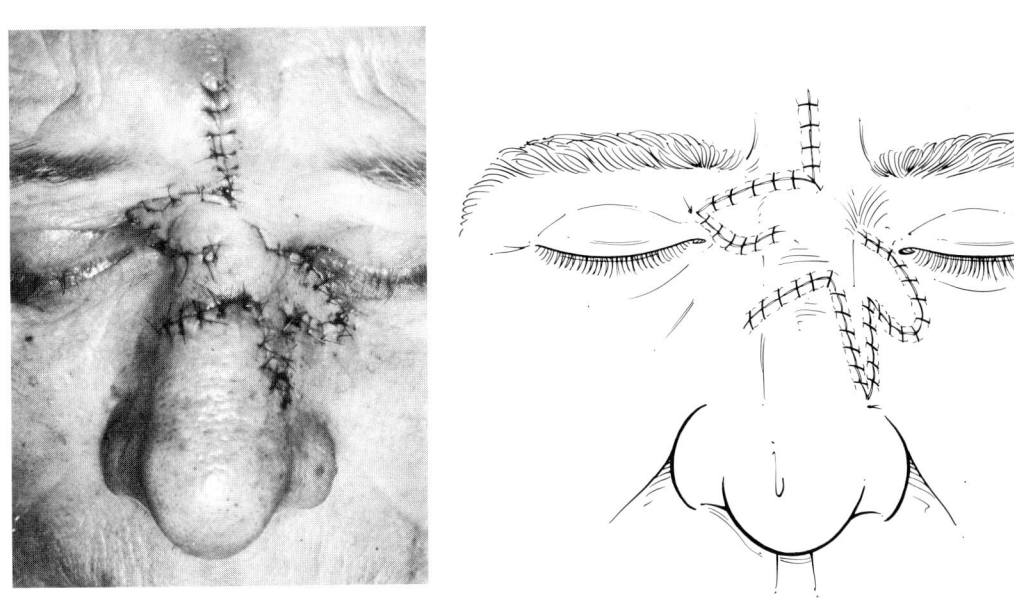

The flap is sutured in place with closure of the secondary defect and no resulting deformity.

PROBLEMS

If the flaps are made too small, particularly too narrow, the alar rim may be distorted. If wide undermining of the flap base is not performed, there may be inadequate rotation and again distortion will result. Because the flaps are rounded, pincushioning can occur. The nature of the flap design inevitably leads to a long and complex scar; fortunately, the scar heals well on the nose and has never been a problem for patient or surgeon.

NASOLABIAL FLAP

A lateral nasal reconstruction (favored by the inexperienced) is the nasolabial flap. It is simple to design and rapid and elegant to execute, but the long-term result is usually aesthetically unacceptable unless used in the correct anatomic area.

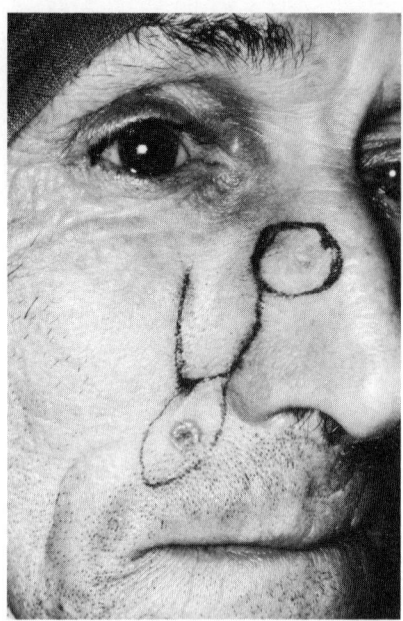

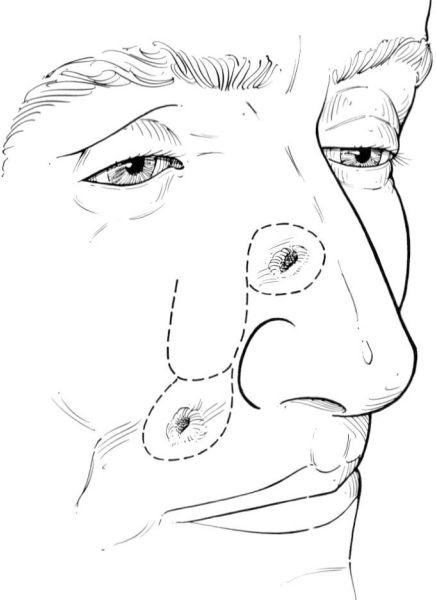

This patient had a basal cell carcinoma on the side of the nose and another in the nasolabial area.

CHAPTER 4
NOSE RECONSTRUCTION

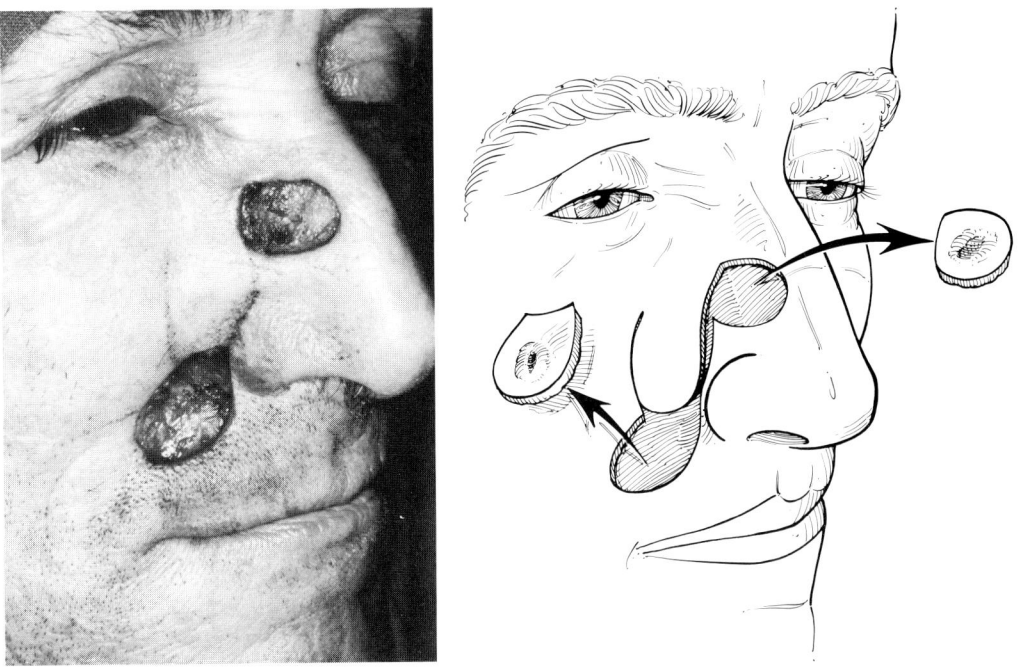

When the tumors are excised, the dog ear of the lower lesion lies in the nasolabial fold.

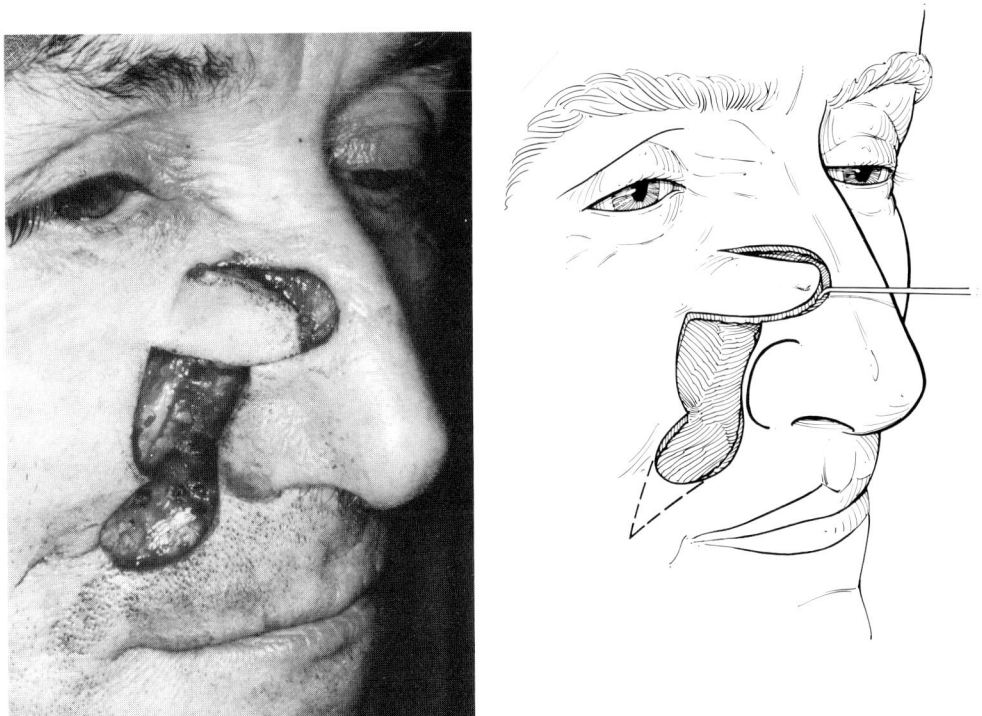

This excess of skin can be used to construct a superiorly based nasolabial flap that can be swung up and medially to close the superior defect.

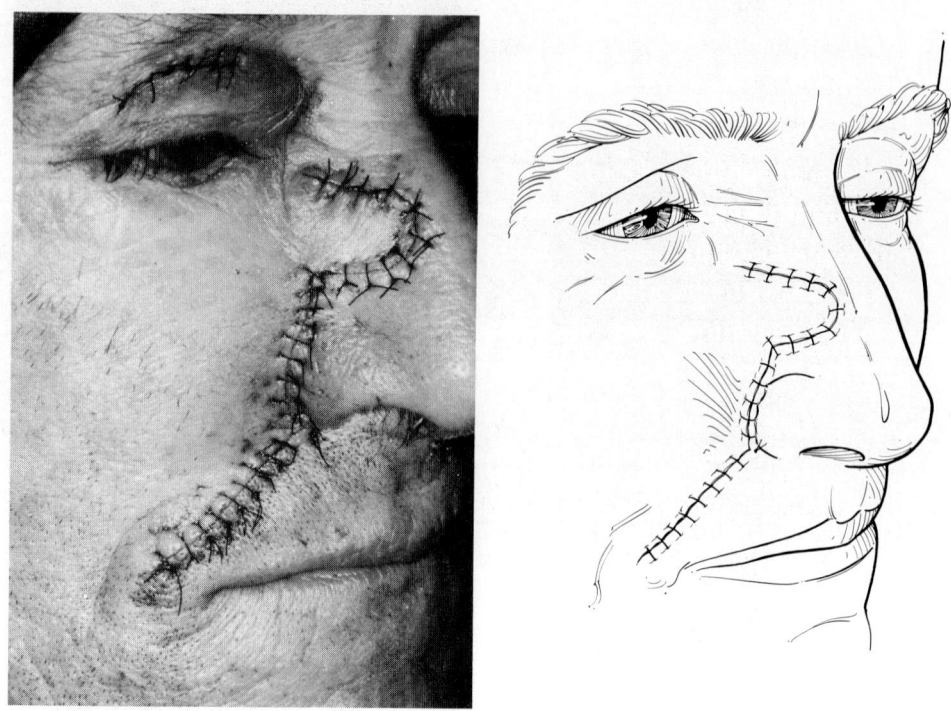

The incisions are well contoured into natural lines, and the flap does not cross a concavity.

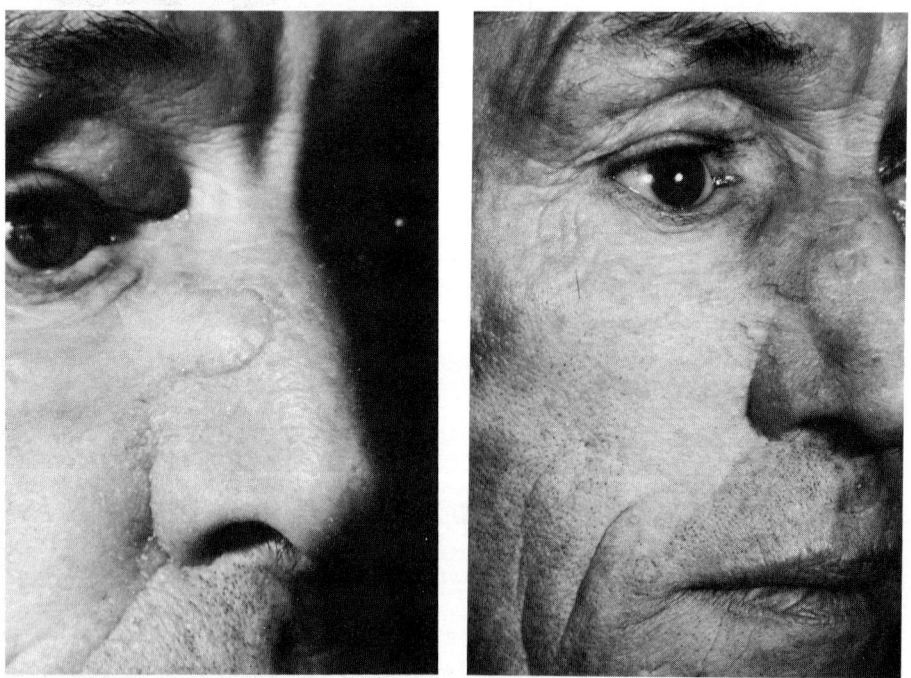

Unfortunately, cheek skin is not the same as nose skin, and often there are texture and color differences, especially in the male. These problems do not improve, even after many years, although the scars do settle extremely well.

CHAPTER 4
NOSE RECONSTRUCTION

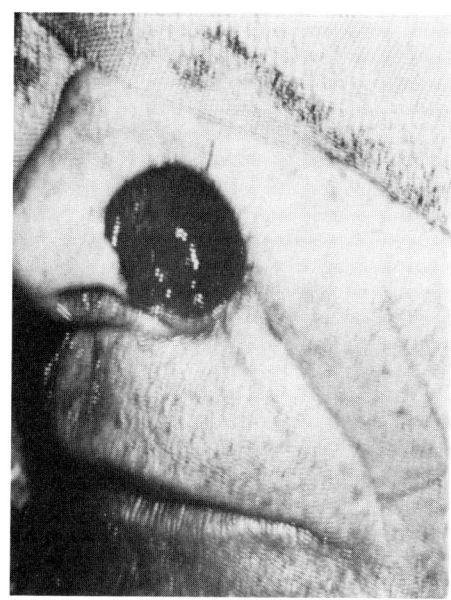 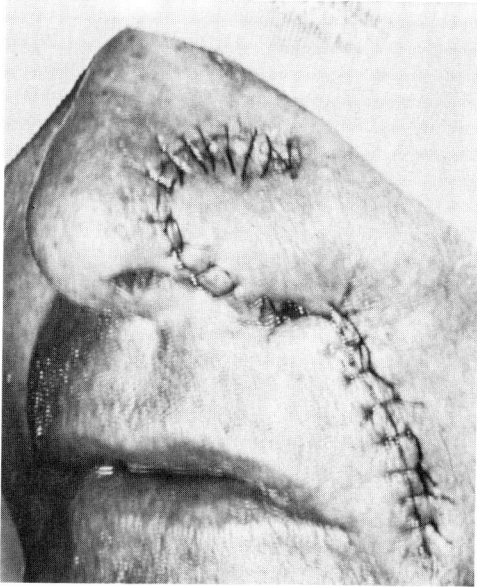

If the nasolabial flap is used low on the nose, the result is usually disastrous. This is well illustrated by the result following excision of a basal cell carcinoma of the alar rim base area. The pedicle is based low and lateral, and the cheek-nose concavity is obliterated.

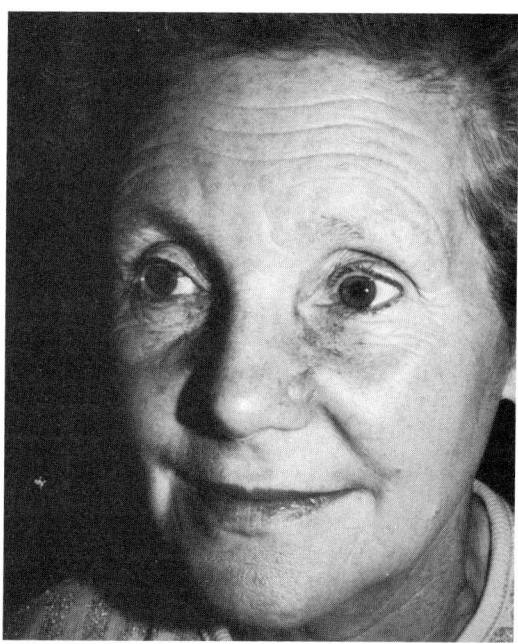

The same problem occurs when a bilobed flap is based in the nasolabial area. In some males, when an inferior flap is used, hairbearing skin will be transferred to the nose—a situation to be avoided.

121

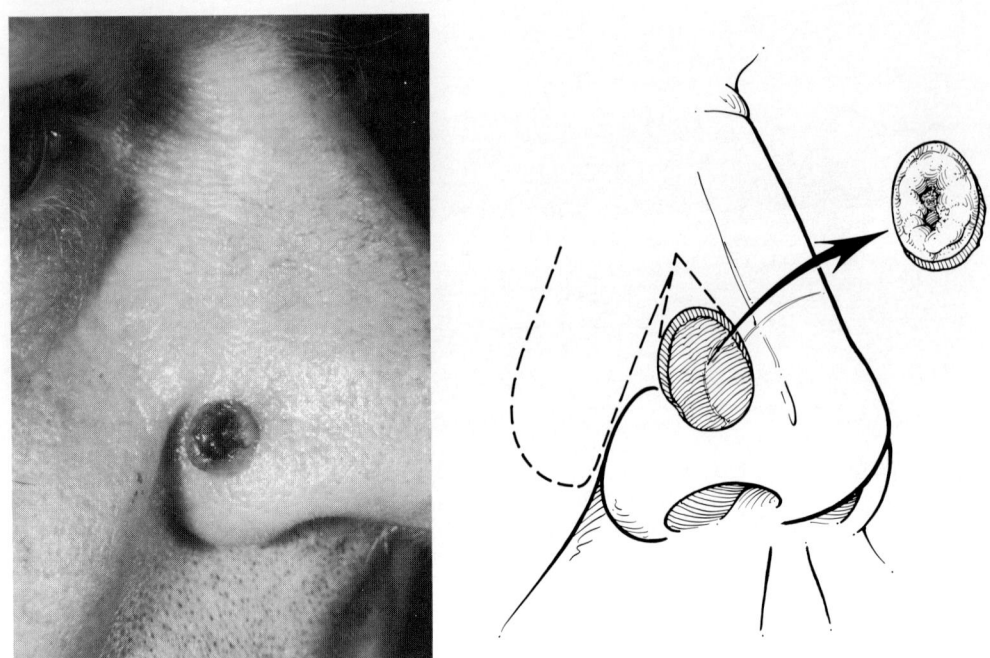

This basal cell carcinoma was excised, and the flap was based high on the side of the nose with a consequently smaller transposition.

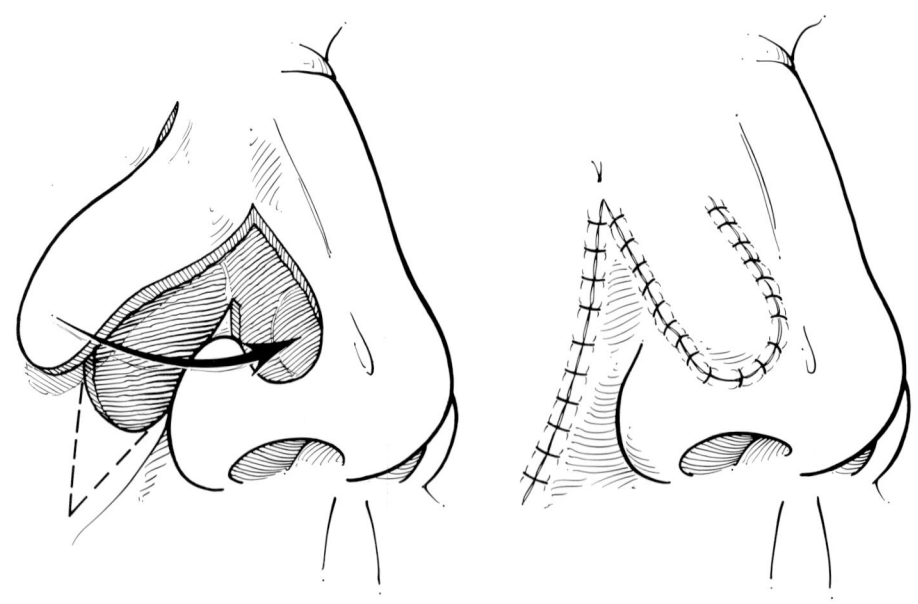

This avoids the cheek-nose concavity but creates another problem.

CHAPTER 4
NOSE RECONSTRUCTION

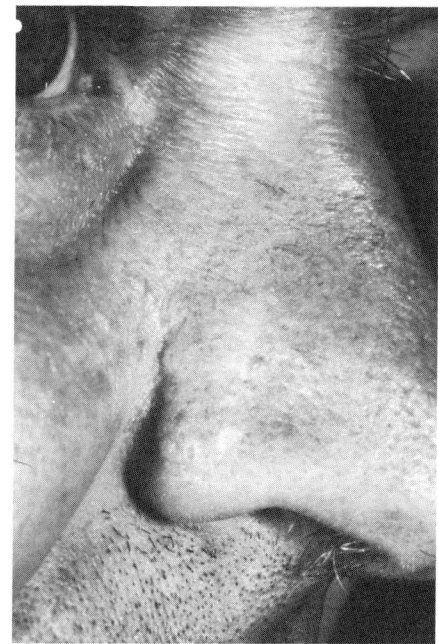

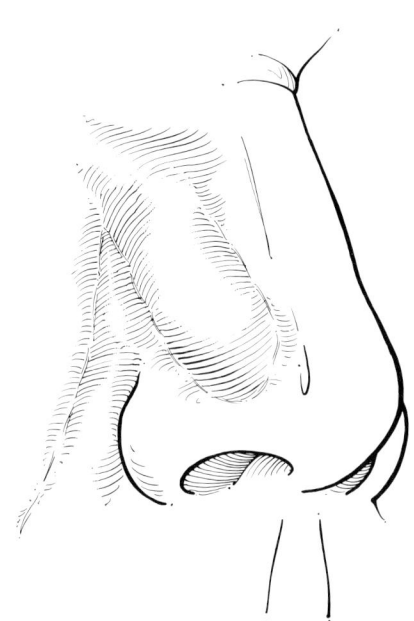

This flap almost always pincushions and looks extremely ugly.

Two-stage nasolabial flaps are possible but unnecessary. They should be used only in exceptional circumstances (e.g., when a larger area is to be reconstructed). Again, in the male, hairbearing skin may be transferred to the nose (see pp. 128-131).

NASOLABIAL ISLAND FLAP

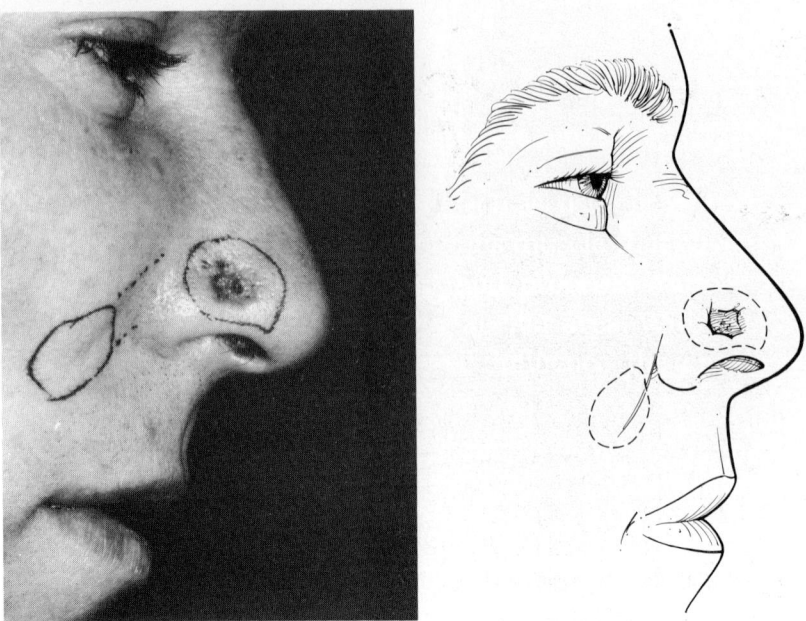

The procedure of taking an island flap from the nasolabial region is elegant to perform. The expected defect after excision of this basal cell carcinoma is measured and drawn on the nonhairbearing part of the nasolabial area. An assessment of pedicle length with a strip of gauze is necessary to ensure that the flap will be long enough to reach and adequately cover the defect.

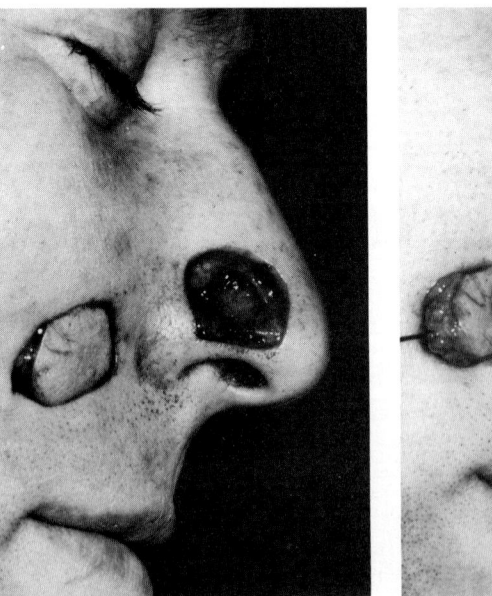 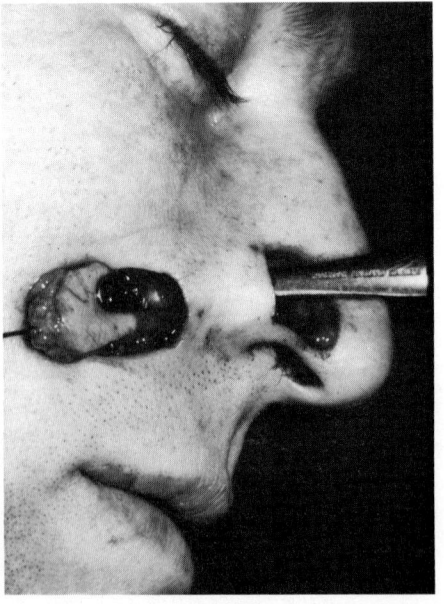

The flap is incised through the skin except at the supramedial area, where the incision is taken only to the subdermal region. The flap is elevated at its required depth. Between the island and the nasal defect, the intervening skin is elevated at the subdermal level to form a tunnel.

CHAPTER 4
NOSE RECONSTRUCTION

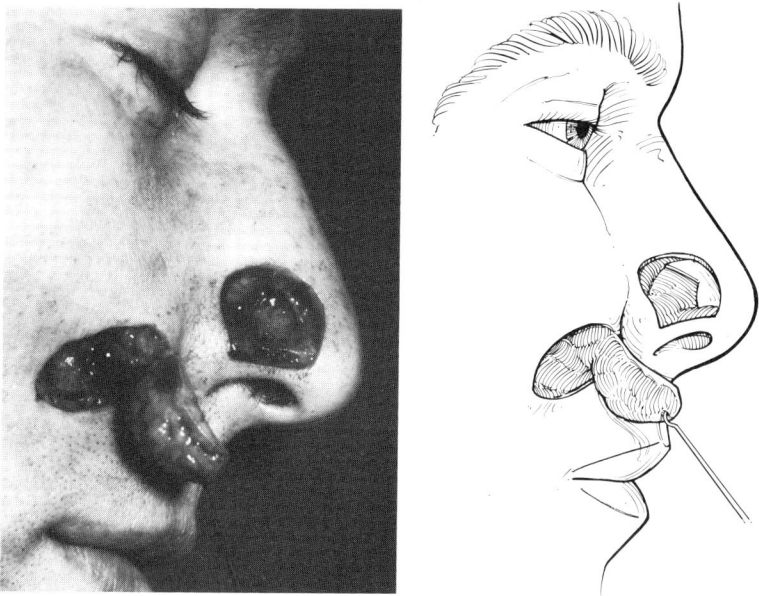

The subcutaneous tissue is divided superficial and deep to the pedicle. The latter is raised off the underlying facial muscles and divided laterally and medially, based superiorly on the lateral pyriform rim.

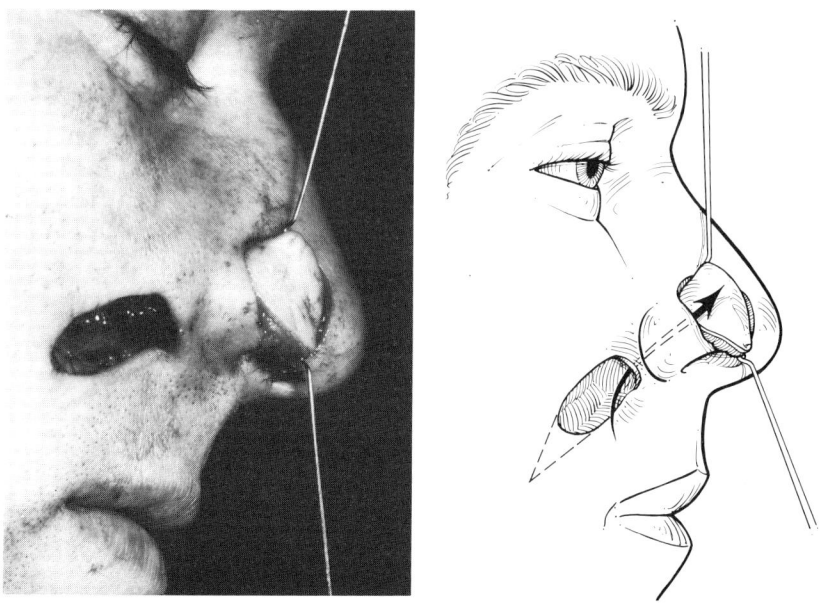

The tunnel is now checked to see that it is spacious enough for passage of the flap and the pedicle. The freedom of the pedicle is assessed. The skin island can now be taken comfortably through the tunnel and sutured into the defect.

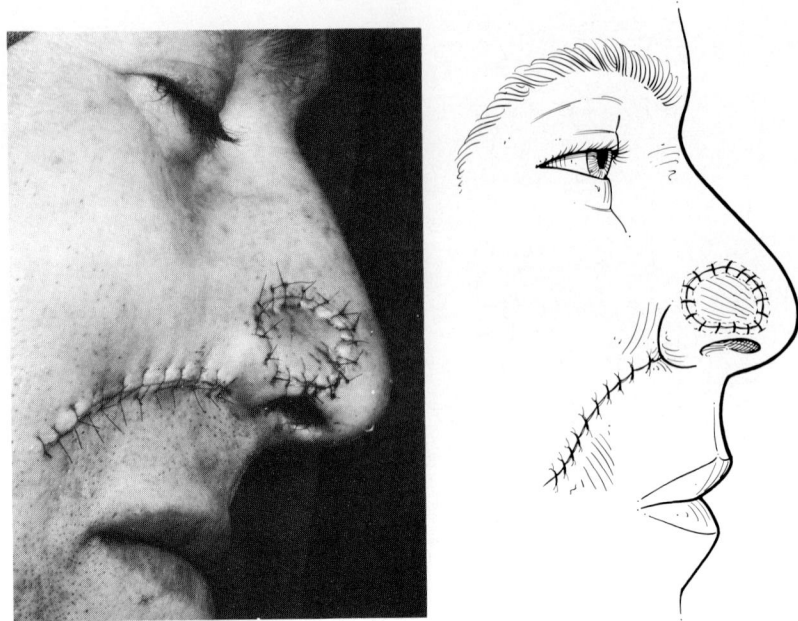

The flap donor defect is closed directly along the nasolabial line.

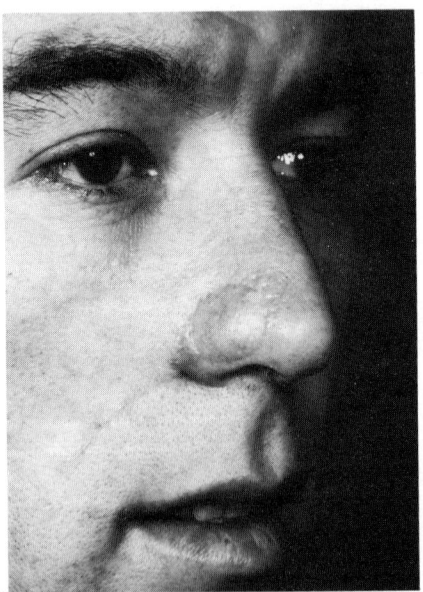
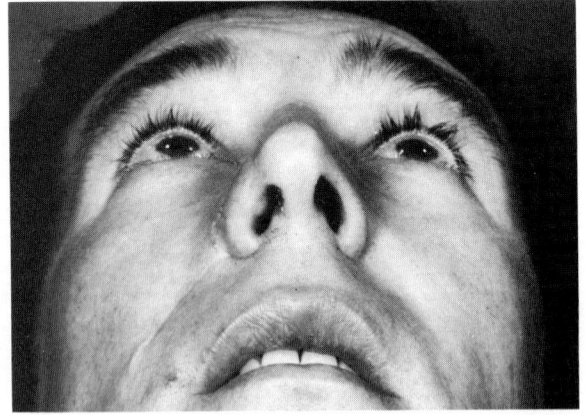

PROBLEMS

The nasolabial island flap gives a nice reconstruction, but it may slightly obliterate the cheek-nose concavity because of the bulk of the subcutaneous pedicle.

CHAPTER 4
NOSE RECONSTRUCTION

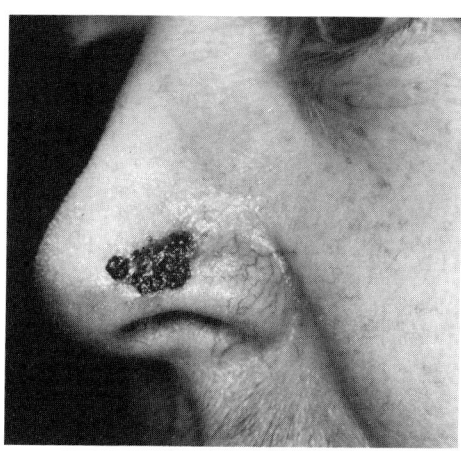

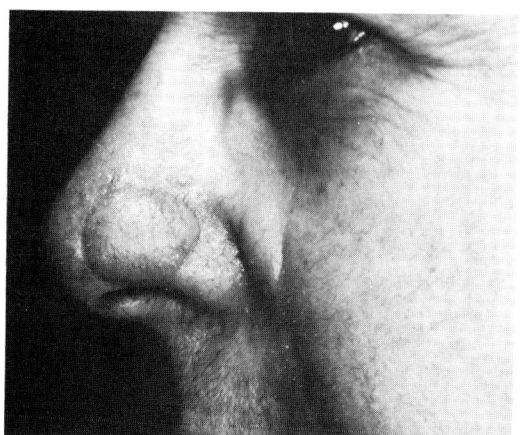

In addition, the flap may pincushion, as illustrated by the result for this patient after a nasolabial island flap was used to reconstruct the defect resulting from resection of an alar rim basal cell carcinoma.

RECONSTRUCTION OF CHOICE

For small defects the simple Banner flap is ideal, although in some regions with double contour reconstruction the rhomboid flap may be more satisfactory. In larger defects the surgeon need look no further than the bilobed flap. The only possible complication that may occur, apart from one caused by poor design, is pincushioning, a defect that may require later revision. All other flaps are either too complicated or may cause problems difficult to solve.

☐ Nasal Tip

In the nasal tip area the skin is smooth, red, thick, and sebaceous, especially in males. These characteristics make the area unsuitable for replacement with full-thickness skin grafts, even those described as "ideal" from the postauricular or nasolabial area. Only neighboring nasal skin usually will suffice. In some males the tip skin may be hairbearing to a variable degree.

NASOLABIAL FLAP

Two-stage nasolabial flaps may be used, especially if the alar rim and nasal lining need to be reconstructed.

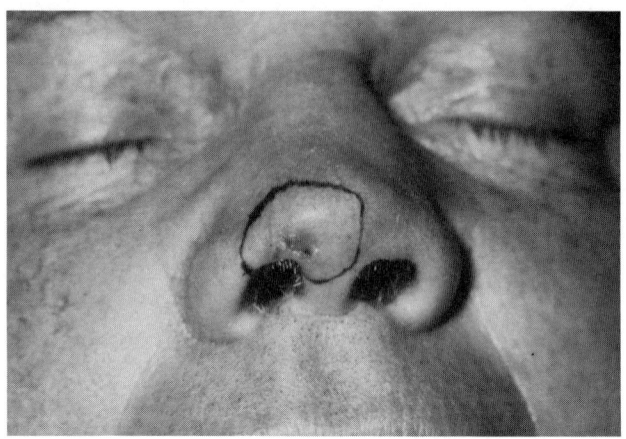

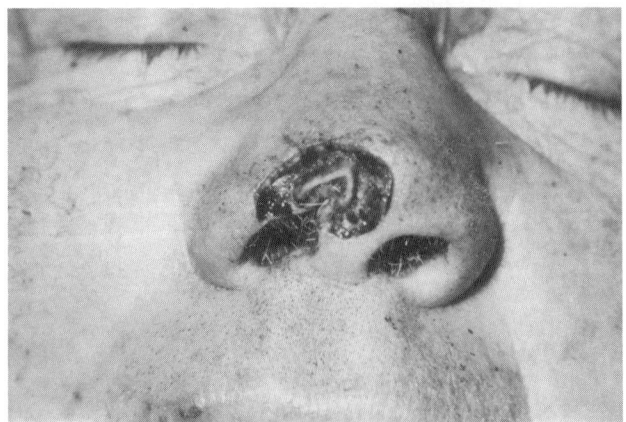

This approach was used for reconstructing the defect following excision of a basal cell carcinoma involving both the outer and inner aspects of the alar rim.

CHAPTER 4
NOSE RECONSTRUCTION

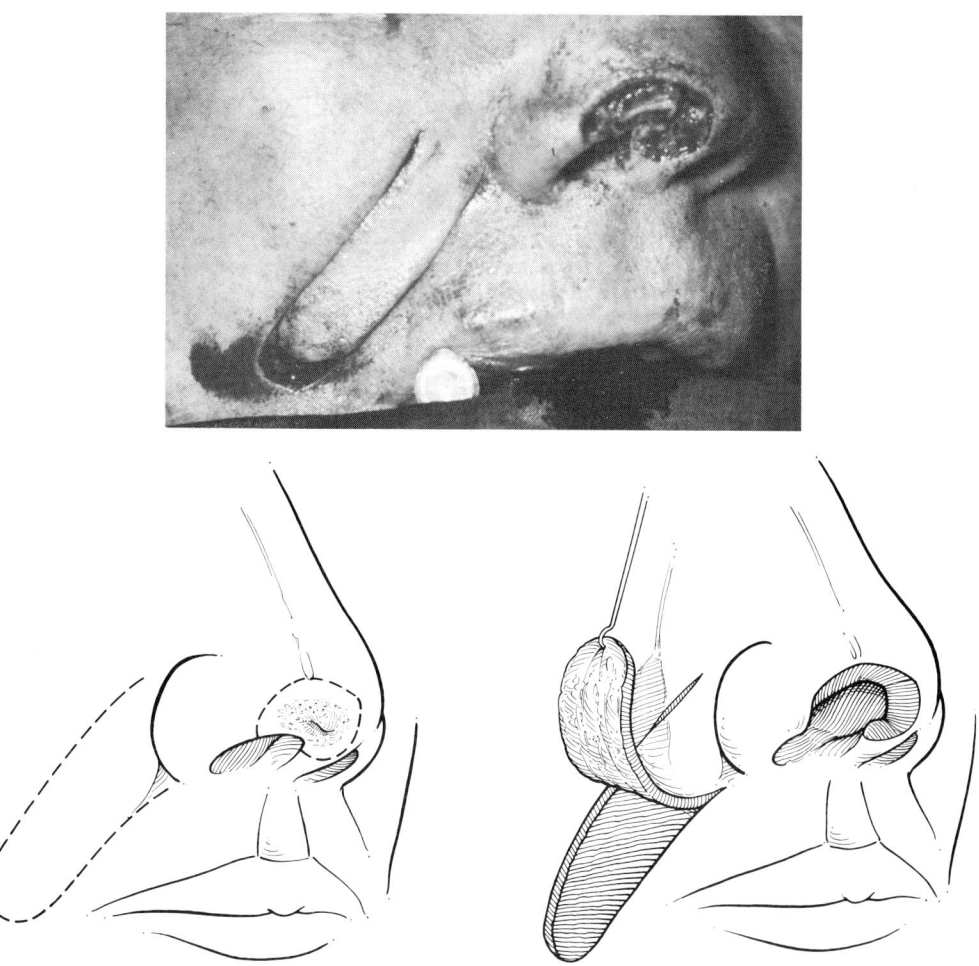

In this situation the flap is designed and elevated based superiorly. To determine if the flap is of adequate length before making incisions, the surgeon can simulate the flap with a strip of gauze and accurately estimate the flap dimensions.

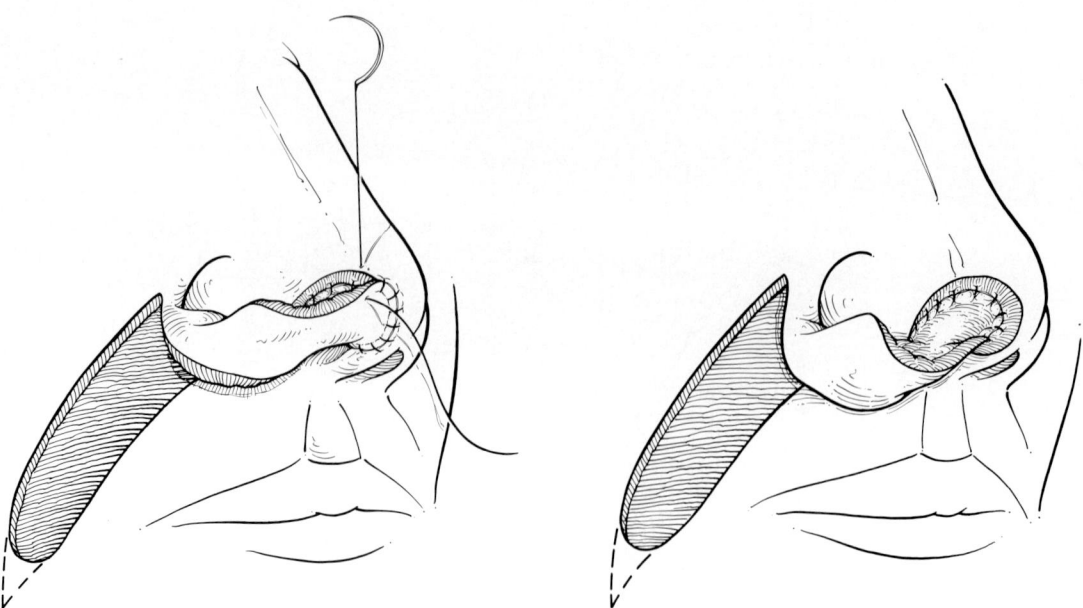

The tip of the flap is rotated, skin inward, and sutured to the intranasal edge of the defect to provide lining. The flap is then derotated; as this occurs, the flap can be sutured to the outer edge of the defect to give full-thickness rim reconstruction.

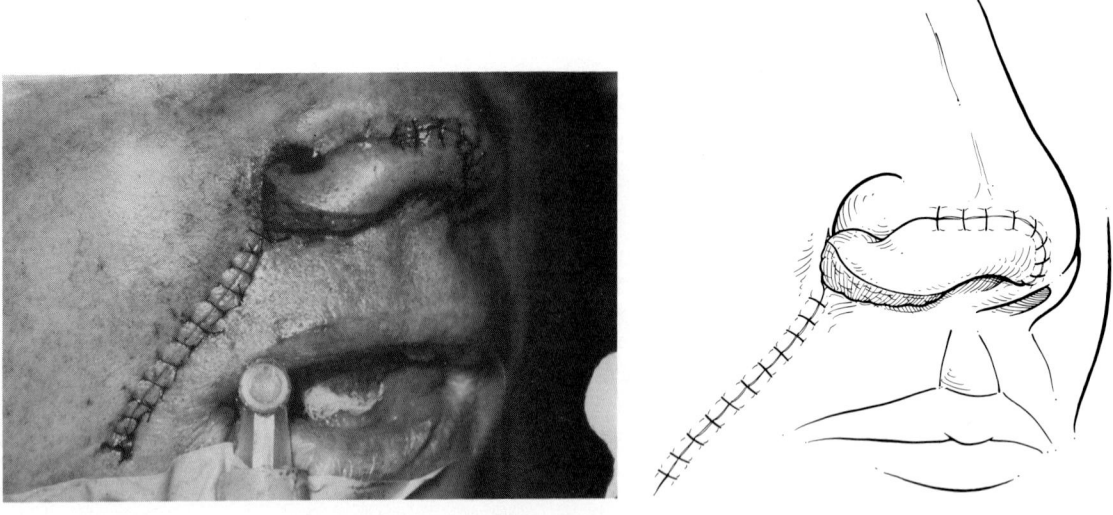

The pedicle is left open; the nasolabial donor site is closed directly.

CHAPTER 4
NOSE RECONSTRUCTION

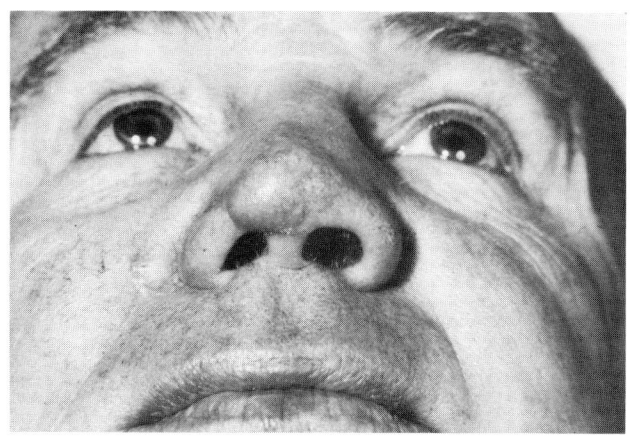

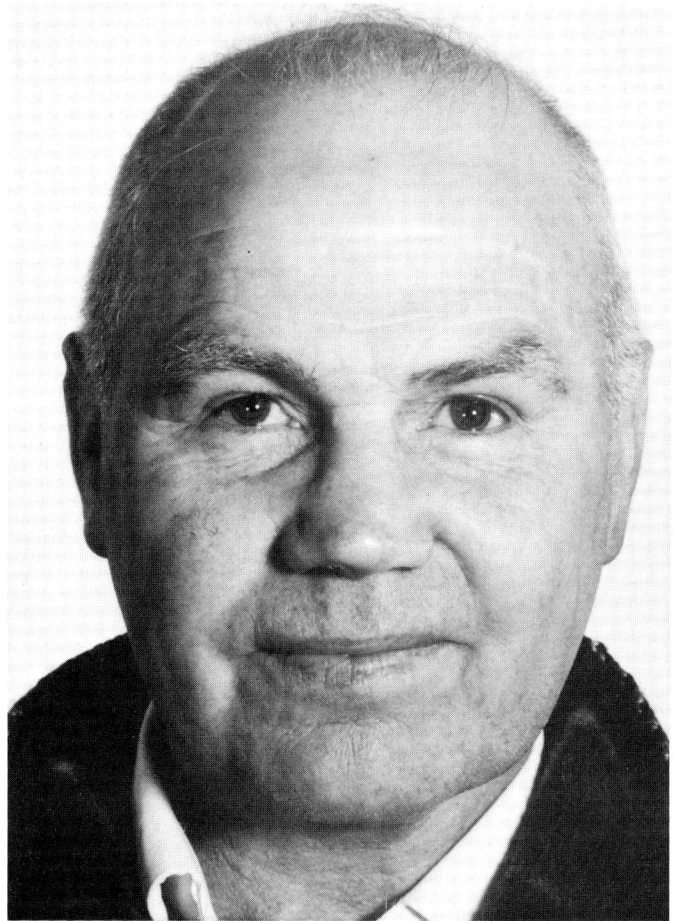

In 10 to 14 days the pedicle is divided, the flap is inset, and the excess of pedicle is trimmed and returned to the nasolabial donor area. The result is satisfactory, but the wrong skin is on the edge of the nose.

PROBLEMS

The nasolabial flap is not recommended for males unless no other type is available. Frequently, the distal end of the flap is composed of hairbearing skin. This leads to the unpleasant consequence of having to shave the nose.

131

RINTALA FLAP

The Rintala flap[15] can be advanced directly downward to resurface nasal tip defects. It has the advantage of providing the most similar type of skin to resurface the nasal tip. The disadvantages are significant and will be discussed later.

Conceptually this is an interesting flap, but in practice it is not particularly useful. In effect, it is a long, random advancement flap.

Flap Design

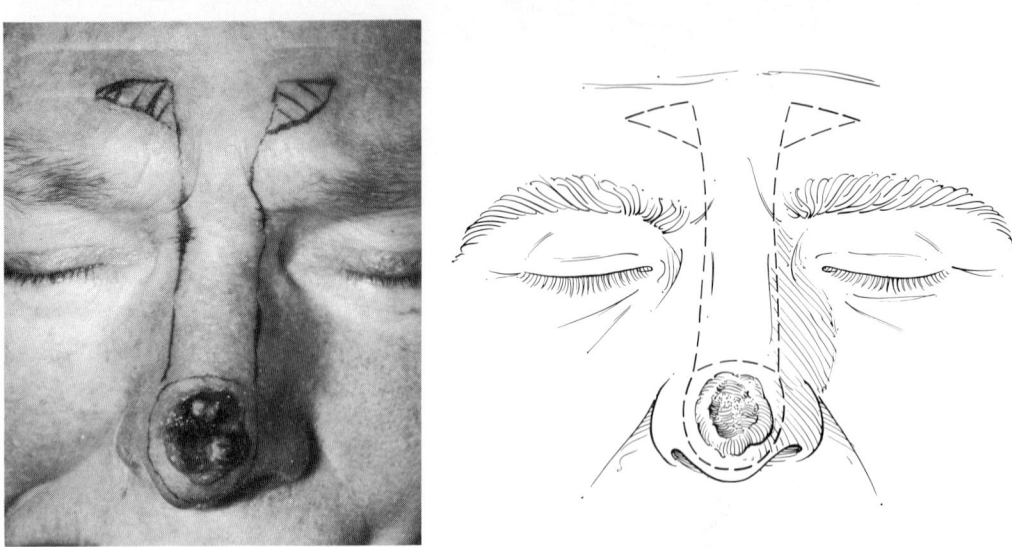

Use of the Rintala flap is illustrated in the resection and reconstruction of a nasal tip basal cell carcinoma.

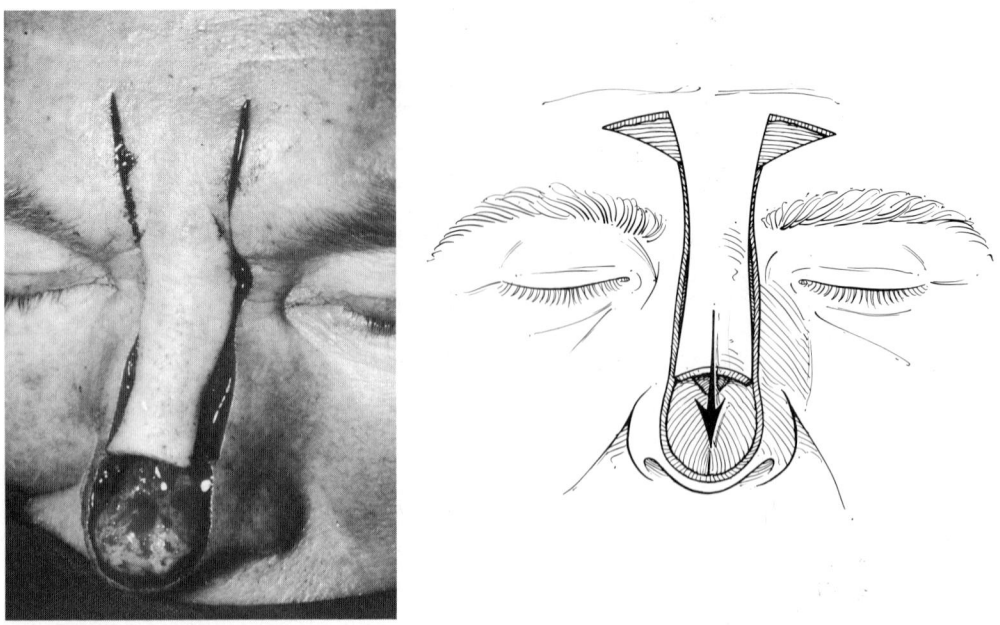

To allow advancement, Burow's triangles are excised bilaterally, lateral to the base of the flap.

CHAPTER 4
NOSE RECONSTRUCTION

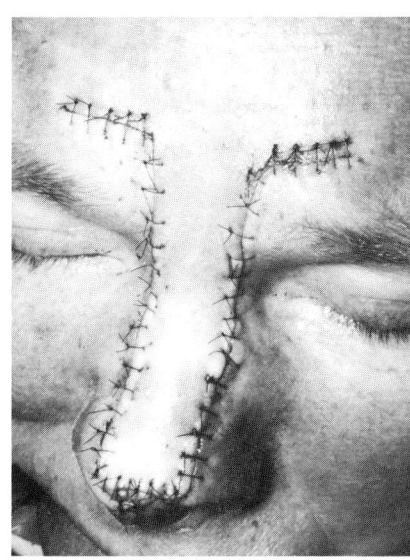
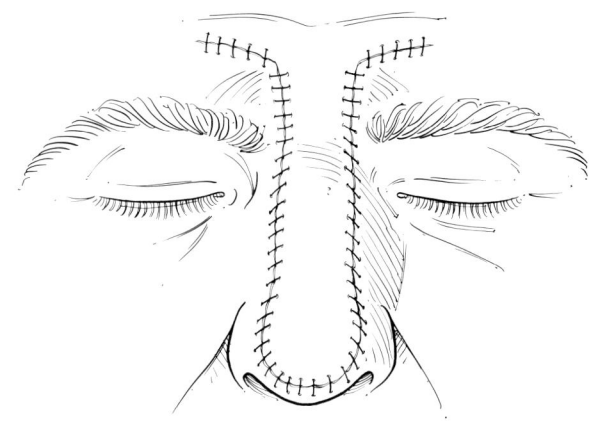

The flap is advanced down the nose to close the defect. A disagreeable degree of tension in the flap always seems to be present at this point. This is noted as blanching.

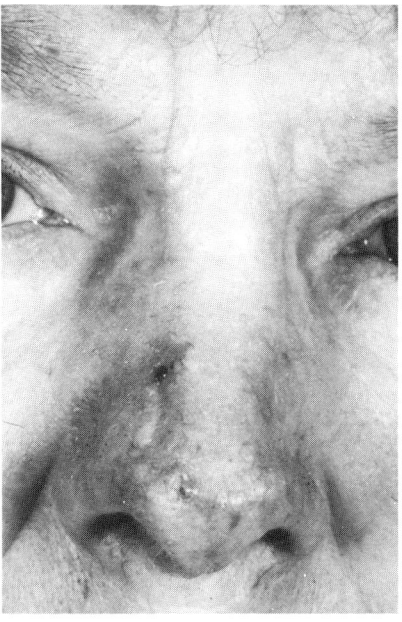

Use of this flap may result in slight nasal shortening. This is not always a bad effect—especially in the older patient, whose nose may droop slightly with age.

PROBLEMS

The Rintala flap has several disadvantages. It may be difficult to achieve sufficient advancement with this flap. There may be some ischemia of the distal end of the flap, which could progress to flap necrosis, delayed healing, and possible scarring. This is present to a slight degree in the patient shown here. The glabellar tissue transferred to the nasal bridgeline may cause an excess soft tissue mass in this area.

The flap can be used for lesions at any level on the central/dorsal line.

BILOBED FLAP

The bilobed flap works well for tip defects of any size, although very small defects can be satisfactorily reconstructed with a Banner flap.

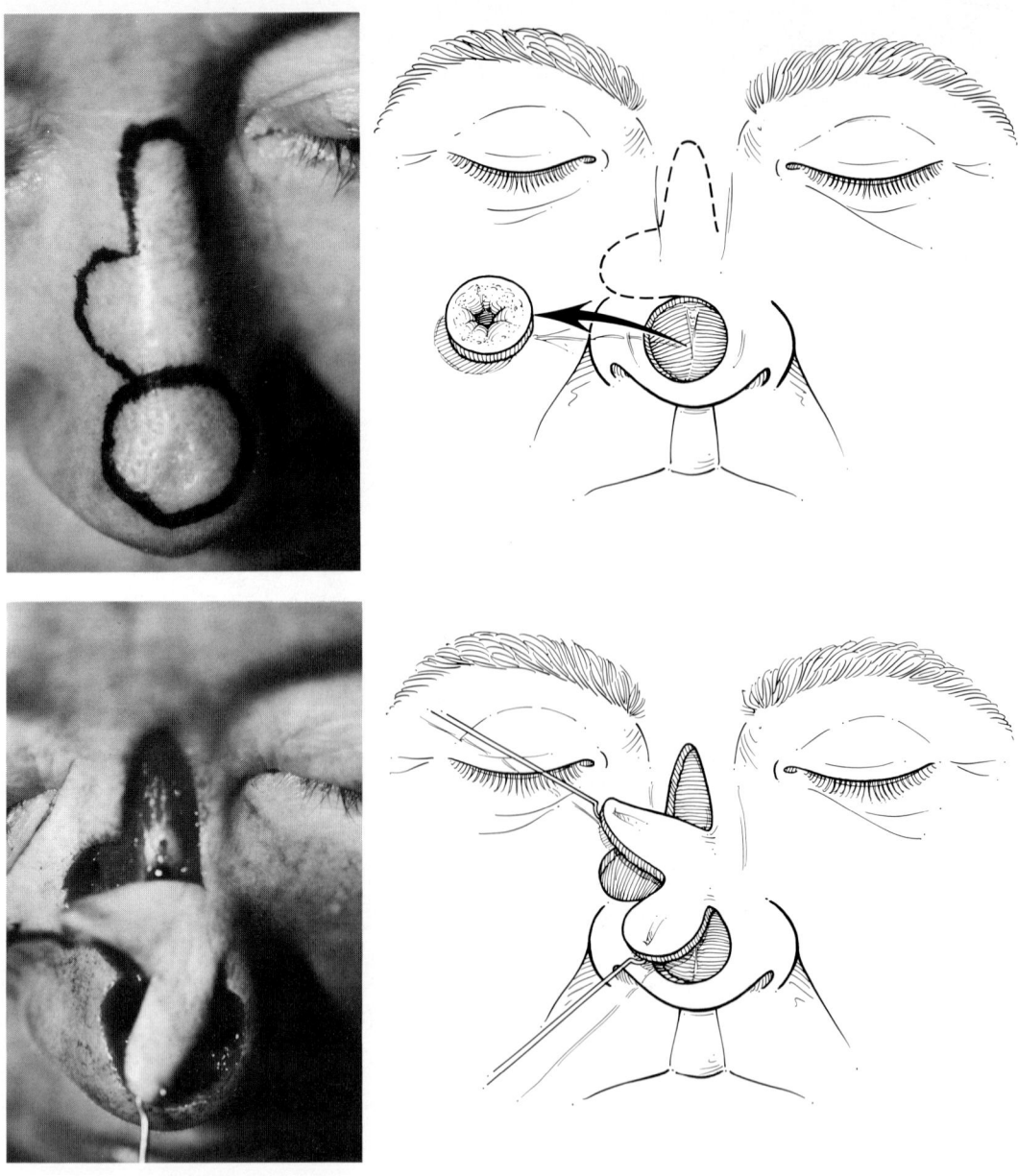

Use of the bilobed flap can be illustrated in this case of basal cell carcinoma of the nasal tip. In contrast to the lateral nasal bilobed flap, the rotation for the bilobed flap is through 180 degrees, with each flap rotating 90 degrees; thus undermining must be adequate.

CHAPTER 4
NOSE RECONSTRUCTION

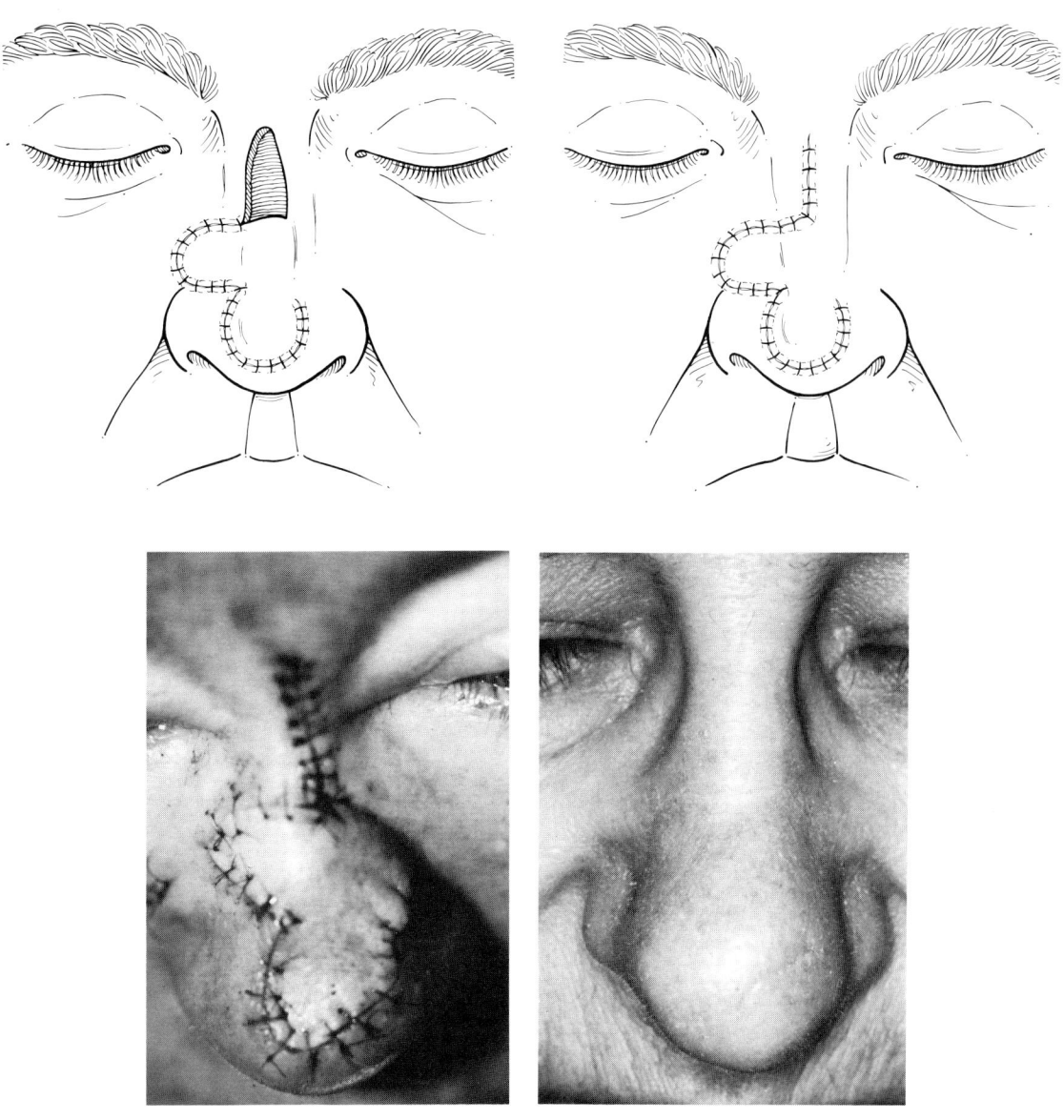

The donor site is the midline glabellar area. (See p. 21 for description of flap design, elevation, and transfer.) The result can be very good, without any disturbance of nasal anatomy. The result after 1 year illustrates how well the nasal scars settle.

OTHER TECHNIQUES

Triangular kite flaps (both unilateral and bilateral), advanced vertically or transversely, have been used in the nasal tip area to reconstruct small defects. Unfortunately, because of the lack of soft tissue underlying the skin, significant flap movement is difficult to attain.

These techniques should be avoided because they result in multiple complex scars.

DIRECT TRANSVERSE CLOSURE

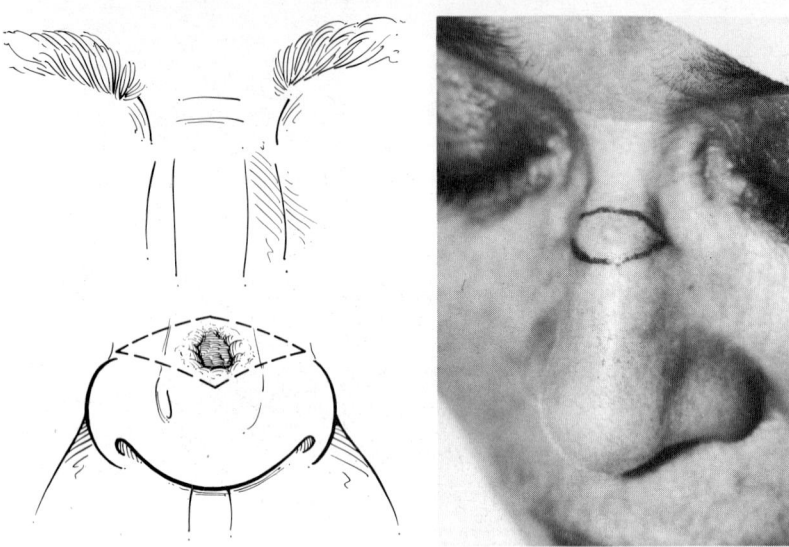

One useful technique with supratip defects is to convert the circular defect into a long transverse ellipse.

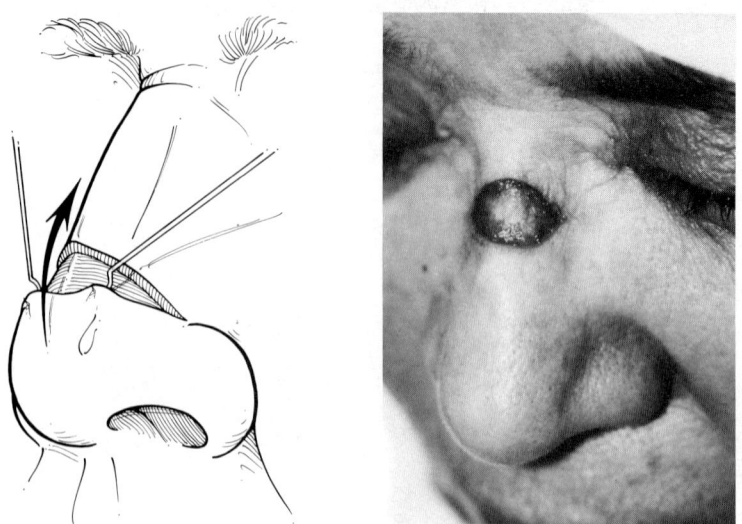

The direct transverse closure should be used only in small to moderate defects in a slightly long nose; some undermining is usually necessary.

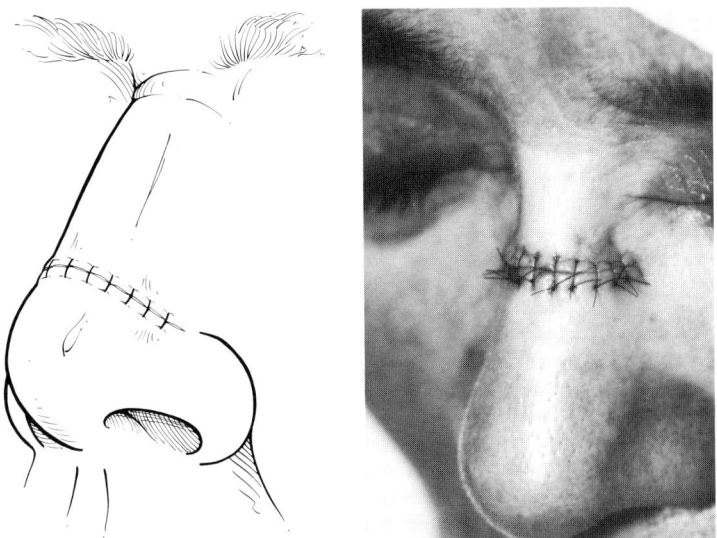

This procedure achieves direct closure of the defect and an aesthetically pleasing nasal shortening.

SURGICAL TECHNIQUE OF CHOICE

The bilobed flap is reliable, easy to perform, and, if correctly designed, does not deform the nose. In addition, it supplies the right kind of skin.

The Rintala flap, for the reasons mentioned earlier, should probably not be chosen unless special circumstances dictate its use.

The two-stage pedicled nasolabial flap may have some place in reconstruction of nasal defects in females. It is useful in both sexes when skin and lining are required.

☐ Columella

The columella, normally fairly bulky, is covered with hairless skin and lies at a lower caudal level than the alar rims. It is a somewhat complex anatomic structure located in a position where it is difficult to transfer tissue. Many complex methods of reconstruction, some multistage, have been developed. Only the simpler and more reliable techniques will be considered here.

NASOLABIAL FLAP

The nasolabial flap is useful in females as a two-stage procedure.

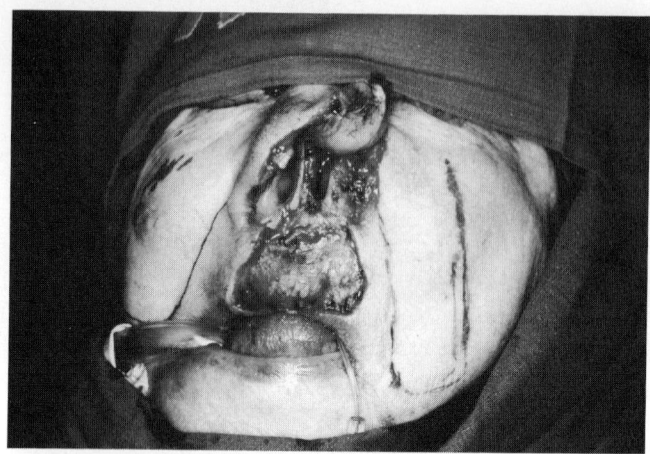

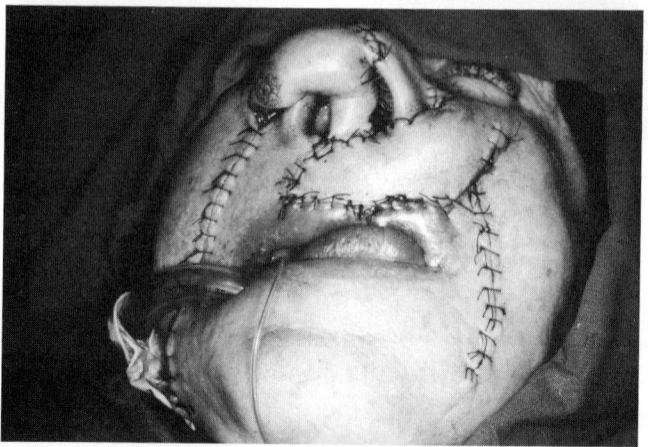

After resection for squamous carcinoma, the columella can be reconstructed with a two-stage nasolabial flap. The columella and the membranous septum are widely resected. A superiorly based (right) nasolabial flap is elevated, and one edge is sutured to one edge of the septal defect; the flap is tubed, and the other edge is sutured to the other side of the defect. Within 10 to 14 days the flap is divided. (In males this flap may transfer hairbearing skin to the defect area.) Although it is possible to do the reconstruction by using the nasolabial skin as an island, this is not recommended because the pedicle may be compressed, which would result in the ultimate loss of the flap. These methods cause a scar in the nasolabial region with some obliteration of the natural contours.

CHAPTER 4
NOSE
RECONSTRUCTION

FORK FLAPS

Fork flaps may be used in cleft lip cases. There is an excess of prolabium and cleft lip scars. Using fork flaps narrows the prolabium and allows scar revision to be accomplished at the same time. In patients with normal lips this would be considered, since the closure of the donor sites of the vertical fork flaps would produce unacceptable scarring of the upper lip.

ALAR RIM FLAPS

The use of alar rim flaps, an often disregarded method, was initially described by Gillies.[4,5] It is a one-stage procedure that transfers nonhair-bearing, well-matched skin to the columella.

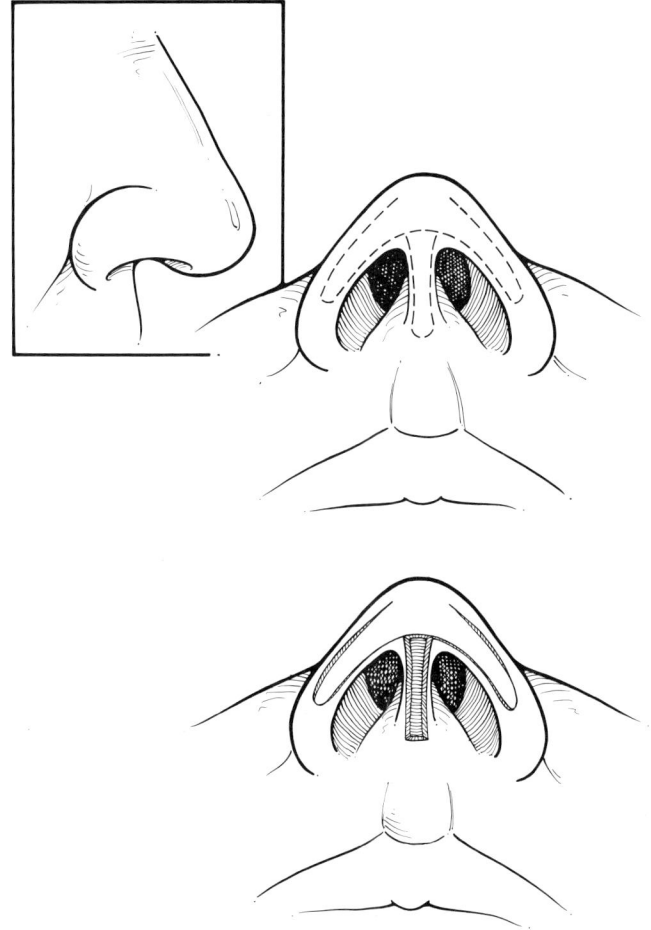

Especially in the male, the alar rims can be wide. It is thus possible to take flaps based on the midline tip area and swing these around to insert them into the defect on the columella. The defect is created; the whole width of the columella should be taken to allow easier insertion of the rim flaps.

139

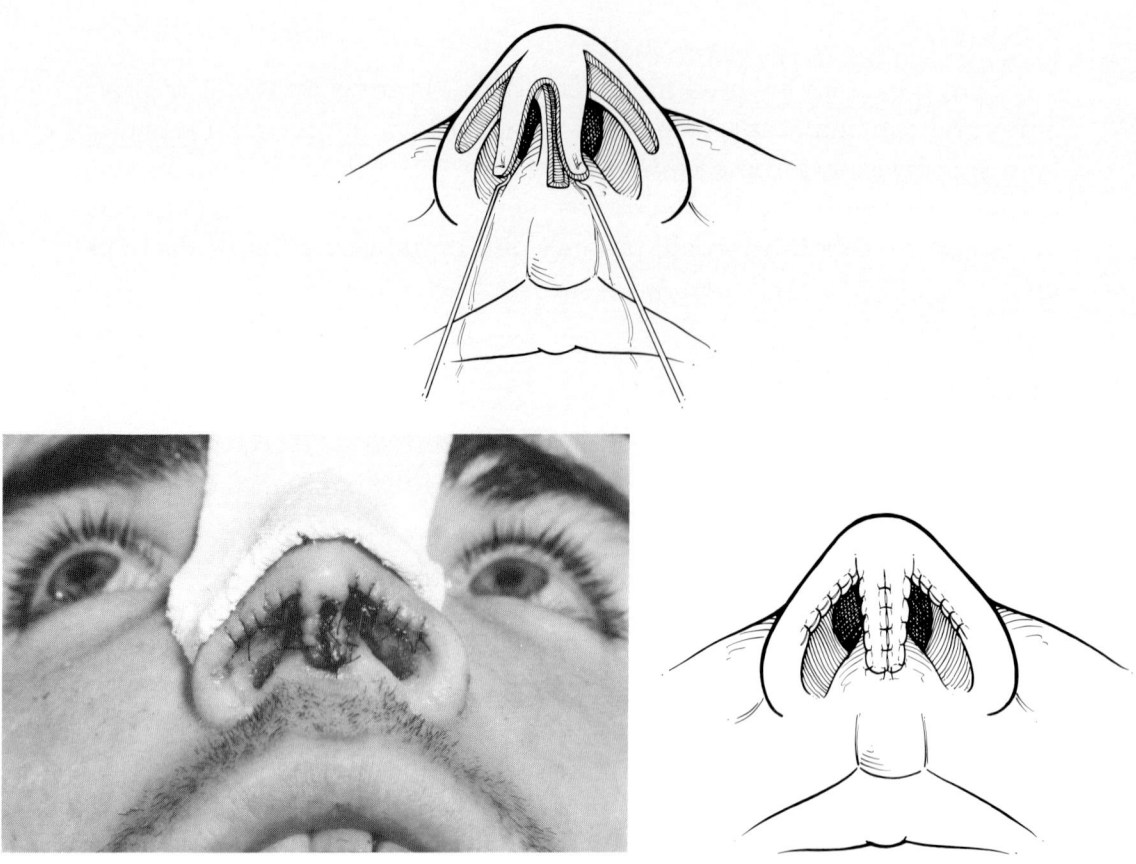

The flaps swing around easily to close the defect; the alar rim donor sites are closed directly.

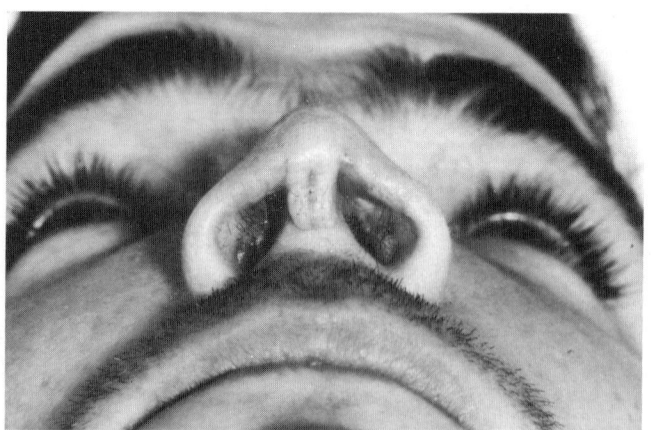

With alar rim flaps the columella can be built up with minimal scarring. For larger defects the surgeon would be forced into using a nasolabial flap or a composite graft from either the helix or the lobule of the ear.

CHAPTER 4
NOSE
RECONSTRUCTION

■ COMPLEX NASAL RECONSTRUCTION

Complex nasal reconstruction is defined as reconstruction of the whole nose or part of the nose. It frequently requires restoration of nasal lining together with specialized areas of the nose, such as the columella, the nostril rim, or the alar base. Reconstruction usually necessitates importation of skin from extranasal areas of availability. Most of this skin supply comes from the forehead and the nasolabial area. The methods used to supply nasal lining will be considered first, and then the techniques for supplying skin cover will be discussed.

☐ Nasal Lining

The nasal lining presents a very specific problem and thus can be examined separately. The four basic ways to supply nasal lining are the following:

1. Skin graft
2. Local in-turned flaps
3. Nasolabial flaps
4. Cheek axial flaps[7,8]

SKIN GRAFT

When a flap (usually forehead) is being prepared for nasal reconstruction, a skin graft can be placed under that area where lining will be required.

PROBLEMS

The skin graft is a simple way of providing lining, but it involves two problems: deficiencies of skin take and contraction of the skin graft. An additional disadvantage is that immediate reconstruction cannot be accomplished because skin graft take is not sufficiently reliable. The skin graft method is used infrequently.

LOCAL IN-TURNED FLAP

The local in-turned flap is used particularly in total or subtotal nasal reconstruction.

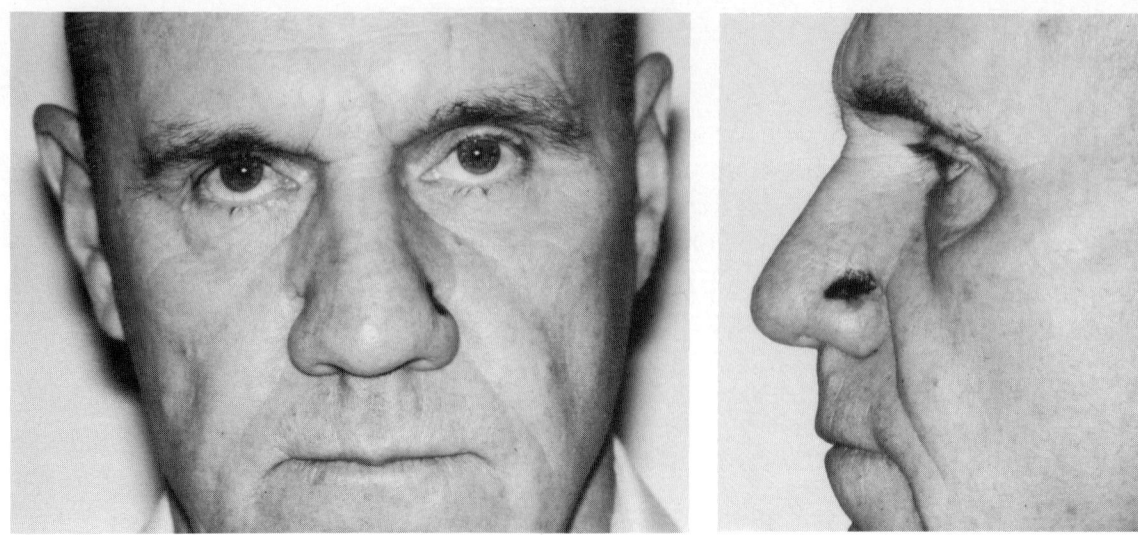

The patient shown here has undergone full-thickness resection of the side of the nose for malignant melanoma.

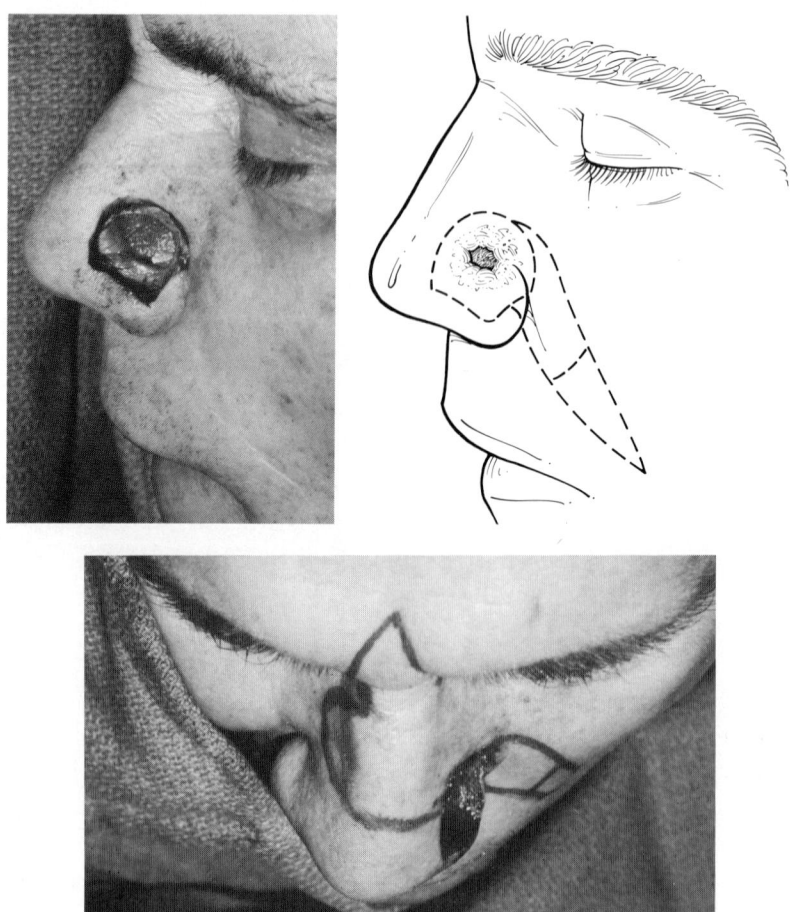

The planned closure is a Herbert in-turned skin flap for lining, a bilobed flap for external cover, and a sliding triangular nasolabial flap to restore the normal anatomy of the alar base area.

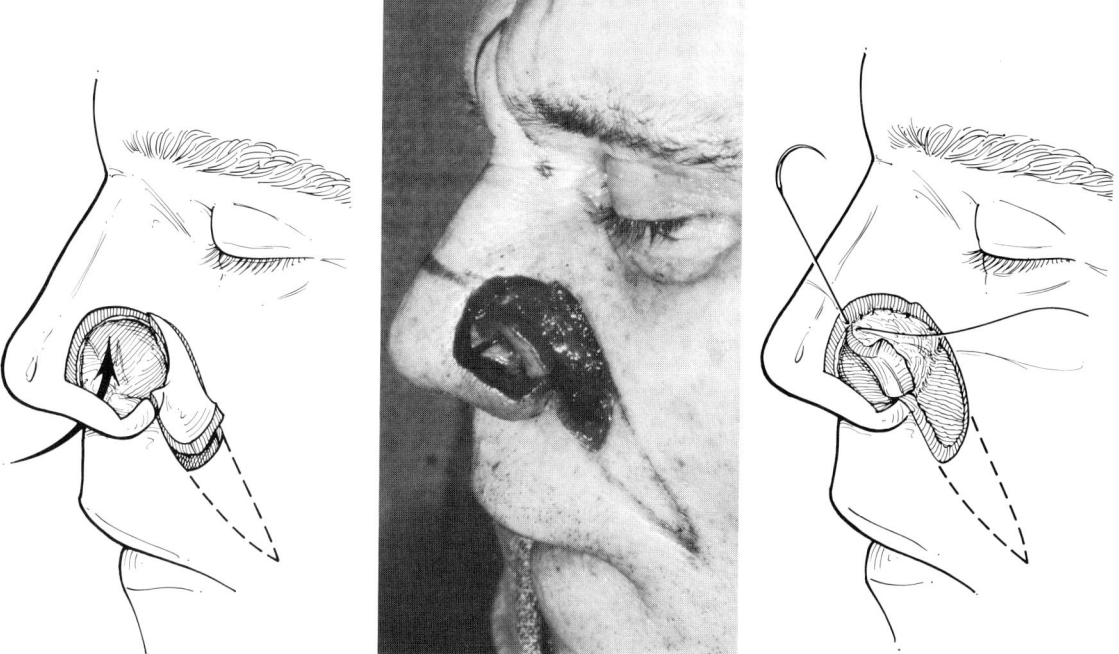

The full-thickness defect is created, and the planned flap is raised based on the pyriform aperture; the flap will be turned in to reconstruct the mucosal defect.

The blood supply along the edge of the pyriform aperture is adequate to vascularize these flaps. Important technical points are to raise the flaps laterally at the subdermal level and as the pyriform edge is approached to go vertically through the fat to the periosteum (if required). The periosteum is incised and can be dissected off the lateral rim of the pyriform fossa. This dissection allows medial shift of the flap; otherwise mobility is not sufficient to allow comfortable suturing in the midline.[6,7]

In secondary reconstruction there is a continuous skin mucosal pedicle, albeit with a scar on it. Although this scar extends across the total base of the pedicle and in theory should cause flap blood supply problems, in practice this does not occur.

In immediate reconstruction the local in-turned flap can be used if the resection has not been taken down to the periosteum of the pyriform edge. If this condition is met, the in-turned flap is used as a skin island and is usually safe, but the reconstruction is less satisfactory; the pedicle is too far laterally.

Gradually by suturing, the intranasal defect is closed securely.

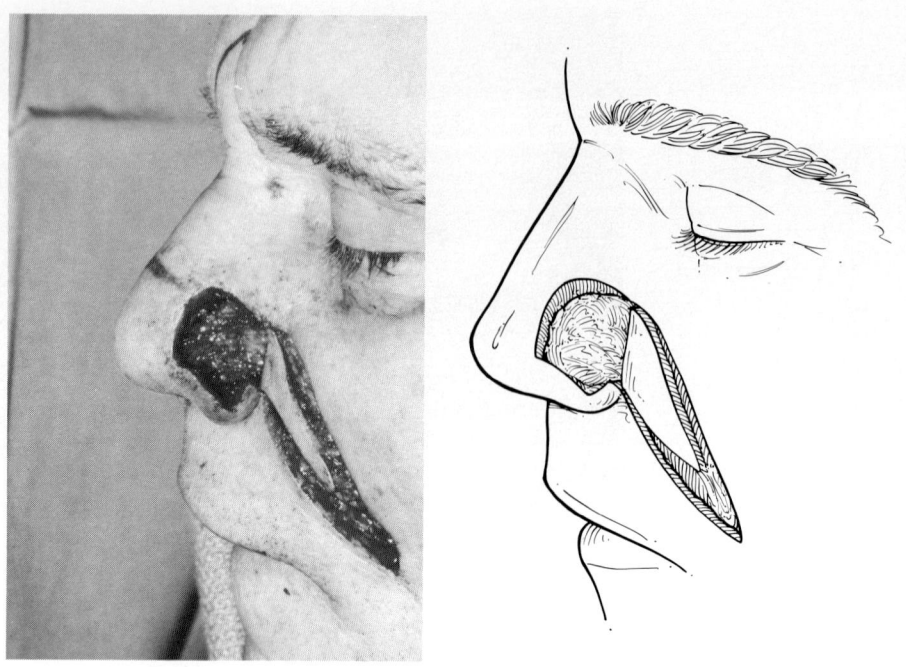

The triangular flap is raised on a subcutaneous pedicle and moved medially to be sutured around the alar region; the secondary defect is closed directly (the V-Y principle).

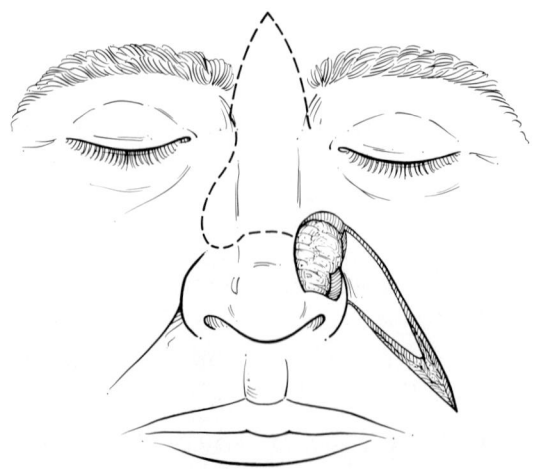

The skin defect on the nose will be closed with a bilobed flap.

CHAPTER 4
NOSE RECONSTRUCTION

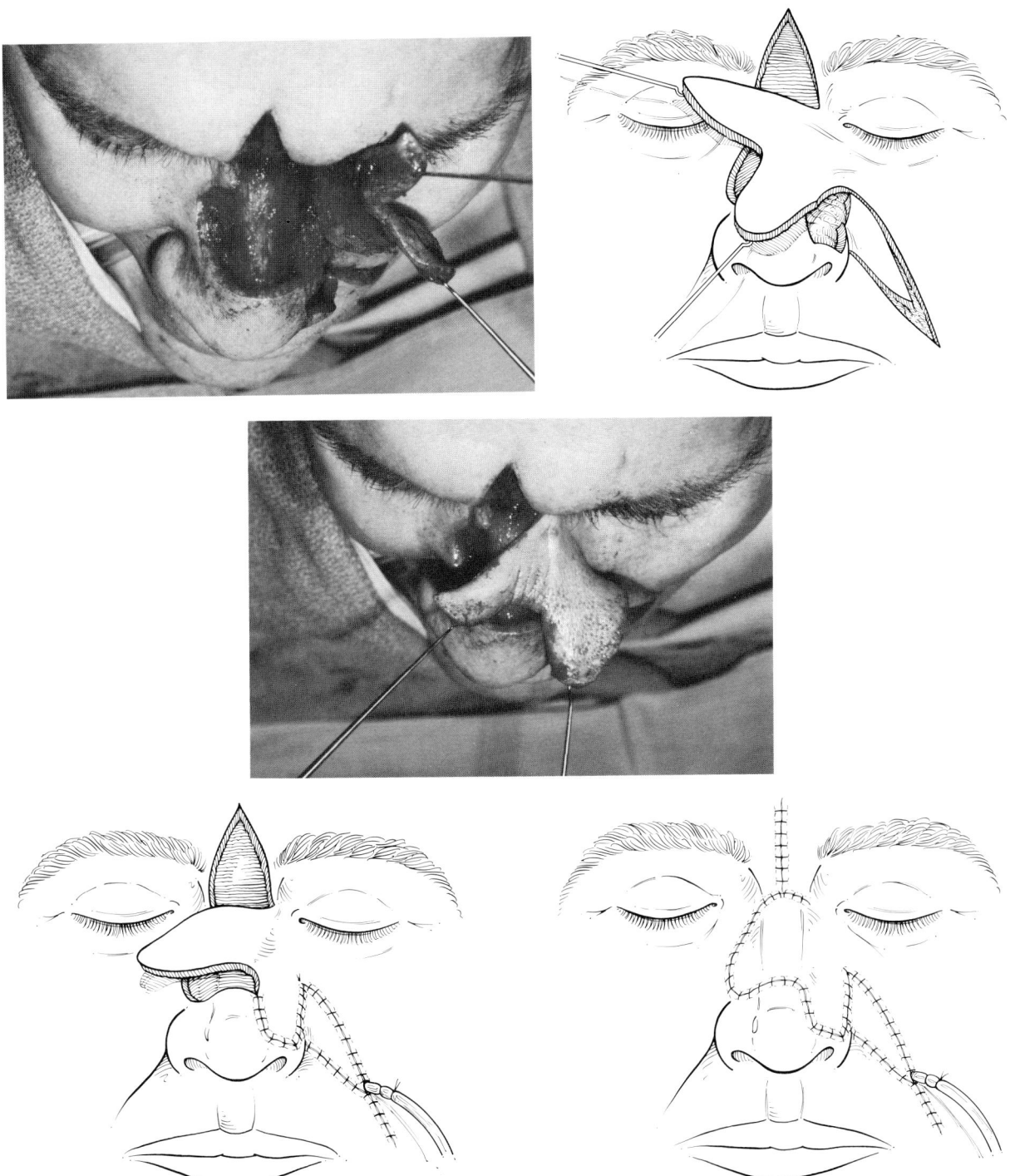

Because the flap has been widely undermined, closure is achieved without difficulty or tension.

145

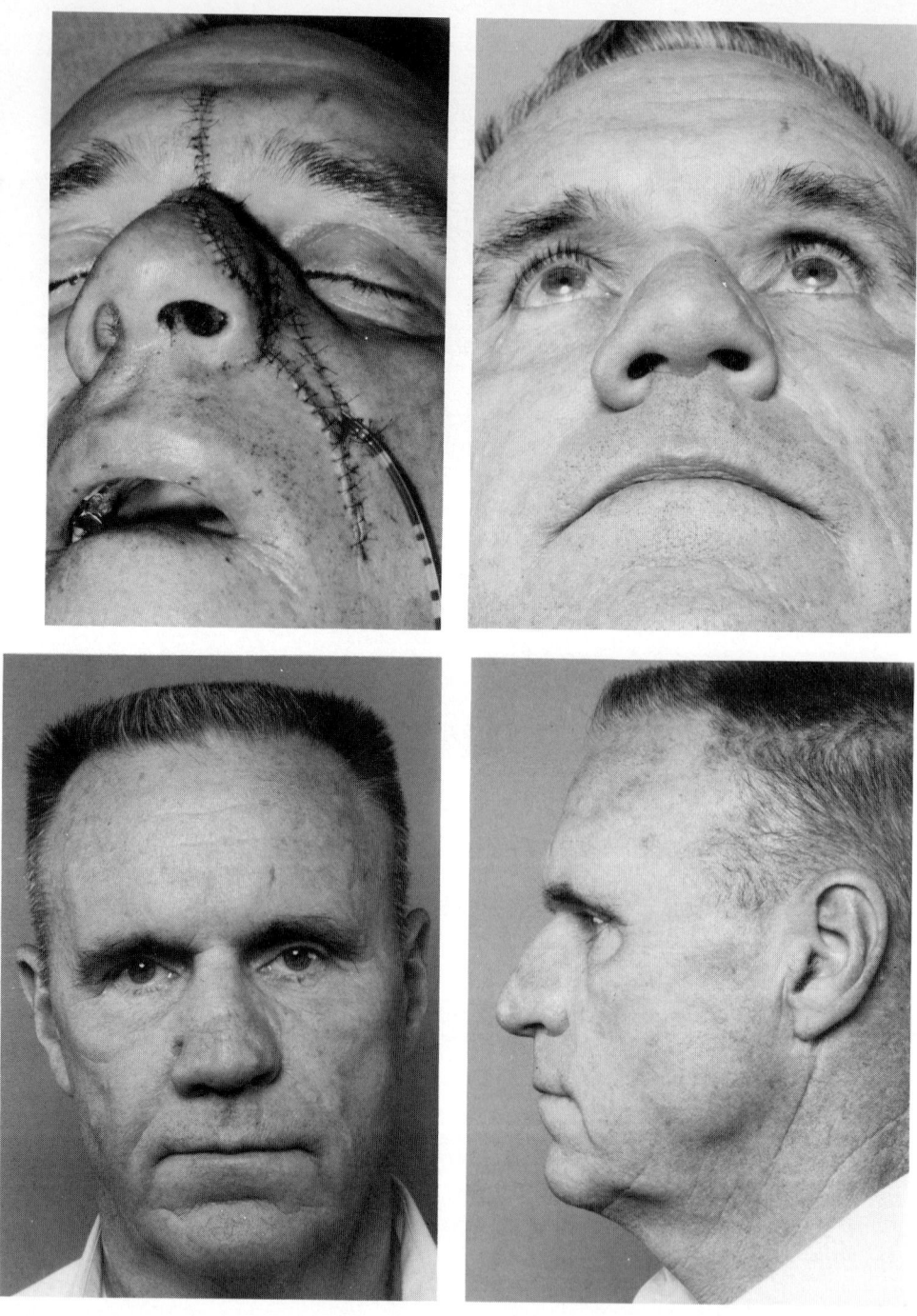

After some initial pincushioning, the flaps settle and the result is satisfactory.

PROBLEMS

If the cheek is tight, it may not be possible to raise a large enough flap to provide sufficient lining. Failure to handle the pedicle properly will result in ischemia and flap necrosis. Pincushioning of the skin reconstruction may occur.

NASOLABIAL FLAP

Nasolabial flaps are usually best used when the lining defect is not over extensive in the vertical dimension, although in loose-skinned individuals a larger amount of skin can be harvested from the nasolabial region with direct closure of the donor site.

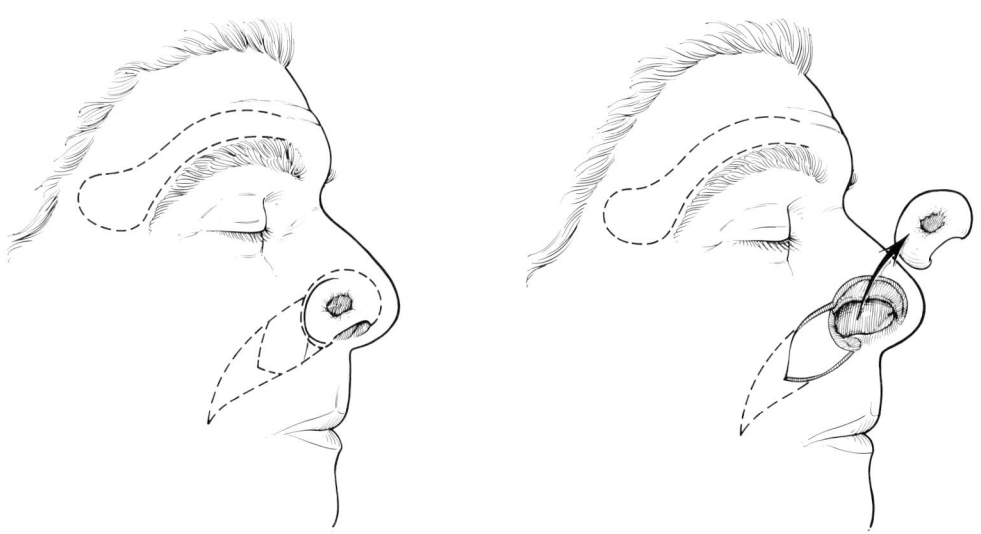

The patient shown here had a full-thickness resection for basal cell carcinoma. Lining was provided by an island nasolabial flap and cover using a Schmid forehead flap (see pp. 172-177).

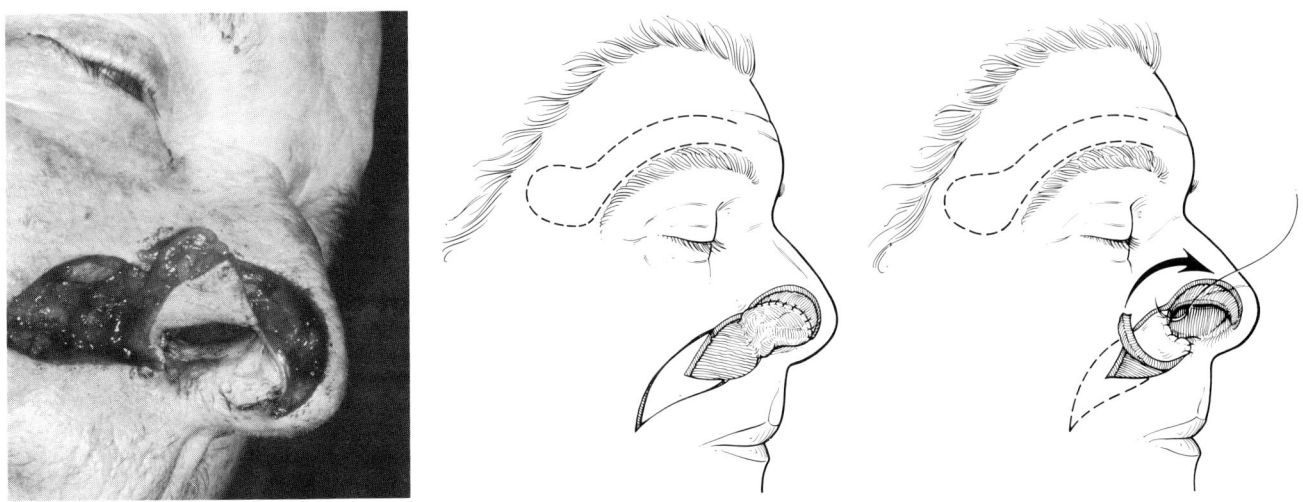

The nasolabial island was lifted on its medial subcutaneous pedicle, turned over, and sutured into the mucosal defect.

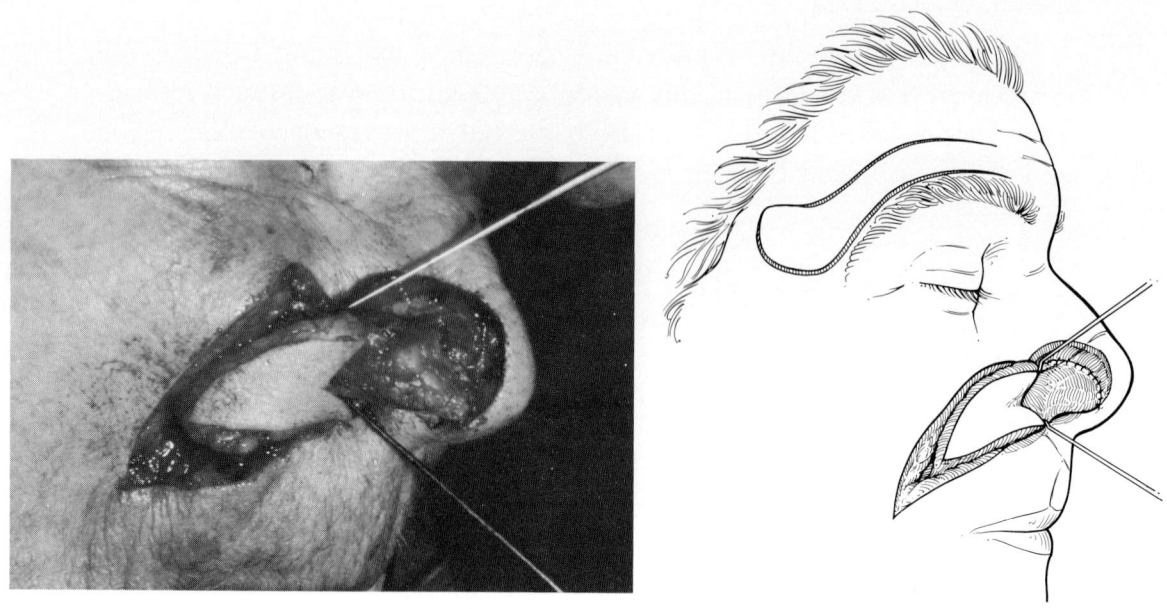

The nasolabial donor site was closed with a sliding island flap.

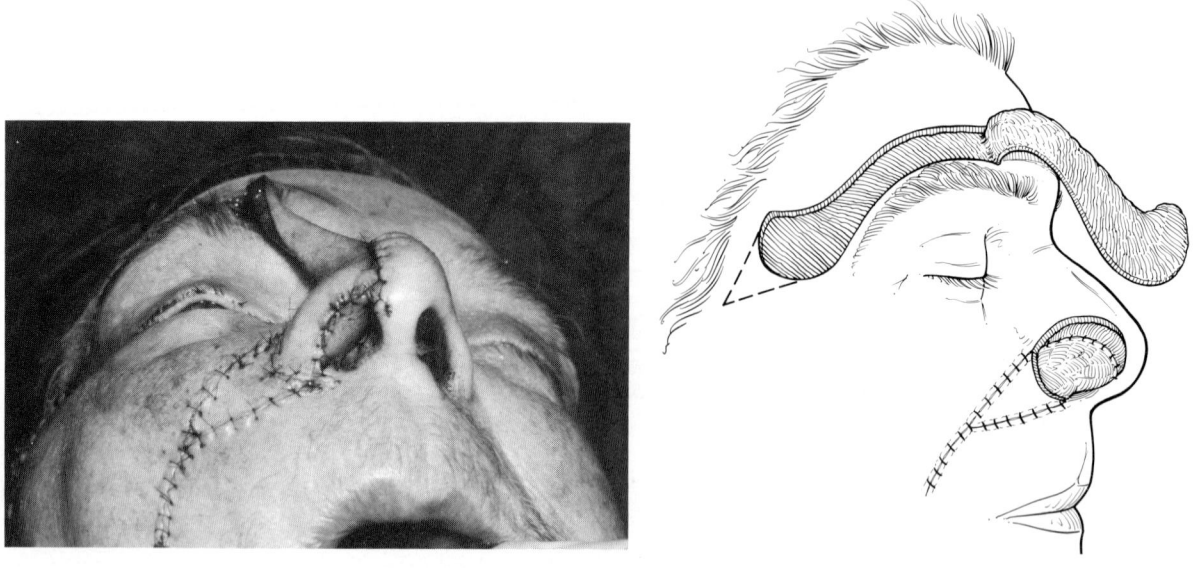

The donor site was closed directly.

CHAPTER 4
NOSE RECONSTRUCTION

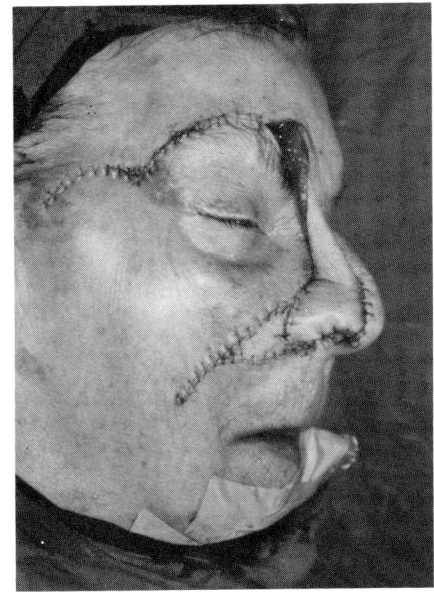

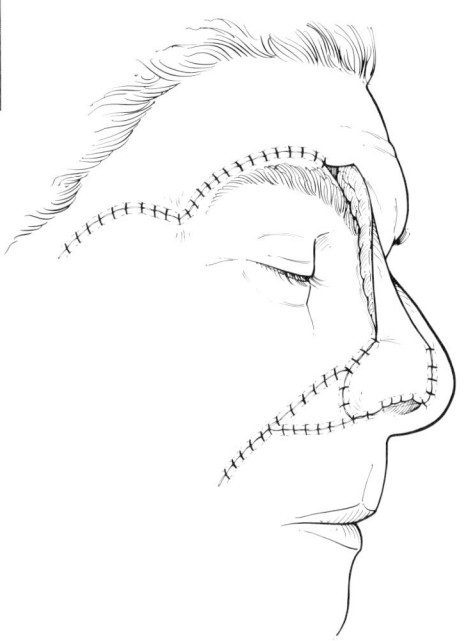

The alar reconstruction was covered with a Schmid forehead flap.

These flaps may be taken on skin pedicles or as islands. For short flaps, the latter is satisfactory. For longer flaps, it is thought that a skin pedicle will give slightly better vascular security.

149

Bilateral Nasolabial Flaps

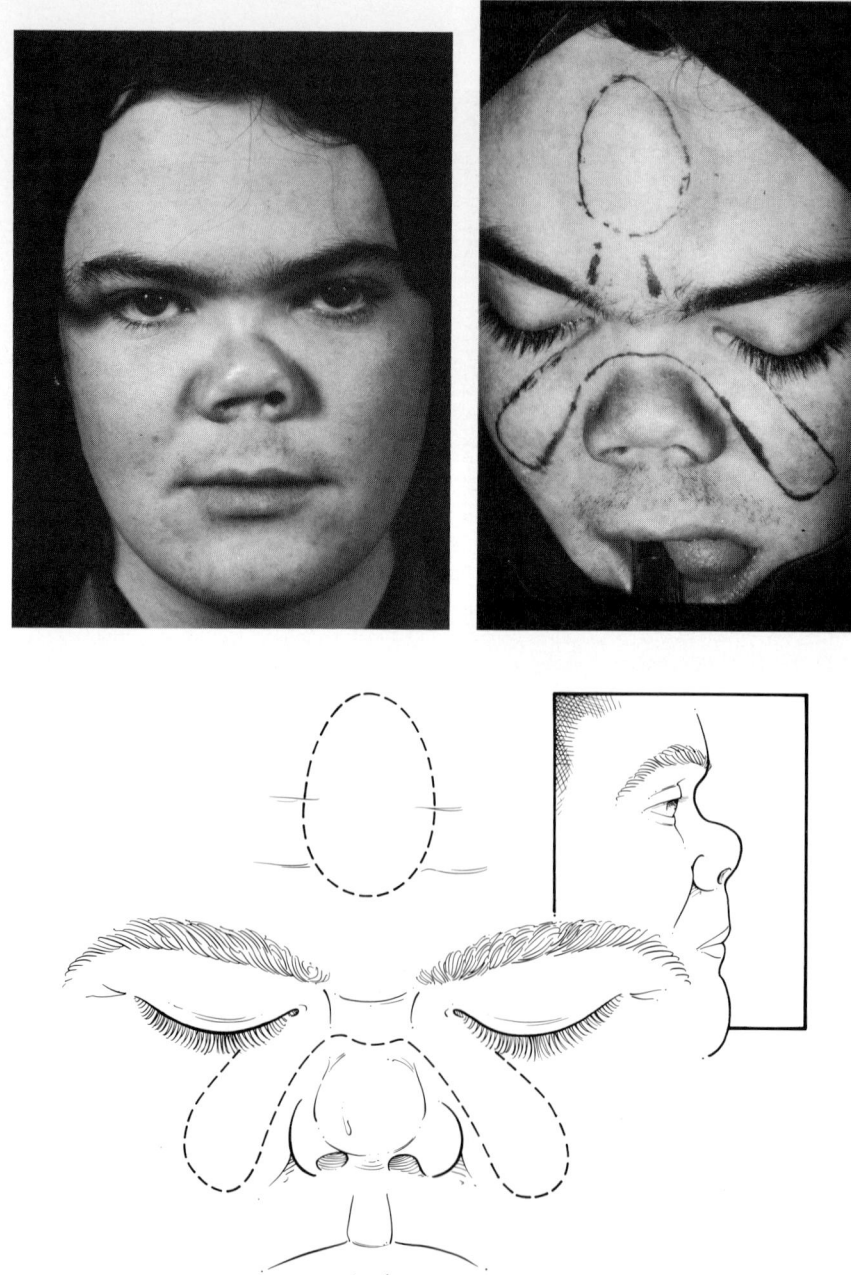

Nasolabial flaps were used in lengthening this congenitally short nose.

CHAPTER 4
NOSE RECONSTRUCTION

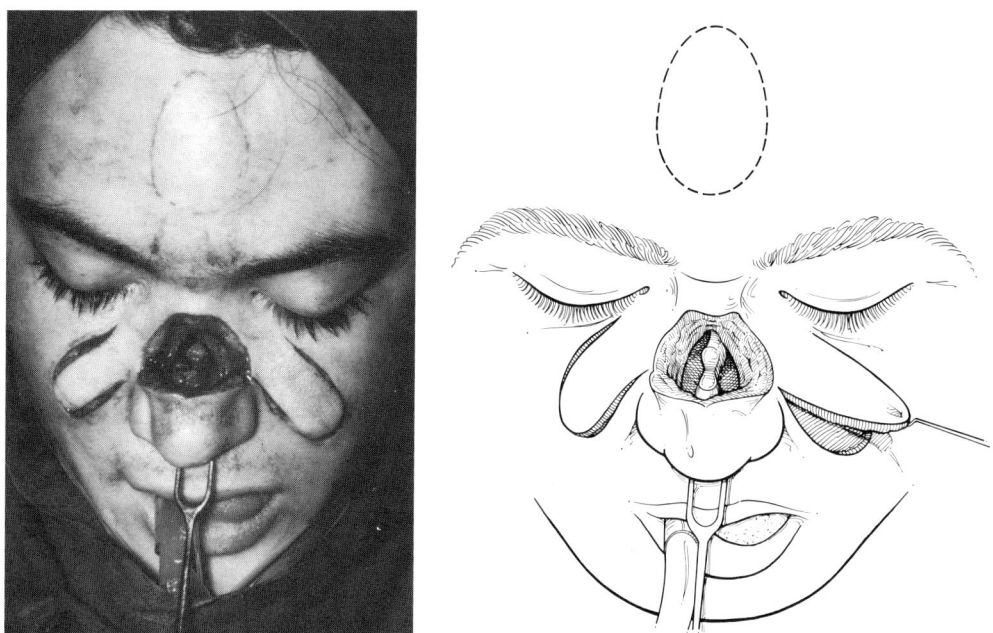

An incision is made through the nasal skin and the septum. This incision is continued posteriorly until the required length for the nose is obtained. The planned nasolabial flaps are elevated to reconstruct the intranasal defect.

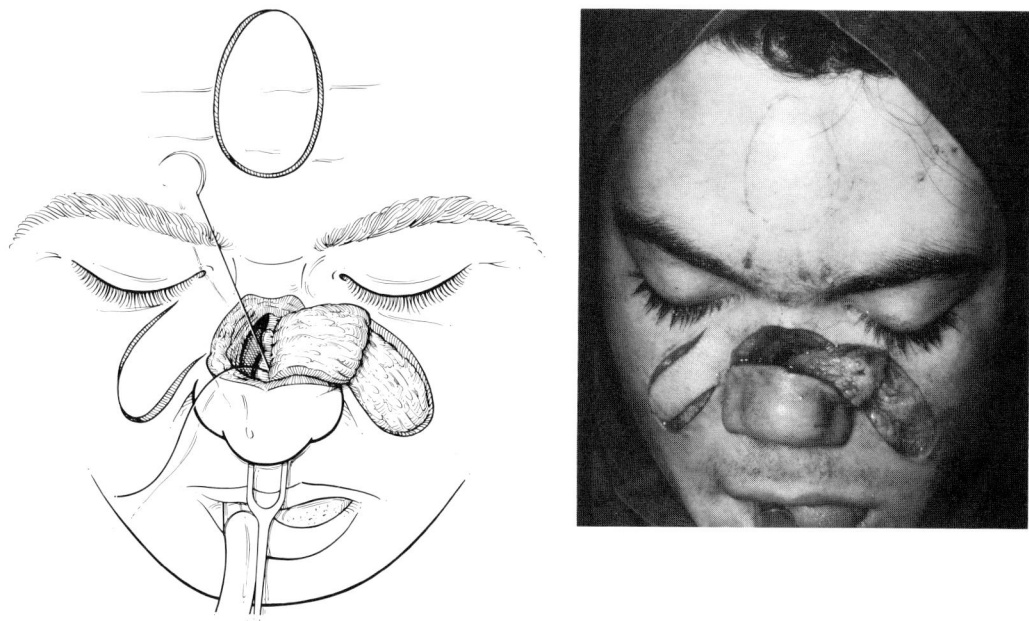

One flap has been used to reconstruct the septal defect on the corresponding side and also the lining of the nasal dome.

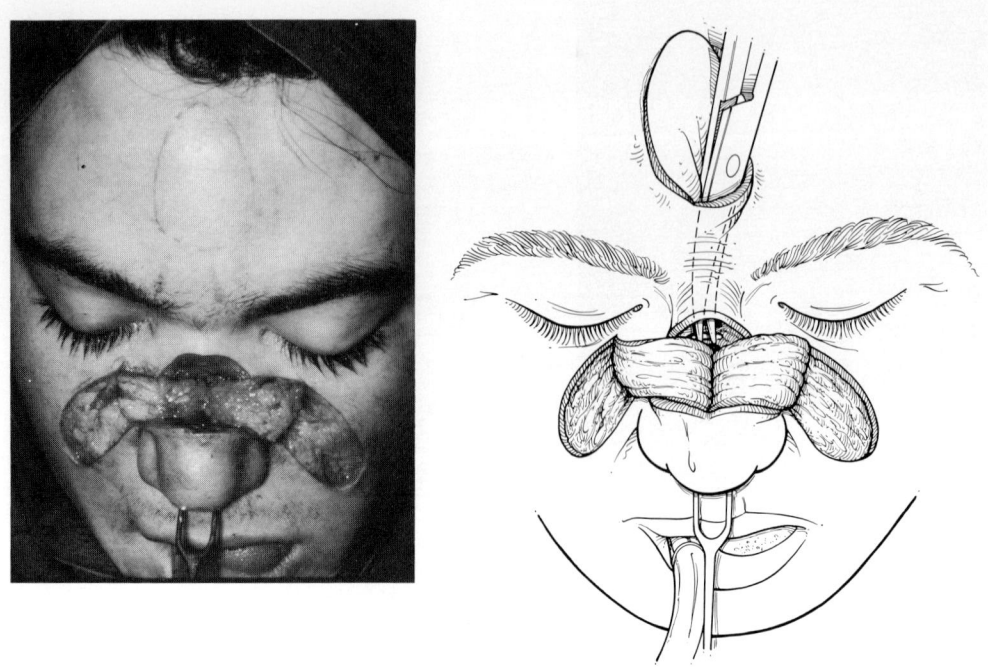

Mucosal reconstruction is completed by turning in and insetting the other nasolabial flap.

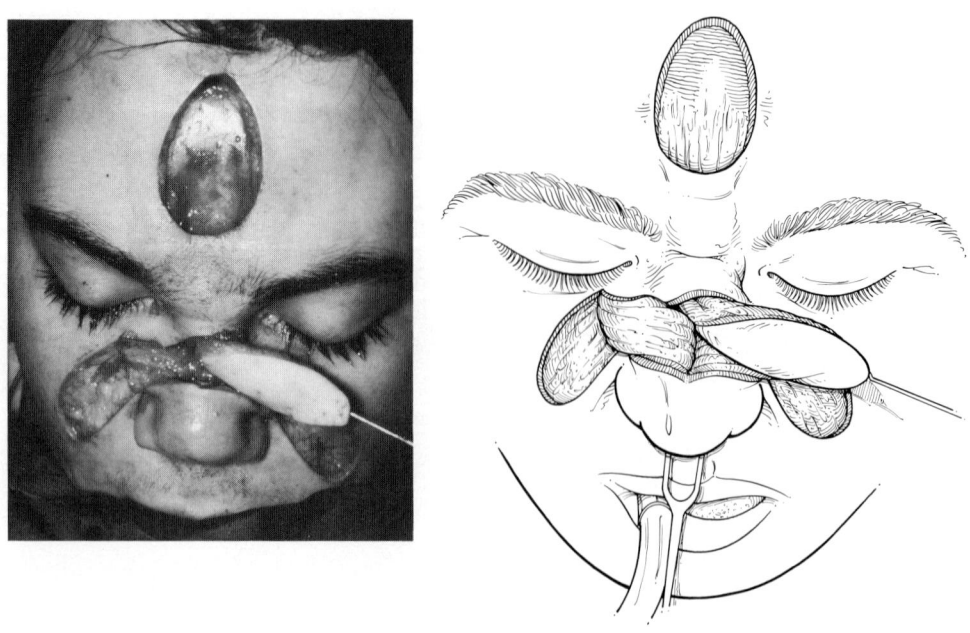

Skin cover is provided by a midline forehead island flap.[9]

CHAPTER 4
NOSE RECONSTRUCTION

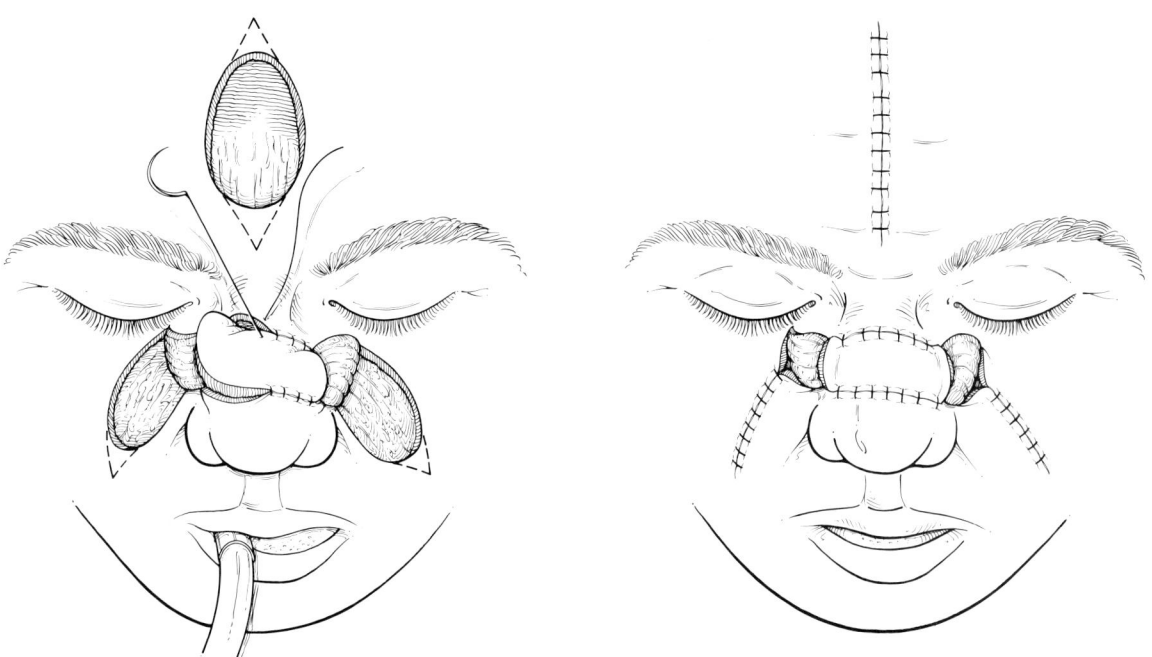

The forehead island flap is sutured to the nasal skin superiorly and inferiorly. Care is taken to avoid compression of the nasolabial pedicles.

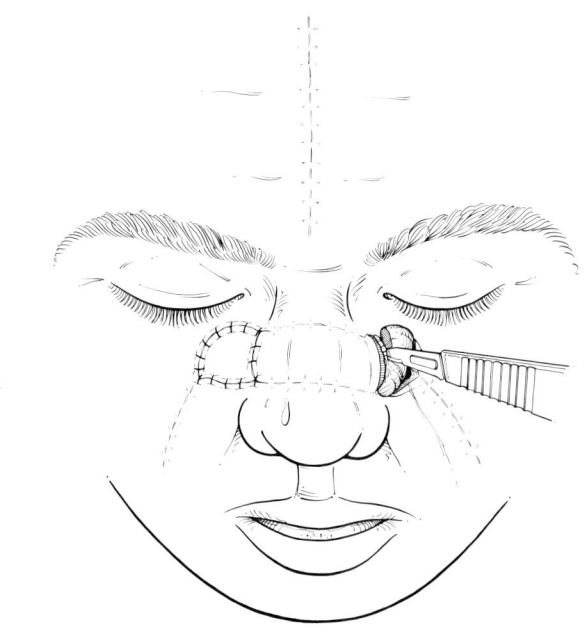

On the tenth postoperative day the nasolabial pedicles are divided. The unused portion of the pedicle is returned to the nasolabial area, and the skin defect on the lateral side of the nose is closed.

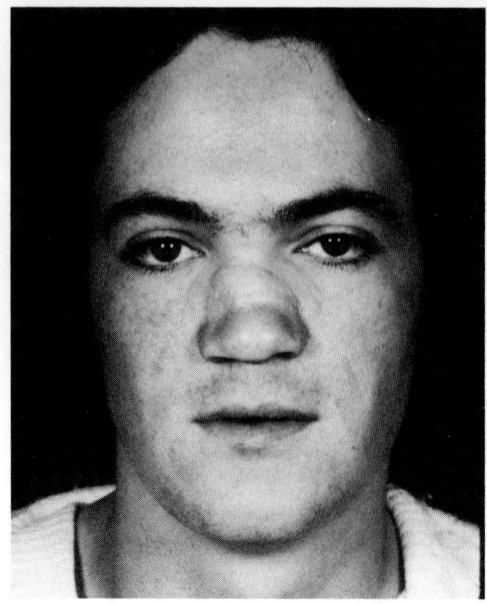

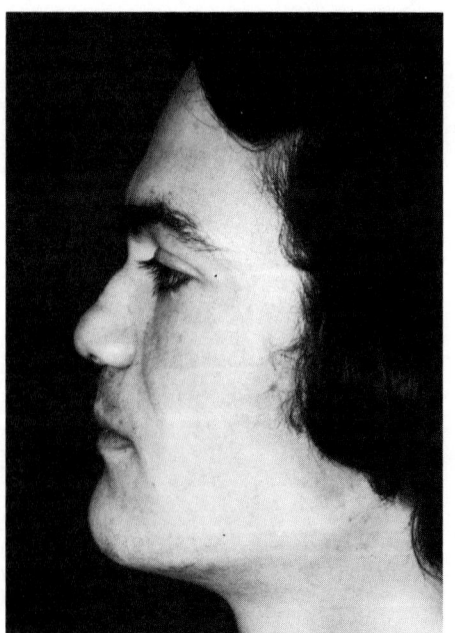

The result is satisfactory.

PROBLEMS

Because of concern about flap vascularity, the nasolabial flap is usually taken with a generous layer of fat. The resulting flap is bulky and will often occlude the airway; trimming can be performed later.

CHAPTER 4
NOSE RECONSTRUCTION

CHEEK AXIAL FLAP

Nasolabial flaps are successful because they are axial flaps, but this was not truly appreciated until the excellent anatomic studies of Herbert and Harrison,[8] which demonstrated that there is a predictable vascular axis situated in the lower third of the pyriform aperture. Thus relatively large flaps can be raised from this area as islands based on this very specific vascular axis.

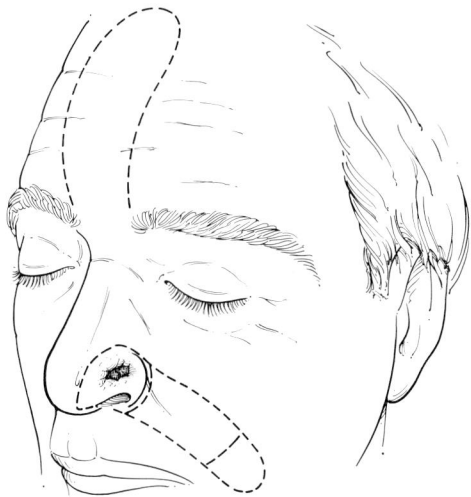

This procedure is planned for a patient with a basal cell carcinoma of the alar rim area requiring a full-thickness resection.

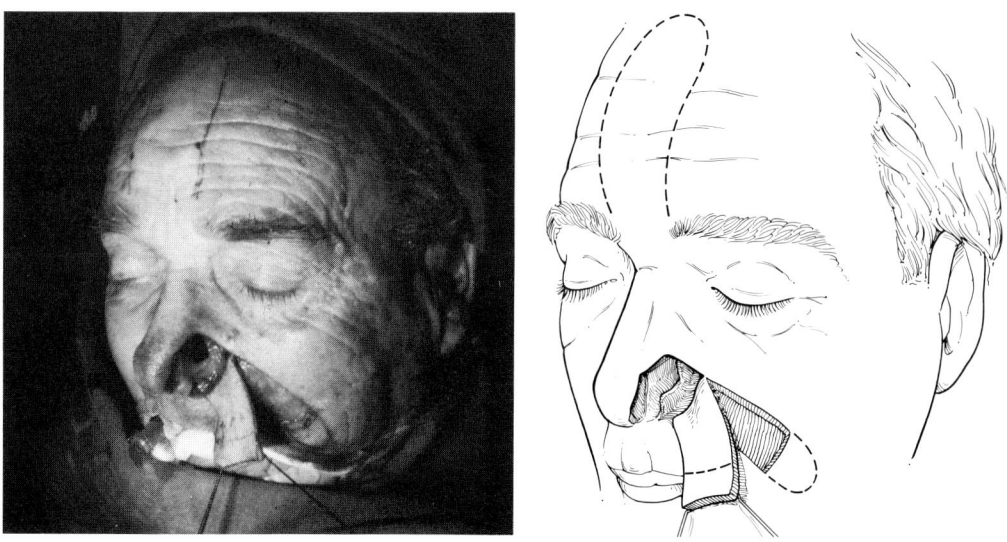

The island is raised and turned in to reconstruct the mucosal defect.

155

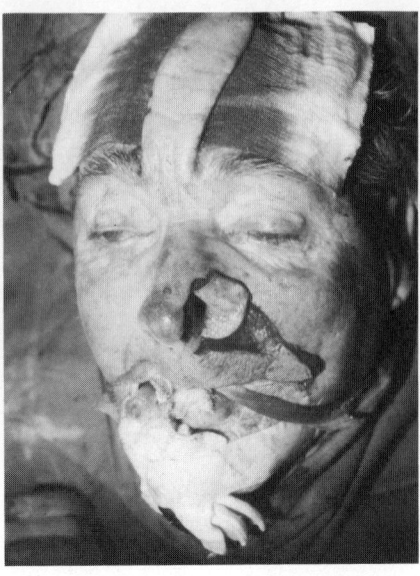
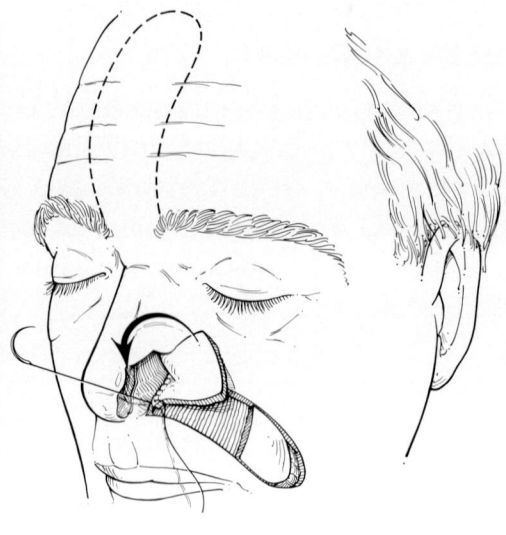

Knowledge of axial flaps has added greatly to the security and versatility of lining reconstruction. It has, however, introduced a complication: how to manage the secondary defect. If this defect is closed directly, the alar base cheek area is obliterated; once lost, it is difficult, if not impossible, to recreate. A method has been devised to deal with this interesting problem. From the caudal end of the cheek defect in the nasolabial area, a triangular island flap with a central subcutaneous pedicle is raised.

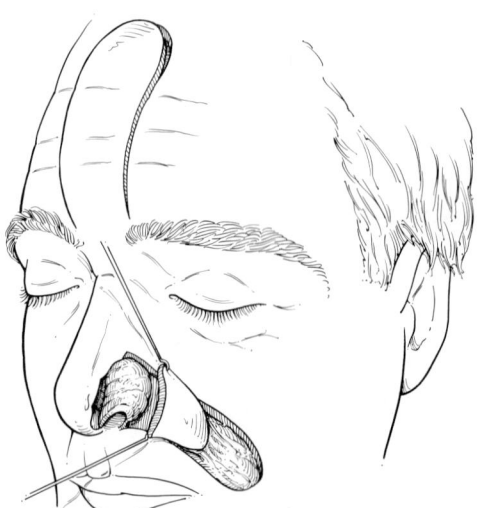

With adequate mobilization, this flap can be advanced and is leading edge sutured deeply with nonabsorbable sutures, which ensures a good alar-cheek concavity when the reconstruction is completed. In effect, this is a V-Y maneuver; the limb of the Y is closed directly in the nasolabial line. There is no doubt that this reliable method of obtaining lining is the one of choice.

CHAPTER 4
NOSE RECONSTRUCTION

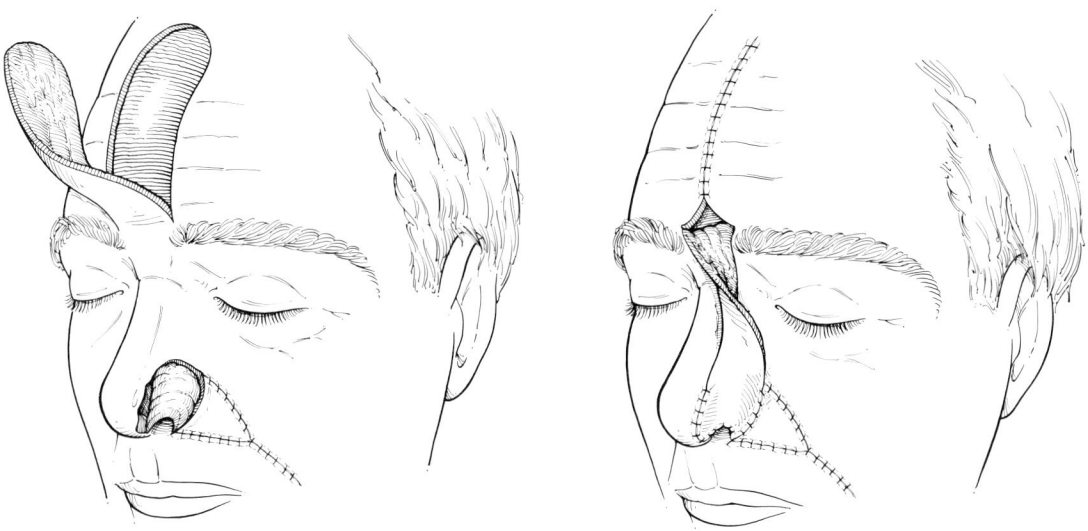

In the case illustrated here, external skin cover was provided by a midline forehead flap.

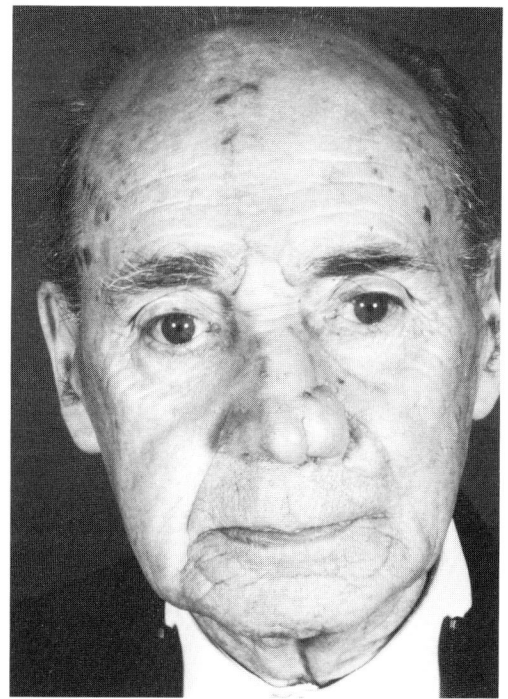

Although initial pincushioning of the flap has occurred, it will eventually settle to give a satisfactory result.

157

SURGICAL TECHNIQUE OF CHOICE

The technique chosen depends on what is left after resection or what is available in the secondary case. Usually in-turned flaps are employed because of shrinkage and problems of "take" associated with skin grafts.

☐ Nasal Skin Reconstruction

Only rarely is tissue from areas other than the face sought for nasal skin reconstruction. However, with the advent of free vascularized tissue transfer using microvascular surgery and the increase in its reliability, this modality of reconstruction may be used more frequently in the future.

The forehead is the time-honored donor site. It can be used in various ways, depending on the size and position of the area to be resurfaced and whether the resurfacing is total or subtotal.

☐ Total Reconstruction

The relatively thin, but stiff, nonhairbearing skin of the forehead provides an excellent medium for nasal reconstruction. The color and texture of this skin is an ideal match. Lining will have been provided by one of the methods described in the previous sections, and on most occasions skeletal support will not be inserted at this point (this will come later, if required).

FOREHEAD FLAP[3,13]

Reconstruction of the total nose requires more skin than may be estimated on initial examination. The clue to planning for nasal reconstruction is to remember the dimensions "3 by 3," referring to the total amount of skin required, which should be 3 inches (7.6 cm) wide and 3 inches (7.6 cm) long. Conveniently, most hemiforeheads, depending on the position of the hairline, are close to these specific dimensions. A bone graft for skeletal support may be inserted at this time, but it is probably wise to leave this until the soft tissue reconstruction has settled and sound vascularity has been established.

The simplest method is the up-and-down forehead flap, based on the contralateral hemiforehead; the vessels are the supraorbital and the supratrochlear. The midline vertical incision is long enough to allow the required hemiforehead to be taken down to the nasal area. The length of this incision determines the position of the scalp incision, which should be placed at such a point to allow 3 inches of scalp above the superior extent of the midline incision to provide a pedicle of adequate width.

CHAPTER 4
NOSE RECONSTRUCTION

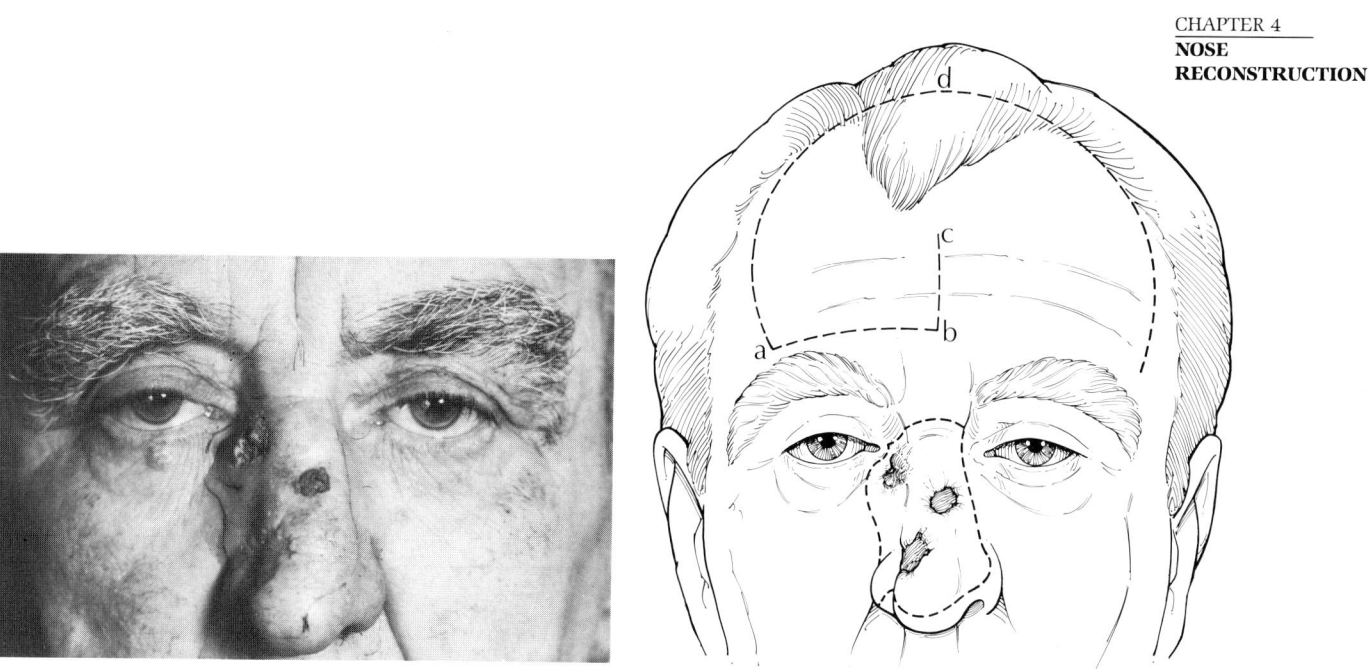

This is illustrated in a patient with multiple squamous cell carcinomas of the nose requiring radical resection. All planning can be done with gauze. If care is taken, the flap should be of satisfactory length and size and the vascularity ensured.

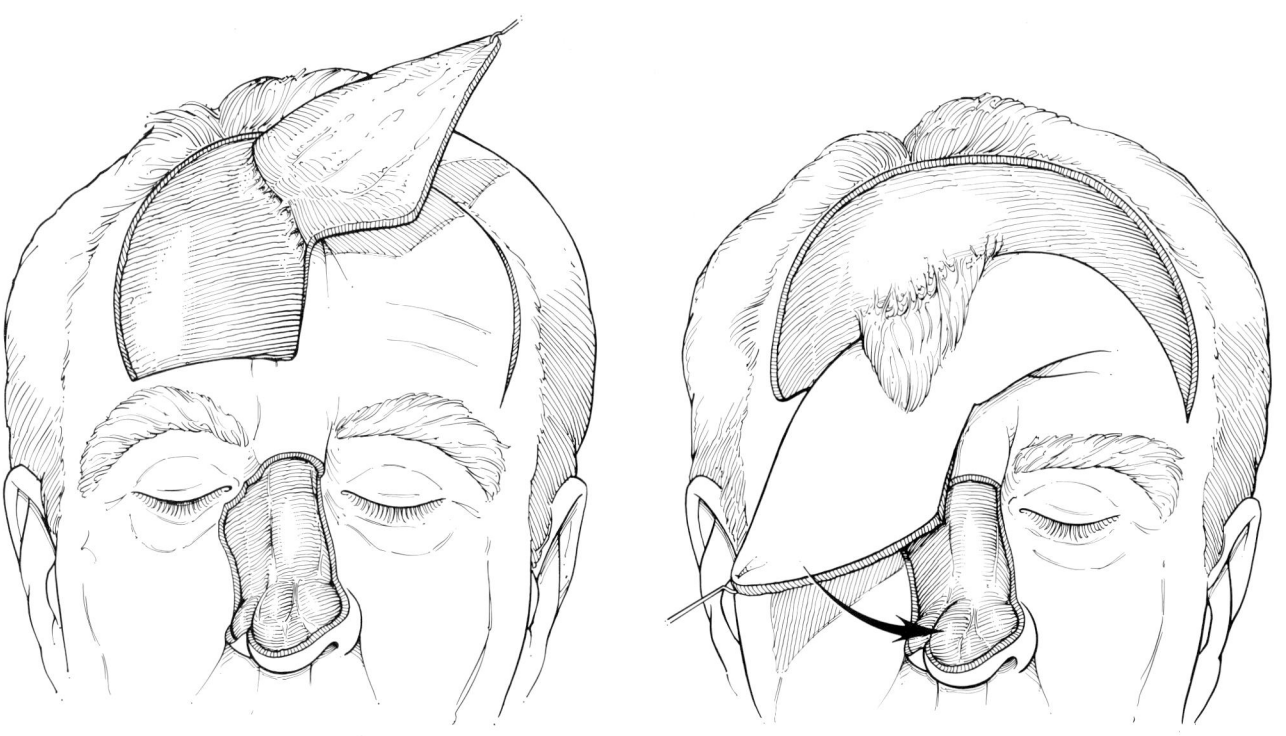

The flap is raised and the pericranium is left intact. The hemiforehead is transposed to the nasal area. If any tension is present, the midline incision may be extended. This allows the forehead to open out and lengthen.

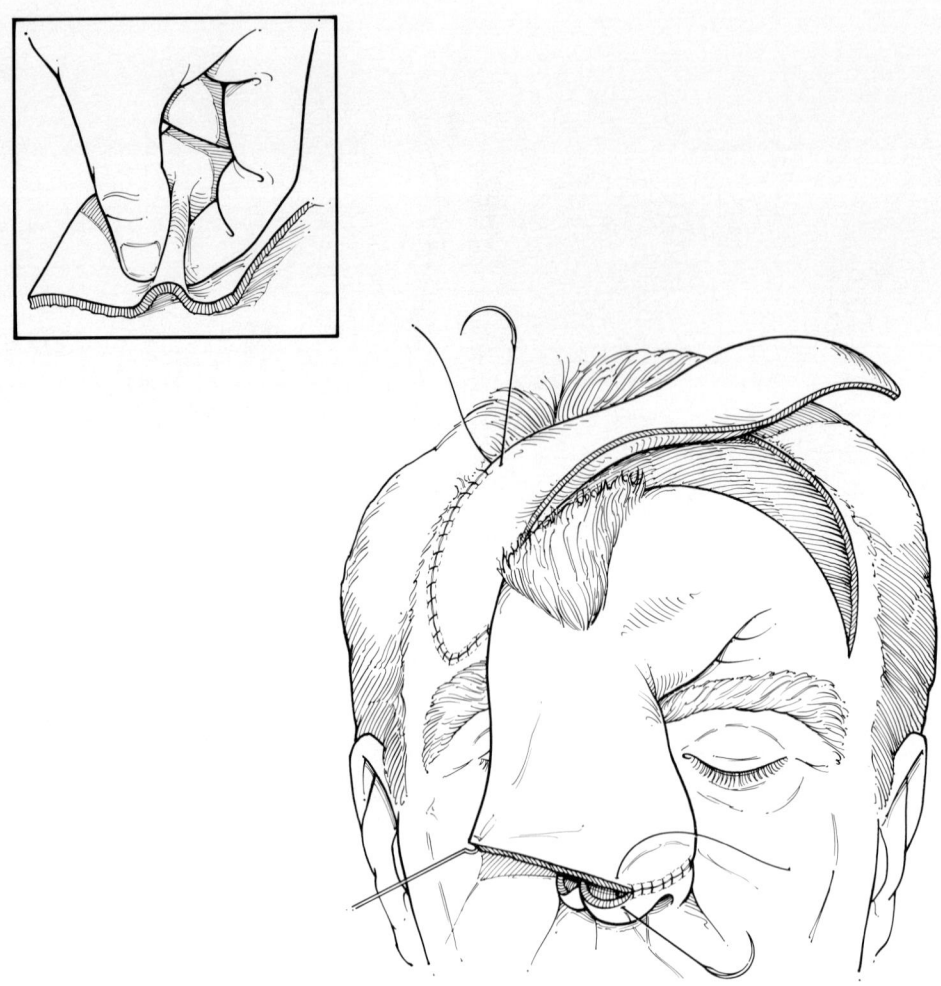

By pinching the lower edge of the flap in the midline, the surgeon can obtain the configuration of the alar margins and the columella. Some strategically placed nonabsorbable sutures can maintain this arrangement. The flap is now sutured into the defect. One useful technique at this point is to suture the undersurface of the flap laterally to any remaining skeleton. This is accomplished by drilling holes in the nasal bones and pyriform aperture edge and by inserting nonabsorbable sutures through these holes to give good apposition of the undersurface of the flap to the nasal bones. In particular, this suturing is advised to ensure a good nose-to-cheek contour. The eyebrow on the side of the flap donor site is hitched up to the pericranium with fine nonabsorbable sutures. This prevents eyebrow ptosis, which gives an asymmetric appearance to the eyes.

CHAPTER 4
NOSE RECONSTRUCTION

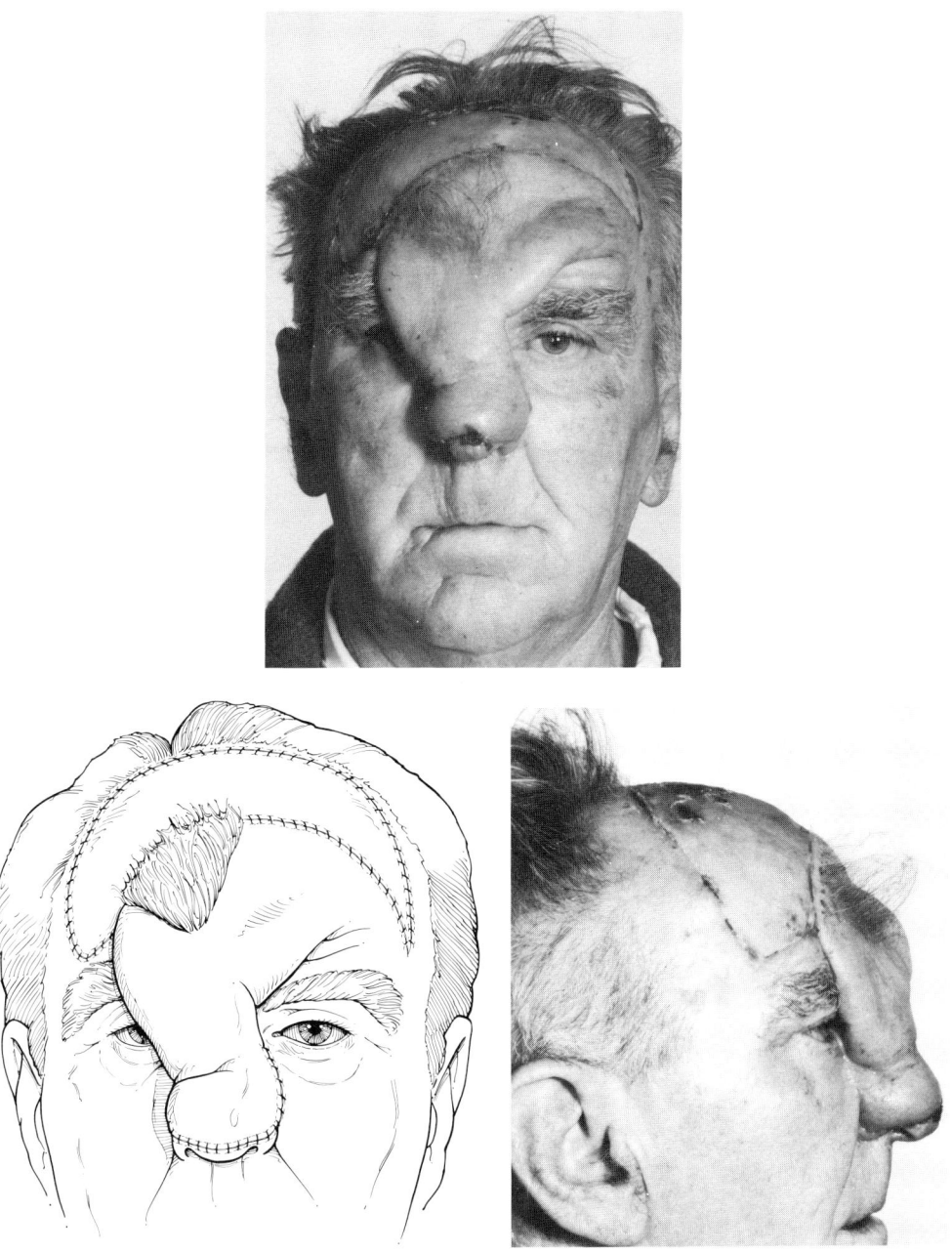

The raw area of the forehead is split-thickness skin grafted, either immediately or in a delayed fashion.

161

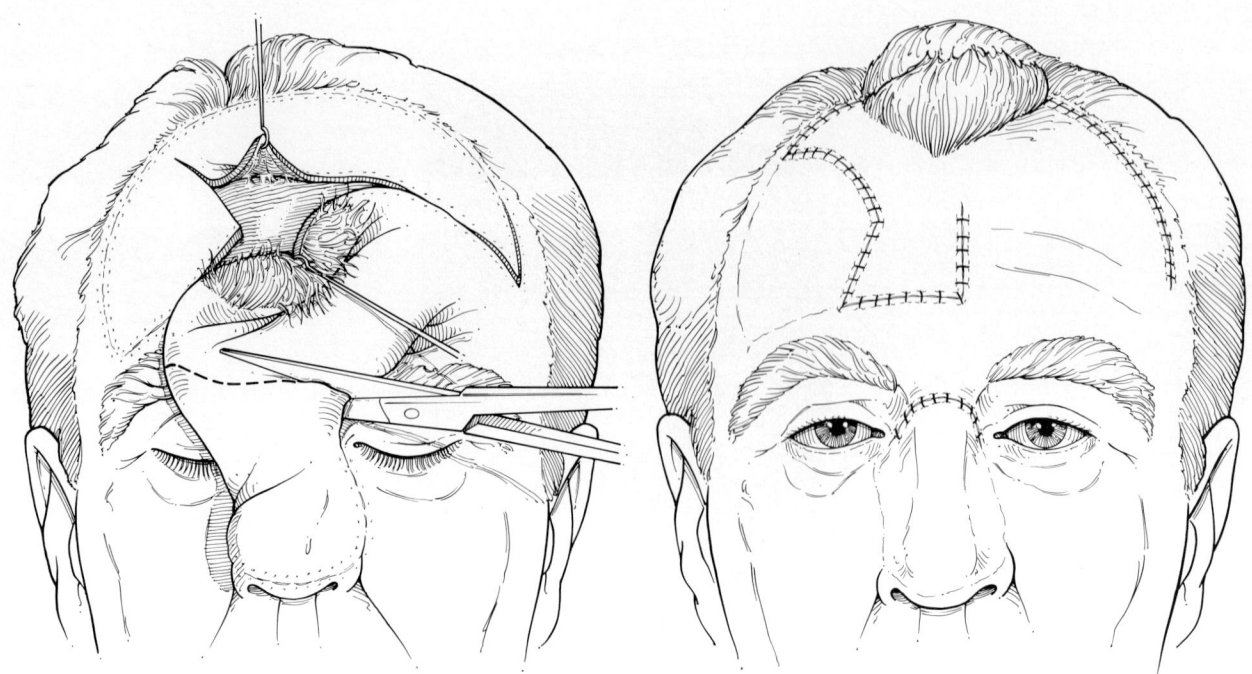

The flap is left attached for 2 to 3 weeks; it is then divided and the unused portion is returned to the forehead.

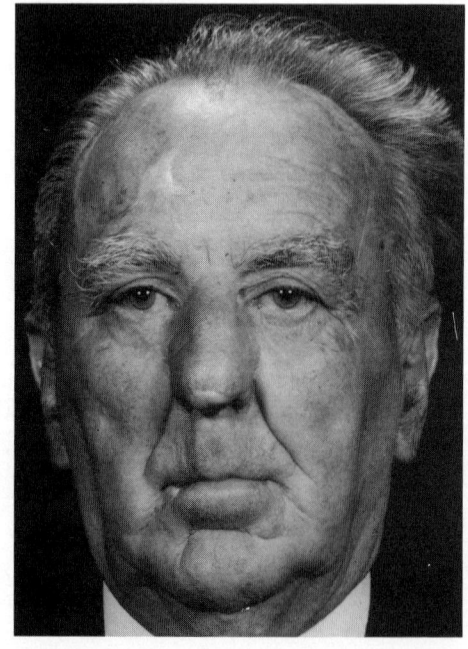

The nose is contoured by thinning the flap superiorly to achieve a reasonable result.

CHAPTER 4
NOSE RECONSTRUCTION

FOREHEAD FLAP AND LOCAL IN-TURNED FLAPS

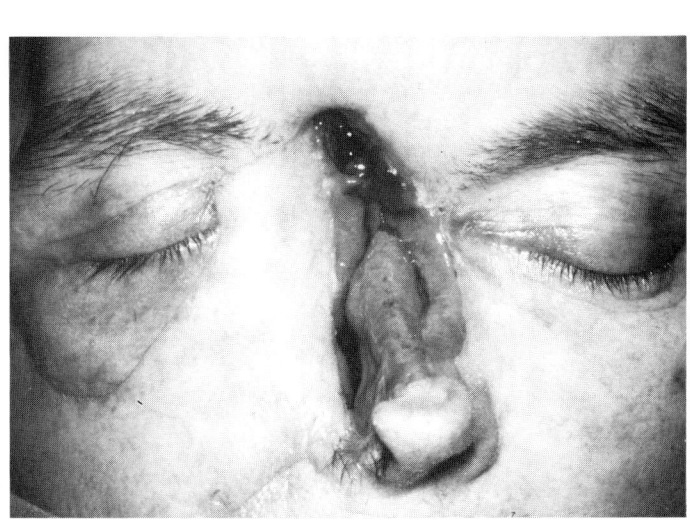
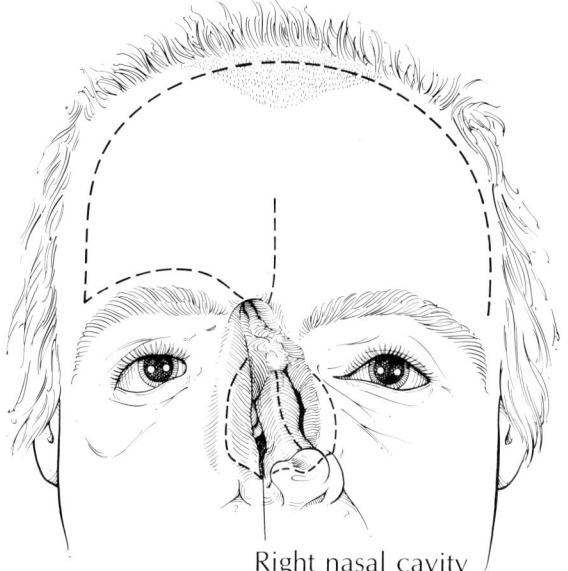

This patient had a secondary nasal reconstruction after resection of the nose for a squamous cell carcinoma. The technique used was basically similar to that presented on pp. 158 to 162. Lining is provided by in-turned local flaps sutured in the midline.

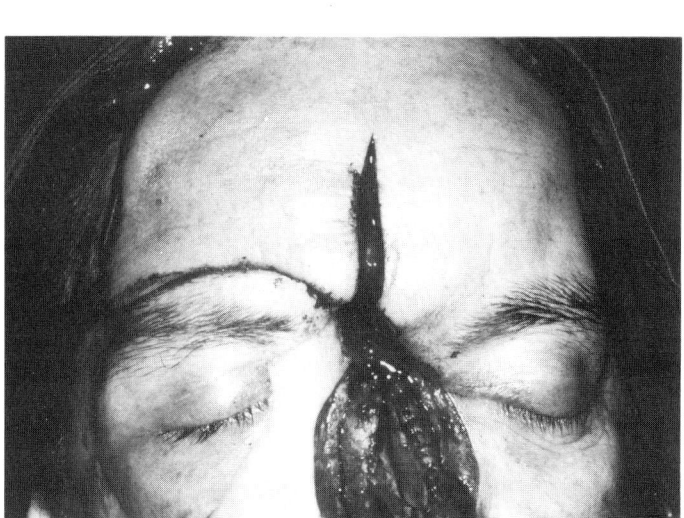
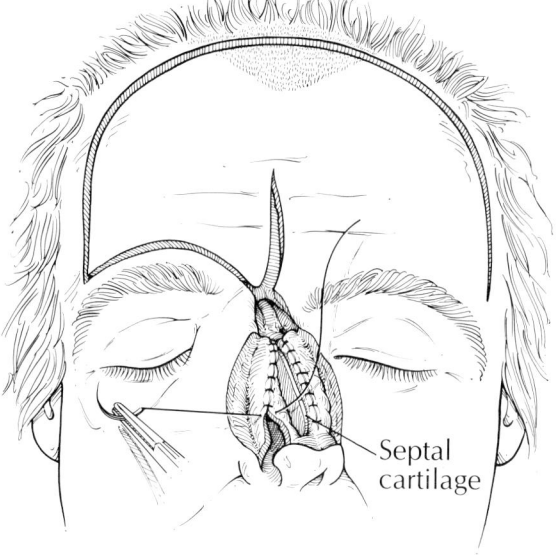

The planned flap is of generous proportions. A surprisingly small amount of paranasal skin needs to be used for mucosal reconstruction.

163

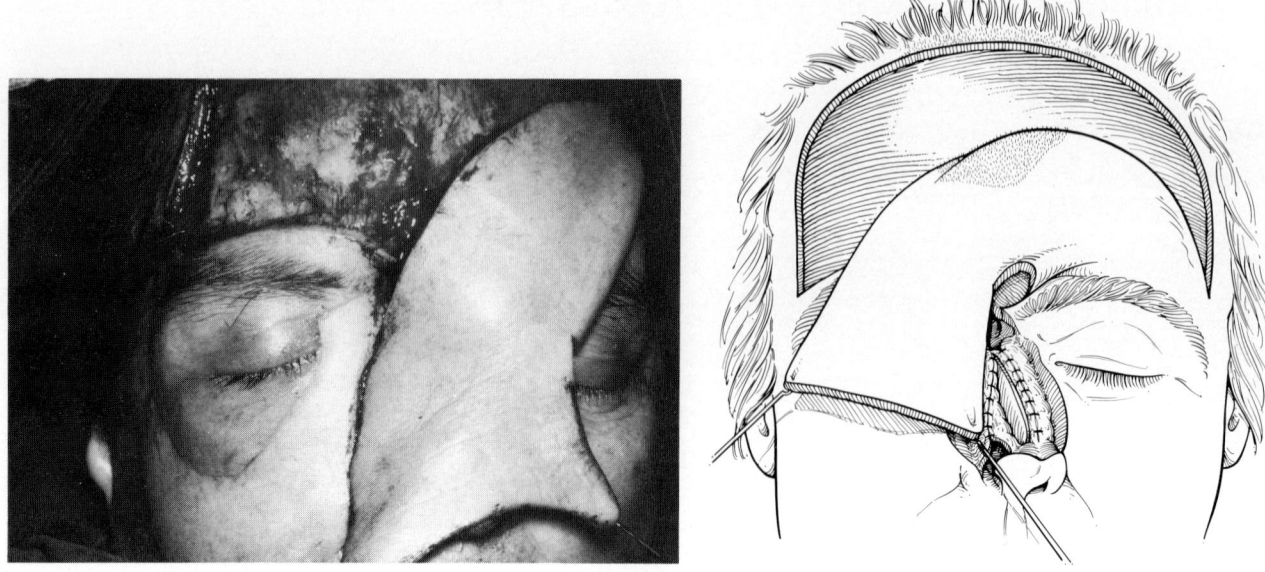

The forehead flap is elevated, as described previously. If planned correctly, flap transposition to the nose can be achieved without tension.

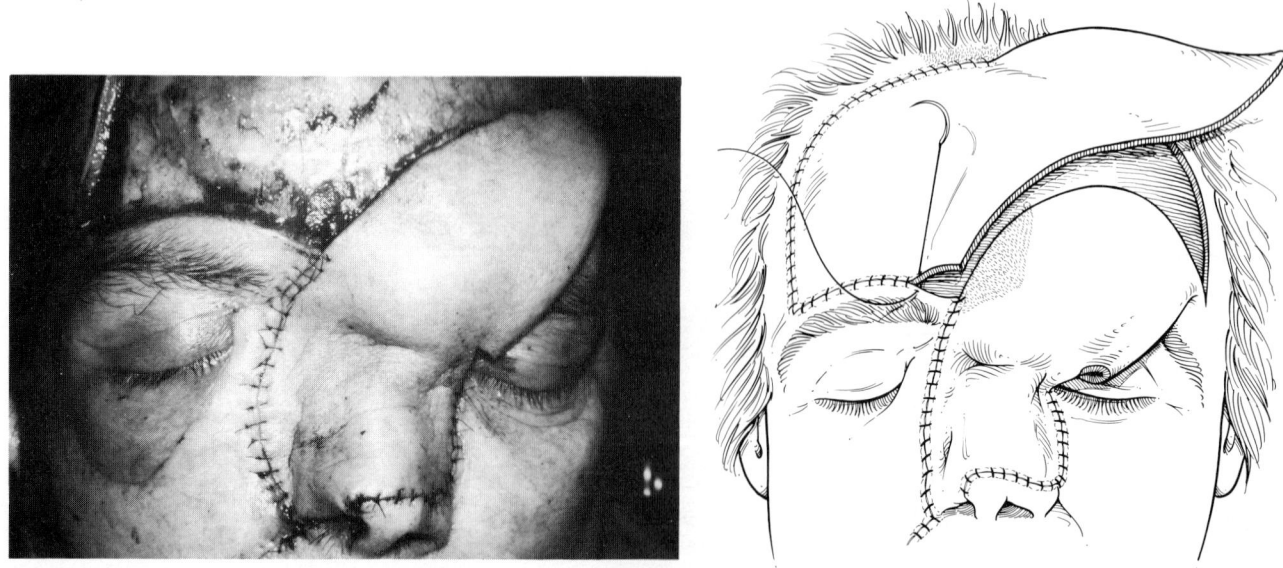

The edges of the flap are sutured to the raw edges of the nasal defect. The forehead is covered with a split-thickness skin graft.

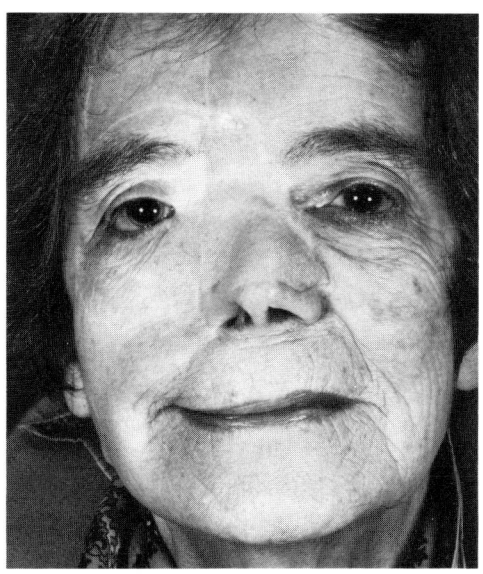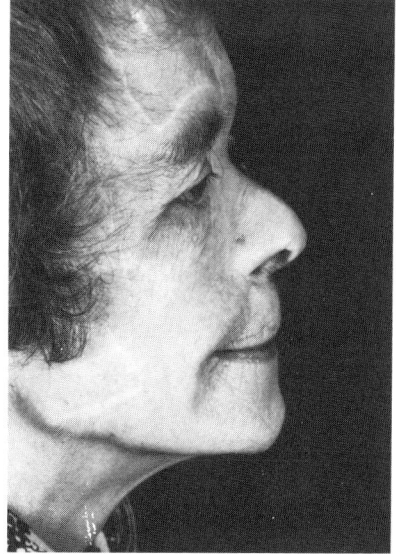

Within 10 to 14 days the pedicle is divided and returned to the forehead. The result is reasonably satisfactory, and the patient does not wish any further surgery. It should be noted that the right-side telecanthus was present before the surgery and resulted from the excision of the penetrating squamous carcinoma of the nasal orbital region.

GALEAL FRONTALIS FLAP

The galeal frontalis flap originated in China. Thus far it has been used infrequently for nasal reconstruction. Undoubtedly, with experience, it will be used more often and with time its value will be assessed. This flap has the advantage of leaving the forehead unscathed.

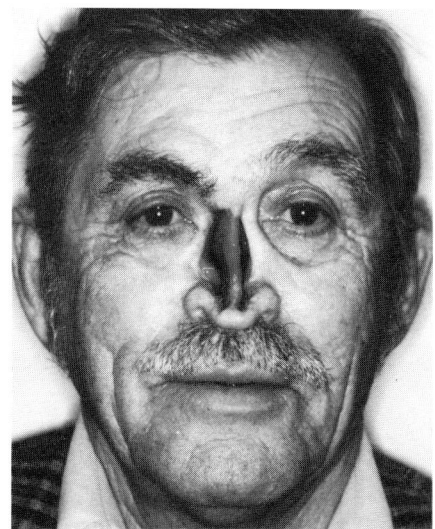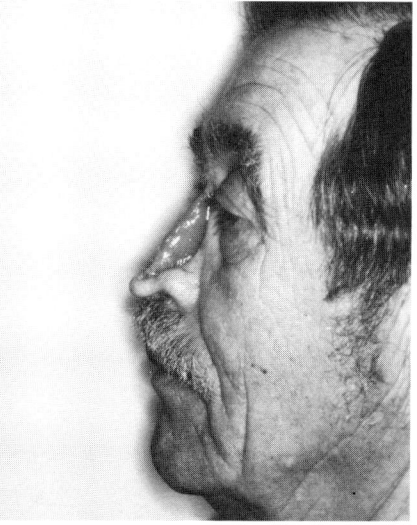

The patient shown here required secondary nasal reconstruction following nasal resection for squamous cell carcinoma.

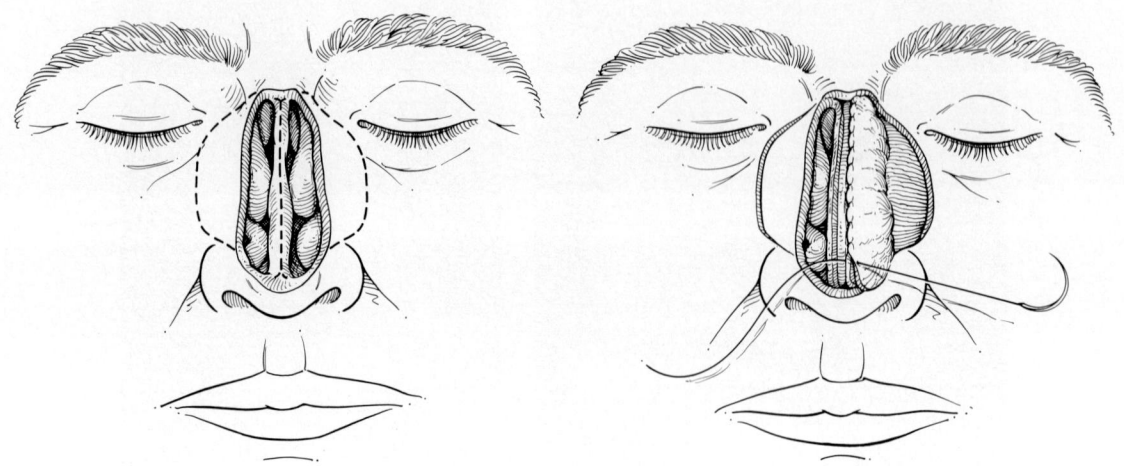

The nasal lining is provided by in-turned paranasal flaps. The septal mucosa is incised in the midline and dissected down on either side of the septum. The edges of the lateral flaps are sutured to the edges of the septal mucosal flaps to give an internal nasal reconstruction.

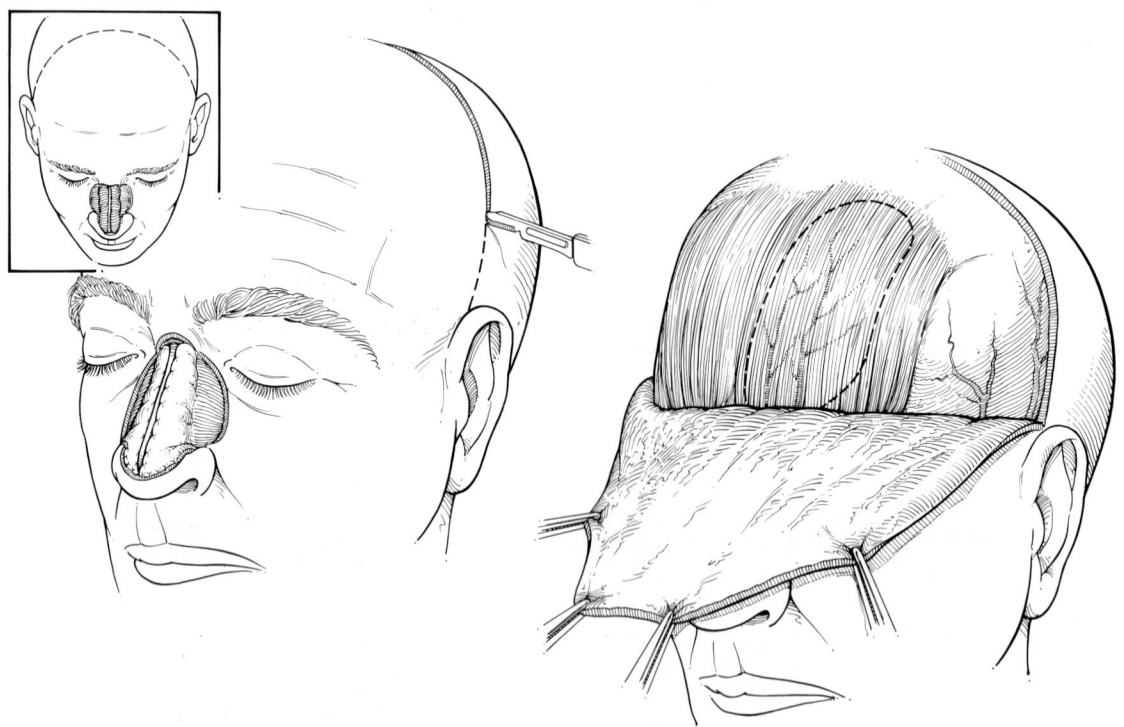

Through a coronal flap or a midline incision, the frontalis and galea are exposed. The dotted line shows the projected flap.

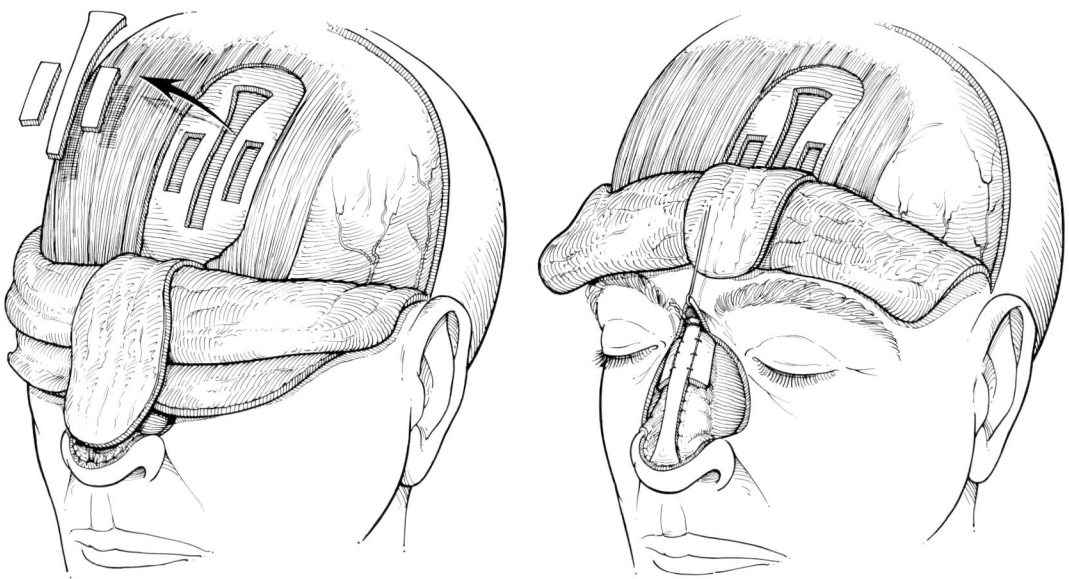

A segment of galea and frontalis, as wide as necessary, can be raised as a flap, extending almost to midskull and based on the supratrochlear and supraorbital vessels. The dimensions of the flap are similar to those of the skin forehead flap described in the previous section. Nasal support is provided by an immediate bone graft, usually outer table of skull.[10]

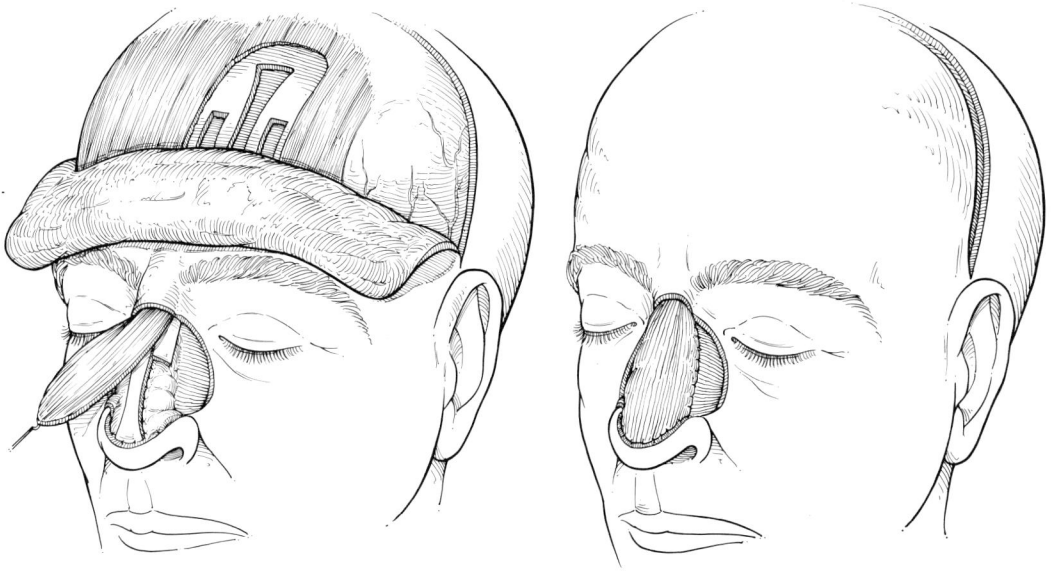

These grafts can be taken from the frontal or temporal area; they are wired in position in the frontonasal area. This reconstruction is covered with the galeal frontalis flap.

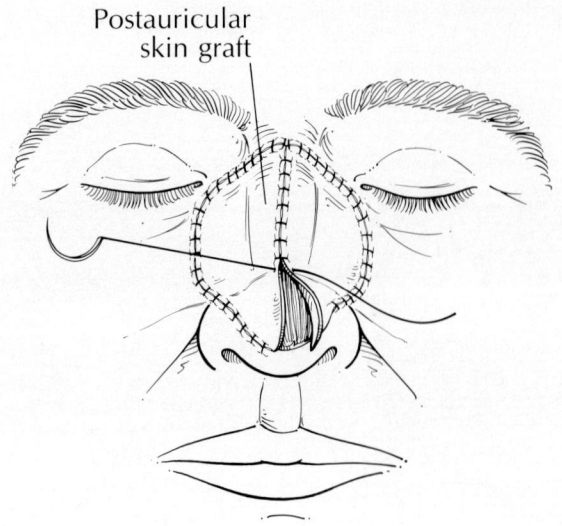

Immediate skin cover is not advised because oozing from the flap is difficult to control. Thus in 24 hours one of the two large postauricular full-thickness grafts can be used to provide skin cover for the reconstructed nose.

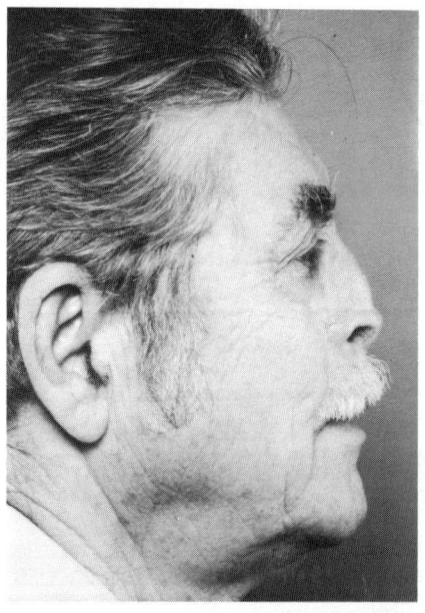
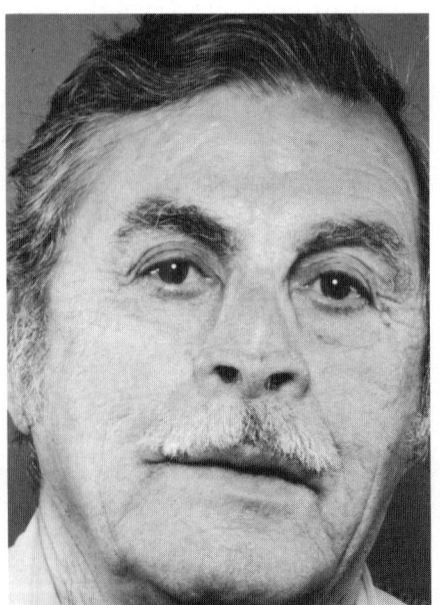

The advantages of this method are lack of obvious scars, no forehead skin grafts, and a thin nasal skin cover.

RECONSTRUCTION OF CHOICE

With the present state of knowledge, the forehead flap is the most reliable method and can give an excellent reconstruction. Unfortunately, the forehead needs to be grafted. This situation may well be obviated by the use of tissue expansion. After the skin has been stretched, the amount of nasal reconstruction can be taken and the defect closed directly without a skin graft. The Chinese method has many attractions, but it must be considered to be *sub judice* at present.

☐ Subtotal Reconstruction

It should be possible to reconstruct a partial nasal defect without creating an appreciable donor site deformity. The areas chosen are chiefly the forehead and the nasolabial area.

FOREHEAD FLAP

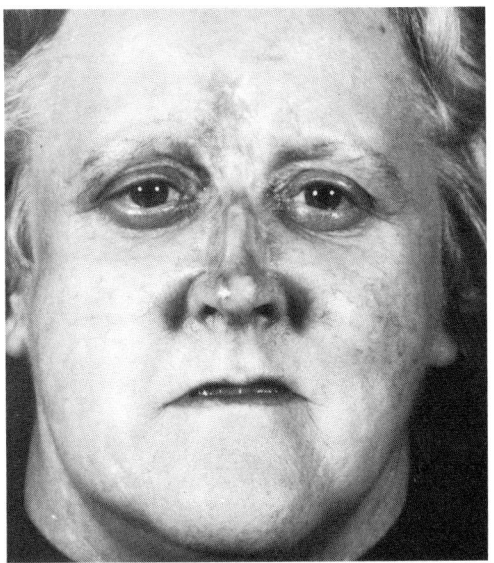

This patient needed partial nasal reconstruction after having had a nasal resection and skin grafting for squamous cell carcinoma.

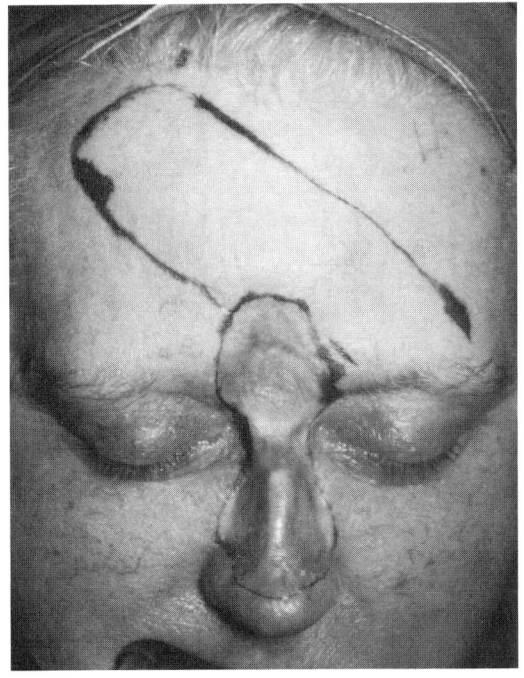
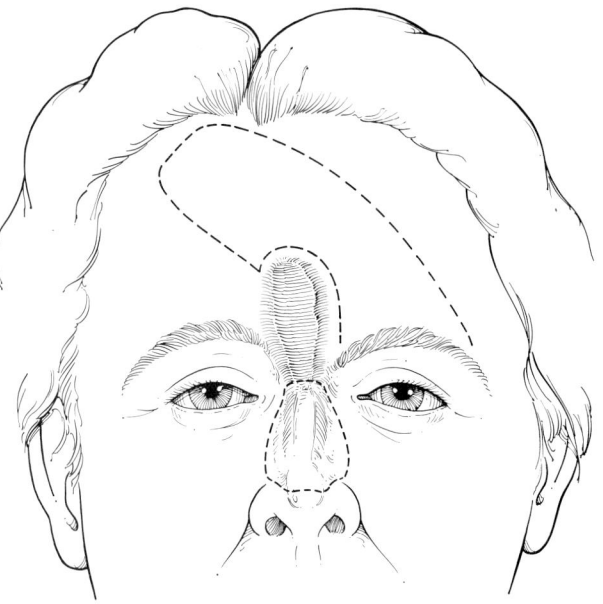

A diagonal forehead flap is planned.

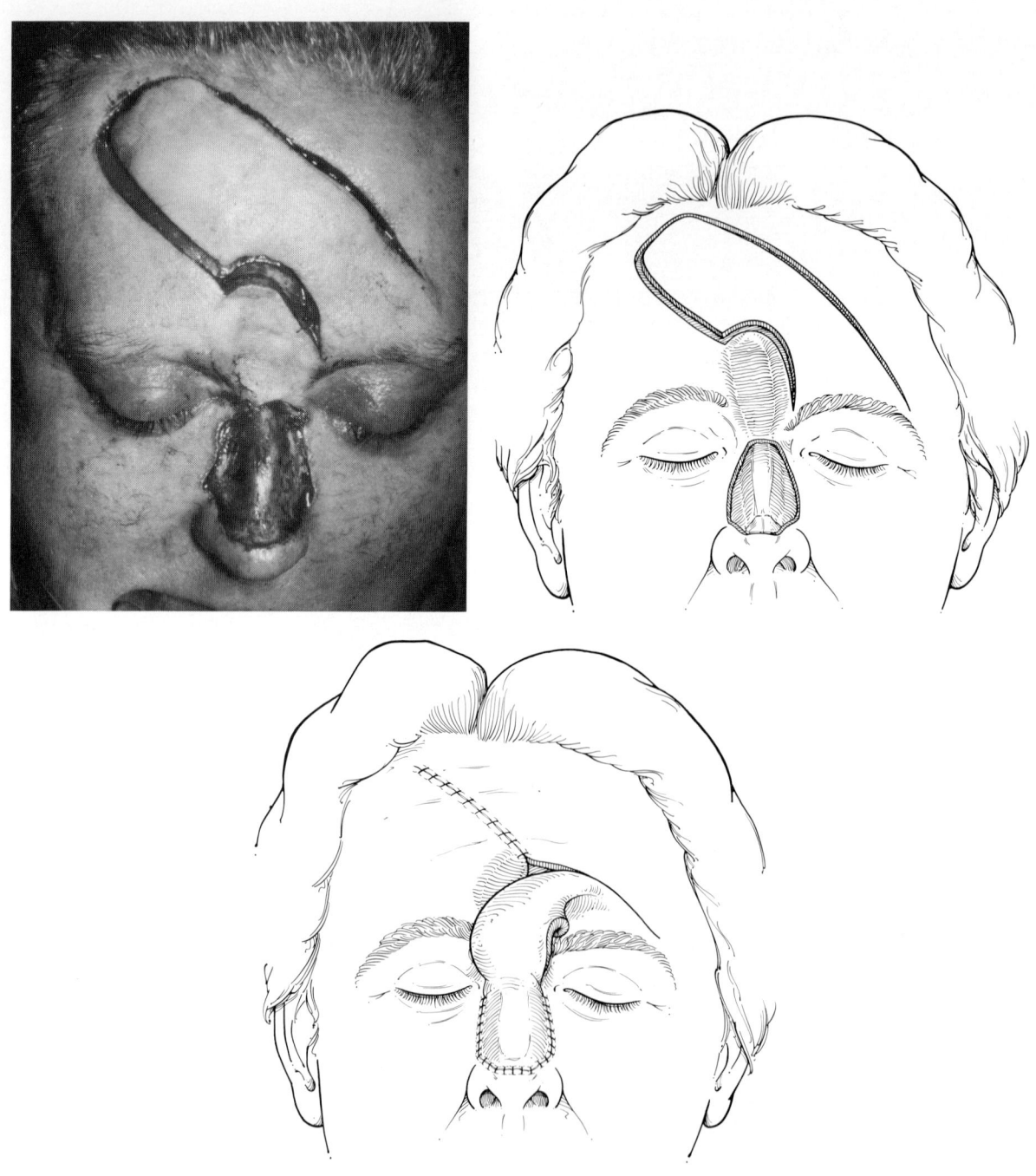

The scarred area of the nose is excised. The forehead flap is elevated and taken down to cover the nasal defect.

CHAPTER 4
NOSE RECONSTRUCTION

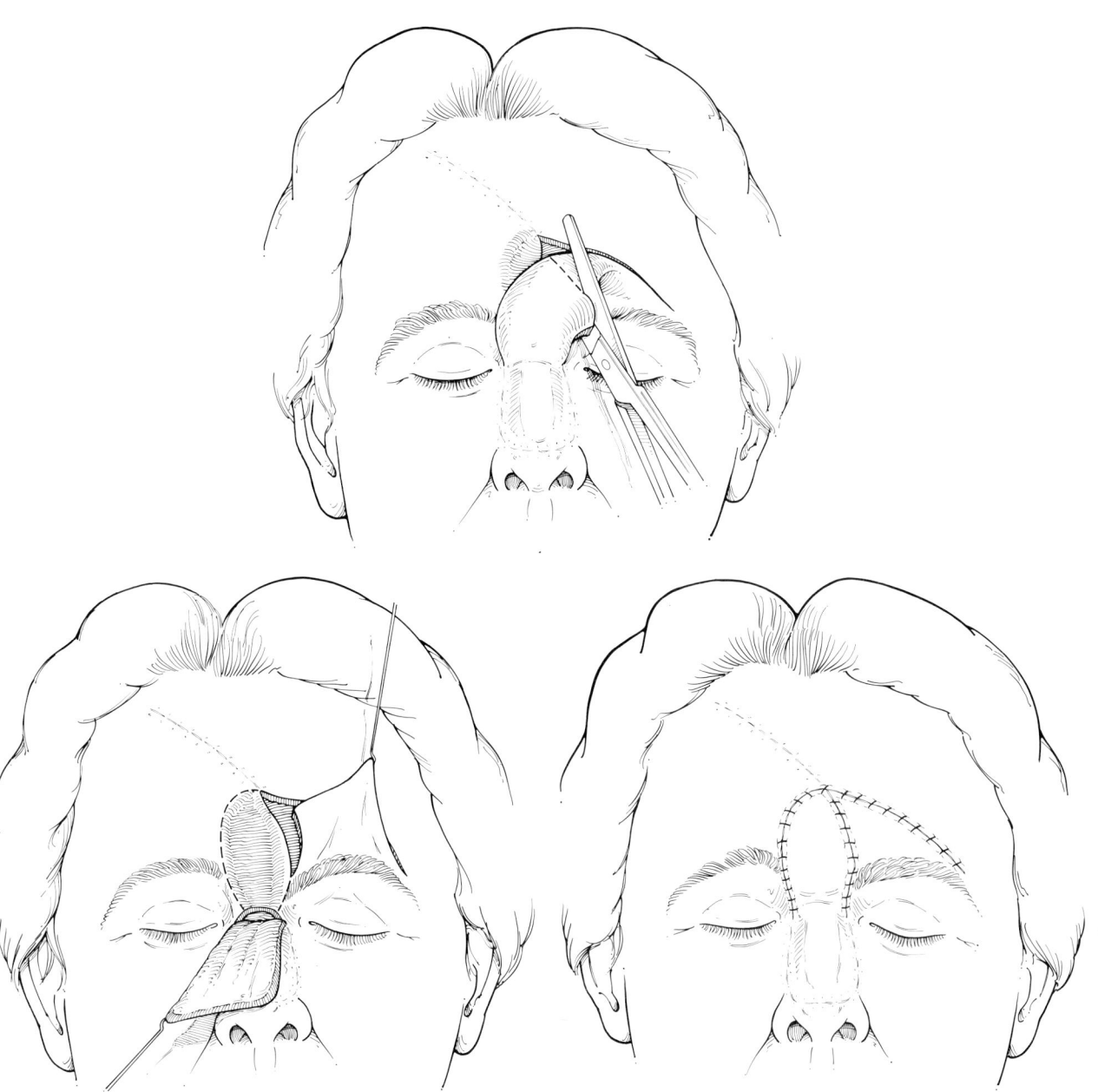

In 10 to 14 days the pedicle is divided, the unused portion of the flap is returned to the forehead, and the nasal flap is inset.

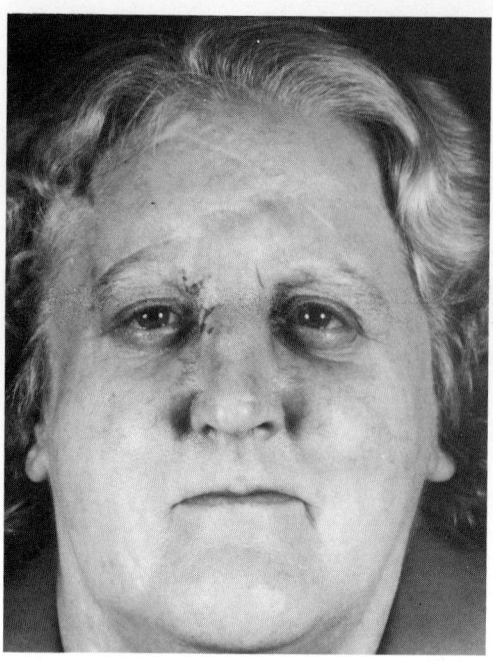

The result of this two-stage procedure is reasonably satisfactory.

SCHMID FLAP

Schmid[16,17] has described an interesting and useful technique designed to minimize forehead scarring and to transfer thin soft skin to the alar area.

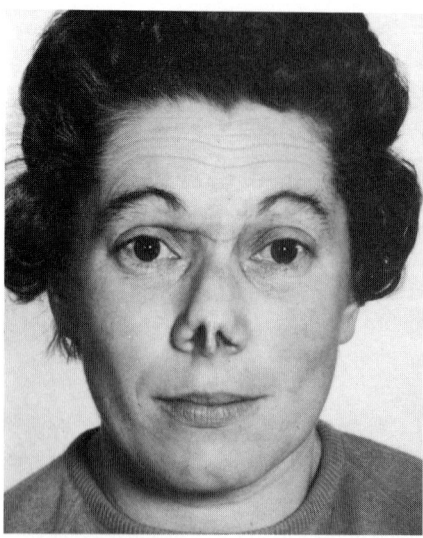 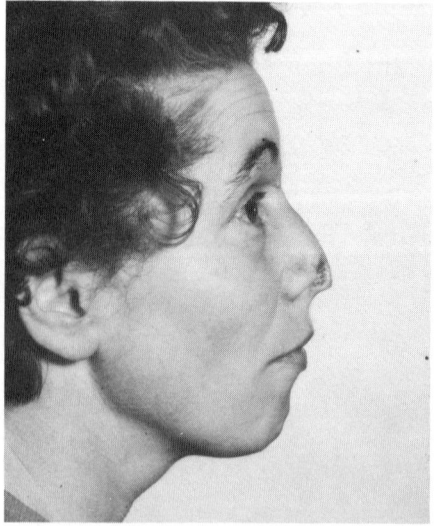

This patient required a subtotal nasal reconstruction of skin and lining. The Schmid flap was considered the best option.

CHAPTER 4
NOSE RECONSTRUCTION

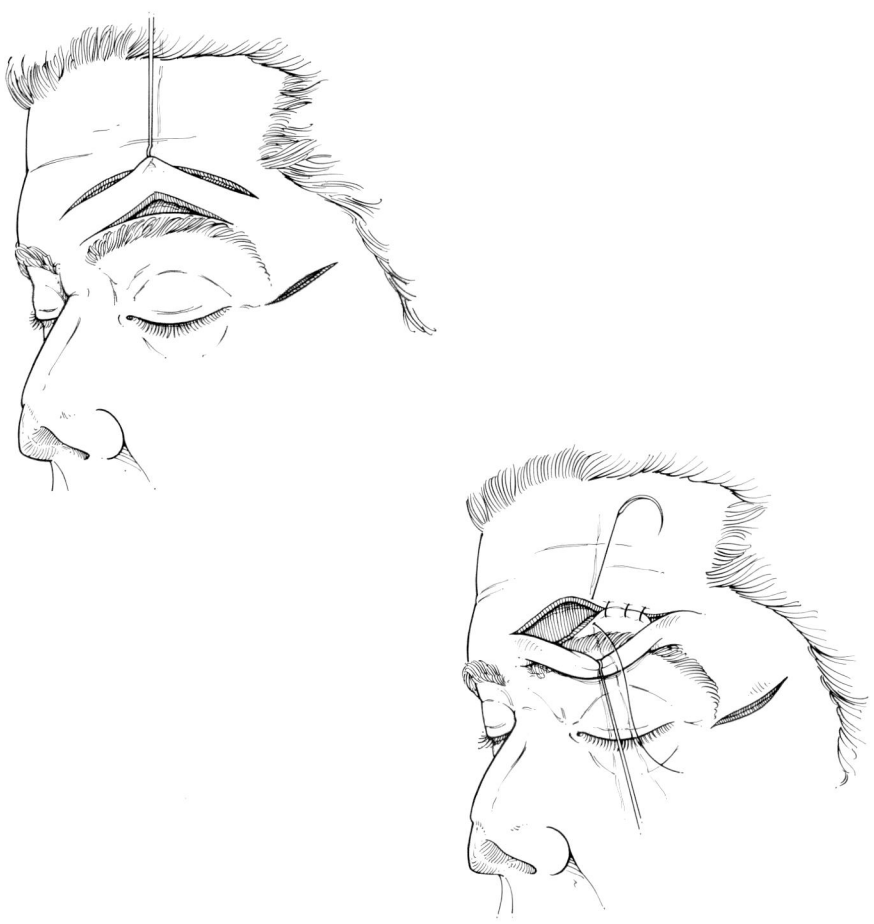

The flap requires an initial delay of 7 to 10 days for complete security, but it can be used as an immediate reconstruction if this is absolutely necessary. The delay should consist of complete raising of the pedicle from its base to the area to be transferred (but not including that area).

Clinical judgment is used as to whether the defect behind the pedicle should be closed and the pedicle left free or whether the pedicle is placed back on the donor site and sutured in position. Any adverse changes in vascularity strongly indicate a conservative approach.

The flap is based on the supratrochlear vessels and is taken horizontally above the eyebrow to the temple area between the hairline and the lateral end of the eyebrow. The pedicle may be tubed, but this is not usually advised. Because the forehead skin is stiff and the pedicle narrow, tubing may compromise the blood supply. It is better to leave the pedicle untubed and raw posteriorly or, for hygiene purposes, to split-thickness skin graft the raw posterior area. Recently pigskin has been used to cover the raw area of pedicles. This provides dry cover for as long as 3 weeks.

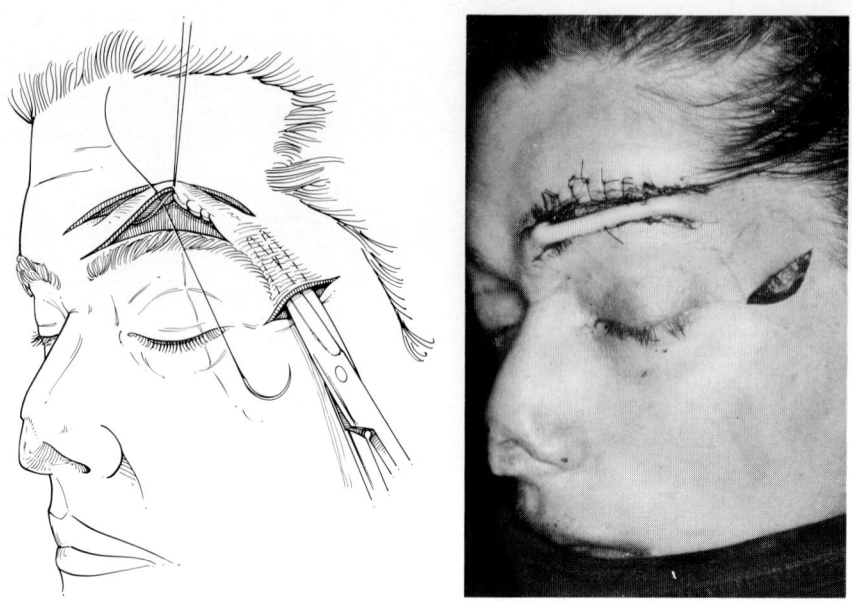

At the distal temporal end of the flap, a pocket is created by scissor dissection. This pocket must be slightly larger than the nostril defect in order to allow for contracture.

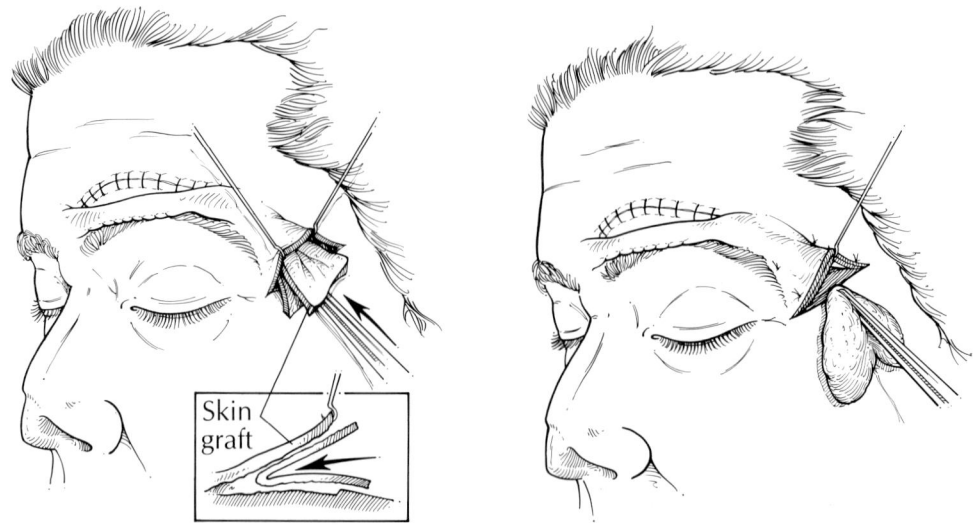

A full-thickness or split-thickness skin graft is inserted into the pocket to cover all the raw areas.

CHAPTER 4
NOSE RECONSTRUCTION

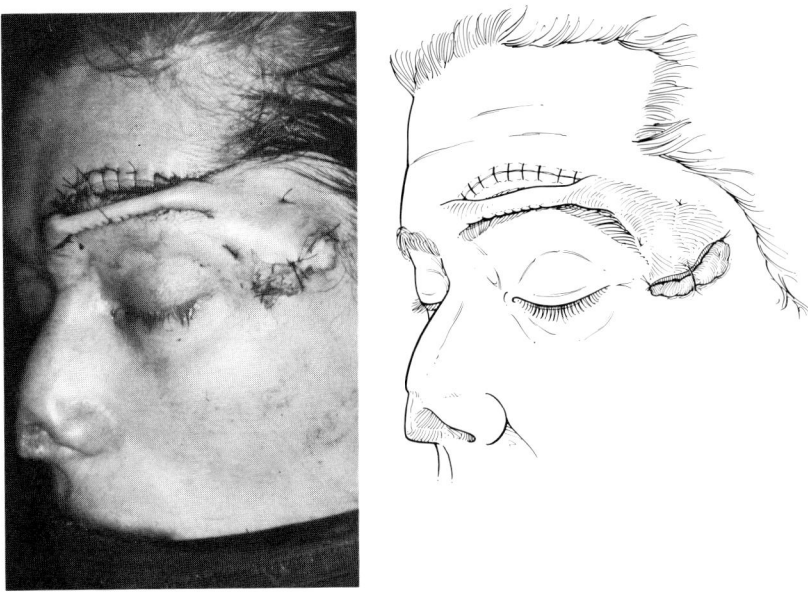

A gauze pack is inserted to prevent hematoma and to facilitate skin graft take.

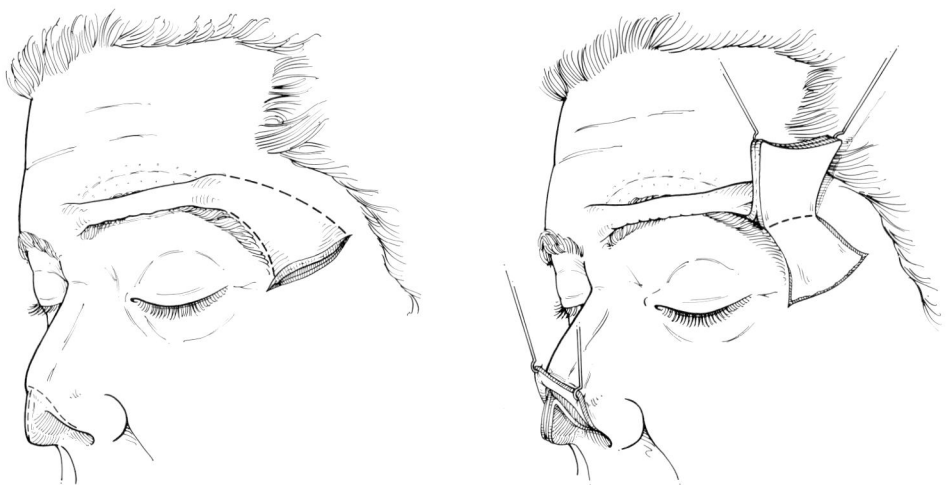

In 10 days the gauze is removed and the distal end of the flap is opened along the lateral edges of the pocket. When this end is opened, there should be skin graft on the flap and on the forehead.

175

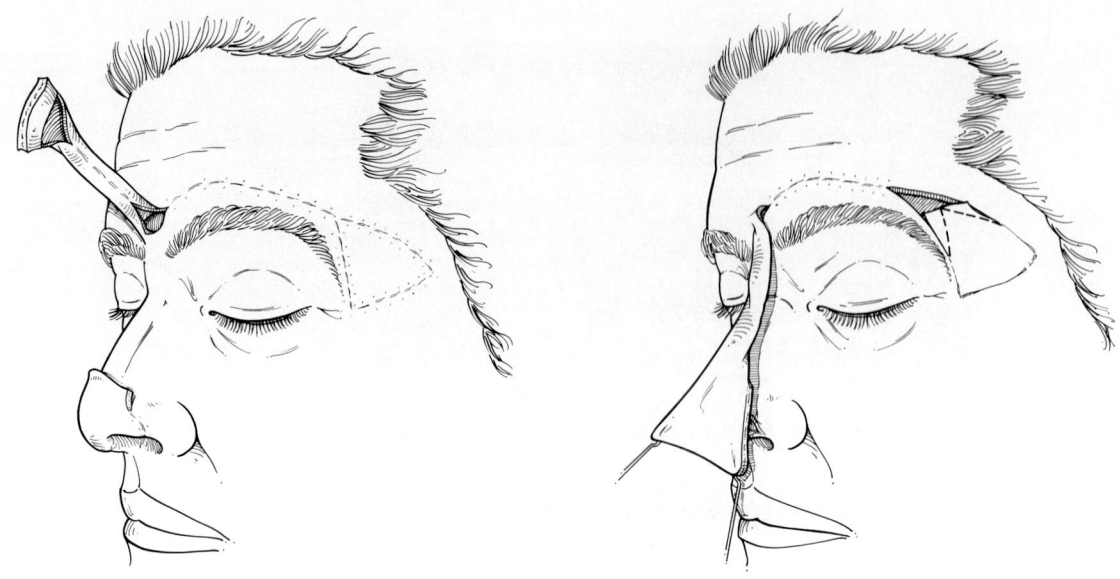

The flap is transferred to the nose; its distal end will reconstruct the nasal tip and the alar defects.

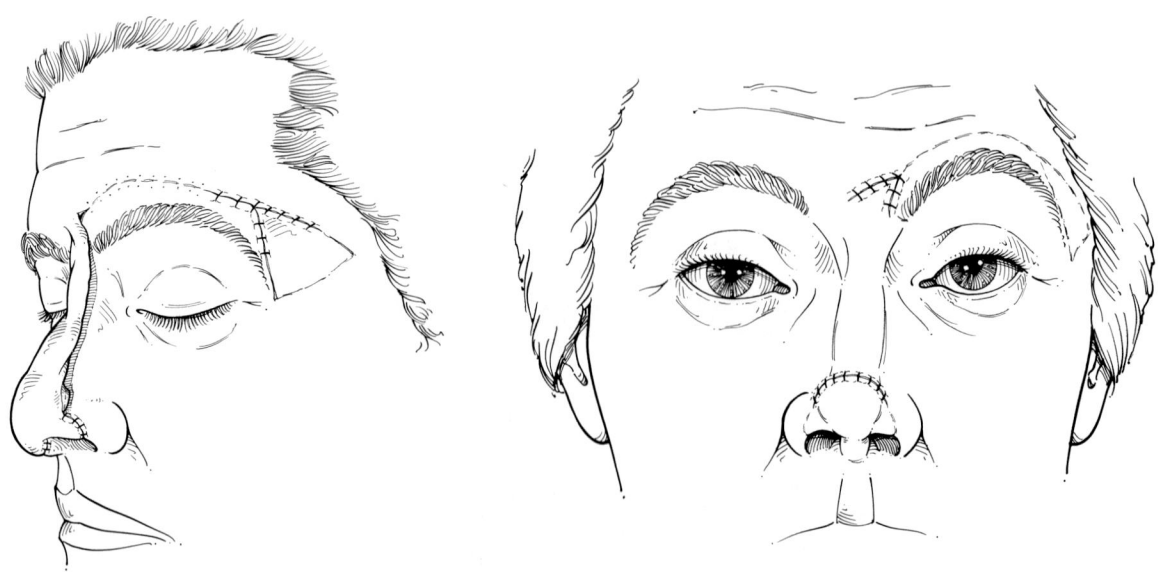

This flap is left for 10 to 14 days and then divided. The unused pedicle is sacrificed and the nasal tip area is trimmed to provide a satisfactory contour.

CHAPTER 4
**NOSE
RECONSTRUCTION**

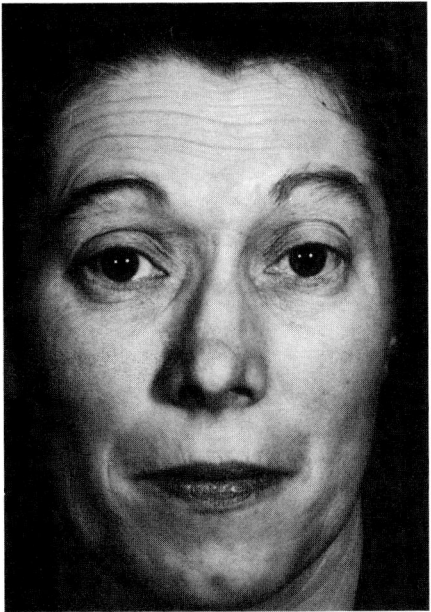

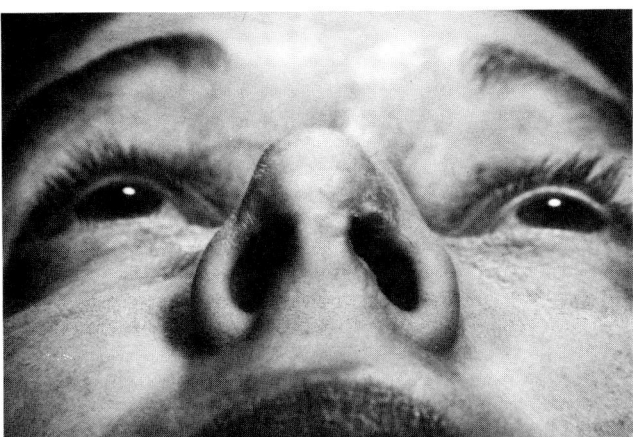

The result should be good, with satisfactory nasal contour, little forehead scarring, and only slight donor deformity.

Bilateral flaps can be used for total nose reconstruction, but this is only possible in older patients with a loose forehead.

PROBLEMS

The blood supply of the Schmid flap is somewhat precarious. Therefore careless handling of the pedicle or failure to delay may cause flap ischemia and necrosis. Occasionally, because of the anatomy of the forehead, it may not be possible to obtain sufficient skin for nasal reconstruction and primary closure. If this is so, a different method should be chosen.

WASHIO FLAP

Washio[18,19] has described a method of nasal reconstruction with the postauricular skin carried as a flap. Indications for use of this flap are alar defects and heminose defects, especially in children. Even in adults enough skin may be obtained from the postauricular and mastoid area to resurface one half of the nose. Through this method skin may be transferred, with no donor site defect and no visible scars.

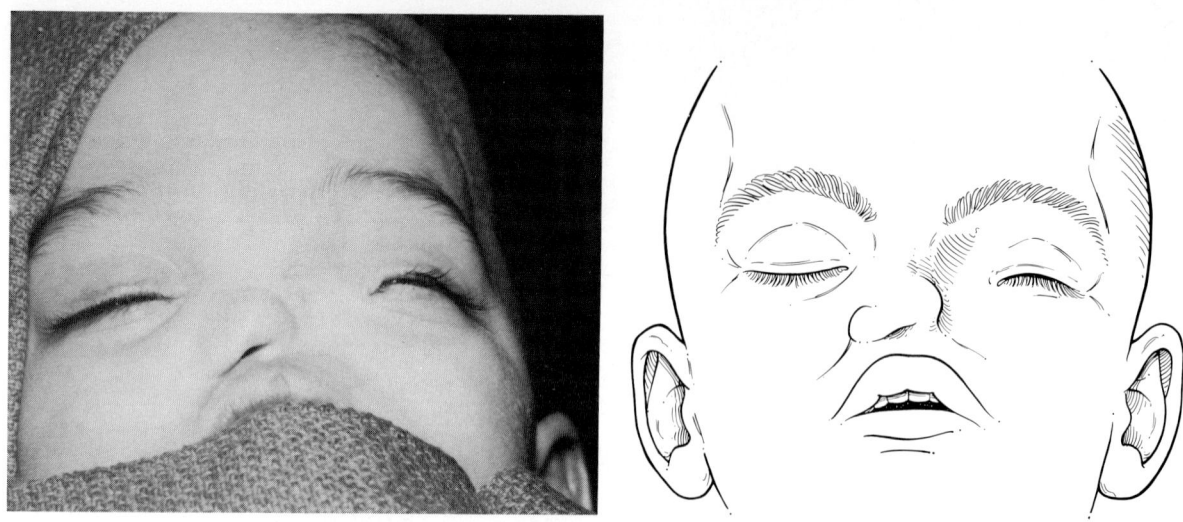

In the patient illustrated here, the Washio flap was used to reconstruct a congenitally absent heminose.

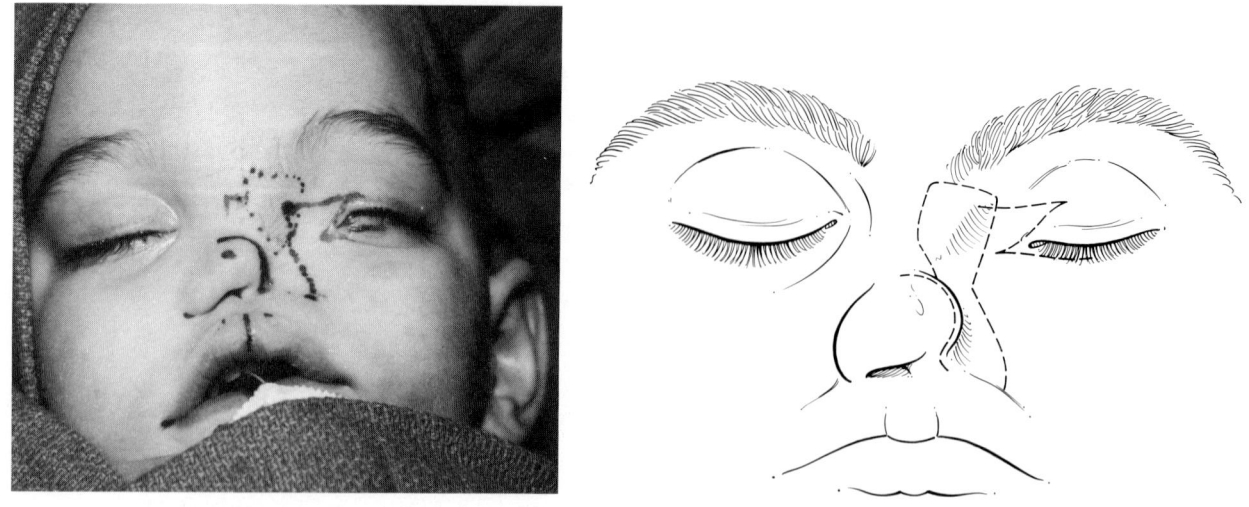

The nostril was initially reconstructed with a local turned-down nasal skin flap. The left medial canthus was repositioned correctly.

CHAPTER 4
NOSE RECONSTRUCTION

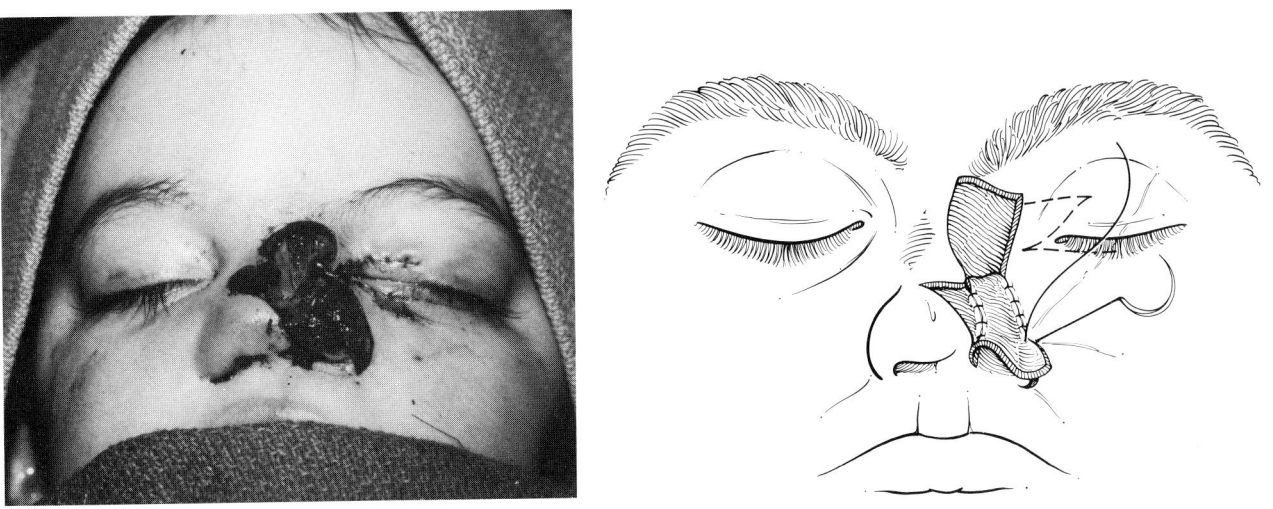

By means of a Z-plasty technique, the upper Z flap was taken from the upper eyelid. The medial canthus is wired in position through transnasal canthopexy technique.

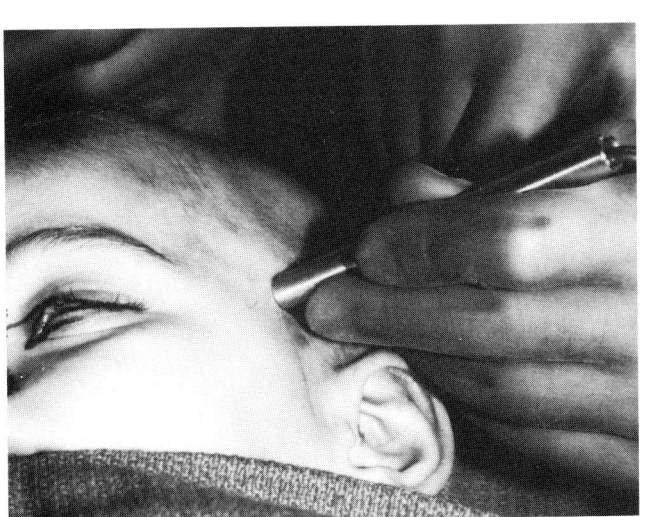 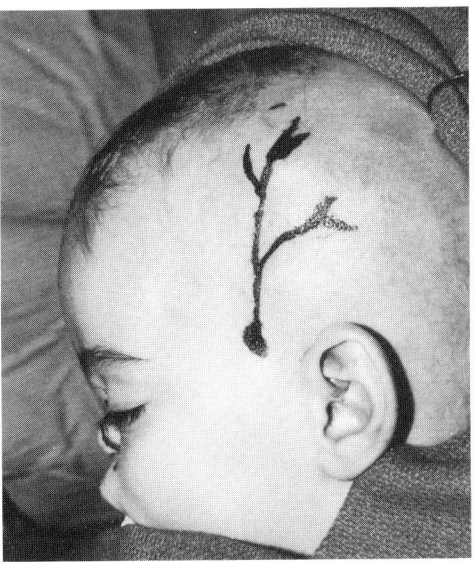

The flap is designed after the temporal vasculature has been mapped out with the Doppler apparatus. The temporal artery and its branches are marked on the skin.

179

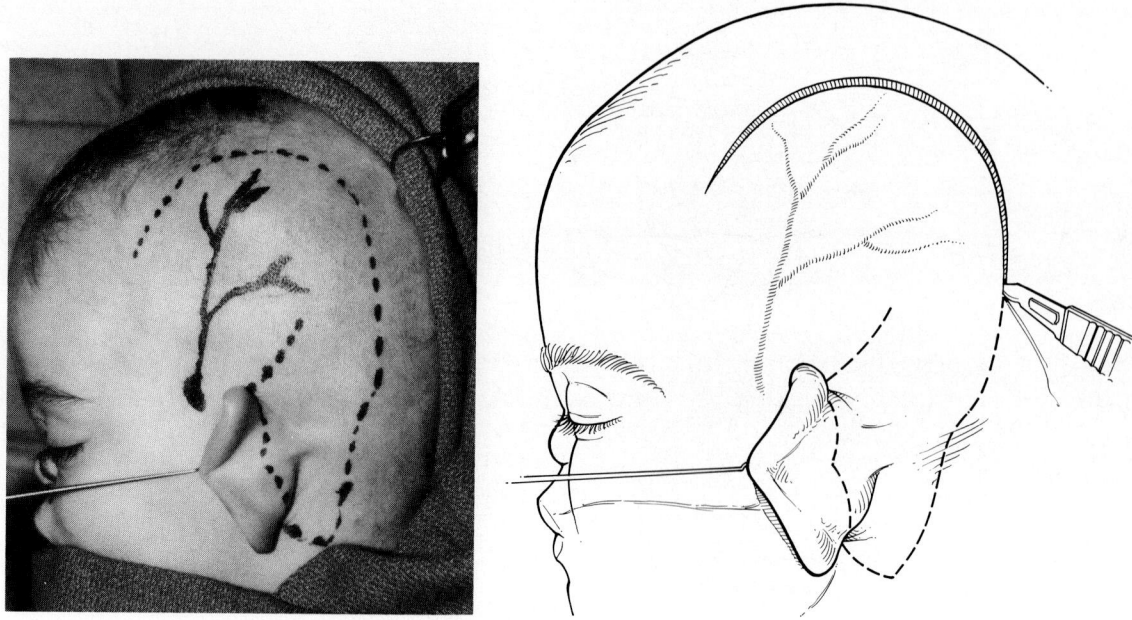

The flap is drawn so that enough postauricular skin will be available for the reconstruction. The concept is similar to the up-and-down forehead flap in that the central incision opens and lengthens the flap.

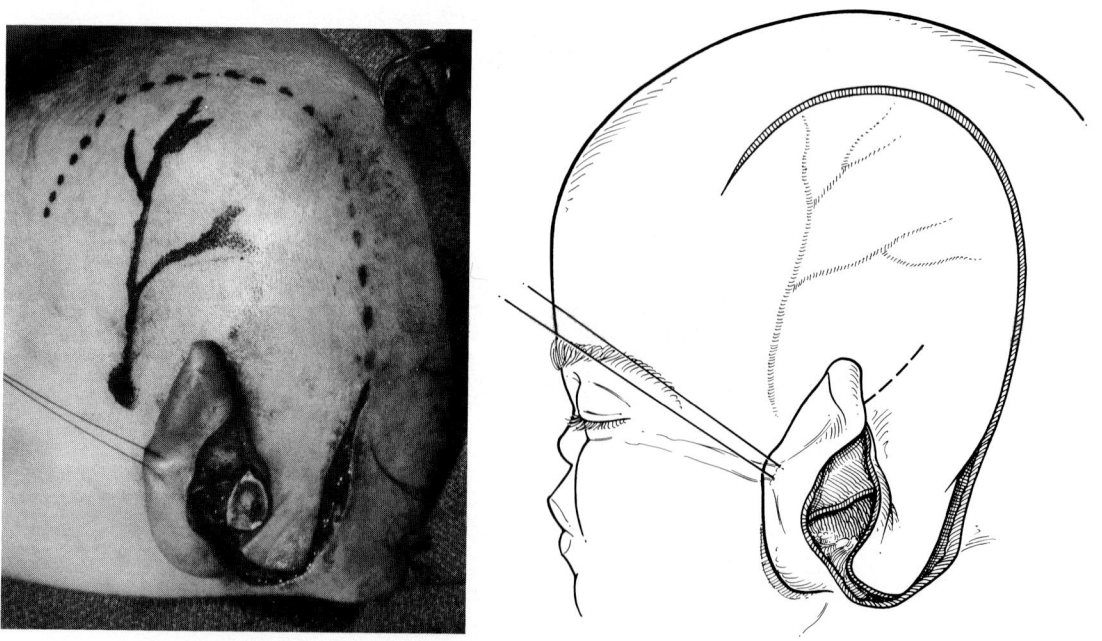

The postauricular and mastoid skin is carried on the end of the flap. The base of the flap is on line between the tip of the helix as it inserts into the face and the temporal hairline vertically above this point. Here the flap is at least 3 inches (7.6 cm) in width. Incisions are then made in the temporal scalp so that the posterior branches of the temporal vessels are included in the flap. Delay is not required but may be considered necessary for vascular security.

CHAPTER 4
NOSE RECONSTRUCTION

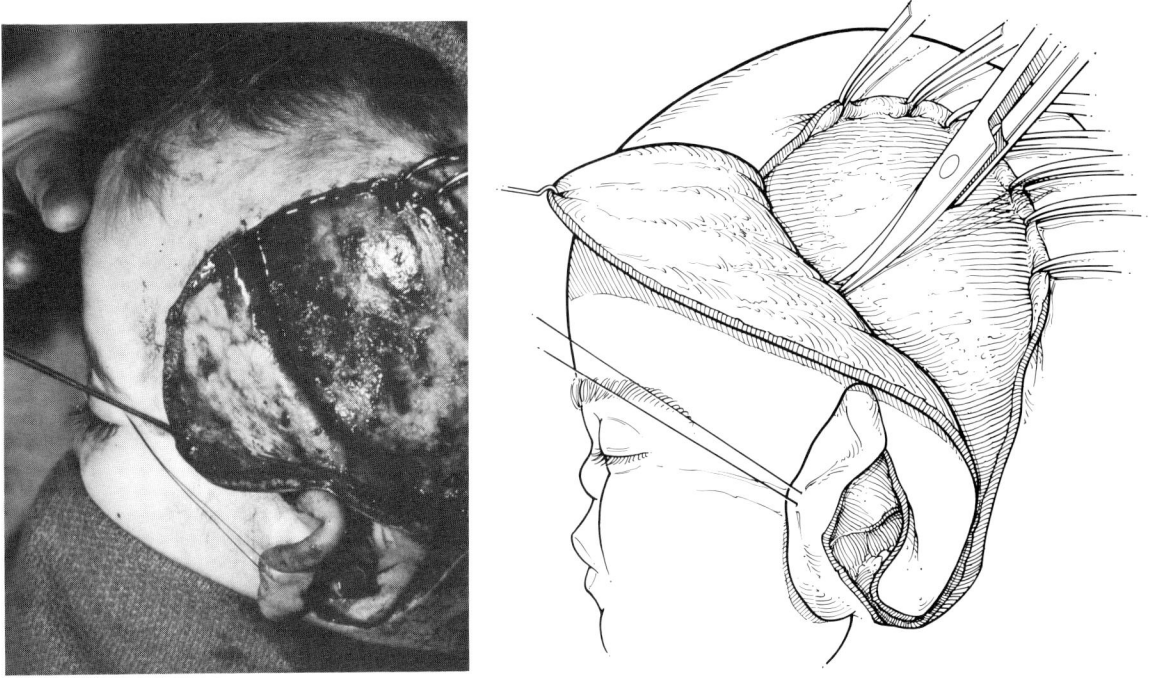

The flap is raised at a subfascial level.

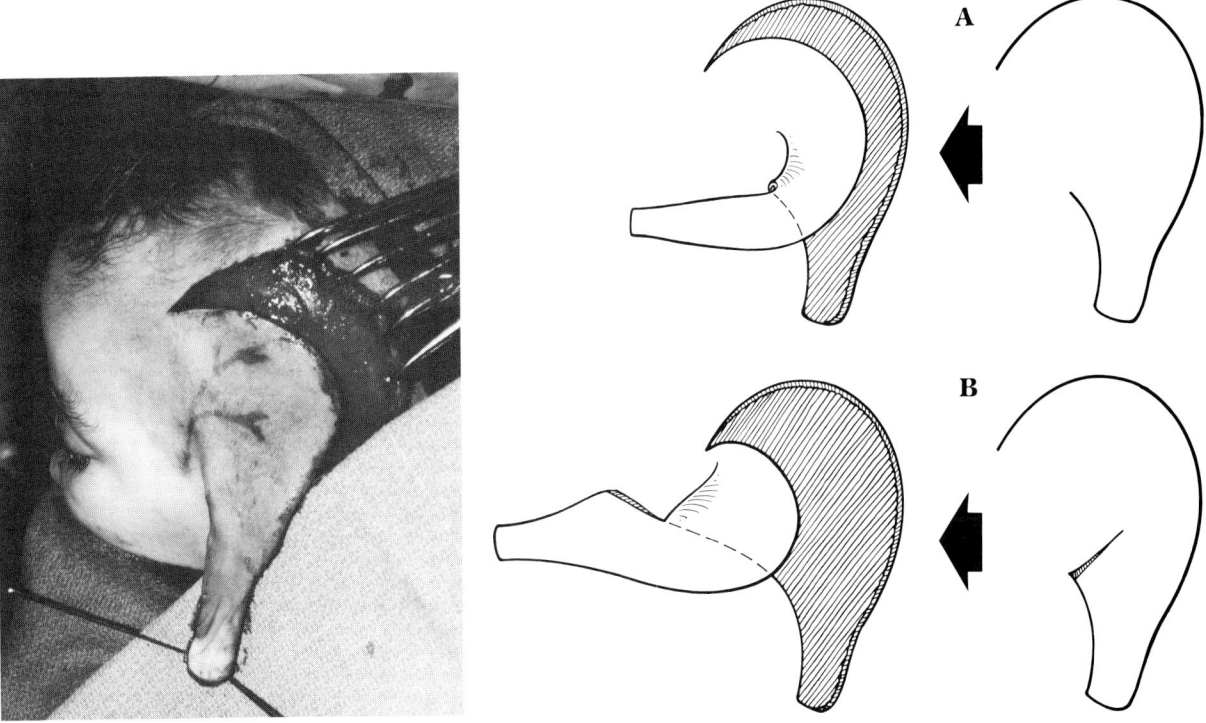

The midline incision is usually conservative and will not allow the postauricular skin to reach the midline.

181

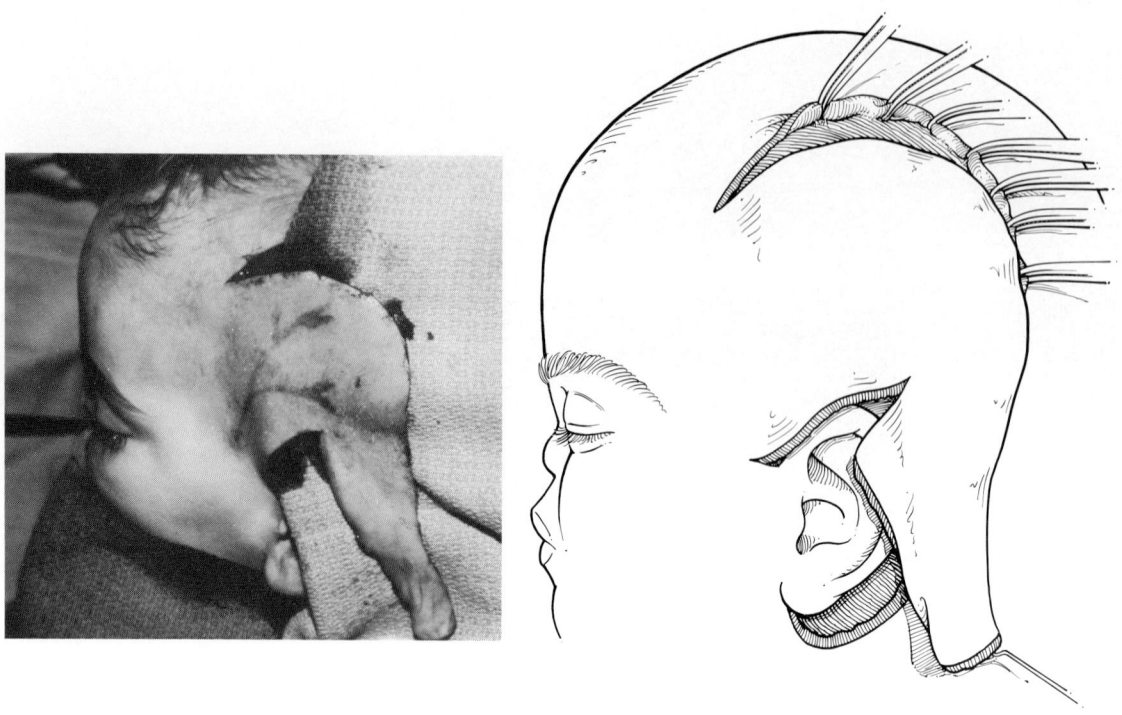

By incising vertically, the surgeon is able to lengthen the flap. To ensure vascular safety, this incising is done with transillumination of the flap; in this way all vessels can be seen and preserved.

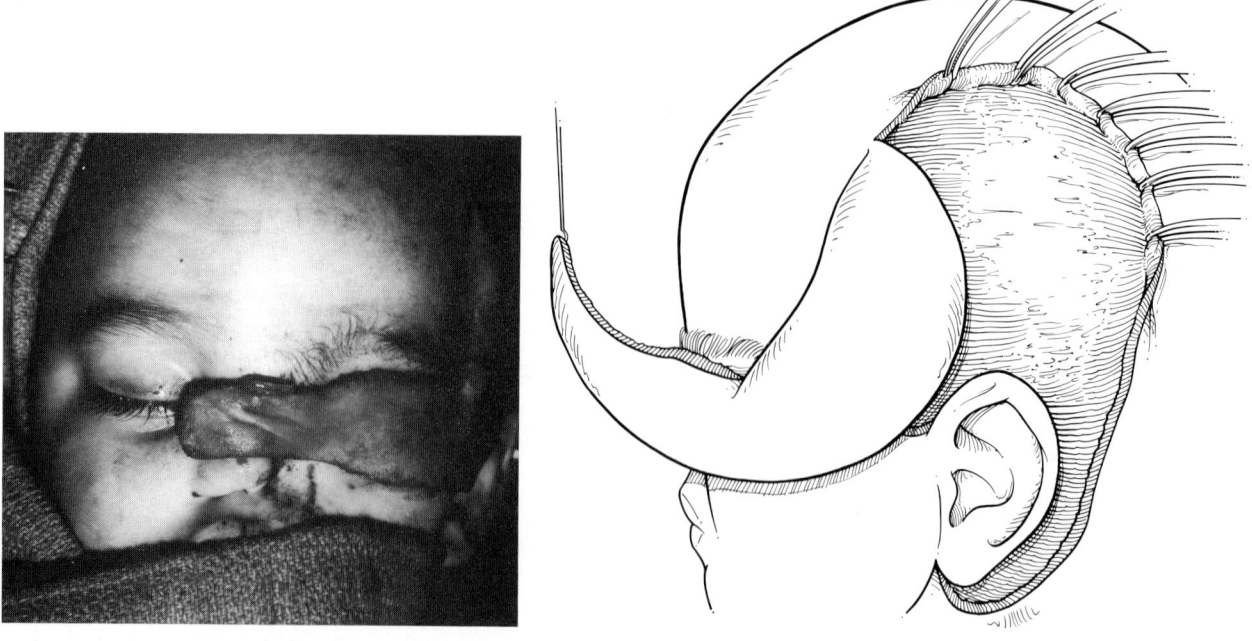

The postauricular skin now lies on the nose without tension.

CHAPTER 4
NOSE RECONSTRUCTION

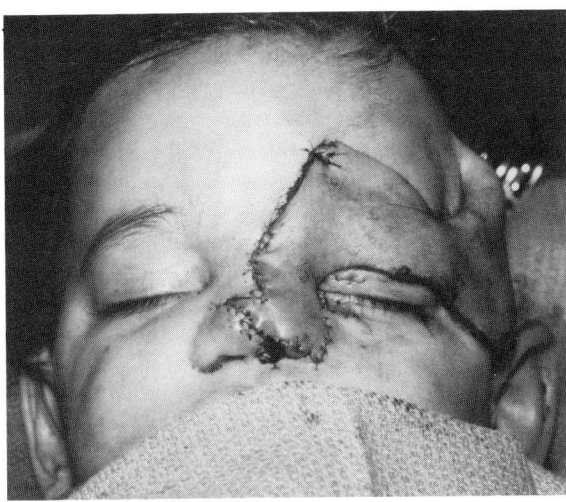 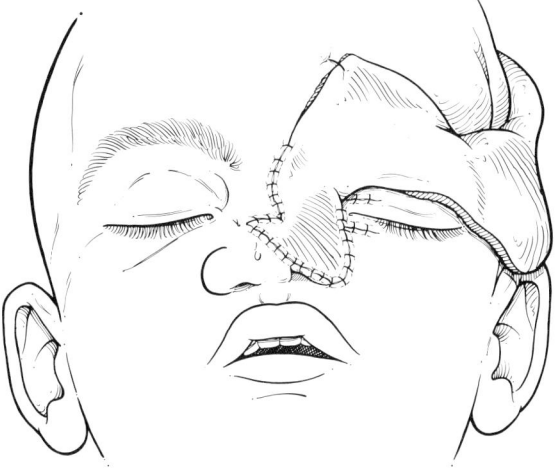

The postauricular skin is then sutured in position to reconstruct the nose.

Between 2 and 3 weeks after the initial procedure, the flap is divided and the unused portion returned. The postauricular defect is always capable of being closed directly. There is no need to skin graft the raw area; dressing is satisfactory until the unused pedicle is returned. Pigskin can be used to resurface the flap pedicle and the donor site. The advantage of this technique is the absence of donor site scars and the transfer of thin skin that is a fairly good color match for the nose.

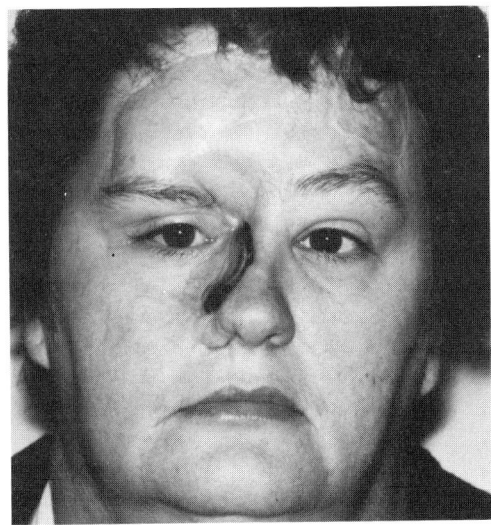 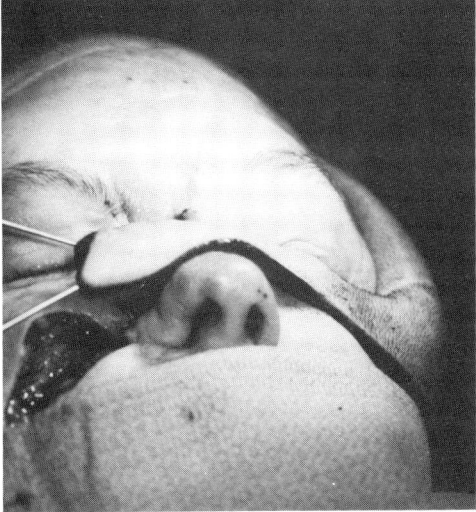

This illustration shows how far the Washio flap can be moved. The postauricular skin has been carried to a defect on the lateral aspect of the nose on the contralateral side following excision and radiotherapy for recurrent adenoceptic carcinoma of ethnoid sinus.

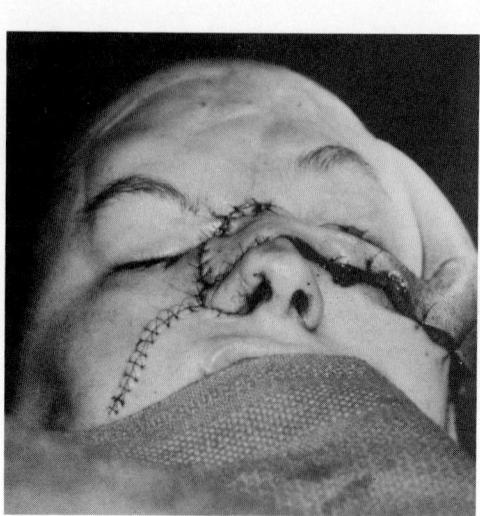
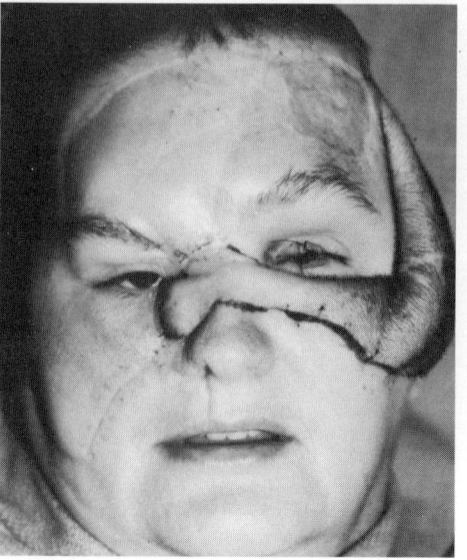

The lining for the defect was provided with an up-turned nasolabial island flap. It can be seen that the forehead had been used for reconstruction in the past and thus was no longer available as a flap.

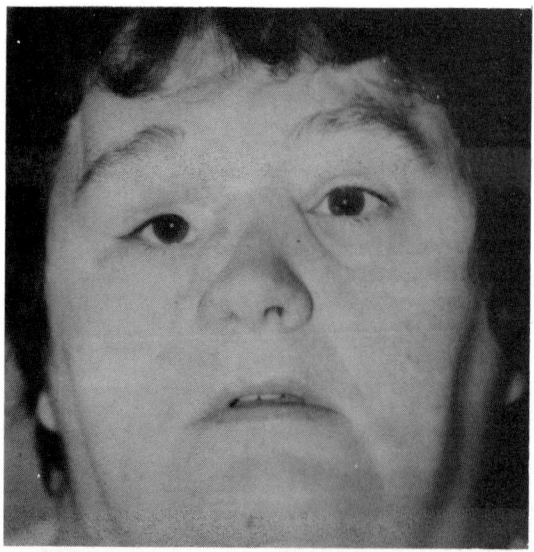

The result of this procedure was satisfactory in terms of reconstruction of this difficult area.

PROBLEMS

The Washio flap must be handled with great care to ensure that the blood supply is sufficient to maintain the postauricular skin. Accurate Doppler mapping is helpful, delay is advised, and tension must be avoided. If these measures are not followed, necrosis of the distal end of the flap and loss of the total reconstruction may result.

☐ Neck Skin

The transfer of neck skin to the nose is a useful technique, especially with extensive facial burns and/or forehead scarring and loose neck skin.

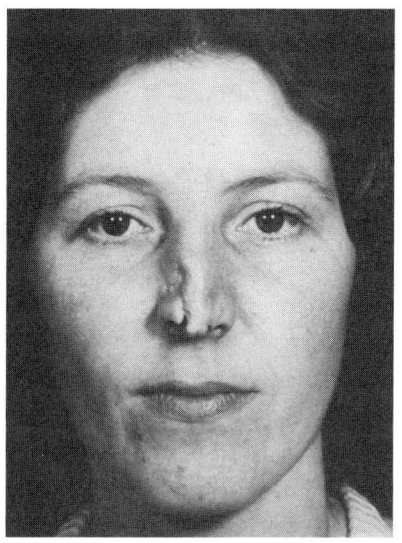
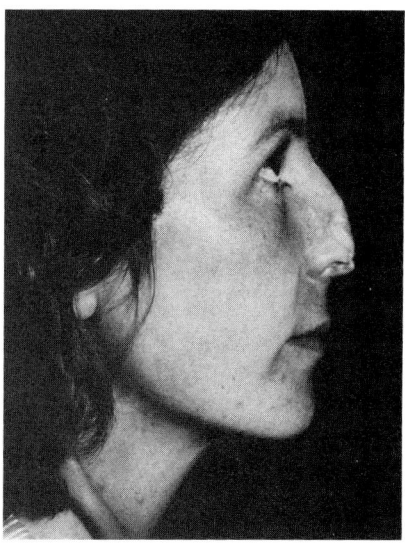

This patient had a full-thickness nasal tip defect and a forehead hemangioma. The trauma had been self-inflicted, and the psychiatrist advised against using the forehead.

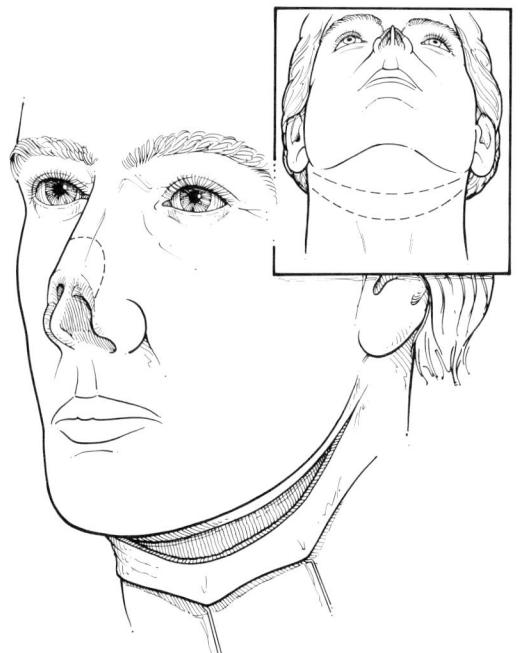
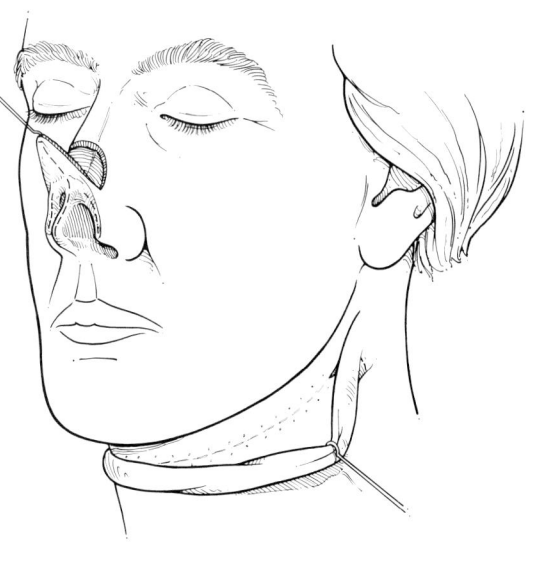

A long-tubed pedicle is raised on the neck, its ends being placed vertically below the earlobes. The pedicle is made as wide as possible, still allowing donor site closure. The donor site is closed directly.

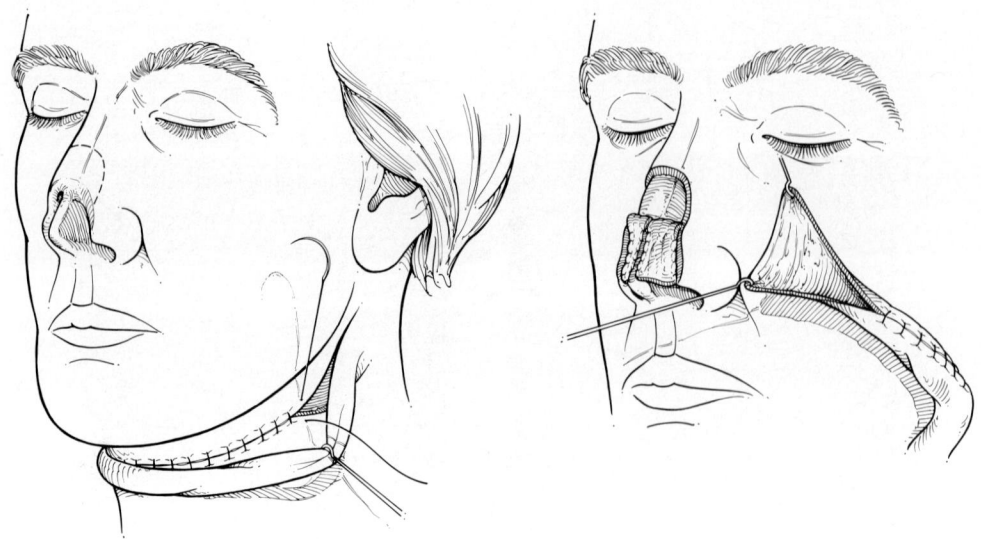

In 10 days one end can be delayed; then, after 7 to 10 days this end is taken up to the nose. Down-turned flaps are used to reconstruct nasal lining. The neck tube is then opened and used to reconstruct the skin defect.

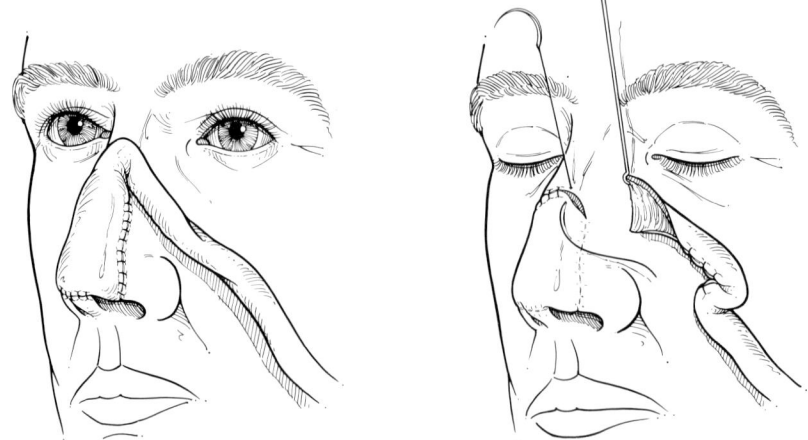

In 2 to 3 more weeks the pedicle is divided at a level that allows enough tissue for total reconstruction of the defect and the flap is inset. The remainder of the pedicle is sacrificed. In subsequent procedures the nasal reconstruction can be sculptured as dictated by the missing nasal skin.

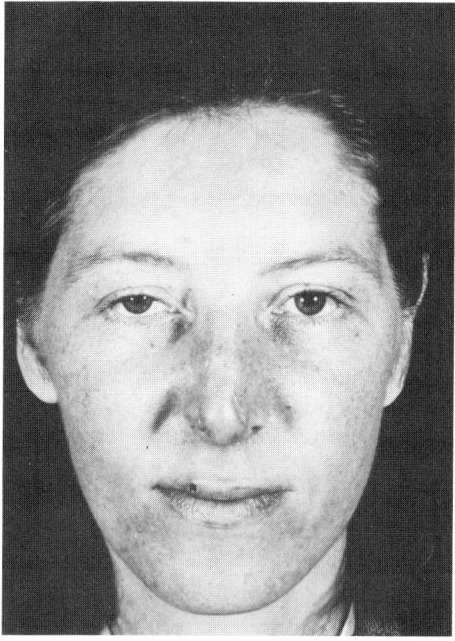
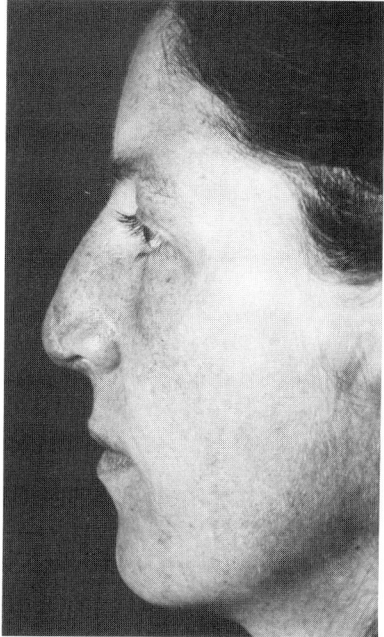

A satisfactory result can be obtained with good nasal contour, skin color, and texture.

PROBLEMS

This long flap must be delayed. If not, ischemia and necrosis will result. The neck scar may be very satisfactory, but in other situations it may be red, broad, and obvious. These problems should be carefully explained to the patient before embarking on this procedure.

☐ Surgical Technique of Choice

Undoubtedly, the forehead flap is simple, rapid, and reliable, but it does have the disadvantage of leaving a scar. With more experience, the Washio flap may become the method of choice for defects up to heminose size. This has been the case in my own practice. The skin is plentiful and thin. Color and texture are quite good, and no donor scar results. However, it is not the most robust of flaps in terms of vascularity; thus it must be planned carefully and subsequently handled with care. In the future, tissue expansion techniques may be used more frequently to provide more skin in the forehead and retroauricular areas for nasal reconstruction.

■ COMPLICATIONS

The only significant complication is loss of the flap. This is unusual, but if it occurs, the flap is removed, and another method of reconstruction is chosen. Occasionally, the skin may be lost, but some subcutaneous tissue is maintained and a skin graft can be applied to gain healing and to allow time to plan future surgery.

REFERENCES

1. Barron, J.N., and Emmett, A.J.J.: Subcutaneous island flaps, Br. J. Plast. Surg. **18**:51, 1965.
2. Esser, J.F.S.: Gestielte lokale nasanplastik mit zweizipfligem lappen, Deckung des Sekundaren Defektes vom ersten zipfel durch den zweiten, Dtsch. Z. Chirurg. **143**:385, 1918.
3. Gillies, H.D.: Plastic surgery of the face (Frowde, Hodder, and Stoughton), London, 1920, Oxford University Press.
4. Gillies, H.D.: The columella, Br. J. Plast. Surg. **2**:192, 1950.
5. Gillies, H.D., and Millard, D.R.: Principles and art of plastic surgery, Boston, 1957, Little, Brown & Co., Inc.
6. Herbert, D.C.: A subcutaneous pedicled cheek flap for reconstruction of alar defects, Br. J. Plast. Surg. **31**:79, 1978.
7. Herbert, D.C., and De Geus, J.: Nasolabial subcutaneous pedicle flaps. II. Clinical experience, Br. J. Plast. Surg. **28**:90, 1975.
8. Herbert, D.C., and Harrison, R.G.: Nasolabial subcutaneous pedicle flaps. I. Observations on their blood supply, Br. J. Plast. Surg. **28**:85, 1975.
9. Jackson, I.T., and Reid, C.D.: Nasal reconstruction and lengthening with local flaps, Br. J. Plast. Surg. **31**:343, 1978.
10. Jackson, I.T., Smith, J., and Mixter, R.C.: Nasal bone grafting using split skull grafts, Ann. Plast. Surg. **11**:533, 1983.
11. Masson, J.K., and Mendelson, B.C.: The Banner flap, Am. J. Surg. **134**:419, 1977.
12. McGregor, J.C., and Soutar, D.S.: A critical assessment of the bilobed flap, Br. J. Plast. Surg. **34**:197, 1981.
13. Meyer, R., and Kesselring, U.K.: Reconstructive surgery of the nose and orbit. In Sisson, G.A., and Tardy, E.M., editors: Plastic and reconstructive surgery of the face and neck, New York, 1977, Grune & Stratton, Inc.
14. Reiger, R.A.: A local flap for repair of the nasal tip, Plast. Reconstr. Surg. **40**:147, 1967.
15. Rintala, A.E., and Asko-Seljavaara, S.: Reconstruction of the midline skin defects of the nose, Scand. J. Plast. Reconstr. Surg. **3**:105, 1969.
16. Schmid, E.: Reconstruction of the orbit and lids, Trans. Int. Soc. Plast. Surg., London, 1959. Edinburgh, 1960, E & S Livingstone Ltd.
17. Schmid, E.: Nasal reconstruction. In Gibson, T., editor: Modern trends in plastic surgery, London, 1964, Butterworth & Co. (Publishers) Ltd.
18. Washio, H.: Retroauricular temporal flap, Plast. Reconstr. Surg. **43**:162, 1969.
19. Washio, H.: Further experience with the retroauricular temporal flap, Plast. Reconstr. Surg. **50**:160, 1972.

CHAPTER 5

CHEEK RECONSTRUCTION

> Blessings on thee, little man
> Barefoot boy, with cheek of tan.
>
> JOHN GREENLEAF WHITTIER
> *The Barefoot Boy*

> Have you not a moist eye, a dry hand, a yellow cheek, a white beard,
> a decreasing leg and an increasing belly?
>
> WILLIAM SHAKESPEARE
> *Henry IV*

As the poets indicate, the cheeks, probably more than any other area of the face, show a variation from individual to individual. Furthermore, as the individual ages, the cheeks change in character. Full, fresh rosy cheeks or plump polished cheeks do not remain so forever. With age they sag and they change in color and shape. The latter change has consolations; more skin is available for the reconstructive procedures that are more frequently required in this age group.

ANATOMY

Skin

Because of its color and texture variation, the Caucasian cheek offers the greatest challenge in reconstruction. The skin over the malar area is thick, highly colored, and shiny; in many people there is an almost telangiectatic appearance in this region. The preauricular skin is pale and thin and of a matt surface texture. The lower cheek skin is less pale than the preauricular skin and not so red as the malar skin; it is intermediate in texture. With age the skin may become more yellow, although in some individuals the malar skin becomes redder often with a shade of purple. In the male the beard area must be carefully observed. All of these factors should be considered when flaps are being planned. The wrong skin in the wrong place will mar an otherwise excellent result.

Musculature

Under the skin lies the investing fascial layer of the head and neck area, the superficial musculoaponeurotic system (SMAS). This fascial layer is located between the skin and the deeper structures, such as the parotid gland, the facial nerve branches, and the muscles of the face.[1] In the neck it is continuous with the platysma muscle.

Deep to this layer lies the parotid gland and its duct, the facial nerve branches emerging from the gland, and the superficial layer of facial muscles. These muscles are the orbicularis oculi, levator labii superioris alaeque nasi, levator labii superioris, levator angulioris, zygomaticus major and minor, depressor angulioris, depressor labii inferioris, and orbicularis oris. The deep muscle group consists of masseter and buccinator.

Nerve Supply

MOTOR NERVES

All the superficial muscles are supplied by branches of the facial nerve (CN VII). The buccinator obtains its motor nerve supply from the lower buccal branches of the facial nerve.

The masseter muscle is supplied by a branch of the anterior trunk of the mandibular nerve, which originates from the third division of the trigeminal nerve (CN V).

SENSORY NERVES

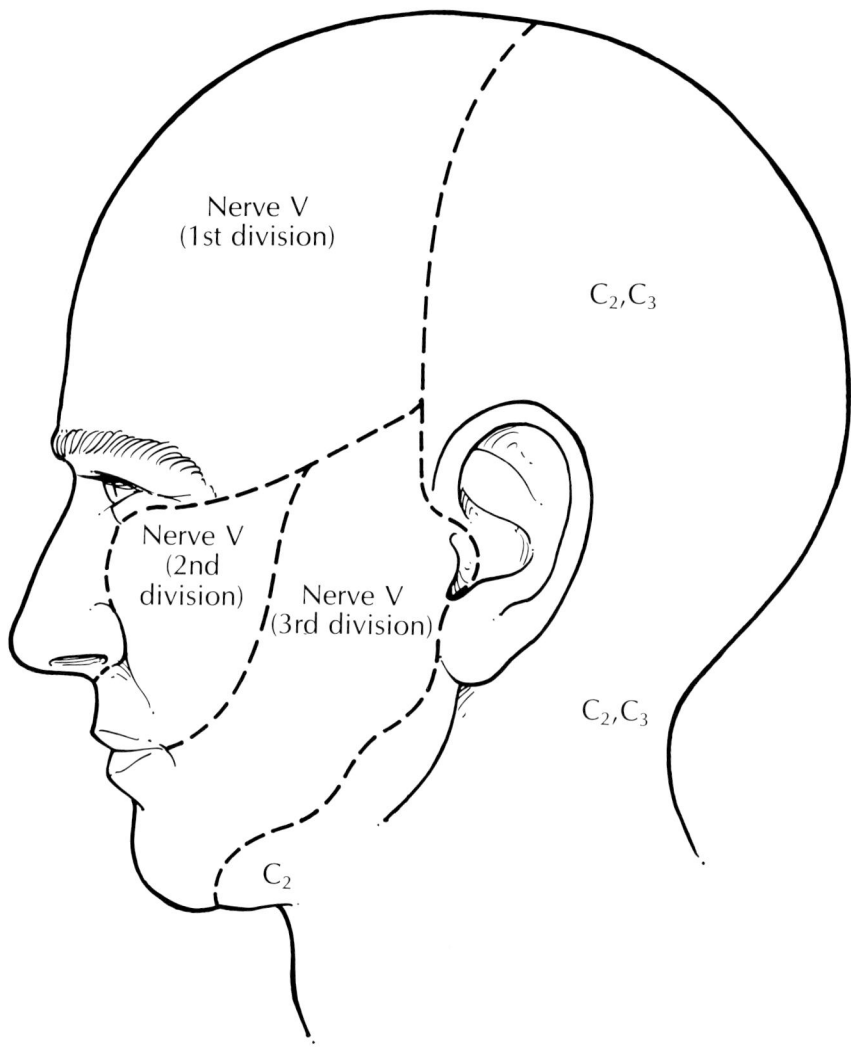

The sensory supply of the cheek is provided largely by the trigeminal nerve. The area from the nose-cheek junction to the line joining the oral commissure to the temporal hairline at the level of the lateral canthus is supplied by the second division through the infraorbital nerve (second division of CN V). The area lateral to this one, extending to the tragus but not incorporating the ear and stopping short of the inferior border of the mandible, receives sensation from branches of the mandibular nerve (third division of CN V). The remaining small lower cheek area and the ear are supplied by the anterior cutaneous nerve of the neck and the greater auricular nerve. These originate in the cervical plexus (CN II and III).

☐ Blood Supply

The arterial supply is largely from the external carotid artery with a contribution from the transverse facial artery, which, like the facial artery, is a branch of the external carotid. The venous drainage is mainly by way of the anterior facial vein.

☐ Lymphatic System

The cheek area is abundantly supplied by a lymphatic drainage system that ends in the parotid nodes, the nodes surrounding the facial vessels, and the submandibular nodes. All of these ultimately drain into the cervical nodes.

■ AESTHETICS

Because of the color and textural variations of facial skin, it is easy to have a poor skin match after flap transfer if due care is not taken. Pale, matt skin in a ruddy polished area is obvious and will remain so. This difference in skin color and texture may be even more striking in the summer, when skin color changes with exposure to the sun. Hairbearing skin transferred to nonhairbearing areas could pose a distressing problem to the patient. Therefore thought must be given to the planning of flaps to prevent these problems from occurring. The surgeon should be constantly studying the aesthetic pattern and variations of the face. In reconstruction of the cheek one important consideration that often may be neglected is to make the thickness of the flap as close as possible to that of the defect. In this way major contour deficiencies may be avoided.

■ PLACEMENT OF INCISIONS

Scars on the cheek may be obvious, and therefore, if possible, they should be placed in the lines of minimal relaxed tension or in the aging lines (see Chapter 1). If planning is satisfactory, few transverse stresses will be placed on the incisions. The resulting scars are narrow and lie in the natural lines of the face, well camouflaged. Occasionally, this ideal situation of scars lying in exactly the correct line may not be possible. This fact must be explained to the patient, and, if necessary, secondary revision can be performed at a later date. Frequently Z-plasties or W-plasties may be employed.

■ AREAS OF TISSUE AVAILABILITY

Local skin can frequently be used to reconstruct cheek defects. The flaps require rotation or advancement of lower facial or preauricular loose skin, which becomes more abundant with aging. The neck is another useful region outside the face. Neck skin is plentiful, has good color and texture, and is easy to move. The forehead may also be used but only in cases of dire necessity. Generally, results with forehead flaps are poor because of the skin's pale color and matt texture. Any significant forehead donor area requires a skin graft that leaves a large cosmetic deformity.

■ AREAS TO BE RECONSTRUCTED

There are several distinct areas in the cheek that have their own particular anatomic characteristics. In each area the skin is different and the contours are unique. For reconstructive purposes the cheek has been divided into the lateral area, the lower cheek, the malar region, the supramedial, and the alar base–nasolabial area. Each will be considered individually from all points of view.

☐ Lateral Cheek Reconstruction

In the male the beard area and the sideburns are definite anatomic features that should not be altered. Pale preauricular skin should not be placed in more highly colored areas. The tragus should not be altered in position and shape.

Fortunately, this is a region where direct closure is usually possible, especially in the older patient. Undermining the skin as in a face-lift produces a generous amount of skin for reconstruction. Occasionally, this is not the case and a local flap is used.

PREAURICULAR TRANSPOSITION FLAP

In this technique the excess of preauricular skin is judged by pinching it between the thumb and index finger. The surgeon can use a length of gauze to simulate the proposed flap and to help him decide whether it is suitable for closure of the defect.

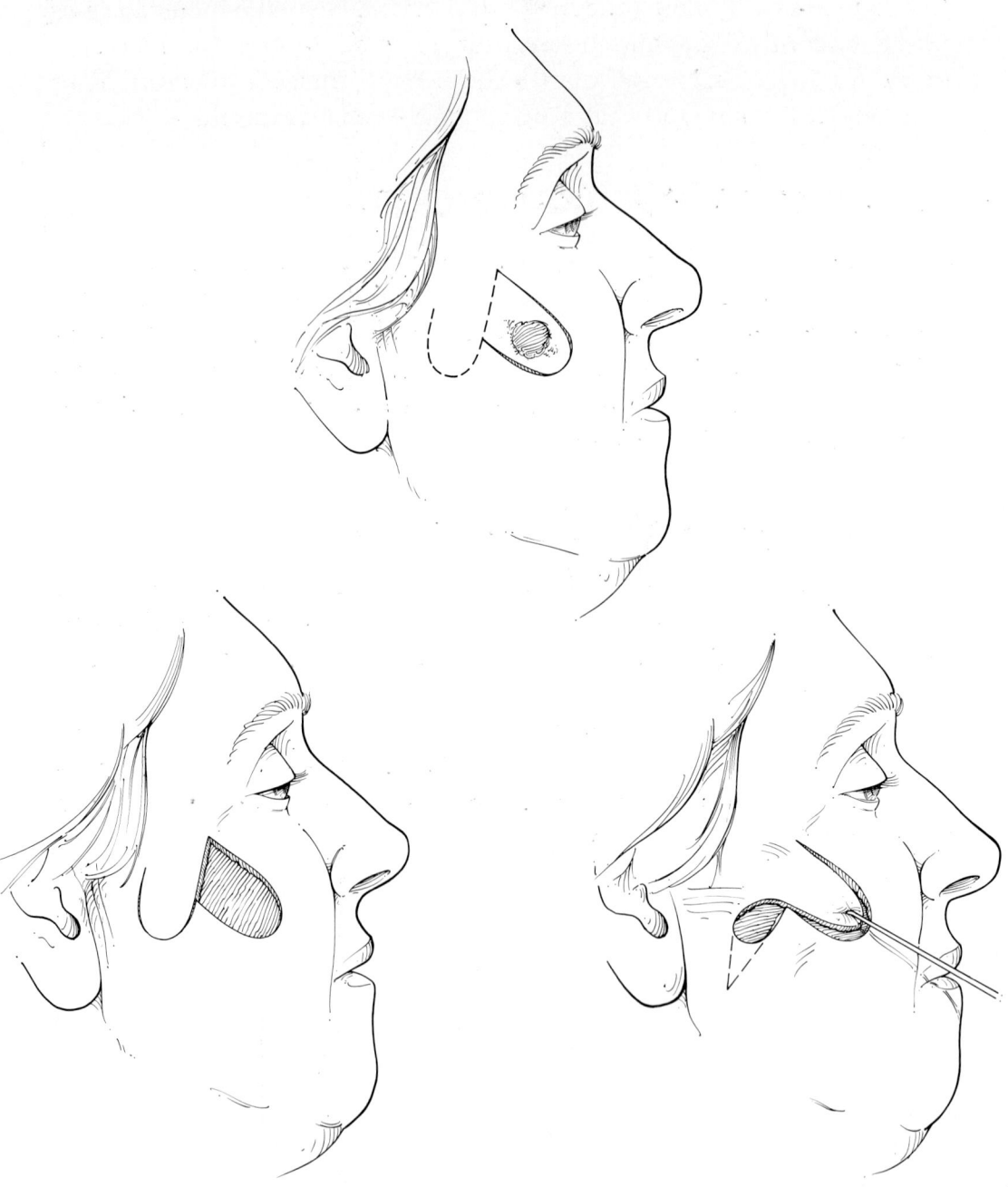

The skin flap is then designed, elevated, and transposed to close the cheek defect. The transposition can be through any range up to 90 degrees.

CHAPTER 5
CHEEK RECONSTRUCTION

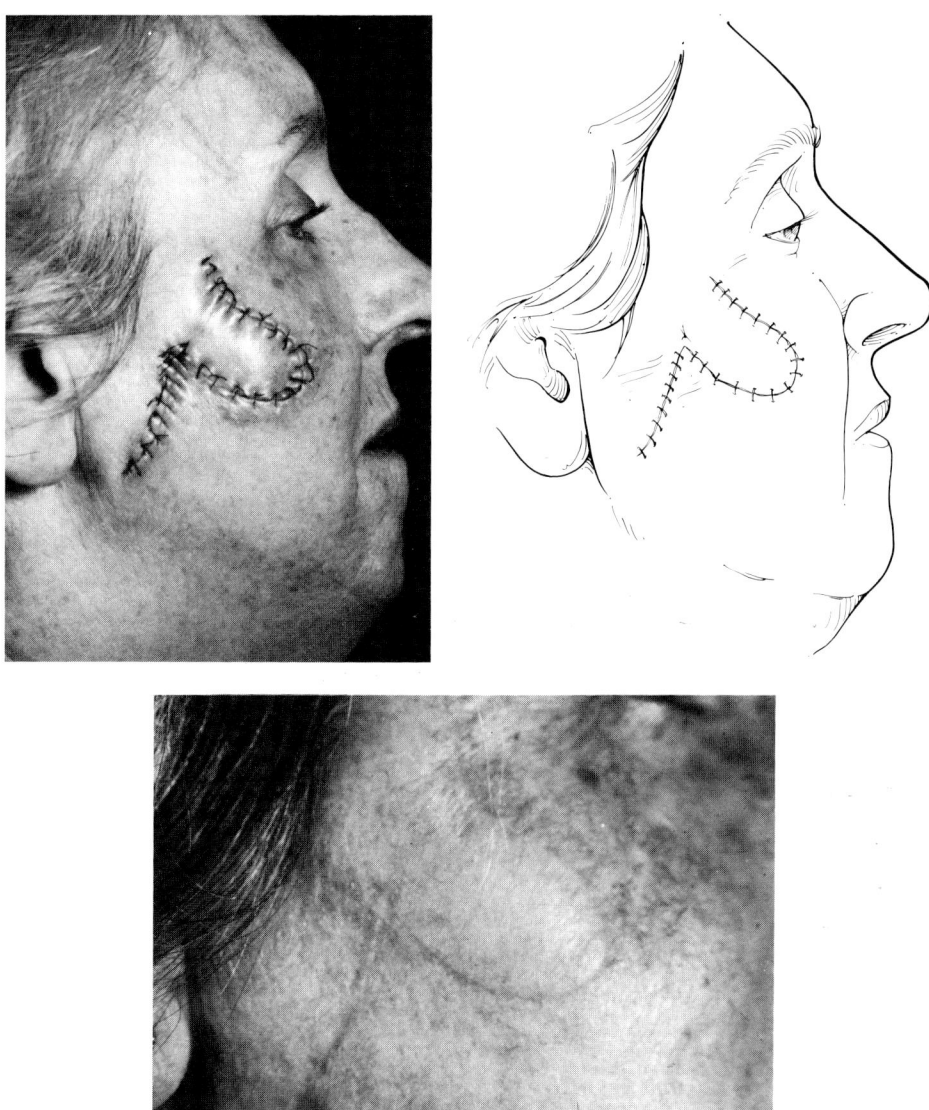

The medial end of the base of the pedicle will develop a standing cone deformity that will require trimming; care should be taken not to compromise the width of the pedicle. The donor site is closed directly.

PROBLEMS

Preauricular skin is thin and pale. Thus it is different from the remainder of the cheek. The latter is thick, highly colored, and in the male, hairbearing. The flap is somewhat obvious when compared with the more florid skin over the malar eminence. It was previously thought that with time this skin would become similar to cheek skin. Experience has shown that this is not the case.

ROTATION FLAP

The rotation flap allows closure of a triangulated defect. The design is simpler than the transposition flap, but undermining and mobilization are more extensive.

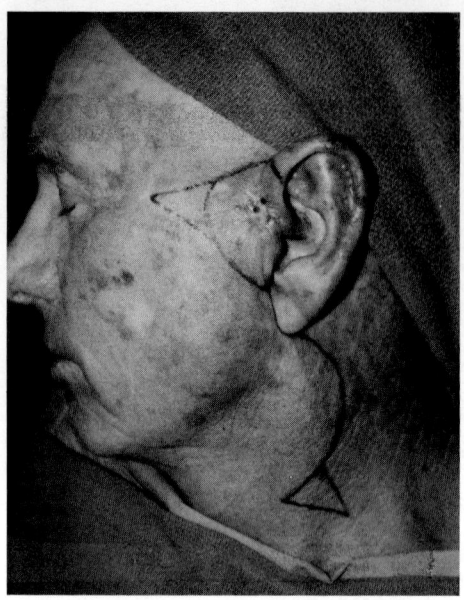

The defect is triangulated with the base laterally or superiorly. If the base is lateral, the skin is rotated from the lower part of the cheek. If the base is superior, the rotation is from the preauricular area. Note that a Burow's triangle has been outlined inferiorly to deal with the standing cone that will develop at that area as a result of the skin rotation.

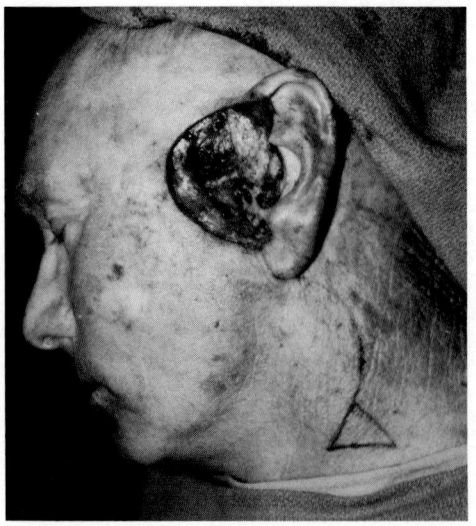

The squamous cell carcinoma has been resected. Only after a frozen section report of total excision will the area be formally triangulated.

CHAPTER 5
CHEEK RECONSTRUCTION

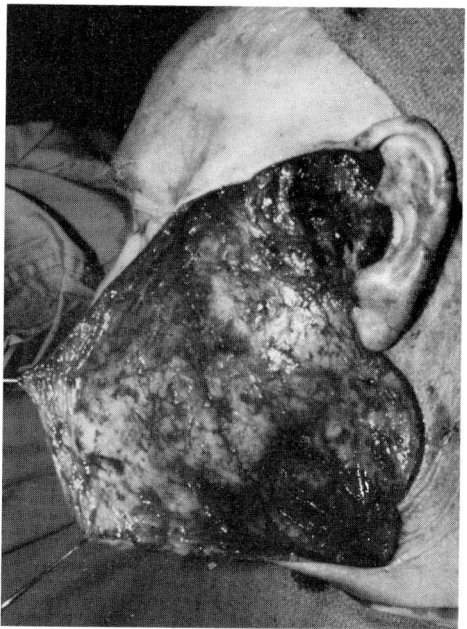

The inferior rotation flap is widely elevated in the face-lift plane.

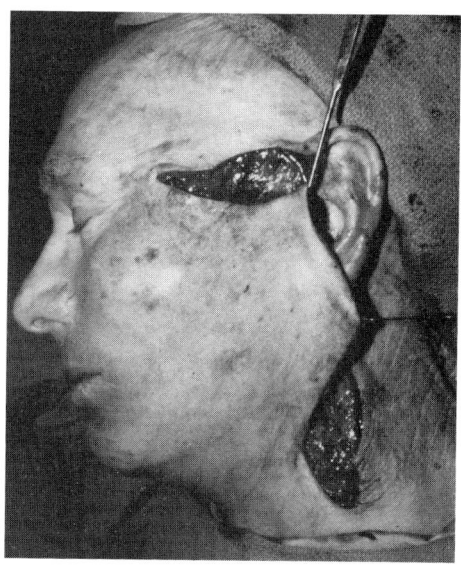

If the flap design and the undermining have been adequate, closure of the post excisional defects occurs without difficulty.

If the base is superior, the rotation is from the preauricular area. As the flap is rotated and sutured into position, excess skin will remain on the cheek side of the flap and result in the development of a standing cone at the end of the arc of rotation. This excess of skin is trimmed as a triangle based toward the flap; in this way the flap itself is not violated. The original vascularity is left undisturbed.

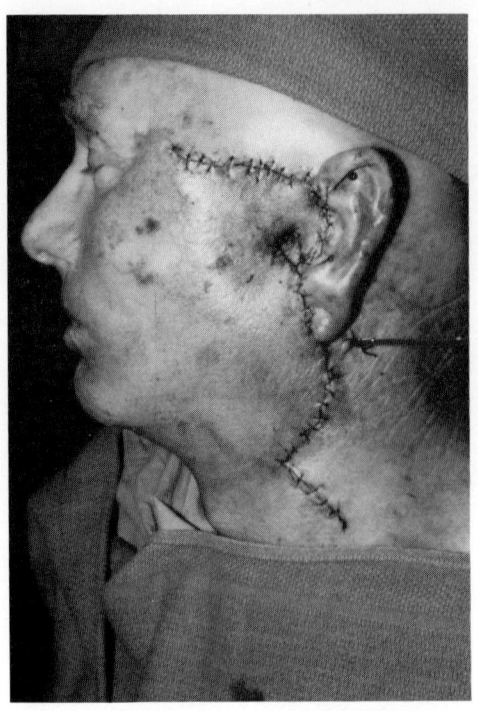

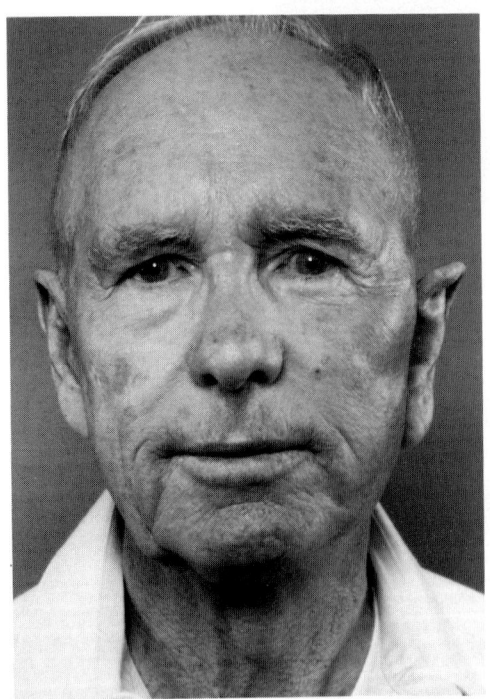
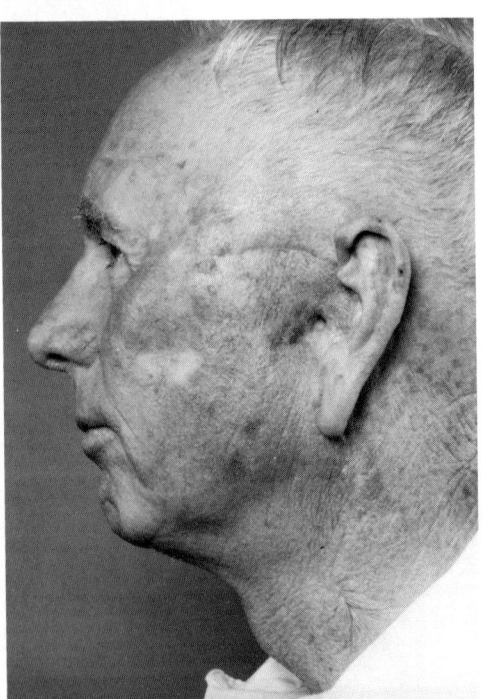

The defect is closed. Burow's triangle has been removed, and the incisions contour well into natural lines on the face and neck.

PROBLEMS

As with the transposition flap, any rotation of preauricular skin anteriorly is a mistake. In the male the line of the hairline will be altered.

BILOBED FLAP

The bilobed flap can be used for small- to moderate-sized lateral cheek defects; undermining and mobilization are less extensive than with the rotation flap, but scarring is more extensive. This flap allows rotation of skin through an arc of up to 180 degrees. The surgeon should judge the practicality of using this flap by assessing how much skin is available in the area from which the second flap will come.

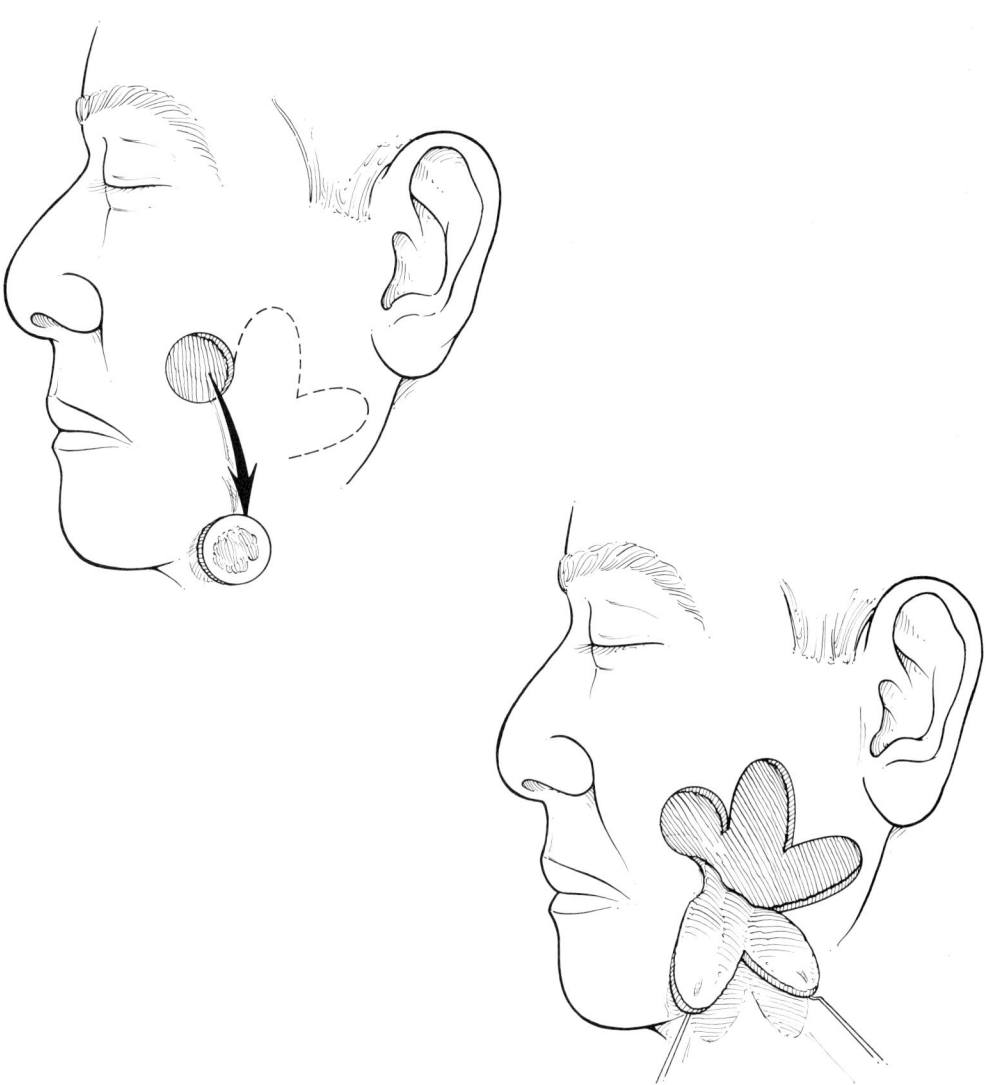

The defect is planned and flap 1, smaller than the defect, is outlined; the axis of the flap is at a 45- to 90-degree angle to the axis of the defect, as dictated by the skin transfer. A still slightly smaller flap 2 is drawn, again at 45 to 90 degrees to the axis of flap 1.

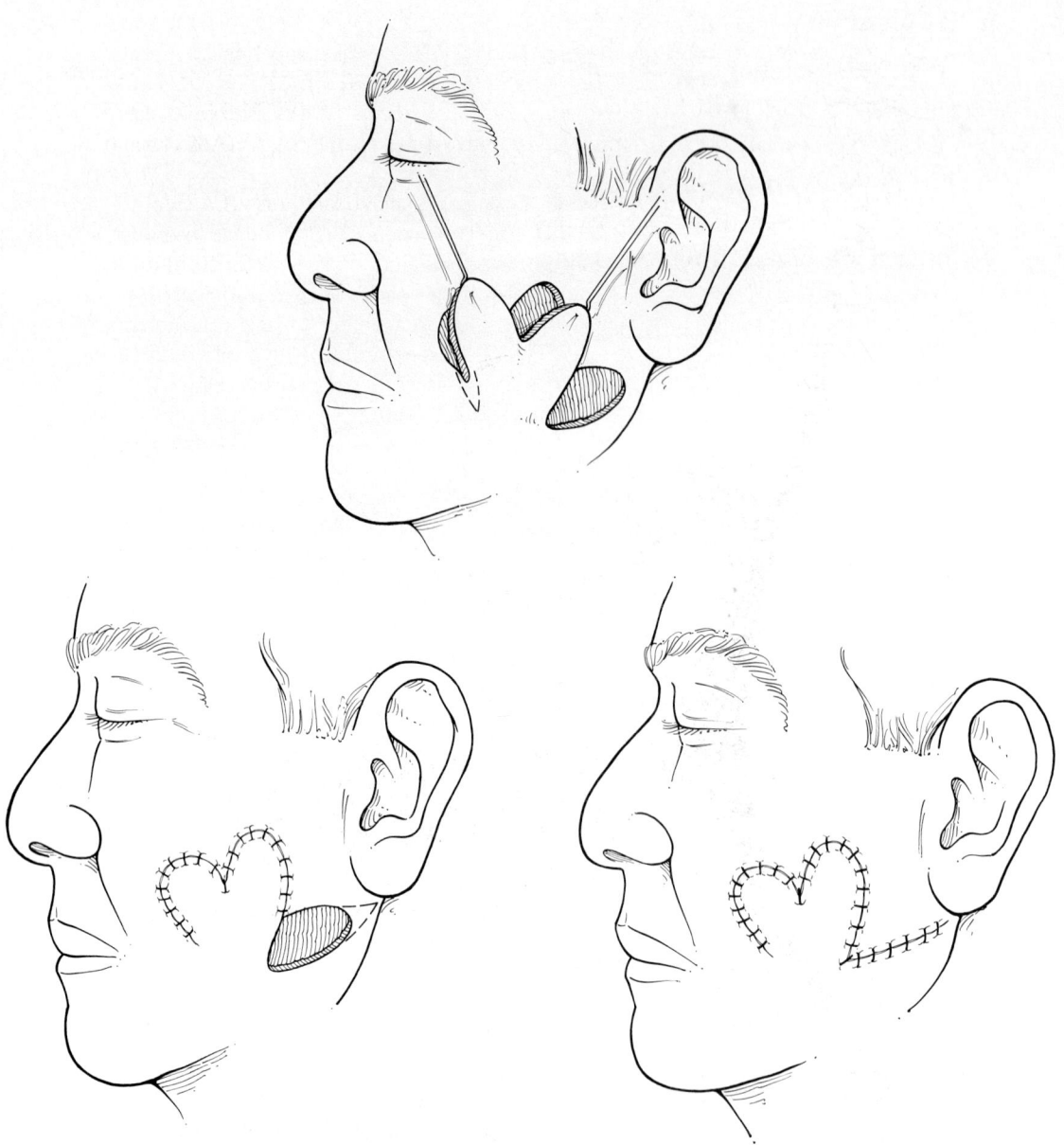

The defect is created and the flaps are transposed. Any necessary trimming is performed, and defect 2 is closed directly.

CHAPTER 5
CHEEK
RECONSTRUCTION

PROBLEMS

As with the preauricular transposition flap the bilobed flap may provide poor skin distribution. More significant is the extensive scarring that results from this procedure in the lateral cheek region. This scarring is obvious and unacceptable; worst of all, it is difficult, if not impossible, to improve. An additional problem results from the pincushioning effect that occurs in some cases and makes the reconstruction very obvious. A second procedure to defat the flaps is required to correct the problem, but it is not always entirely effective.

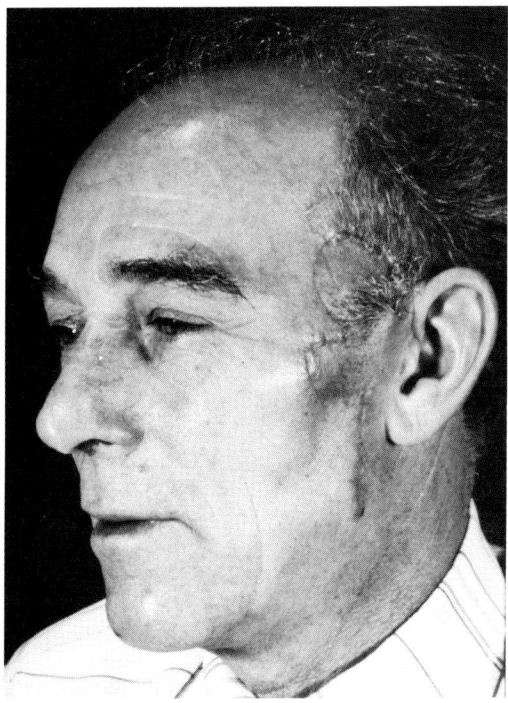
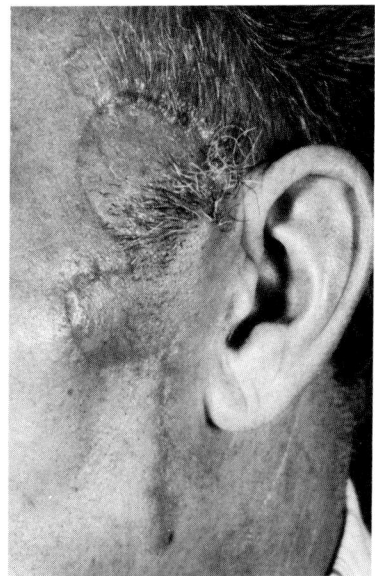

Frequently as depicted here, the hairline may be altered in a way that cannot be camouflaged in the future, a particular problem for the male patient.

201

RHOMBOID FLAP

The rhomboid flap can be used to close defects similar to those already discussed. Its geometric design makes it more rigid than some flaps, but it allows for very exact planning. The planning of the rhomboid is very similar to that undertaken for the transposition flap.

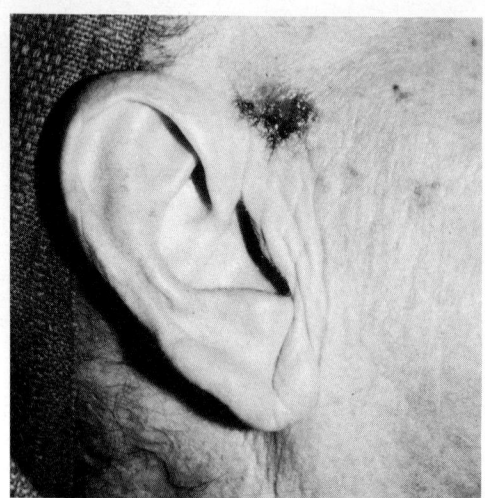 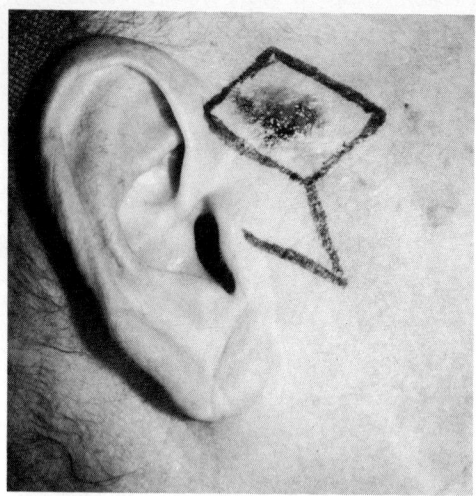

This preauricular basal cell carcinoma is suitable for excision as a rhomboid and closure by means of a rhomboid flap.

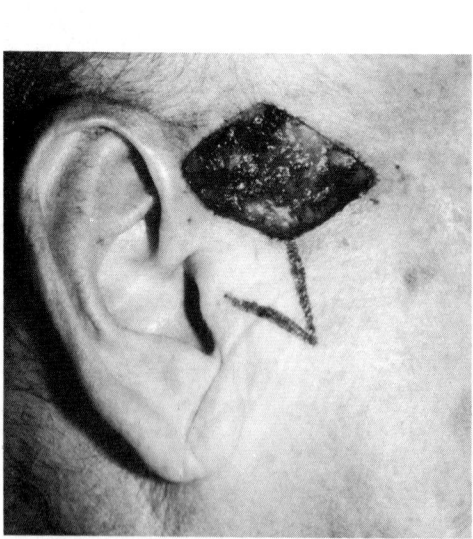 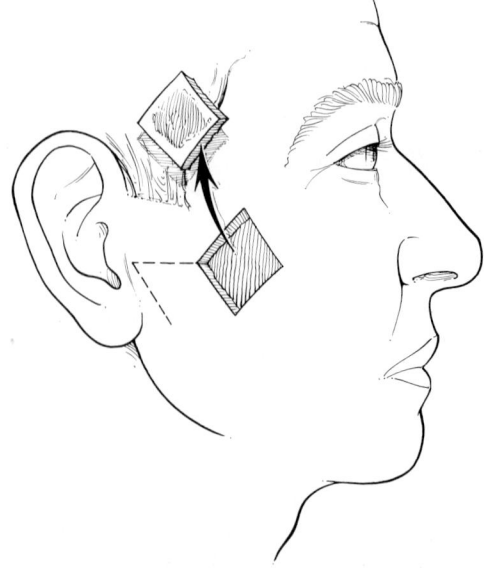

The lesion is excised with the 120-degree angle of the rhomboid placed caudally. Thus an inferior rhomboid flap is designed. Alternatively, as in the diagram above, the flap may come from the preauricular area as a posterior rhomboid moving anteriorly.

CHAPTER 5
**CHEEK
RECONSTRUCTION**

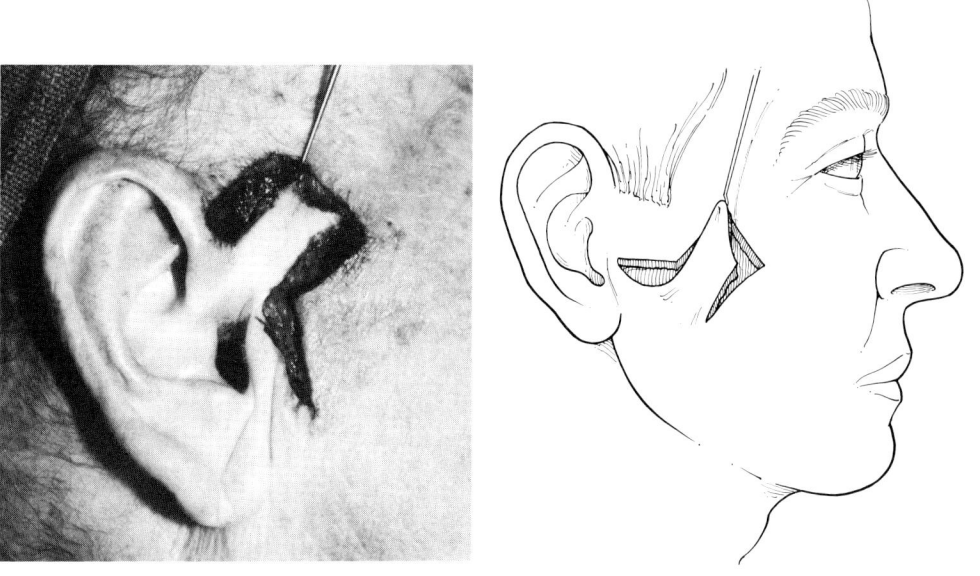

The mobile flap is transposed into the defect without difficulty.

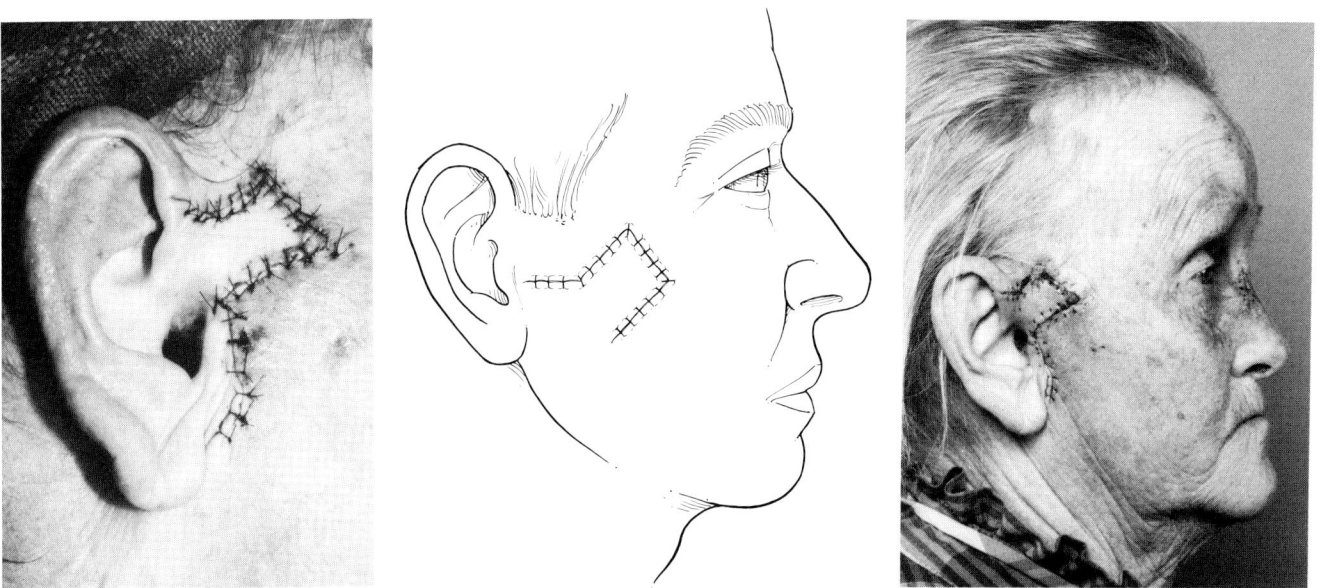

The flap contours well on the face, and the donor incision is in an acceptable position whether the flap moves vertically or horizontally.

PROBLEMS

Poor redistribution of skin and a complex scar pattern mar this type of reconstruction. As with rhomboid flaps in other areas, pincushioning is not a problem.

203

SURGICAL TECHNIQUE OF CHOICE

The most practical reconstruction in most cases is that of an inferiorly based rotation flap. In areas closer to the malar region a laterally based rotation flap may give a very satisfactory result. In some females the preauricular transposition flap may be satisfactory; it should be performed only on those patients having pale, thin skin on all areas on the side of the face. This flap requires less experience in flap planning than the rhomboid flap. Thus the margin for error is greater.

☐ Lower Cheek Reconstruction

The lower cheek is a very obvious area of the face, and therefore scars and contour irregularities are easily noticed. If incisions are taken over the body of the mandible, the resulting scars often stretch, become indrawn, and are difficult to correct. In the male this region is the beard area, and so hearbearing skin is required for its reconstruction.

The loose skin of the neck is a fruitful region for taking local flaps. In planning such flaps the concavity of the neck and the convexity of the area overlying the body of the mandible must be considered. A vertical scar on the neck will contract and cause a band. A similar scar over the mandible will show the problems already mentioned. The neck skin may be slightly paler than that of the lower face skin, and in the male it will often contain less hair.

The excess of skin in the lower face is again posterior and inferior. All local flaps must come from these areas.

CHAPTER 5
CHEEK RECONSTRUCTION

RHOMBOID FLAP

Even large defects can be closed with rhomboid flaps taken from the neck. Accurate closure of the rhomboid defect will always be possible without difficulty.

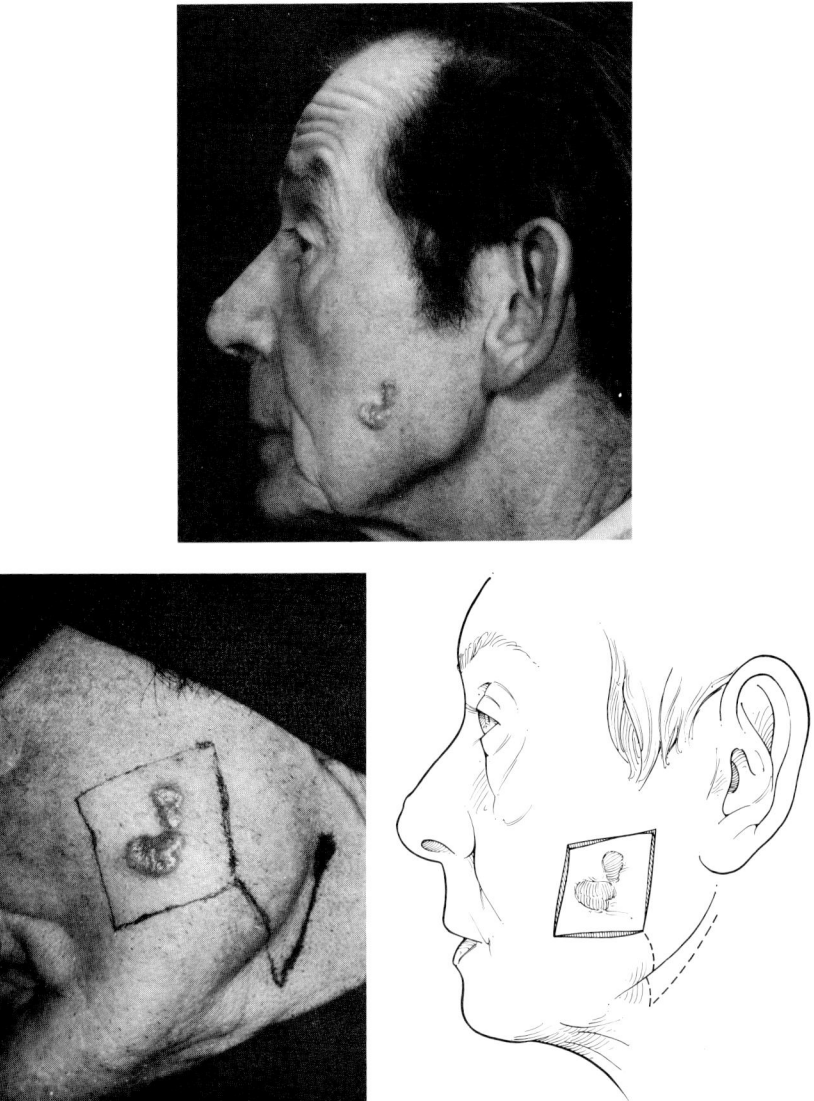

It is better to plan the flap with a donor site that will be closed with a vertical scar. Thus, as this patient with a lower cheek basal cell carcinoma demonstrates, the rhomboid is positioned with the 120-degree angle situated caudally. Unless the defect is very large, a rhomboid flap closure will usually be possible.

205

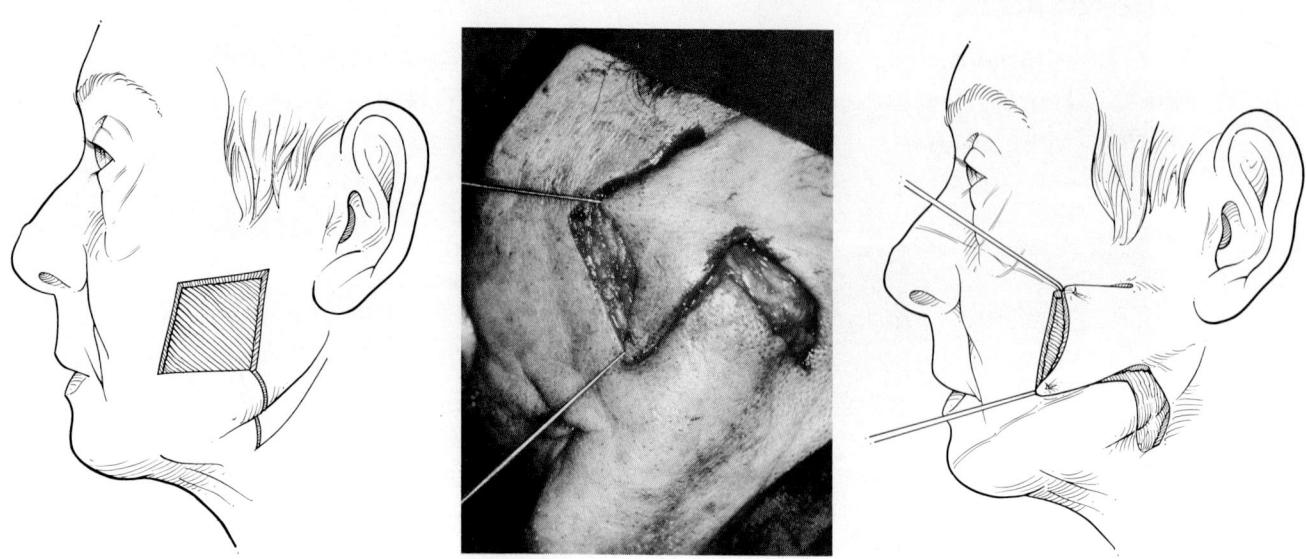

After excision of the basal cell carcinoma, the posteriorly based rhomboid flap is transposed into the defect. The neck donor site is closed directly without difficulty.

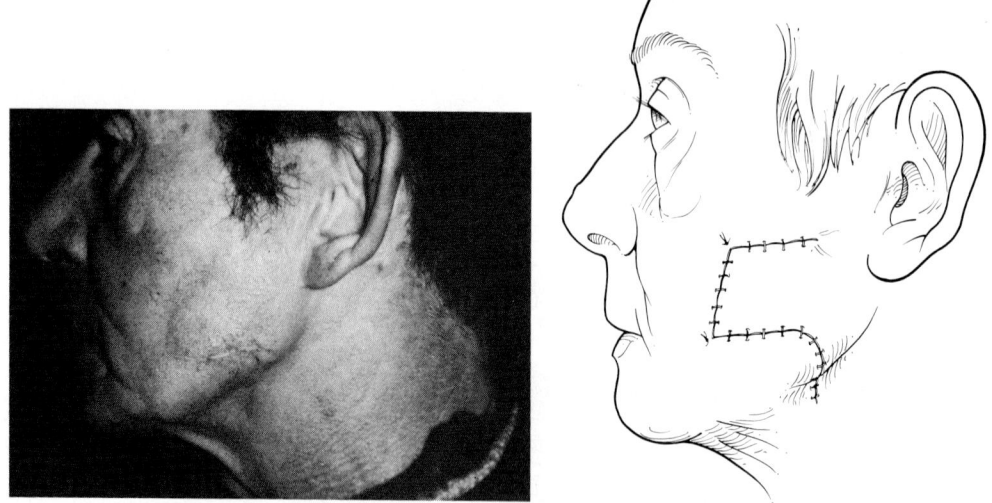

The rhomboid flap is successfully integrated into the face without contour problems and the scar is usually quite acceptable.

PROBLEMS

The scar associated with the rhomboid flap is complex, and if there is a healing problem, it would be obvious. The vertical mandibular scar can become indrawn, and the resulting contour change can make the scar noticeable and difficult to improve.

CHAPTER 5
CHEEK RECONSTRUCTION

TRANSPOSITION FLAP

The transposition flap is indicated for defects similar to those described for the rhomboid flap. Planning is somewhat simpler and a length of gauze can be used in place of the flap to assess dimensions and rotation.

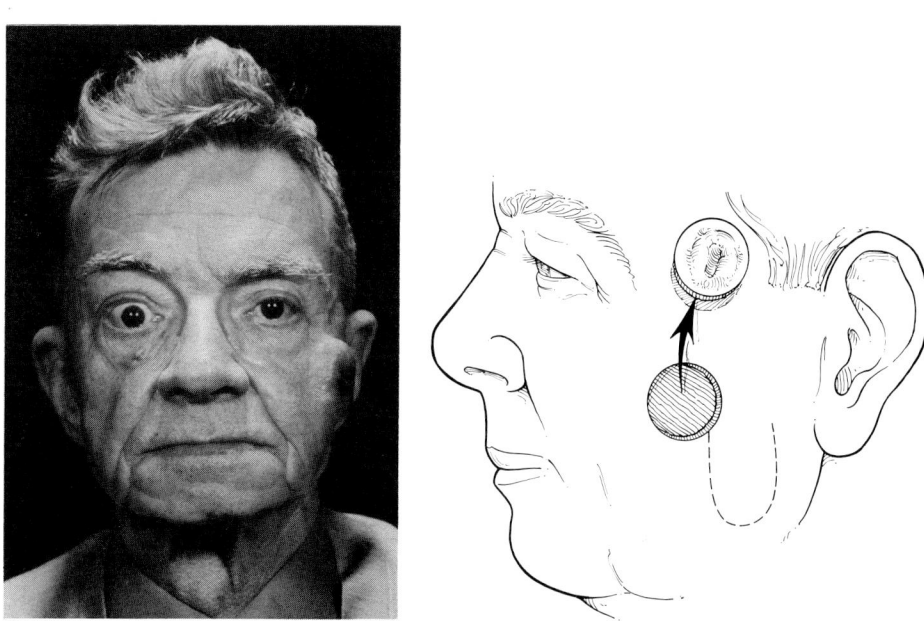

In effect, this is a rhomboid without angles, as can be seen in the reconstruction used for this patient to correct a defect left from resection for a basal cell carcinoma of the cheek. The method of assessment of flap availability is exactly the same, with thumb and index finger used.

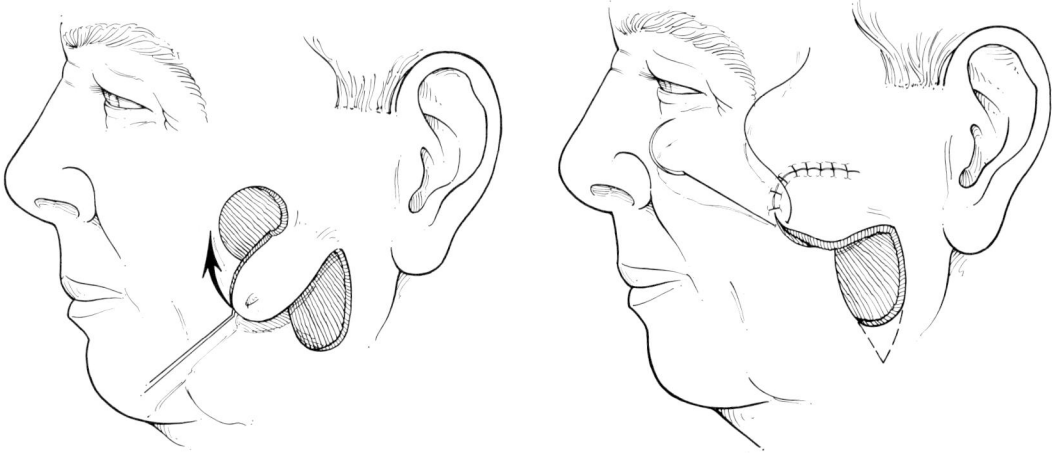

After the flap has been rotated and sutured into position, a standing cone develops at the upper part of the flap base and needs to be trimmed. (For a more detailed description of this flap, see pp. 10-11.)

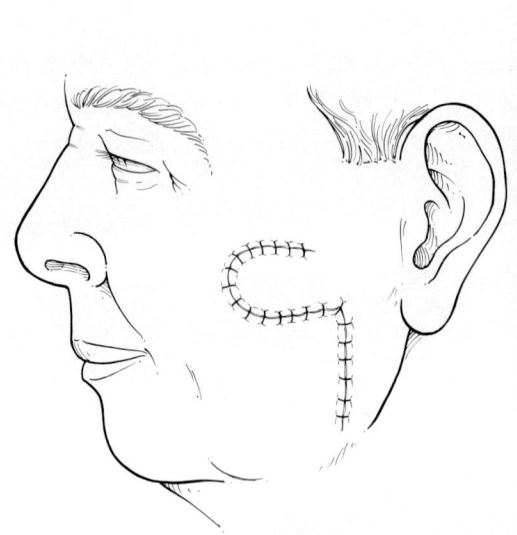
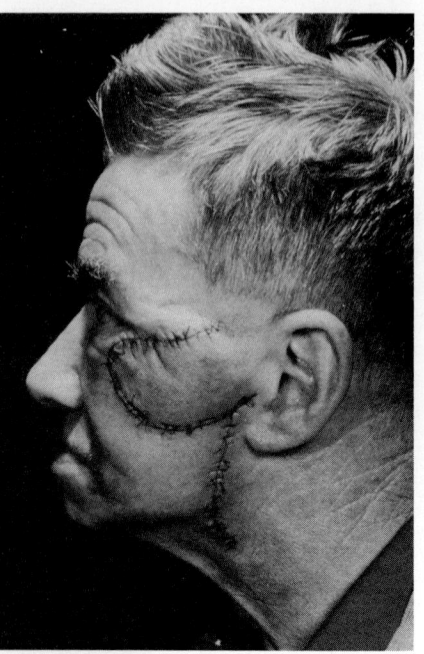
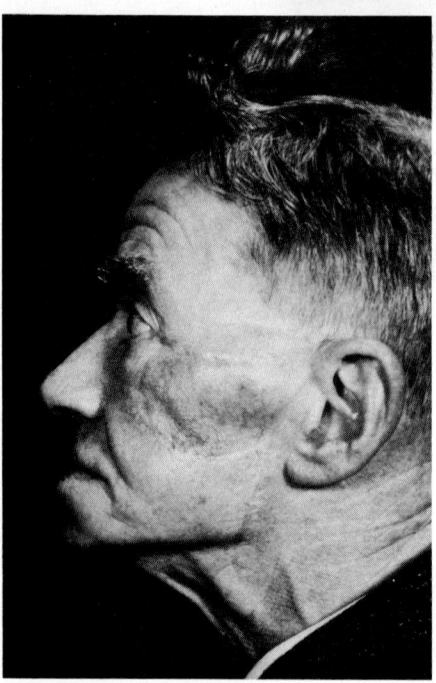

In this particular case, perhaps as a result of the size of the flap and the age of the patient, the flap has contoured well into the face. No pincushioning has occurred, and the scars show little evidence of contracture. There is some degree of color and texture variation in relation to the surrounding skin.

PROBLEMS

The problems with the transposition flap are the same as those of the rhomboid flap, namely, the complex scar and the vertical scar running over the mandible. The transposition flap has the additional risk of pincushioning. When this occurs, the subcutaneous fat of the flap must be thinned, a procedure that may not be entirely successful.

ROTATION FLAP

Fairly large lower face defects can be closed by using a rotation flap, but the surgeon needs to undermine and mobilize more neck skin than is necessary for the rhomboid or conventional transpositional flap. The eventual scar is less complex, yet it does extend over the mandibular body and may be obvious in this area.

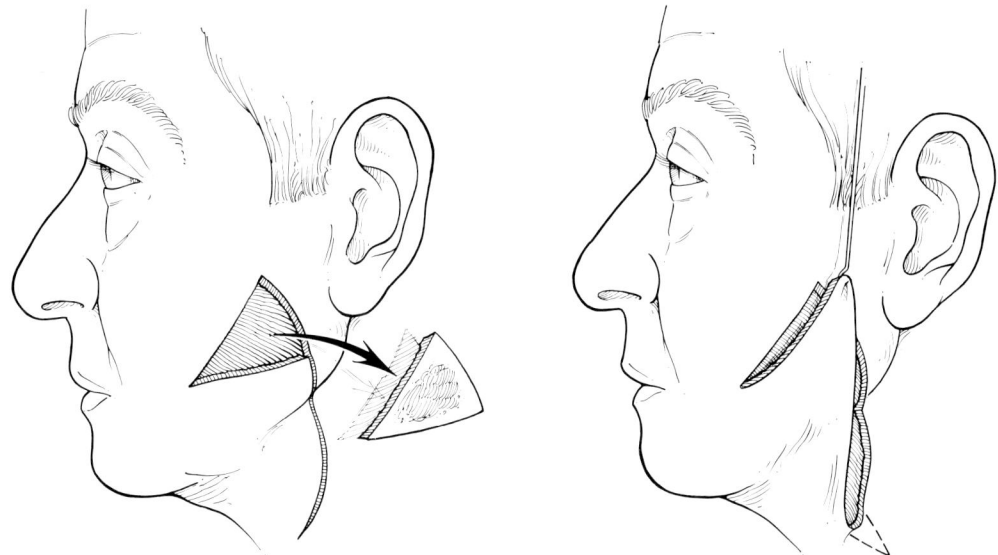

In preparation for the use of a rotation flap, the surgeon triangulates the defect. The flap design is taken down onto the neck. As in all neck-to-face flaps, care must be taken to avoid damage to the mandibular branch of the facial nerve. As a precaution the surgeon must be certain to dissect above the platysma. If the facial vessels are seen, then the nerve is nearby. As the flap rotates upward, an excess of skin develops on the outer edge of the skin incision.

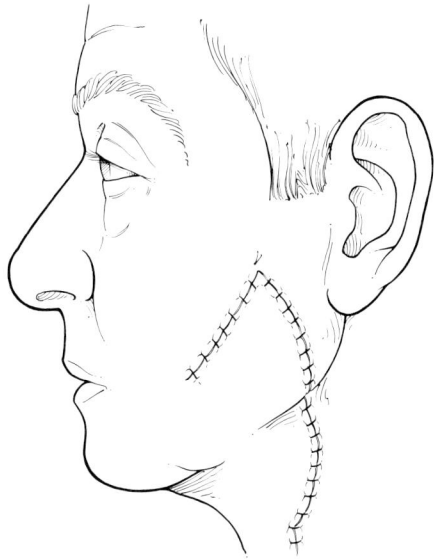

After suturing of the flap is complete, the excess should be trimmed in a direction away from the flap base.

PROBLEMS

The rotation flap has not been a very satisfactory type of reconstruction. It always seems to result in a degree of downward pull. In addition, the flap often pincushions, and the neck scars may become obvious. Planning for the rotation flap is not as positive and secure as for the transposition flaps.

SURGICAL TECHNIQUE OF CHOICE

The rhomboid flap is now considered to be the procedure of choice. Planning is accurate and the scar is acceptable. The transposition flap is very similar to the rhomboid flap in terms of basic concept, but pincushioning is encountered more frequently.

The rotation flap, often used in the past, does not always transfer skin as efficiently as the transposition flaps. In addition, because of the more extensive undermining required, there is a greater chance of damaging the mandibular branch of the facial nerve.

☐ Malar Region Reconstruction

The malar region is a difficult area to reconstruct. It has a convex contour and is highlighted by illumination from any direction. Therefore scars are obvious and contour defects stand out very clearly. The skin texture in this area is smooth and shiny; the color is often red and telangiectatic. The skin is not usually hairbearing, a characteristic that precludes the use of skin from distant areas of the face. In addition, there are several distinct landmarks—lower eyelid, lateral canthus, and temporal hairline—that should not be disturbed in any reconstruction.

RHOMBOID FLAP

The rhomboid flap may be used for small defects. It has the distinct advantage of allowing the excision defect to be placed in such a way that the rhomboid flap can have skin of exactly the correct color and texture. It is constructed as described on p. 16.

CHAPTER 5
CHEEK RECONSTRUCTION

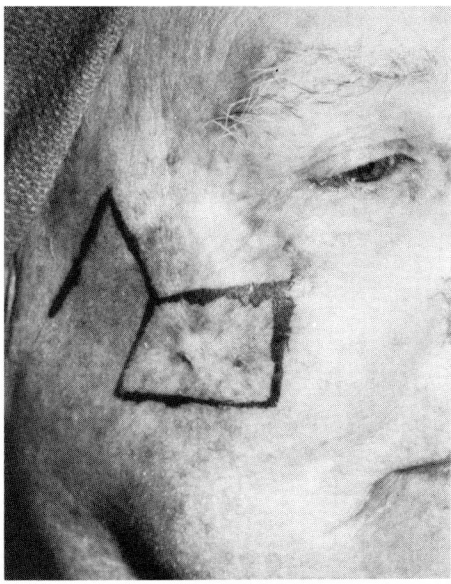

This elderly patient's recurrent basal cell carcinoma of the malar area was suitable for rhomboid excision under frozen section control.

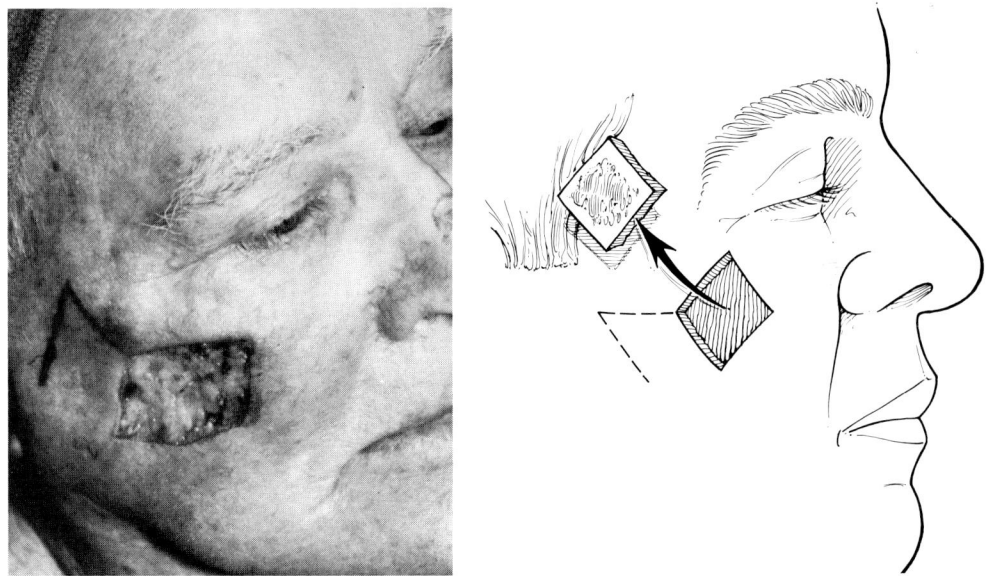

The donor rhomboid was placed laterally with a planned vertical closure. The diagram shows a slightly different, but equally effective, placement of the rhomboid.

211

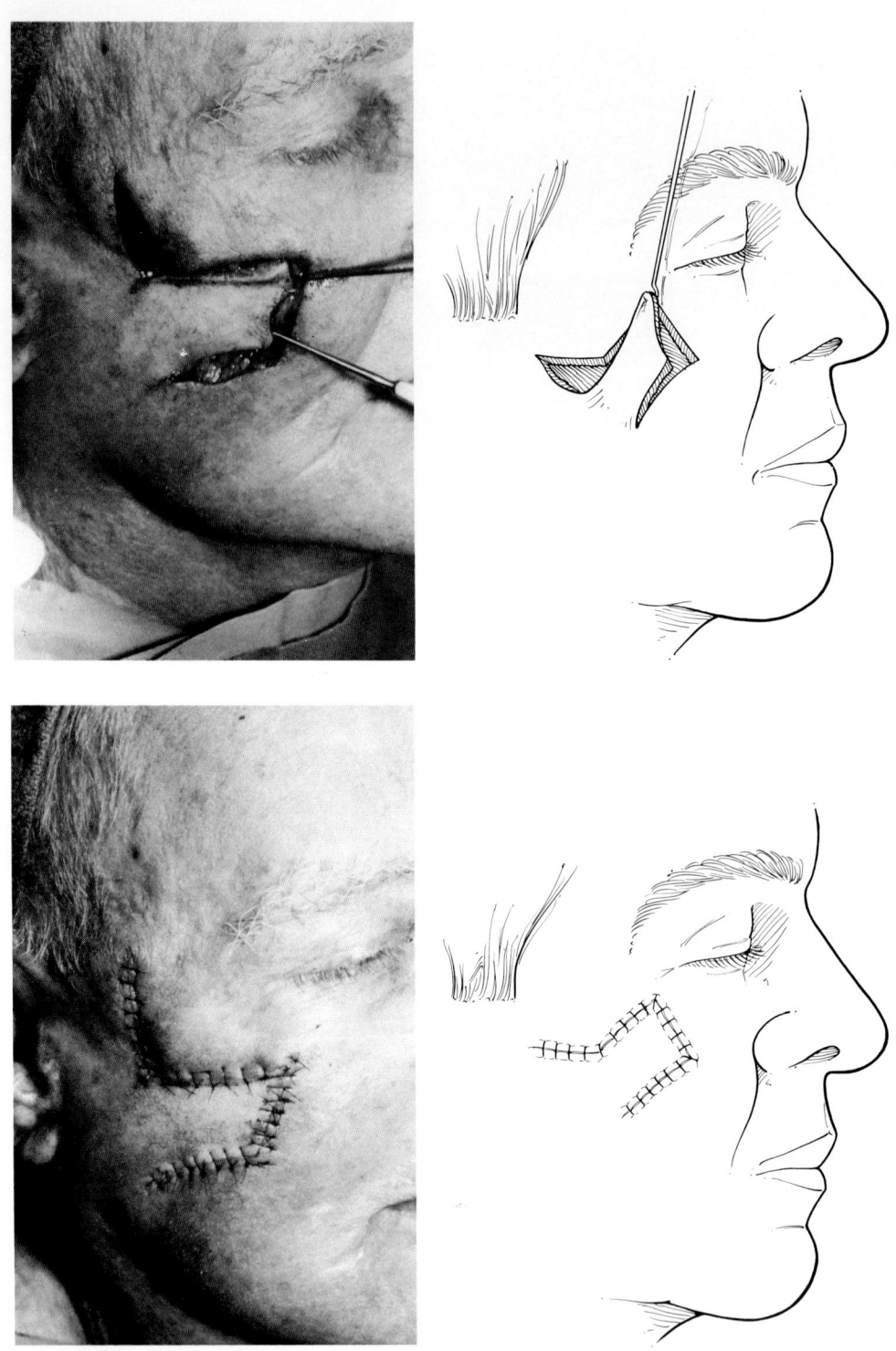

The flap can be rotated into the defect without difficulty. The donor site closes directly.

CHAPTER 5
CHEEK RECONSTRUCTION

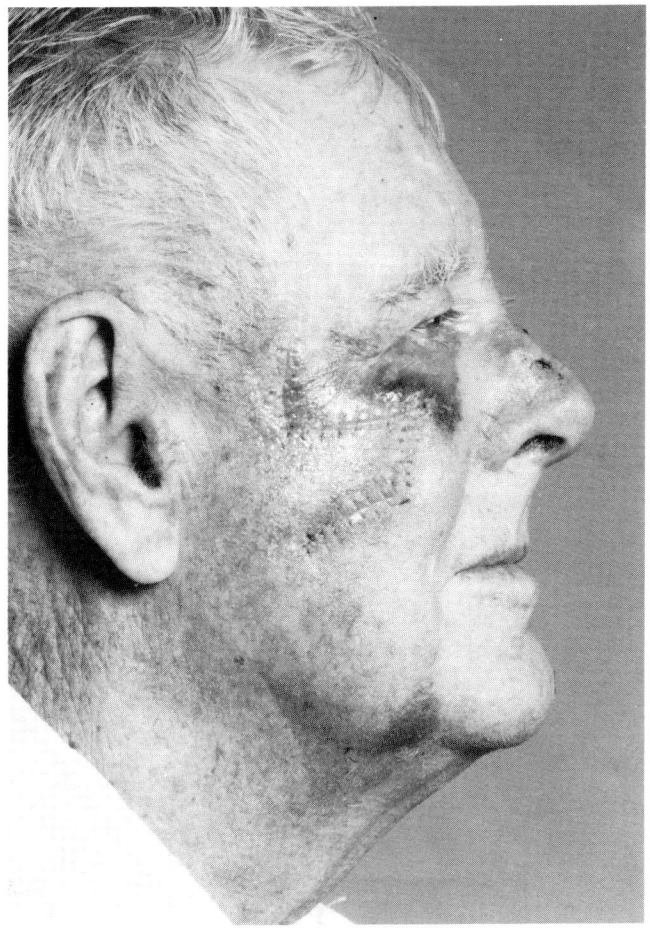

Early postoperative result shows reconstruction without disturbance of local anatomy.

PROBLEMS

Only small defects can be dealt with by means of the rhomboid flap, and the complicated scar can be very obvious. The lower lid and canthus may be pulled down slightly.

BILOBED FLAP

The bilobed flap is used for only small defects because of the extensive scarring and potential change of the hairline or beardline if large flaps are raised. Planning, which can be precise, is performed in exactly the same manner as described on p. 21.

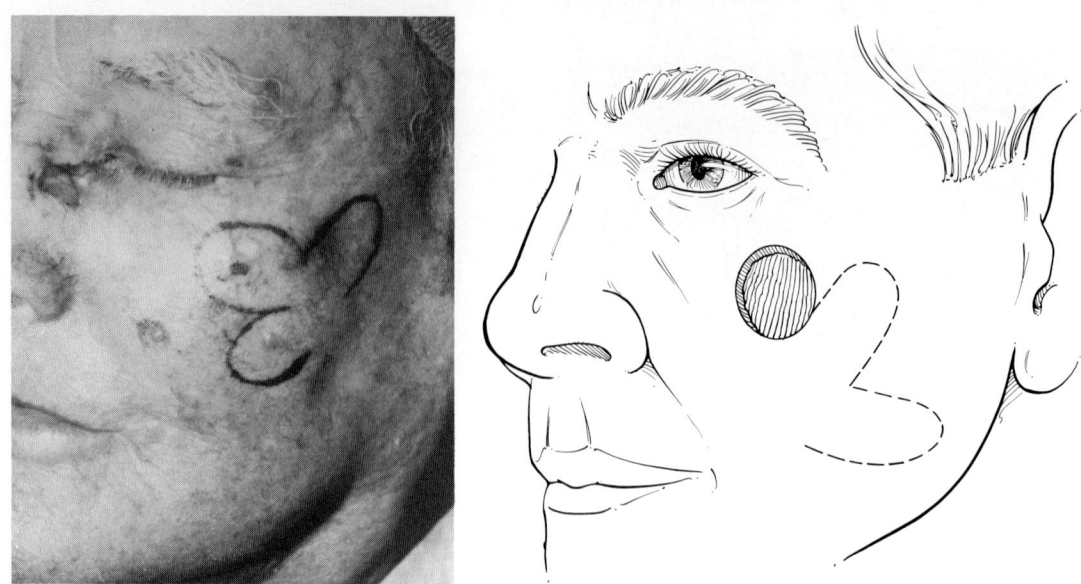

Although the diagram shows the ideal situation, the patient illustrated here with two basal cell carcinomas on the left cheek had a modified bilobed reconstruction. The flaps are outlined; the two lower flaps are each excisional flaps.

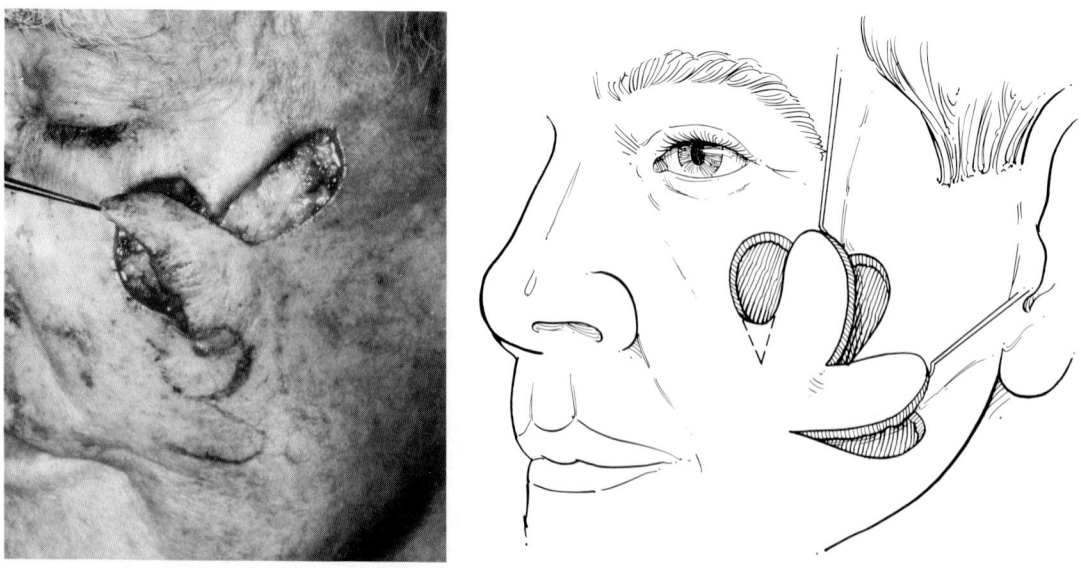

After excision of the upper lesion, the first flap is rotated down for assessing the dog ear that will form.

CHAPTER 5
CHEEK RECONSTRUCTION

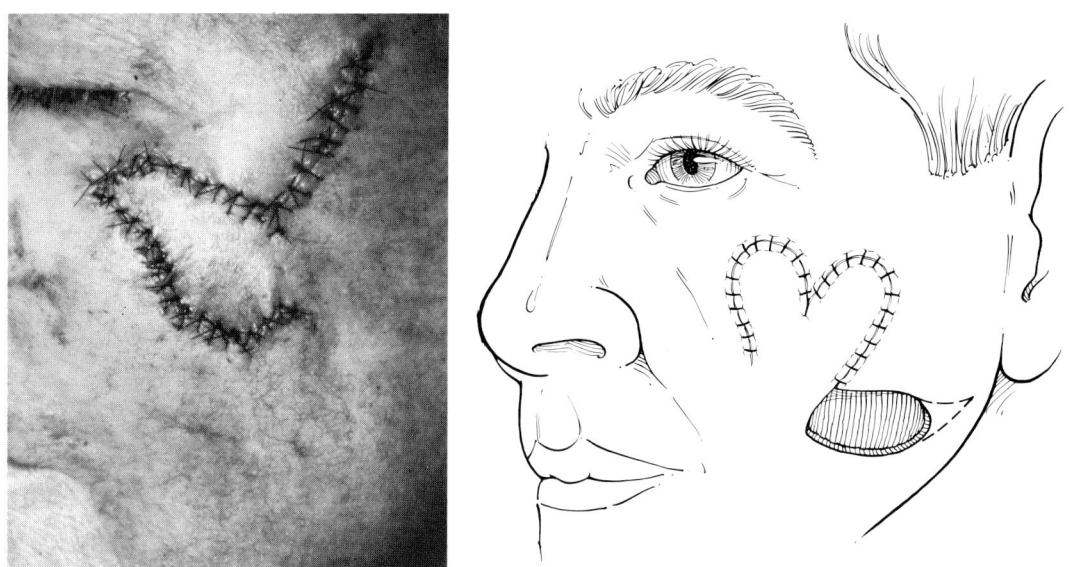

The second lesion is resected, and the defect is covered with a mini flap constructed from the dog ear of the first flap. This is a modified bilobed reconstruction.

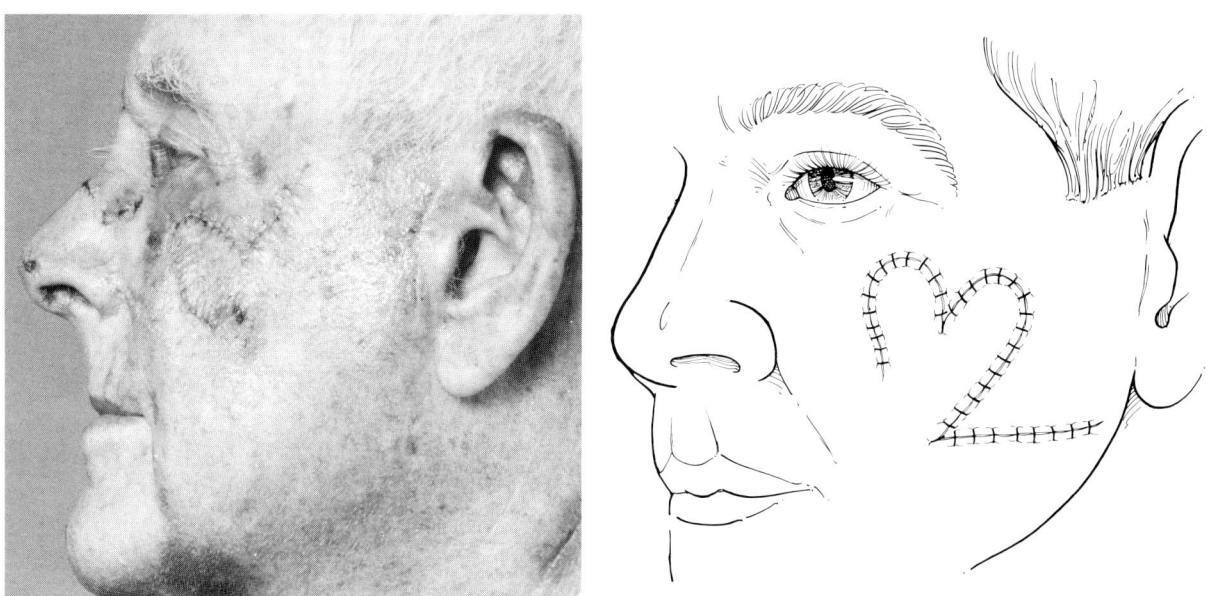

Early result showing good contours and no distortion of anatomy.

PROBLEMS

The scar associated with the bilobed flap is complicated and obvious, and pincushioning of the flaps may occur. Perhaps even more problematic in the male is the chance of bringing hairbearing skin into a nonhairbearing area. Both the bilobed and rhomboid flaps tend to bring paler skin from the lower face into the ruddy malar area, thus making the reconstruction obvious.

TRANSPOSITION FLAP

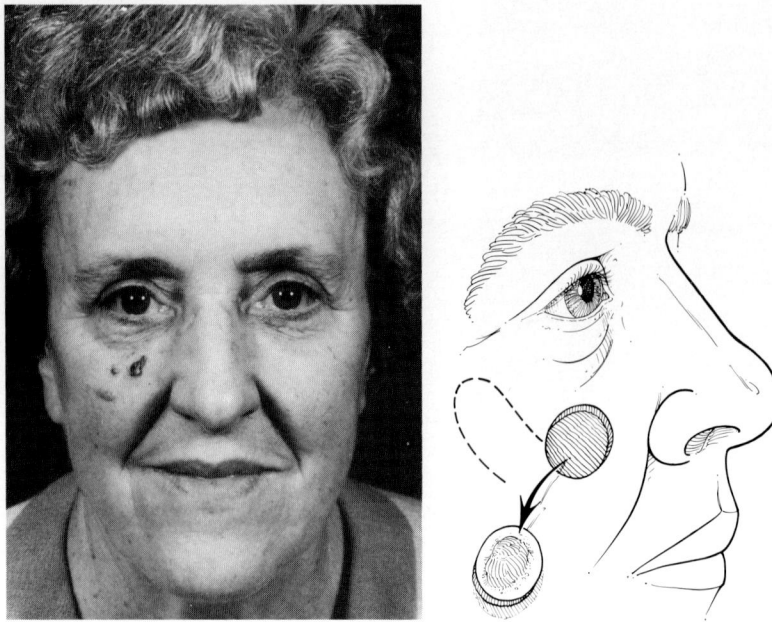

The transposition flap is planned by using a length of gauze to determine the correct flap length and width and the feasability of direct closure of the donor site.

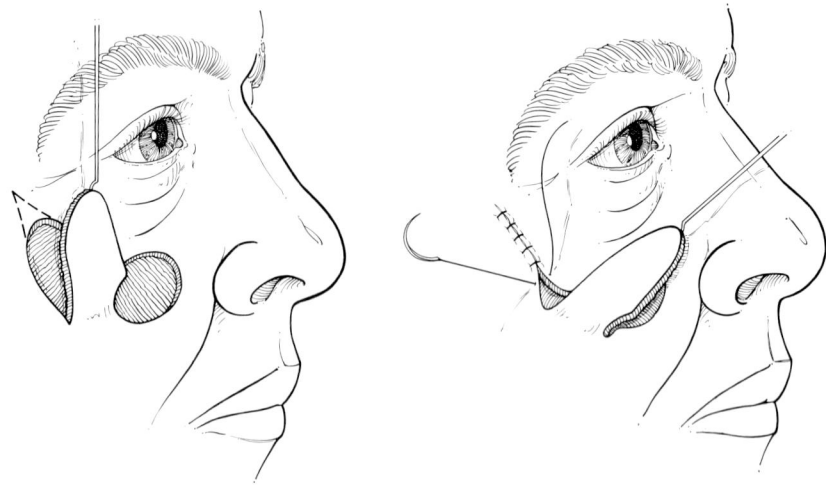

After planning, the flap is elevated. It should rotate effortlessly and be comfortably sutured into position.

CHAPTER 5
CHEEK RECONSTRUCTION

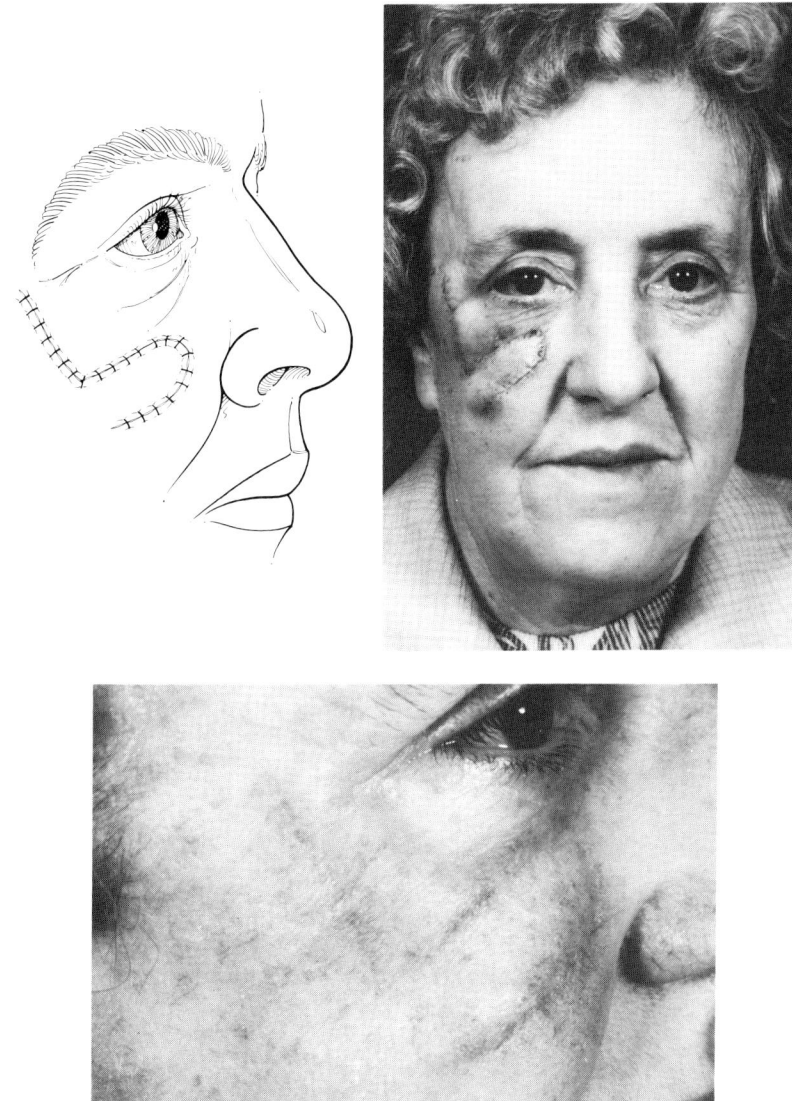

PROBLEMS

The patient illustrated here demonstrates the problems encountered with the transposition flap. The area of available skin tends to leave a donor site at right angles to the ideal minimal tension lines in this region. Furthermore, the color of the flap may differ from that of the skin it replaces, and flap pincushioning may occur.

LATERAL CHEEK ROTATION FLAP

This rotation flap is used for defects of virtually any size. It transfers skin based on the loose skin of the preauricular area and sometimes from the lower face and neck. The laxity allows medial movement of lateral cheek skin. The larger the defect, the more extensive is the undermining and mobilization required.

The defect is triangulated, and then a lateral cheek flap is designed for closure. The flap must be of adequate size; if not, there will be pulling down of the lateral end of the lower eyelid, which results in problems ranging from a slight increase in scleral show to frank ectropion.

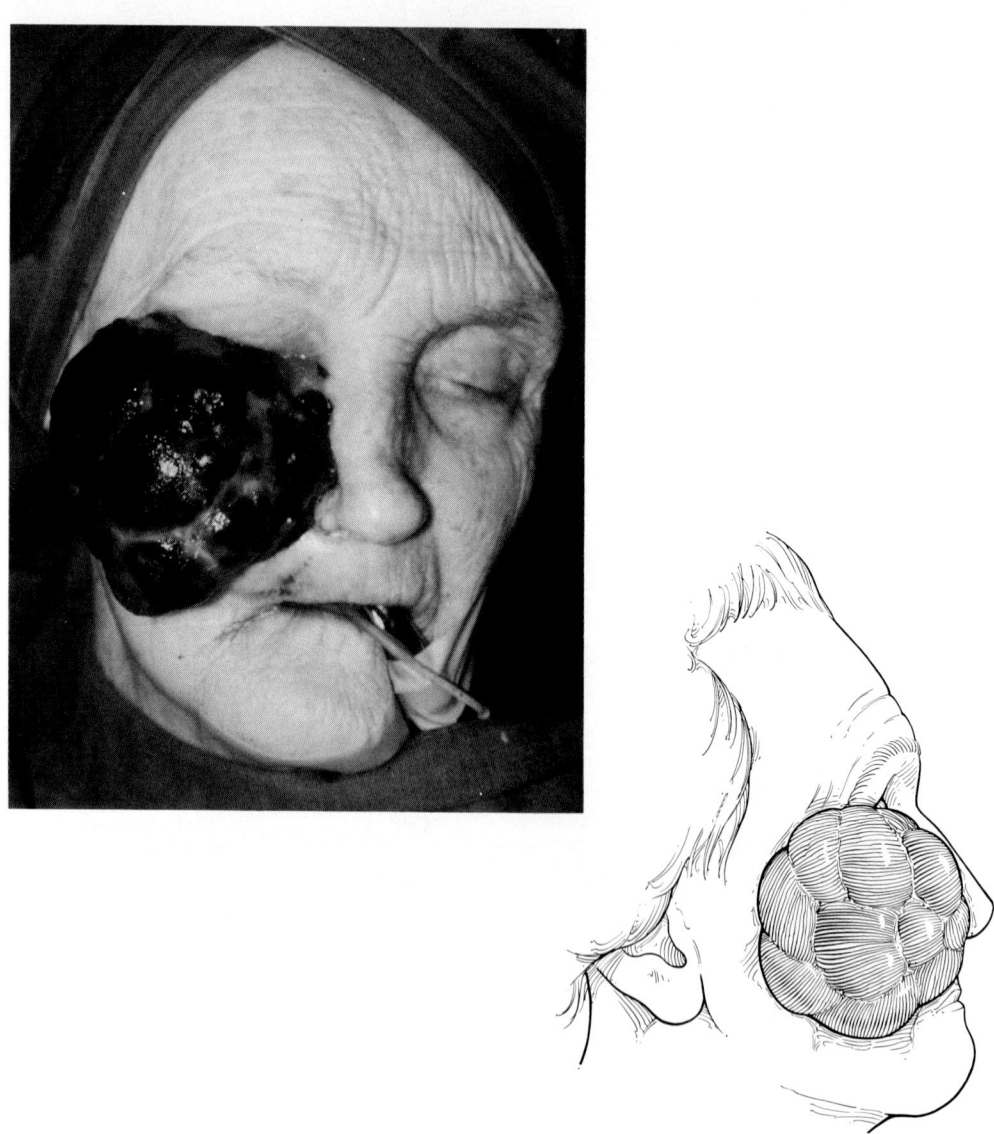

CHAPTER 5
**CHEEK
RECONSTRUCTION**

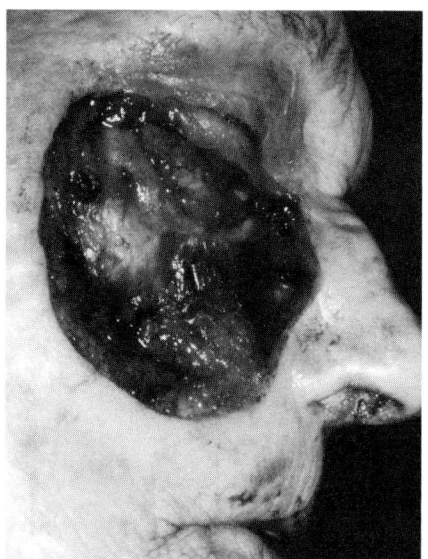

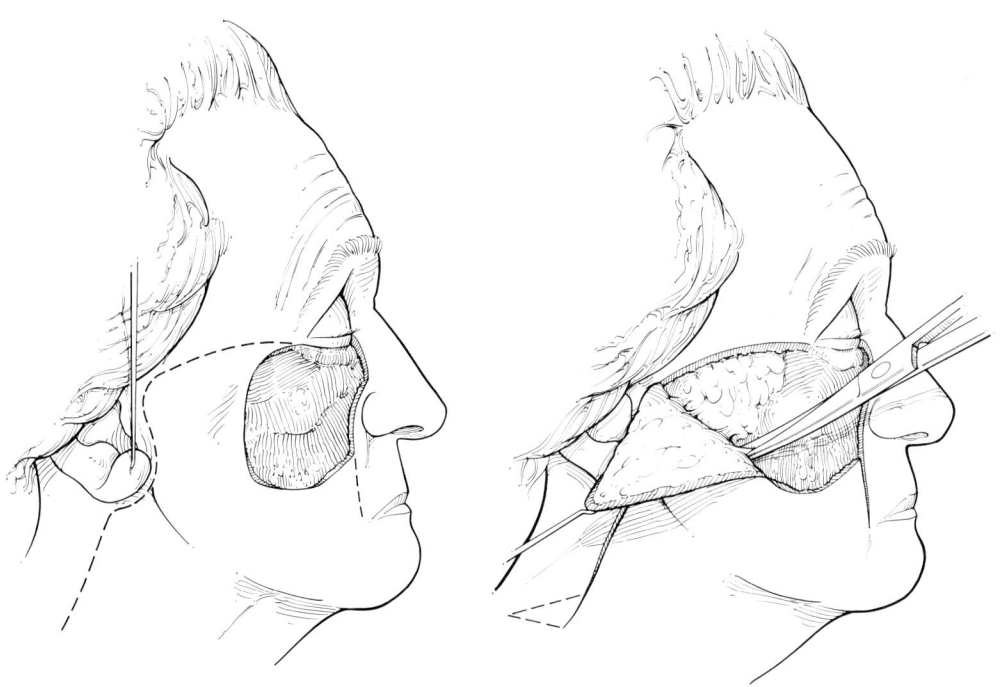

In moderate to large defects, such as the one created in this patient, who had a large exfoliating malignant melanoma excised, the cheek flap incision runs laterally, upward, then down in the preauricular area, and continues down into the neck.

219

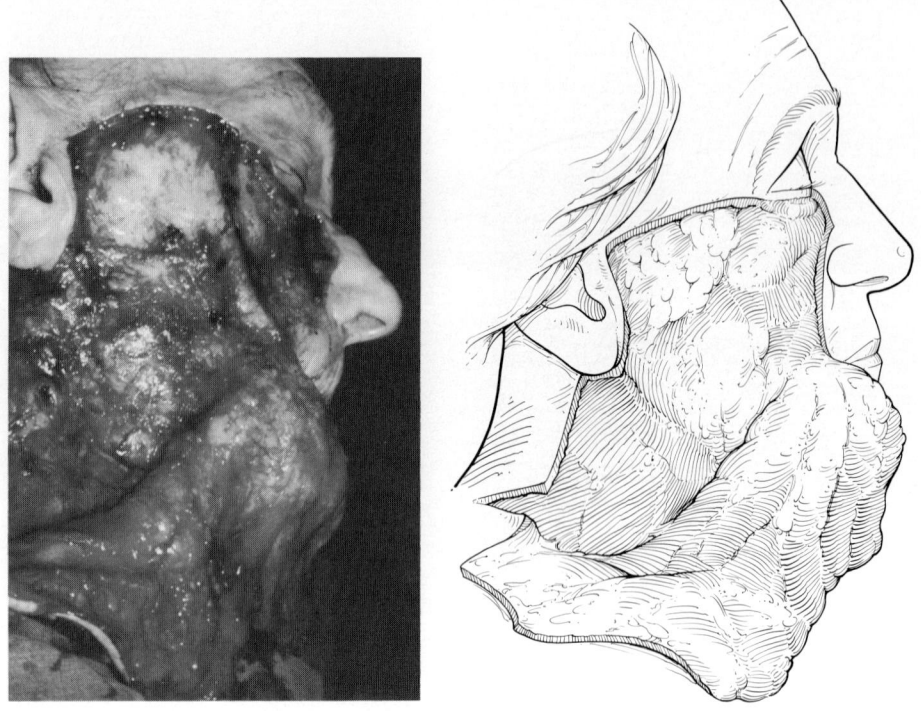

The whole cheek is elevated in the face-lift plane.

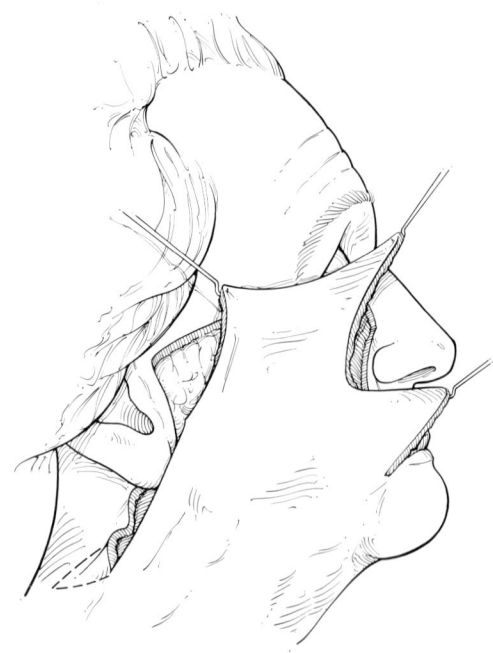

Adequate flap closure is tested by pulling on the flap with hooks.

CHAPTER 5
CHEEK RECONSTRUCTION

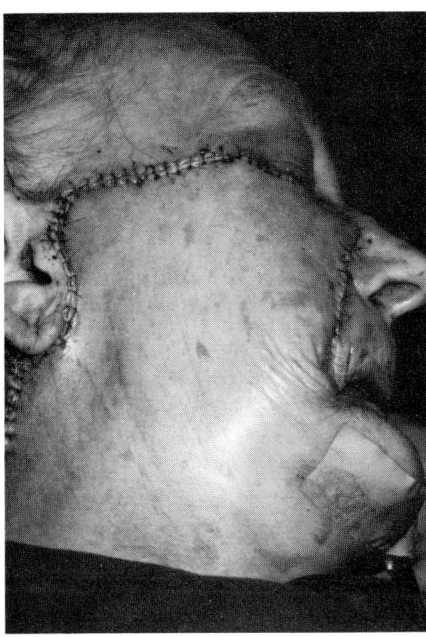 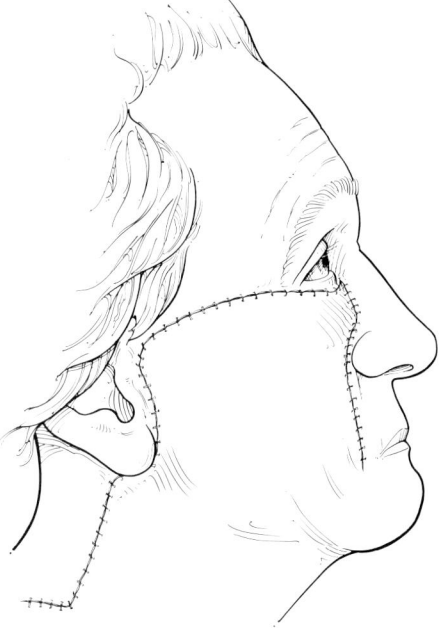

When enough advancement has been gained, medial closure is effected. The remainder of the flap incision is closed. The donor defect is closed by advancement of temporal and preauricular skin and drains are inserted. The resulting dog ears on the cheek, at the base of the vertical incision, and on the neck usually require excision.

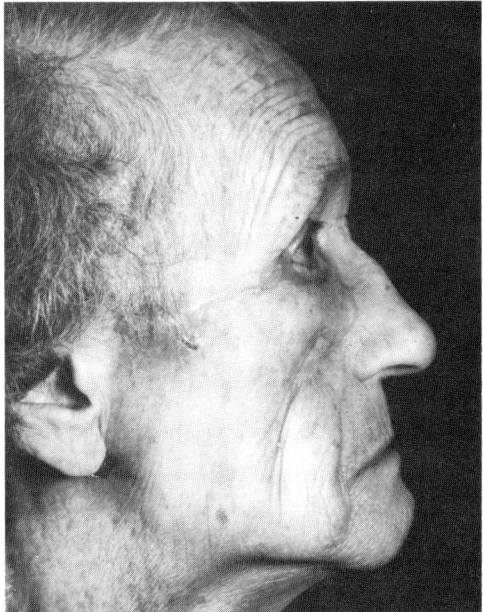

The deep surface of the flap should be anchored to the soft tissue, preferably including the periosteum over the malar area. This procedure will help prevent dragging down of the eyelid.

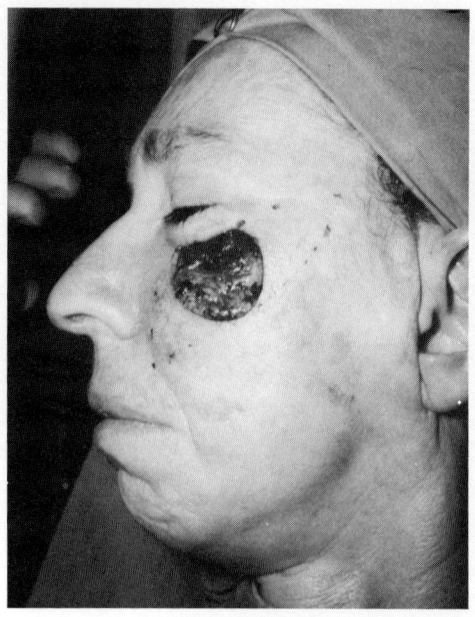
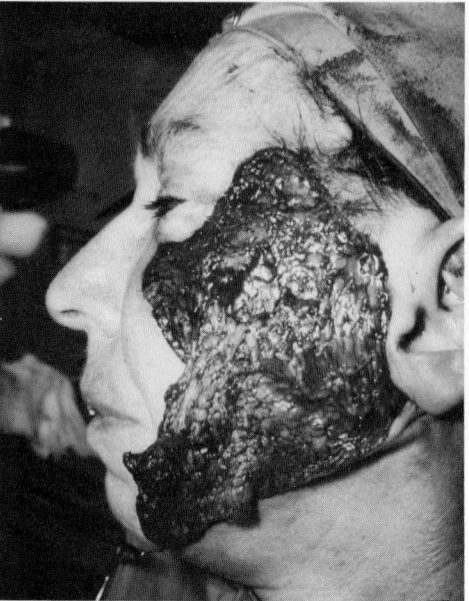
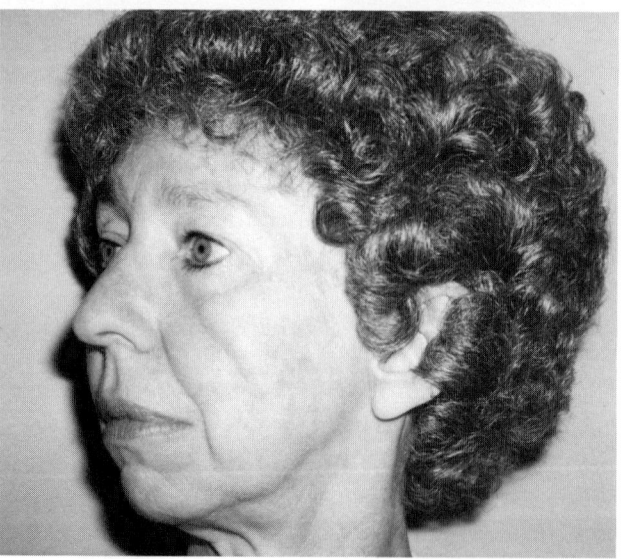

This patient illustrates the reconstruction of a smaller defect. In spite of the dimensions of the defect, in the cheek region a large flap is necessary in order to achieve a satisfactory reconstruction.

PROBLEMS

In the male, some shifting of hairbearing skin to a nonhairbearing area will occur. The sideburn will need to be trimmed or shaved higher to disguise this. As shown on p. 225, after excision of a large port wine stain, hairbearing skin has been shifted to totally resurface this patient's lower eyelid, a situation that required later excision and full-thickness skin graft replacement. Poor flap design may cause some degree of ectropion of the lower lid. If the undermining and the dimensions of the flap are inadequate, ischemia and loss of the tip of the flap may result. Hematoma can produce the same effect. It can also cause pincushioning associated with fibrosis, a problem that usually resolves itself with time.

SURGICAL TECHNIQUE OF CHOICE

If well designed, the rotation flap is an excellent form of reconstruction in the cheek.

The rhomboid flap can be used for small lesions, but the complexity of scarring associated with it and the bilobed flap makes both methods generally unacceptable. On balance, the rhomboid flap is preferable to the bilobed flap.

☐ Supramedial Cheek Reconstruction

The supramedial cheek area is difficult and fascinating to reconstruct because of its anatomic complexity. Several significant anatomic landmarks and important functional structures are located in proximity to one another. The skin in this area is thin and nonhairbearing. The medial canthus, the punctum, the caruncle, and the medial end of the lower lid—all lie just above this region and can be deformed if any skin loss takes place. The resultant scarring and contracture can cause obvious ectropion and troublesome epiphora. The patient may experience bouts of conjunctivitis.

To reconstruct the supramedial cheek area, the surgeon can use skin lateral or superior to the defect. Occasionally, when the defect is small, donor tissue may be taken from an inferior position.

LATERAL ROTATION FLAP

The lateral rotation flap can be used to close defects of any size. It is extensile in that the preauricular and neck skin can be mobilized as necessary to obtain the required shift of skin.

Feasibility for using this flap should be assessed by pushing the cheek skin medially with all the fingers of the hand; the expected success of the flap is judged according to the movement of the skin and the excess amount that develops in front of the fingers. If this excess is at least equal to the defect, reconstruction with a lateral rotation flap should be possible.

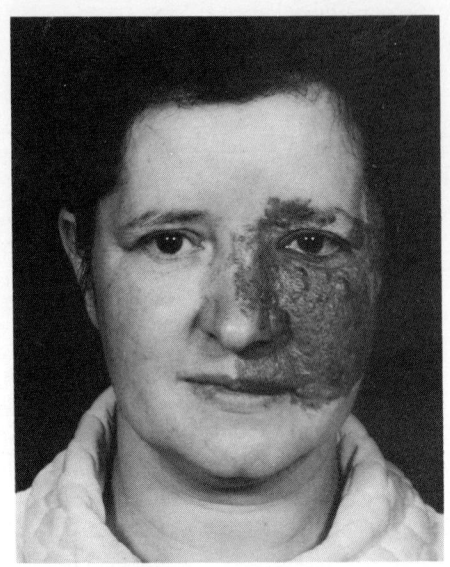
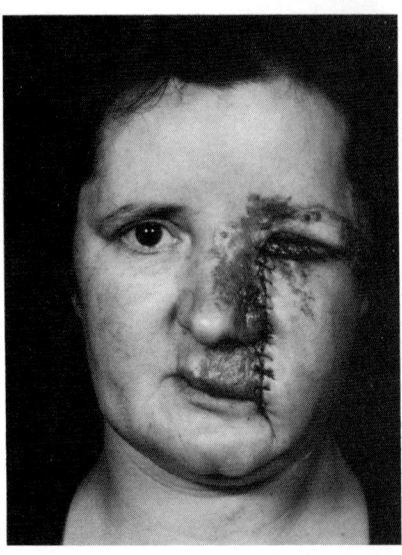
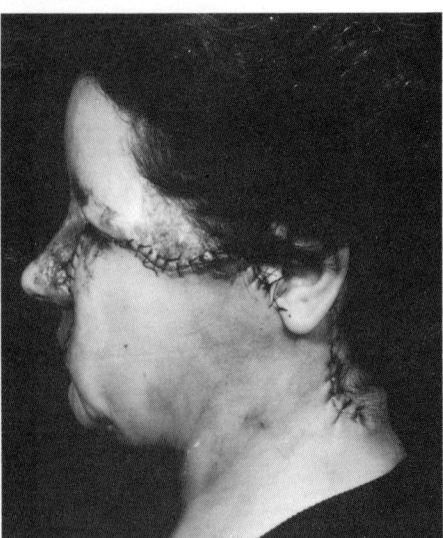

The patient shown here required a large rotation flap to close a defect resulting from excision of a nodular port wine stain. The technique used is similar to that illustrated on pp. 218 to 221.

The defect is triangulated with the base superior. An incision is made laterally and then taken down the preauricular area, around the earlobe, and down the neck, and a skin flap is fashioned. The incision and the undermining continue until the defect can be closed comfortably. Usually a small drain is inserted under this type of flap to prevent hematoma.

CHAPTER 5
**CHEEK
RECONSTRUCTION**

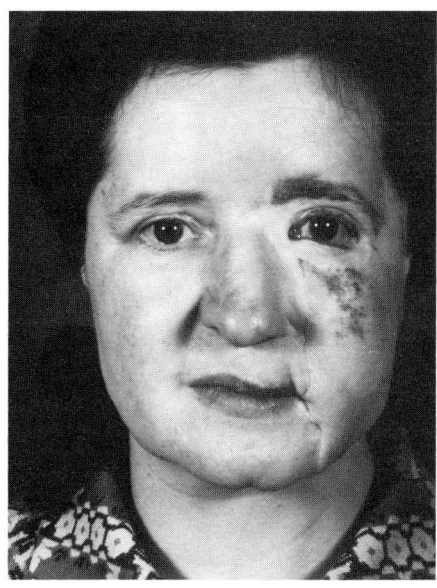 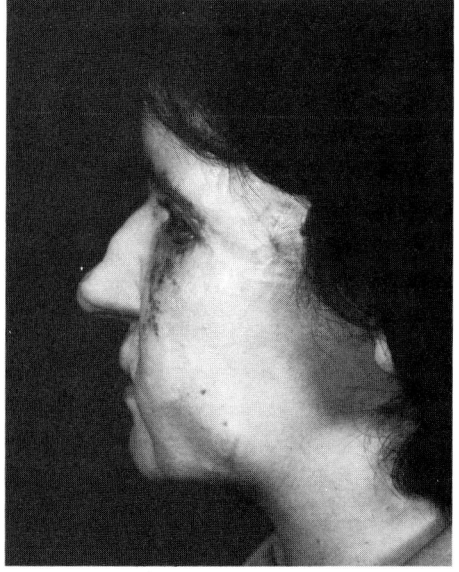

With this technique the surgeon can reconstruct large defects with satisfactory results.

PROBLEMS

The scar parallel to the eyelid margin is not a desirable feature. It may be obvious and cause lid edema or slight ectropion in the elderly patient.

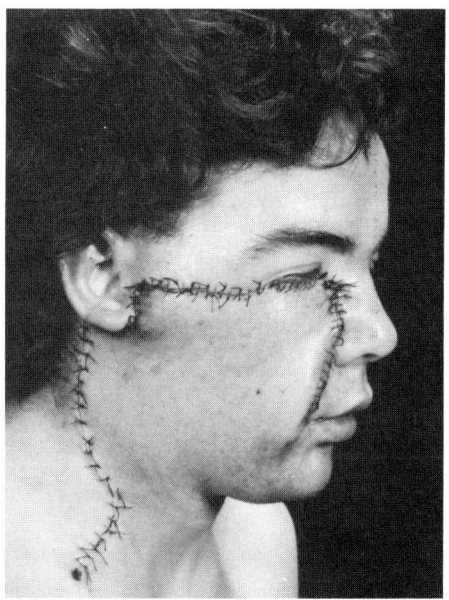

As shown here, hair may be transferred to a nonhairbearing area. Hematoma should be prevented at all costs. It causes tension and may lead to ischemia and loss of the tip of the flap. Similarly, a flap that is too small to effect comfortable closure may suffer a similar fate. To prevent cheek sagging and ectropion, suturing the undersurface of the flap to malar periosteum is strongly recommended.

INFERIOR ROTATION FLAP

By using the planning method described for the lateral rotation flap, the surgeon can judge the amount of excess skin available for upward movement.

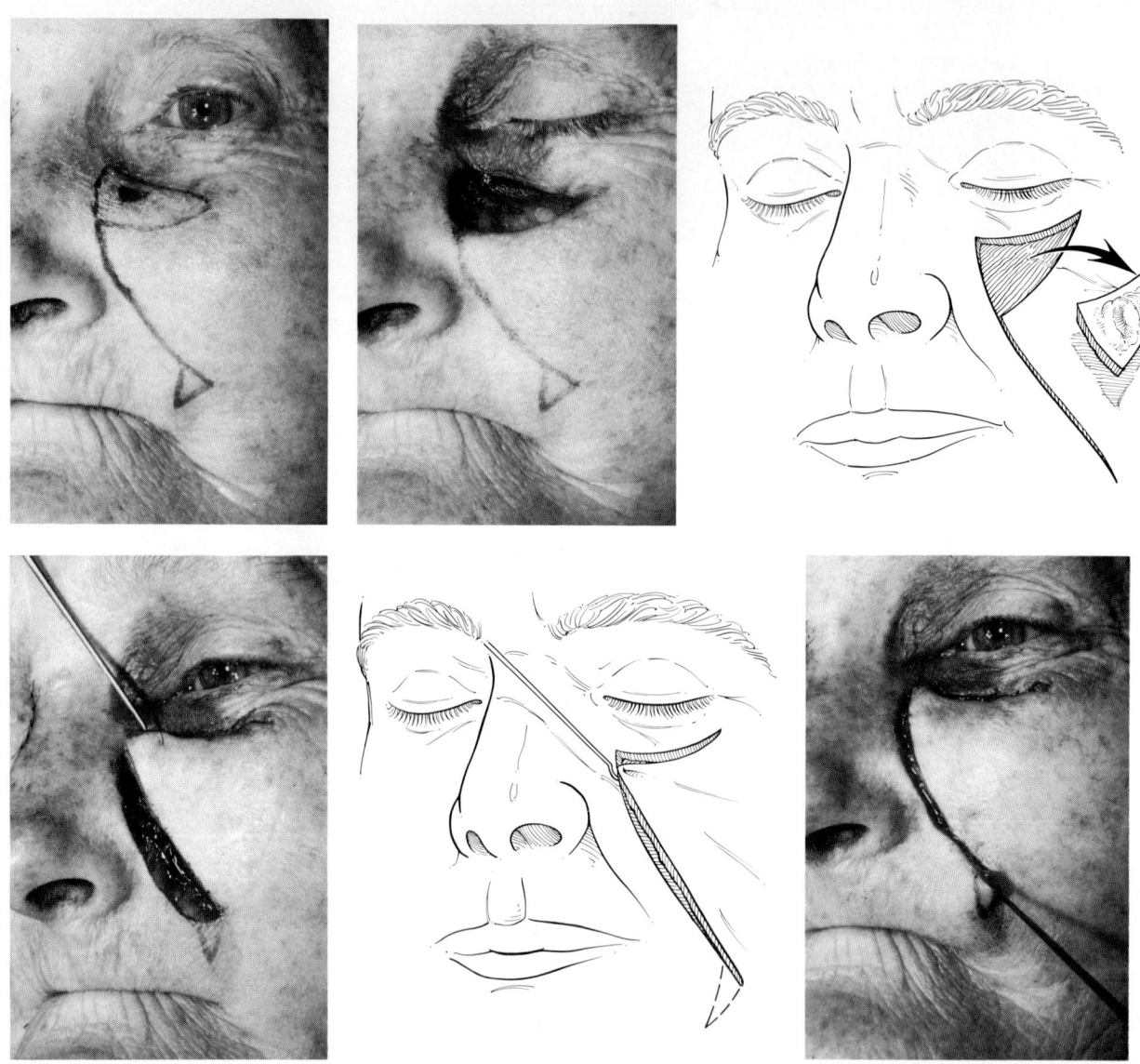

The defect is triangulated, and the flap is planned so that it rotates upward along the nasolabial fold. The flap is elevated, and the incision is taken far enough to allow the rotation to proceed to obtain comfortable defect closure. A dog ear or Burow's triangle is excised from the caudal end of the incision.

CHAPTER 5
CHEEK RECONSTRUCTION

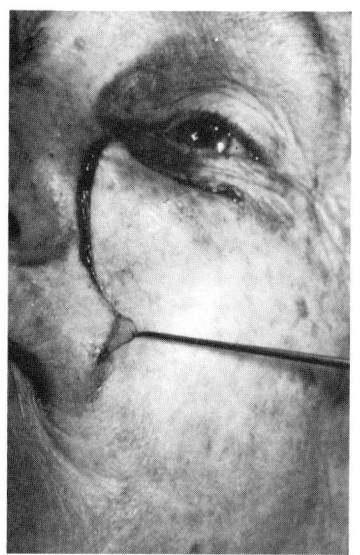
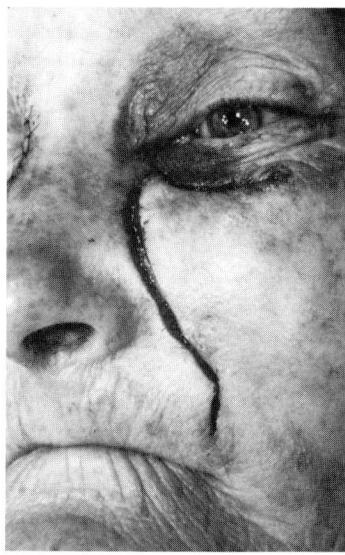
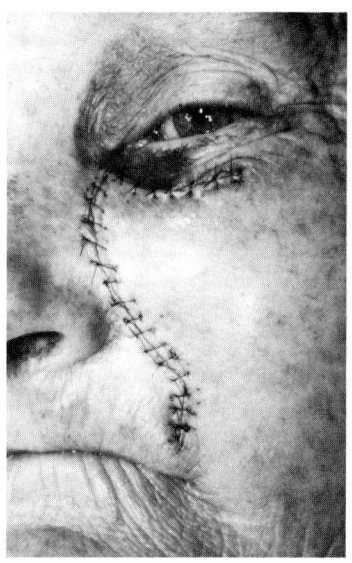
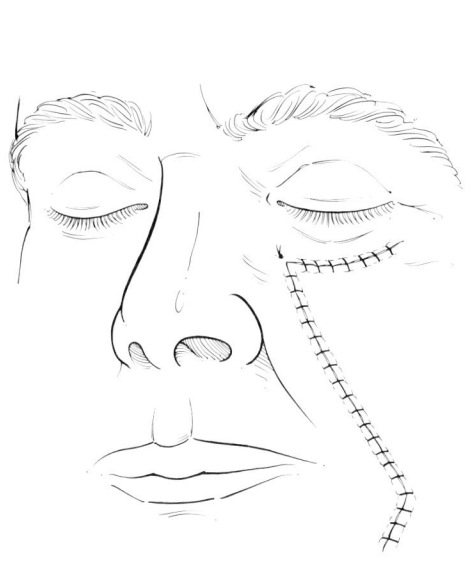
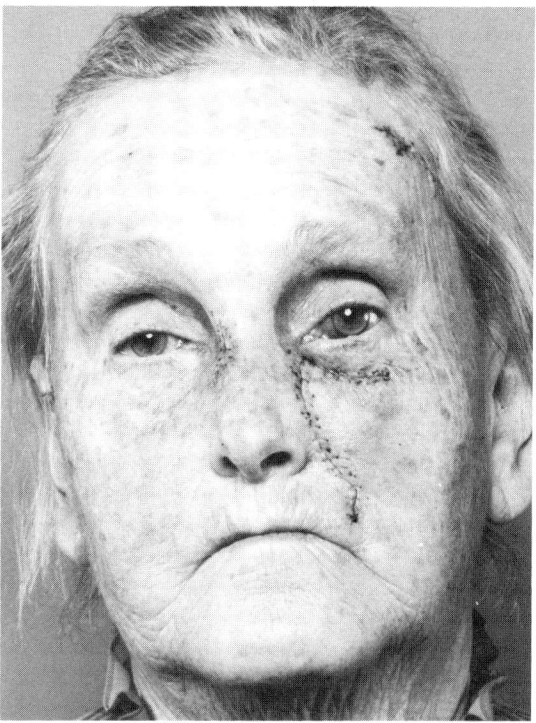

The line of defect closure falls comfortably within the nasolabial line and is aesthetically very acceptable, although there is a slight distortion of the palpebral aperture.

PROBLEMS

All indications are that the inferior rotation flap should be an ideal flap. The rotation is in good line, and in the older patient plenty of tissue should be available.

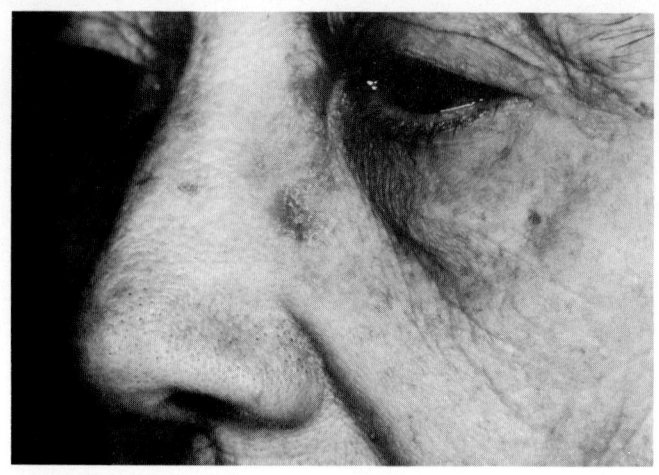

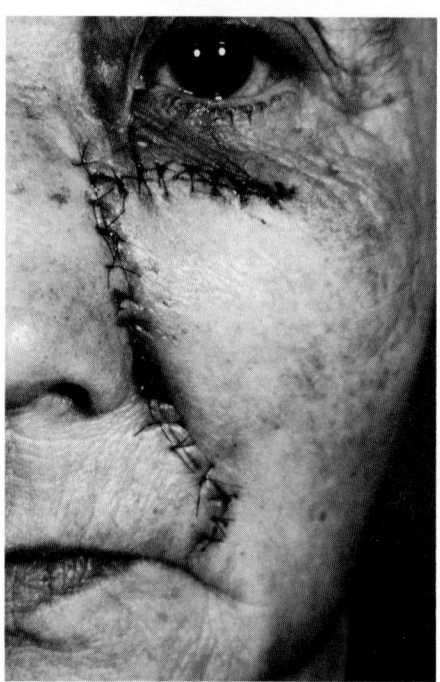

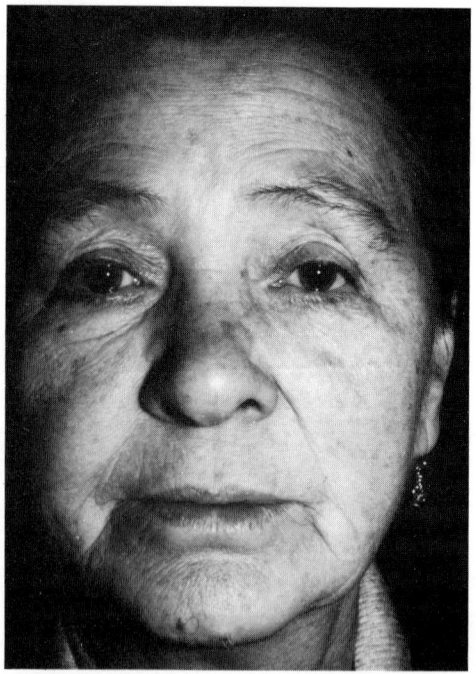

In reality, in spite of its popularity, this type of flap is a poor one. Gravity works against it. Pincushioning often results and emphasizes the nasolabial fold, causing facial asymmetry. Even if the flap is well planned, the scar parallel to the lid margin may cause lid edema and ectropion, as described earlier. However, in the elderly patient, it is a rapid and secure method to use.

ADVANCEMENT FLAP

The advancement flap can be used to close moderate-sized defects. It is pleasant to use because it involves a more limited dissection than the rotation flap to obtain the required amount of skin advancement for defect closure.

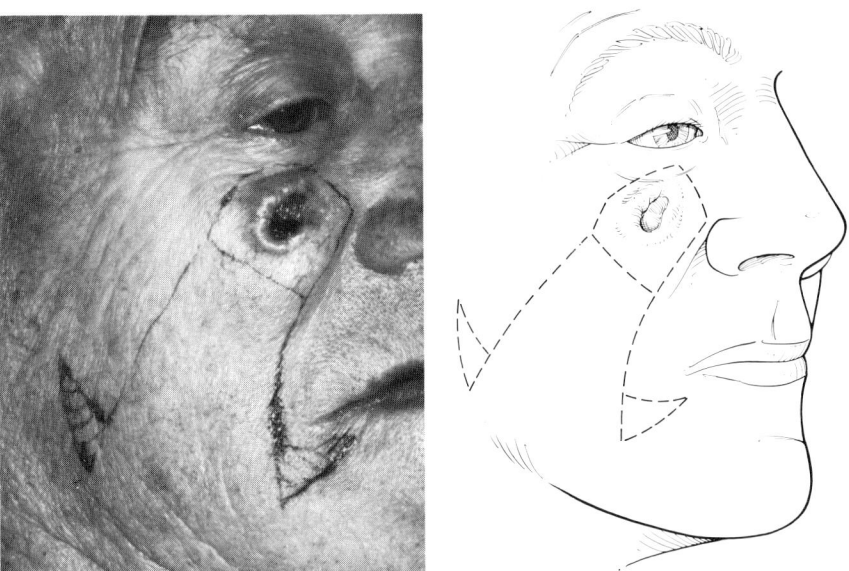

The excision is planned as a square or a rectangle. From the sides of the defect, two parallel lines are drawn along the line of the nasolabial fold.

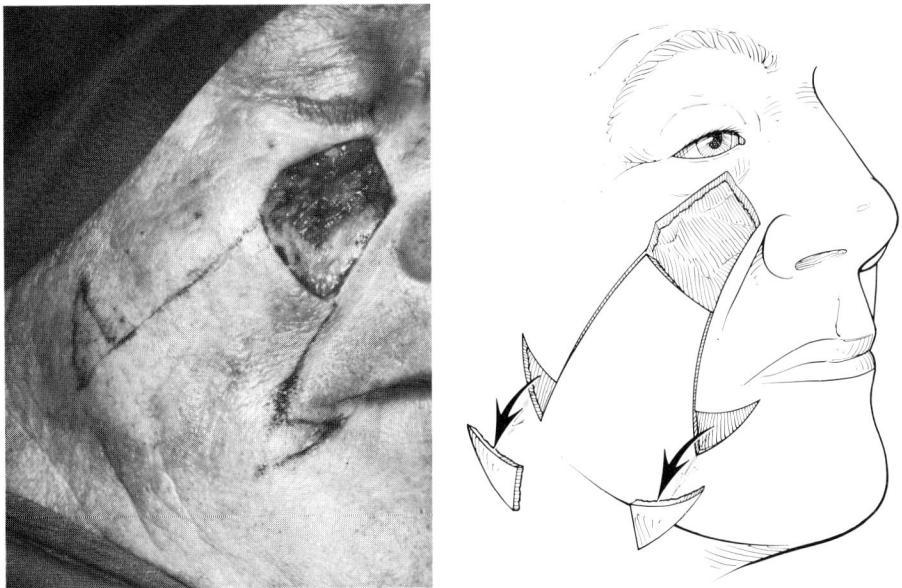

The lesion is excised and the long flap between the lines is designed and elevated.

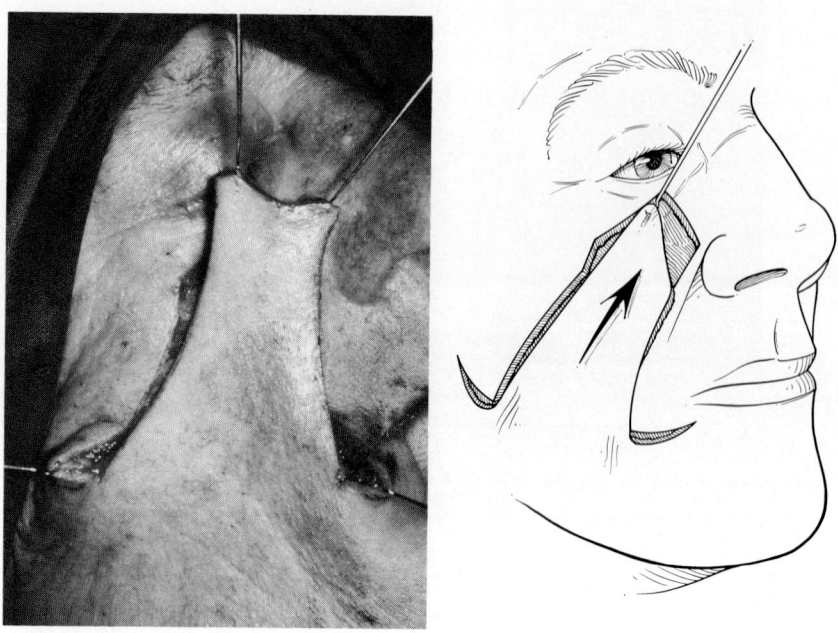

Advancement is judged by gently pulling on the flap with hooks until the defect can be closed comfortably.

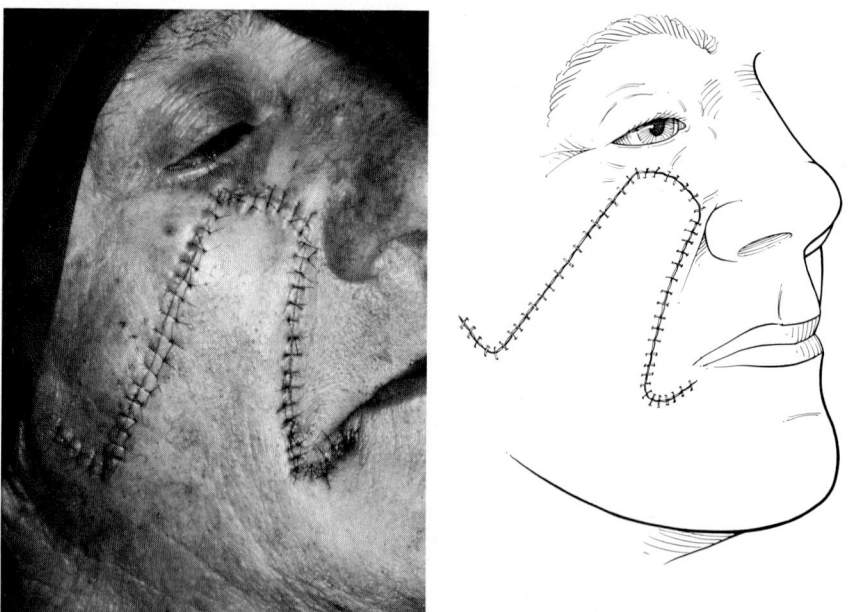

As the flap is sutured, excesses of skin appear on either side of the flap base. These standing cones are excised as the so-called Burow's triangles.

CHAPTER 5
CHEEK RECONSTRUCTION

PROBLEMS

With this technique there may be minimal pulling down of the lower lid, a problem that does not merit correction. Apart from this, no problems have been encountered with the advancement flap.

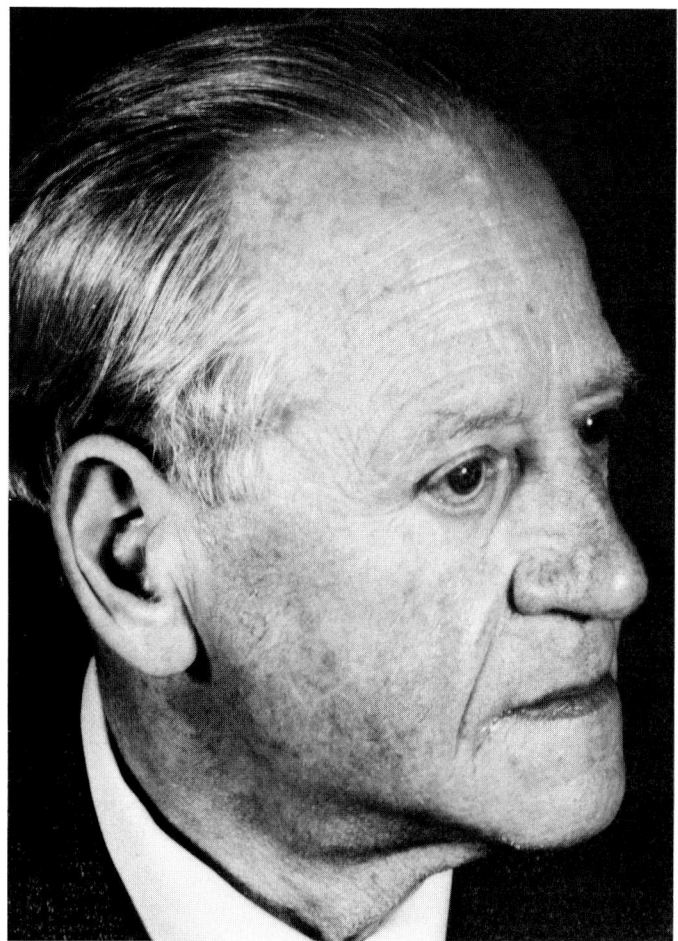

The scars situated in the nasolabial line are not particularly noticeable. Perhaps because of the square design of the flap, pincushioning does not occur.

HORIZONTAL ADVANCEMENT FLAP

This patient with Merkel's cell tumor illustrates the use of a transverse advancement flap to close a post excisional defect in the supramedial portion of the cheek.

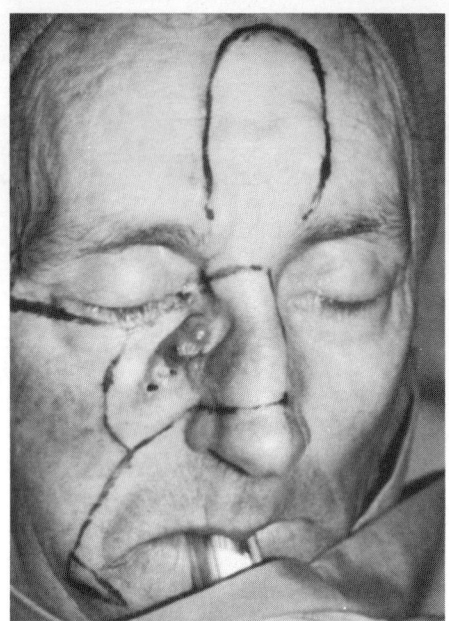
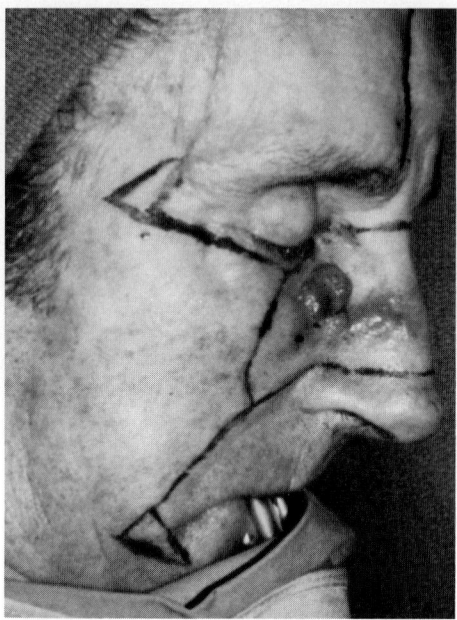

The flap is planned in exactly the same way as the preceding flap. The lateral margins of the flap are placed under the lid margin and in the line of the nasolabial fold.

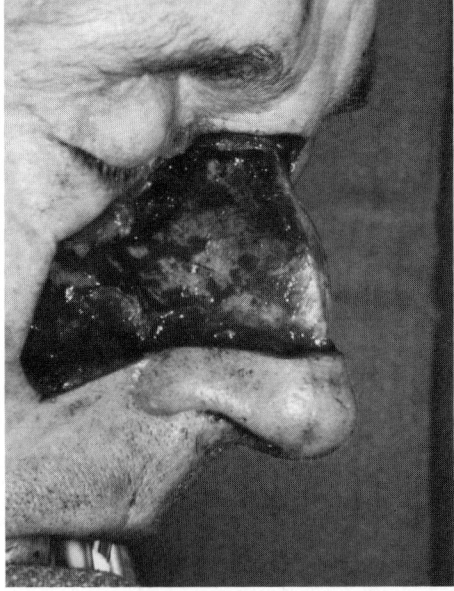
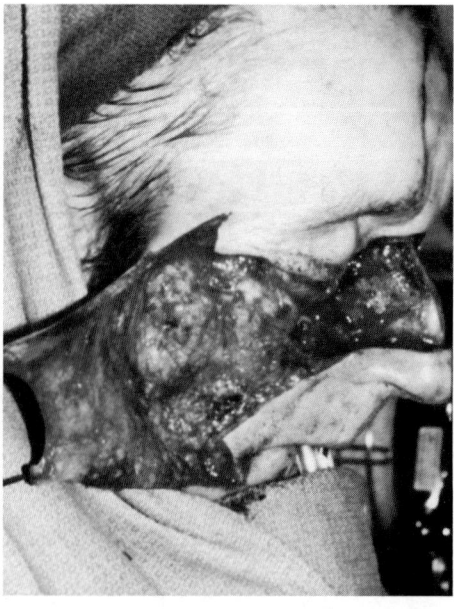

The defect is created by resection of the tumor, and the cheek advancement flap is elevated with excision of Burow's triangles at its base.

CHAPTER 5
CHEEK RECONSTRUCTION

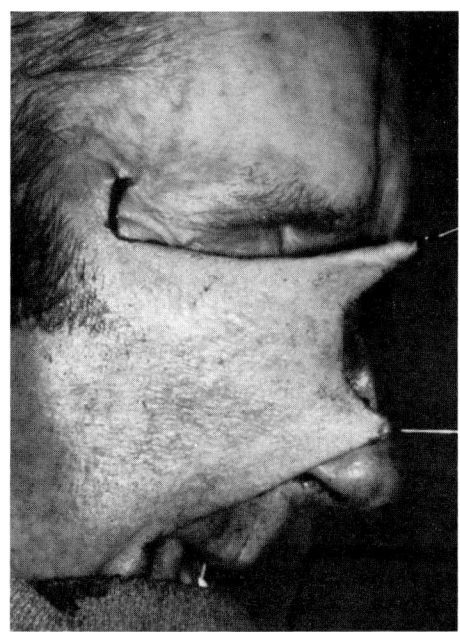

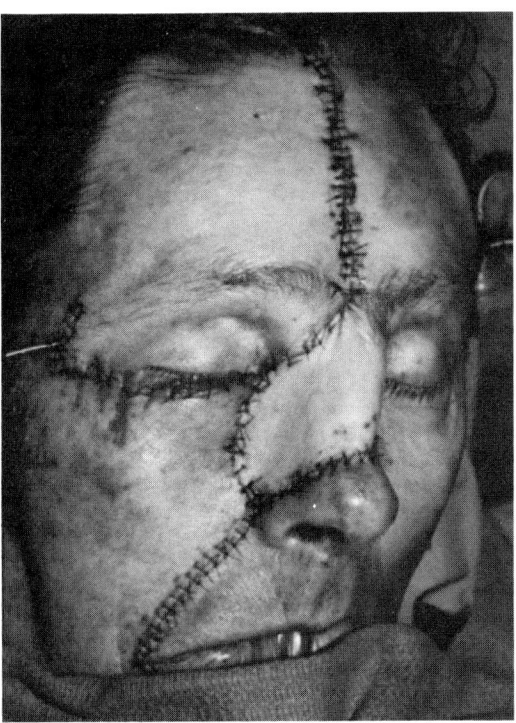

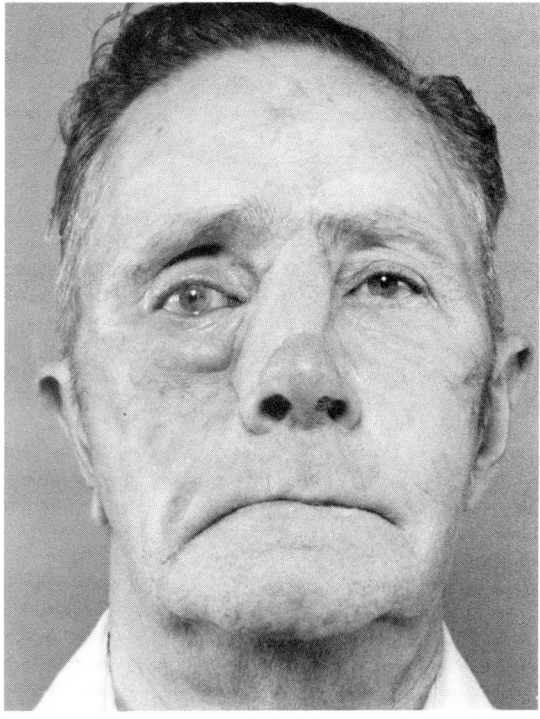

The nasal portion of the defect is closed with a vertical midline forehead flap. The great advantage of this method is the reduced amount of dissection required to close the defect as compared with that needed for a large cheek rotation flap.

PROBLEMS

No problems have been encountered with this type of flap. The deep surface of the flap should be anchored to the zygomatic periosteum to prevent sagging and ectropion of the lower lid. A drain must also be placed under the flap to prevent hematoma.

VERTICAL TRIANGULAR ADVANCEMENT FLAP

This is a large kite flap that can be used in the supramedial cheek area, but it is better suited for a defect located slightly lower than the ones being discussed in this section. It is also best reserved for smaller defects. The flap has the advantage of requiring very limited dissection and manipulation to obtain significant skin advancement.

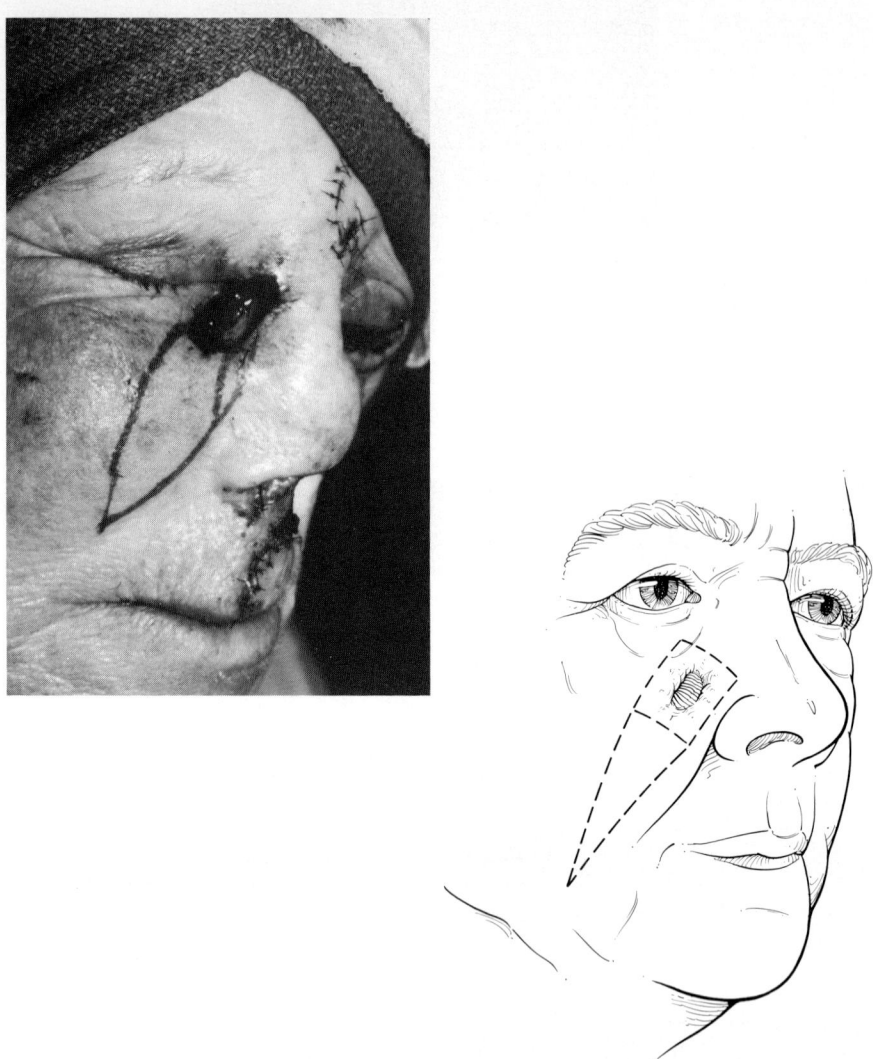

The excision is planned as a square. From the inferior side of the square, a triangle is drawn on the nasolabial line. The length of the triangle is approximately twice the length of the side of the square.

CHAPTER 5
**CHEEK
RECONSTRUCTION**

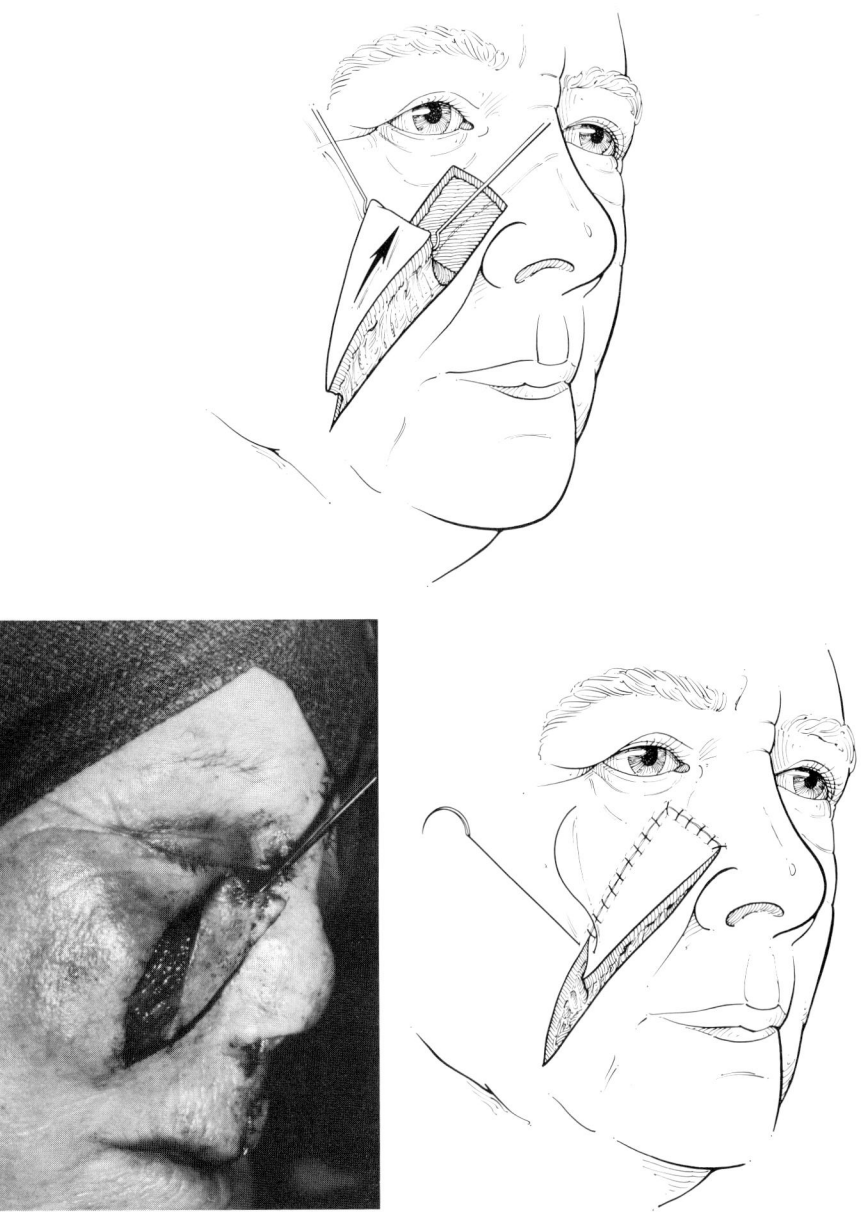

The lesion is removed and the triangle is incised down to subcutaneous fat. In most older patients the amount of advancement of the triangle on this subcutaneous pedicle is sufficient to gain closure.

235

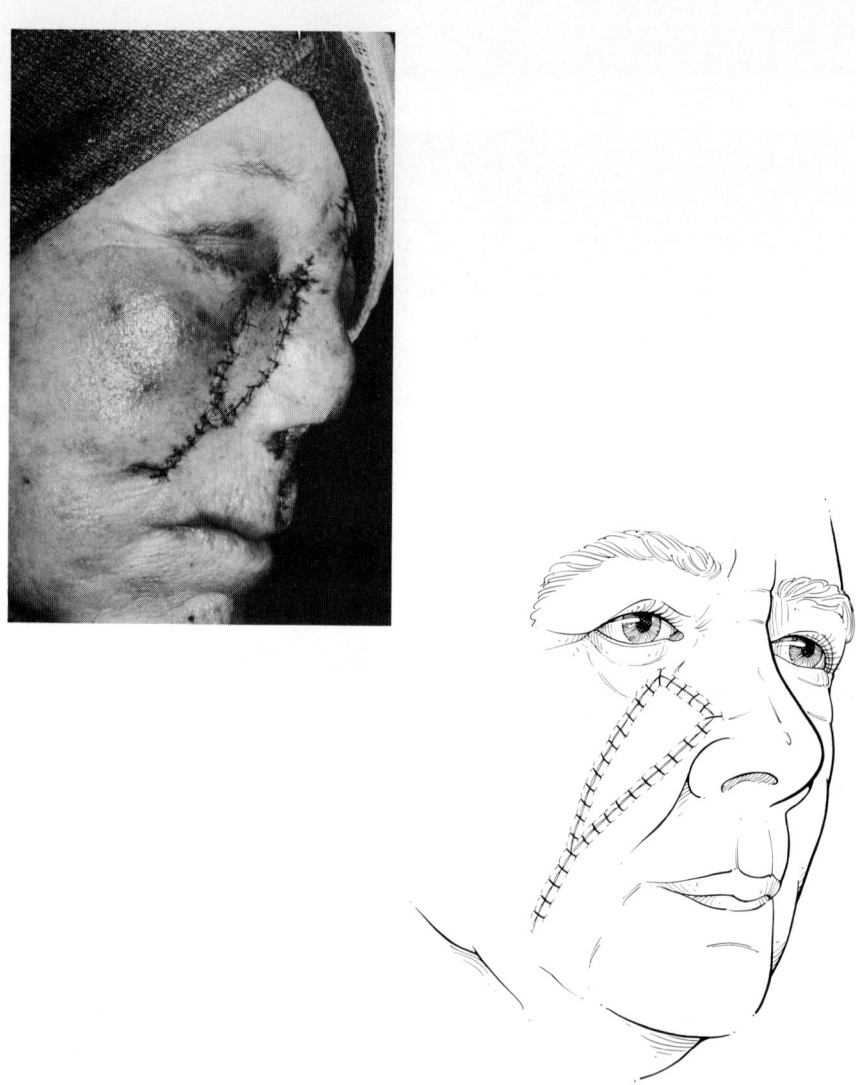

The secondary defect is closed in a V-Y fashion.

PROBLEMS

Pincushioning of the flap may occur, but this usually settles spontaneously. If it does not settle, the resulting island of skin can be difficult to correct and may require several episodes of fat contouring. No other problems have been noted.

CHAPTER 5
CHEEK RECONSTRUCTION

NASOLABIAL TRANSPOSITION FLAP

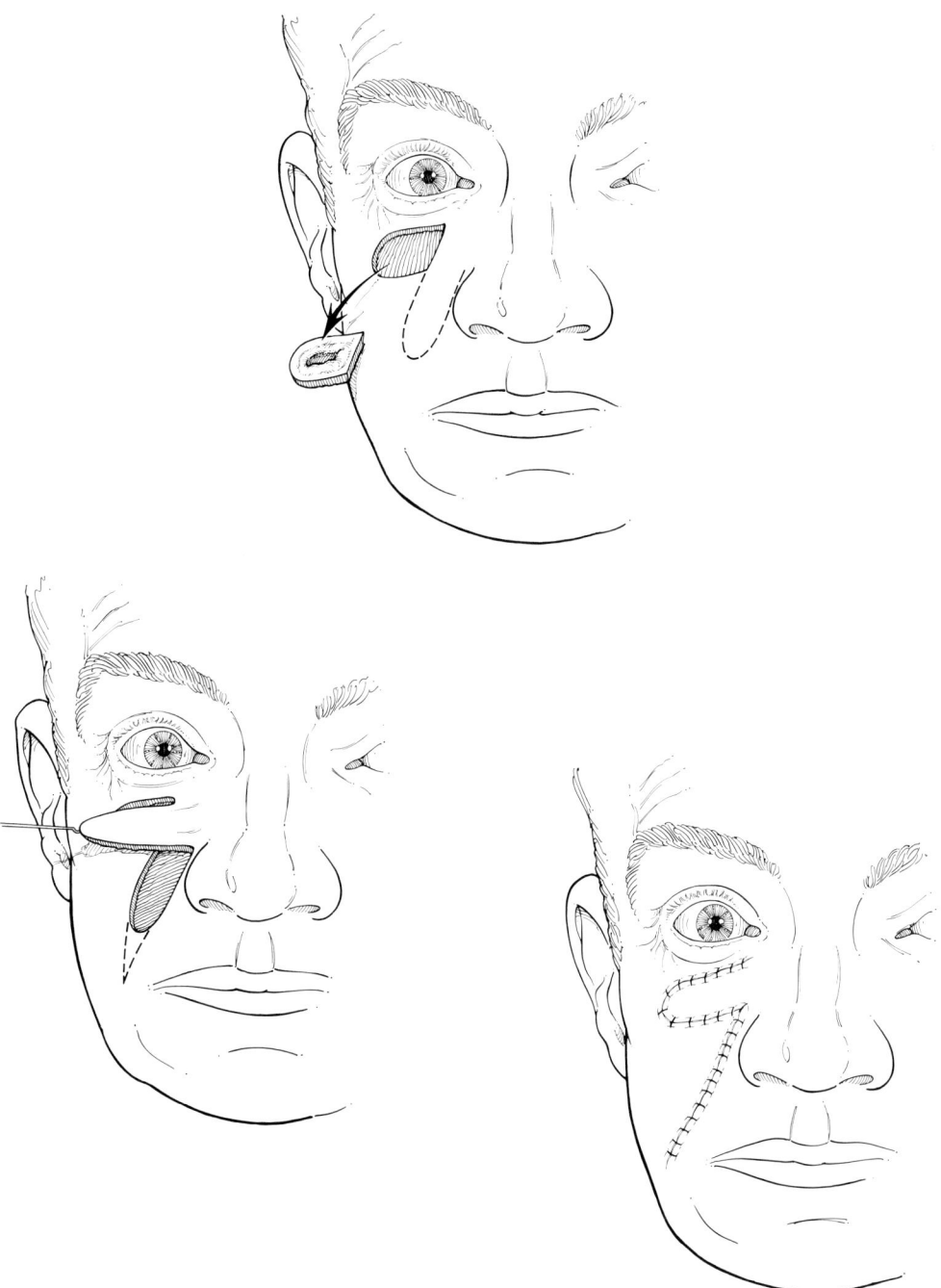

The nasolabial transposition flap is a useful flap that may be applied for closure of defects of the upper cheek. The donor site of the nasolabial fold is plentiful. The flap is based superiorly and is transposed at 90 degrees to close the defect. The donor site is closed directly.

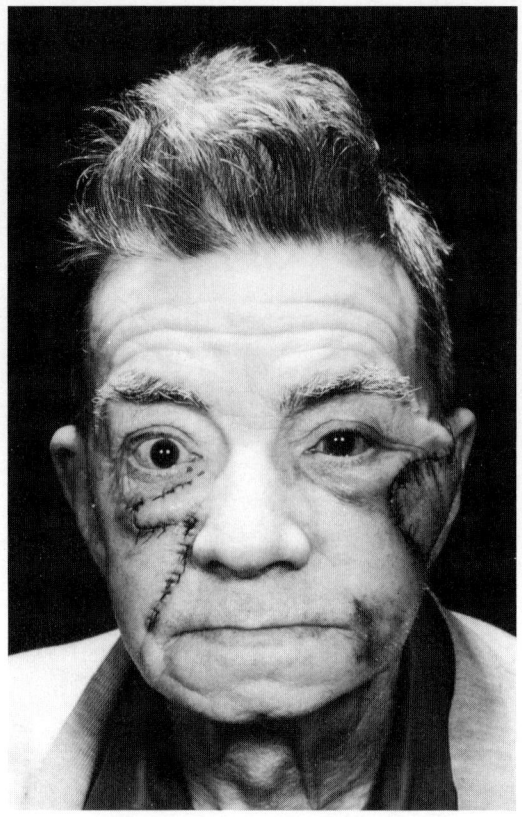
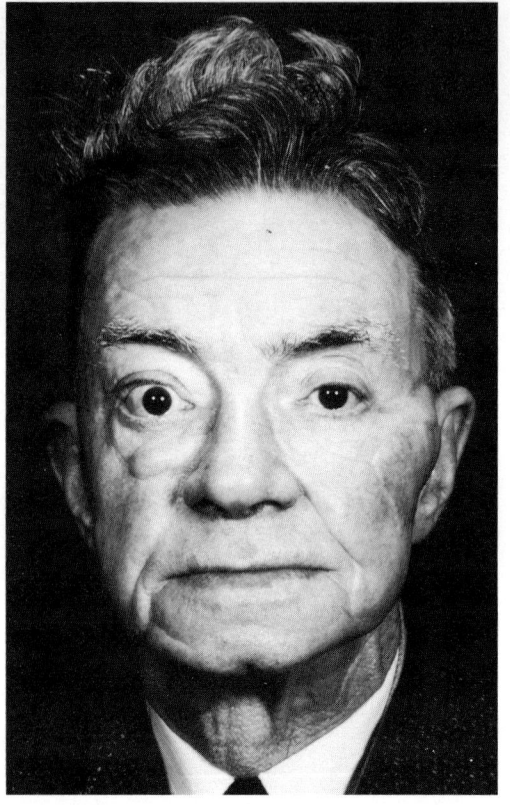

The patient illustrated here had a basal cell carcinoma of the right cheek that was reconstructed in this fashion. Proptosis of the right eye was present before surgery; this appearance was not the result of the reconstructive surgery.

PROBLEMS

Bunching of the flap and some flattening of the nasolabial fold are possible problems resulting from the use of this technique. (This can be seen in the preceding illustration.) Nevertheless, it is a useful reconstructive approach.

CHAPTER 5
CHEEK RECONSTRUCTION

TRANSVERSE TRIANGULAR ADVANCEMENT FLAP

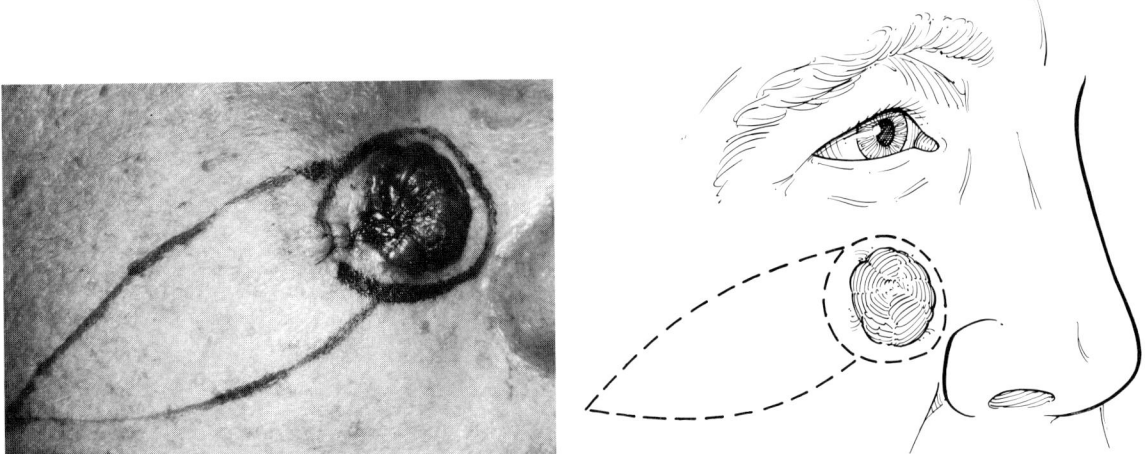

In the patient illustrated here, a pigmented basal cell carcinoma has been removed from the paranasal area. It is possible to plan a transverse triangular island flap that is advanced in a V-Y fashion to give satisfactory closure of the excisional defect.

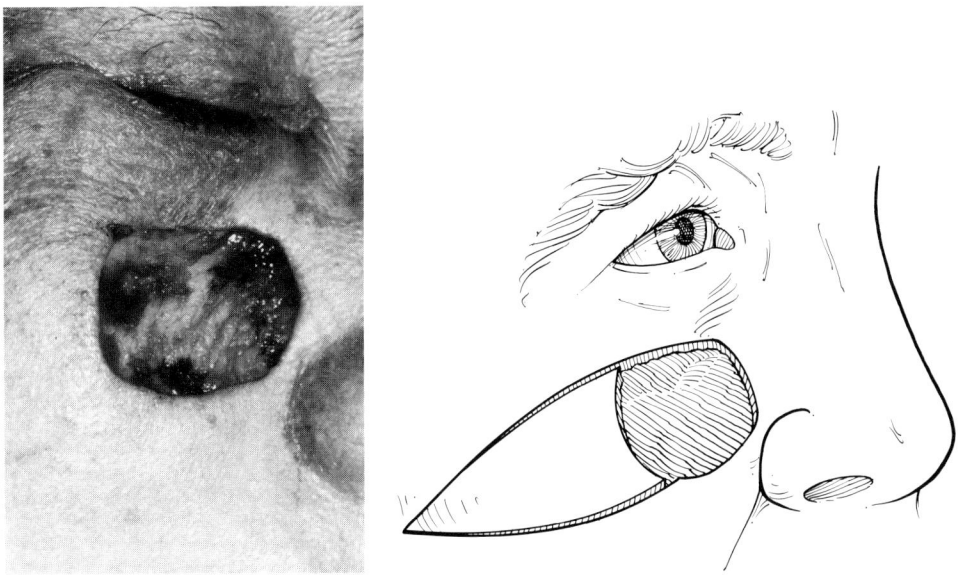

After excision of the lesion, the transverse triangular flap is incised down to the underlying subcutaneous tissue.

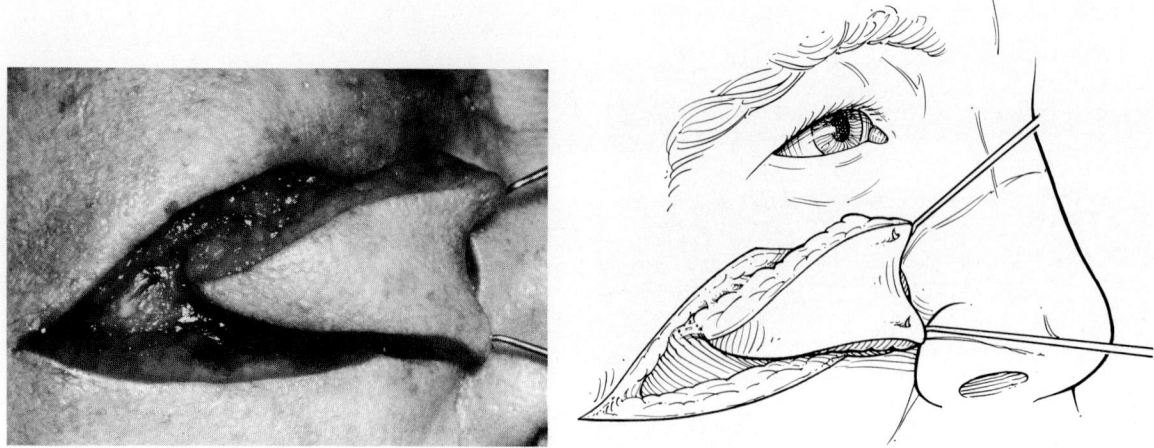

The flap is mobilized on its subcutaneous pedicle until the required medial movement can be achieved.

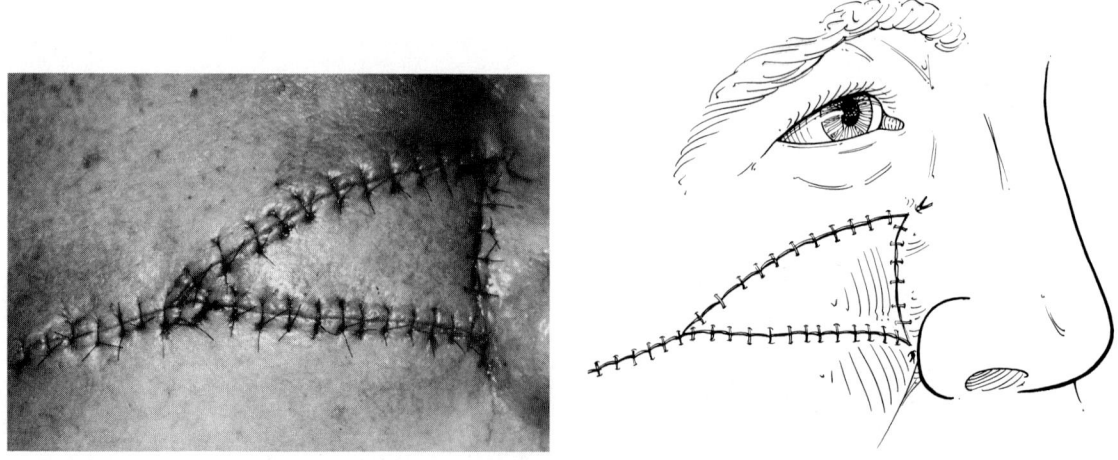

The closure is in a V-Y fashion, with care taken to be sure that the medial edge of the triangular flap lies in the nose-cheek junction. In this way a satisfactory aesthetic result is obtained.

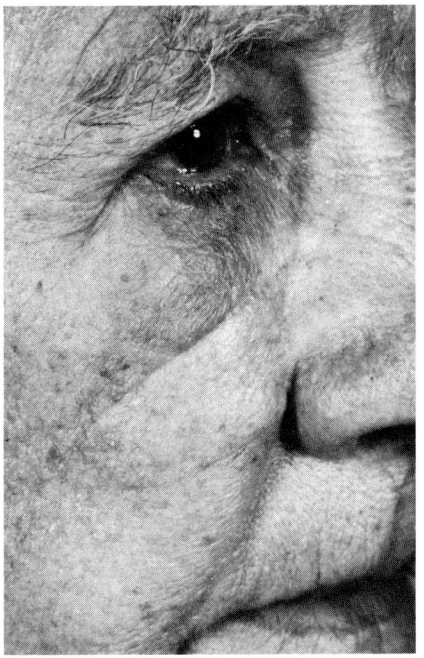

PROBLEMS

The scars resulting from the nasolabial transposition flap are oriented almost at right angles to the ideal skin lines on the face, and therefore they are obvious. The island can pincushion and thus cause an obvious and unattractive contour defect. For these reasons this procedure is rarely indicated.

SURGICAL TECHNIQUE OF CHOICE

The straight advancement flap followed by the vertical triangular advancement flap has given the best results in reconstructing the supramedial cheek area. The scars are in an ideal line and therefore not particularly noticeable. The dissection is more limited than with the other methods. Perhaps because of this, there has been almost no morbidity associated with these flaps. However, not all patients are suitable for this approach, and it may be necessary in some to use the lateral rotation flap in spite of its potential problems.

The latter method is excellent for large defects. For the surgeon with experience in using advancement flaps, this approach to large defects may also be substituted, as shown effectively in the patient on p. 232.

☐ Alar Base–Nasolabial Region Reconstruction

One concern associated with reconstruction in this area is the liklihood of distortion of the alar base. Worse still is the possible obliteration of the complex surface anatomy of the alar base–cheek area. All methods that involve importing bulky flaps or skin grafting procedures tend to cause these problems. Such methods should not be used and thus will not be considered here. Only two methods are worthy of consideration: the nasolabial triangular advancement flap and the perialar crescentic advancement flap.

NASOLABIAL TRIANGULAR ADVANCEMENT FLAP

If the defect lies just lateral to the alar base, the reconstruction must be such that no lateral tension is placed on the alar base; otherwise it will be displaced laterally. The chosen method must not interfere with the natural lines of the alar base cheek junction. If this should occur, the symmetry of the nose would be affected in a most obvious way. The triangular advancement flap fulfills these criteria and requires very little dissection.

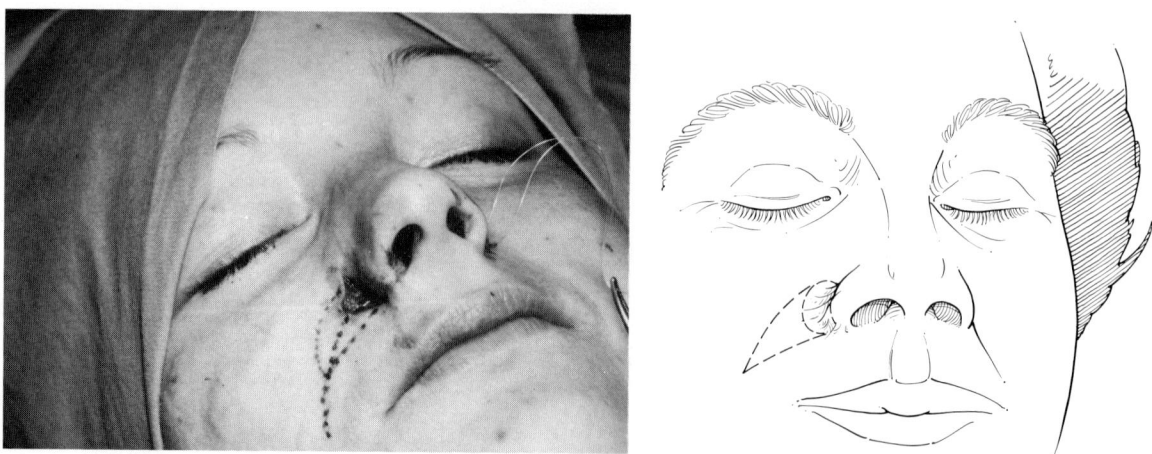

The excision is planned as a wide crescent. The planned reconstruction is a triangle lying along the nasolabial line.

CHAPTER 5
CHEEK RECONSTRUCTION

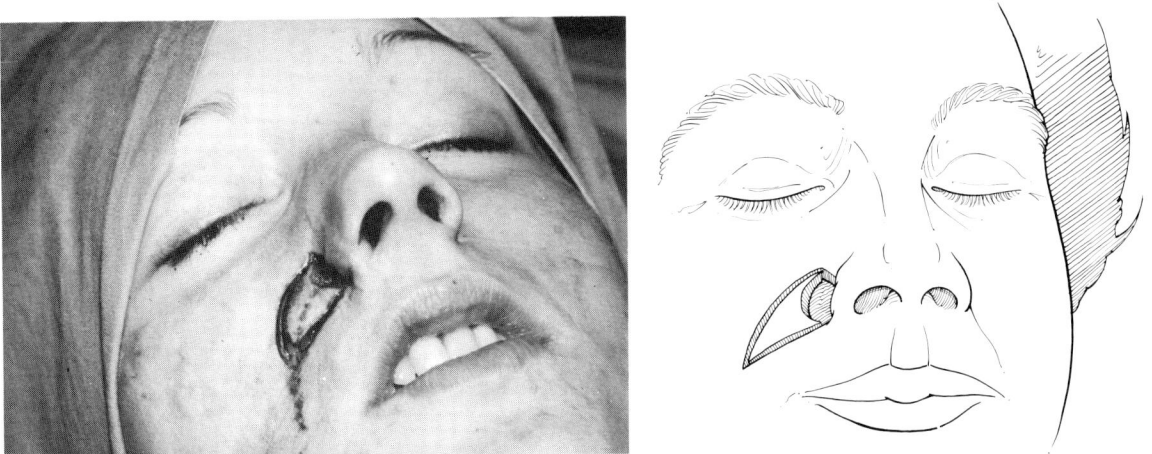

The defect is created, and the flap is elevated as an island on a subcutaneous pedicle.

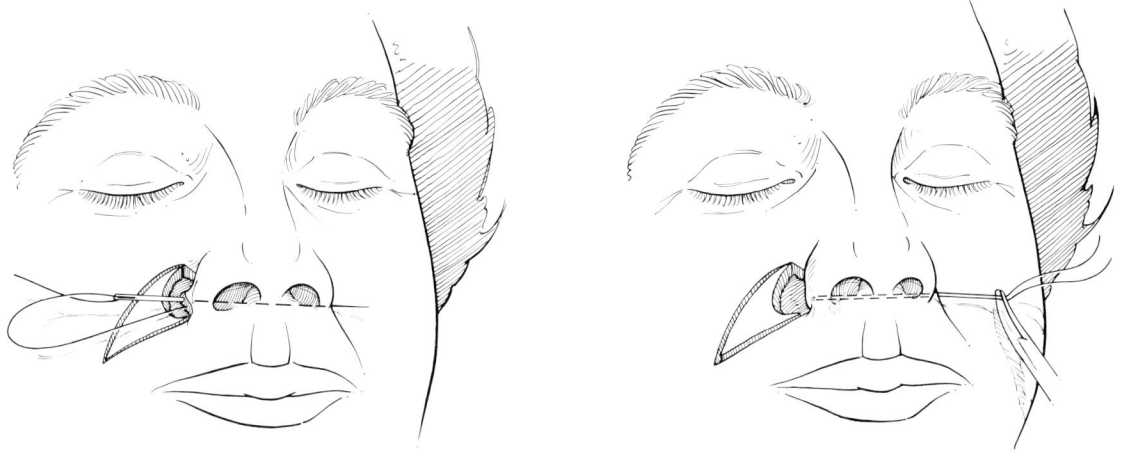

The medial edge of the flap must be fixed deeply in the groove between the alar base and the cheek. This may be accomplished by direct suturing to deep tissue. In an alternative procedure the medial edge is anchored by a suture passed from the medial edge of the triangular flap, under the nose, to exit at the contralateral nasolabial area. The suture is tied tightly enough to create a symmetric alar base region.

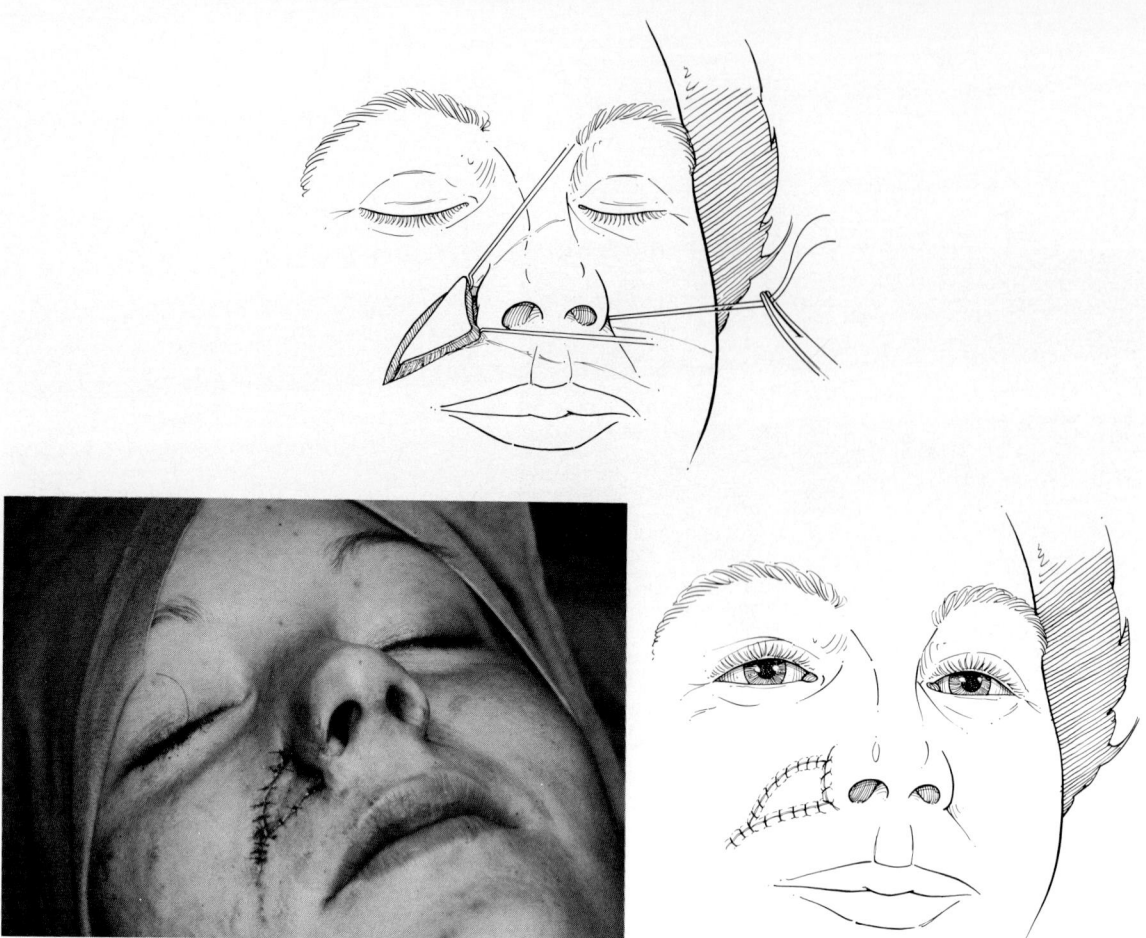

It is not necessary to perform much contouring of this new flap because the concave leading edge of the flap fits neatly into the convex medial edge of the defect. The donor site is closed in a V-Y fashion.

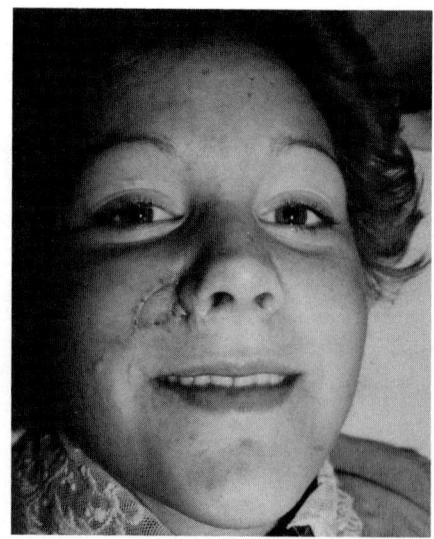

PROBLEMS

It may not be possible to use this flap in large defects because of the difficulty in obtaining enough skin in the transverse dimension. Apart from this limitation and a moderate amount of pincushioning that occurs occasionally, it is an excellent method of reconstruction that ensures good preservation of the complex anatomy of the region.

PERIALAR CRESCENTIC ADVANCEMENT FLAP

First described by Webster,[2] the perialar crescentic advancement flap is undoubtedly one of the most ingenious methods of local skin movement ever devised. With this method superior and inferior dog ears are excised in such a way as to enhance flap advancement. The concept is similar to that of Burow's triangles. Larger defects can be reconstructed with this type of flap than with the triangular advancement flap.

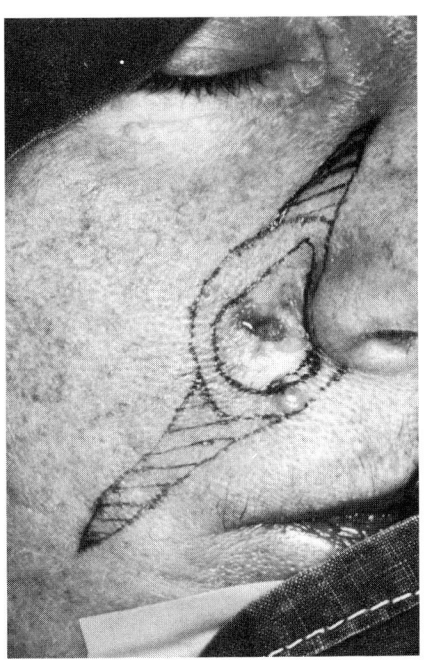

This recurrent basal cell carcinoma just lateral to the alar base will be excised and closed with the perialar crescentic advancement flap, as planned in the illustration above.

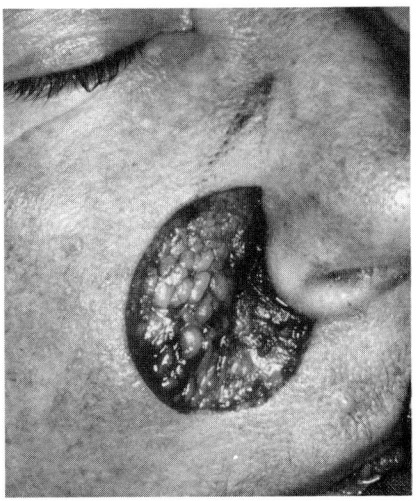

The basal cell carcinoma is widely excised.

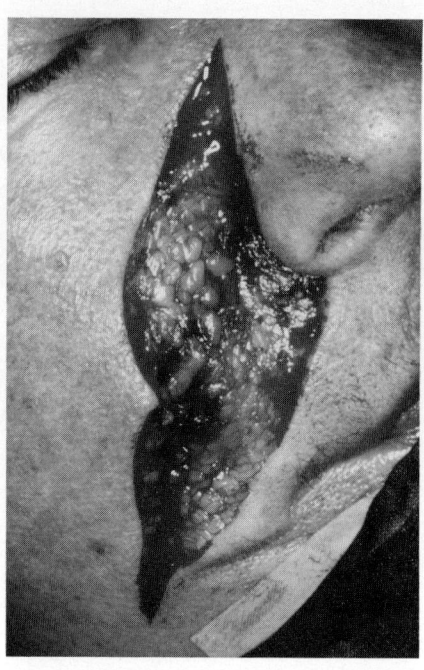

Long ellipses, which are in effect triangles, are excised above and below the defect. The superior excision runs along the junction of the nose and the cheek, often as high as just below the medial canthus. The lower excision extends along the nasolabial line as far as necessary.

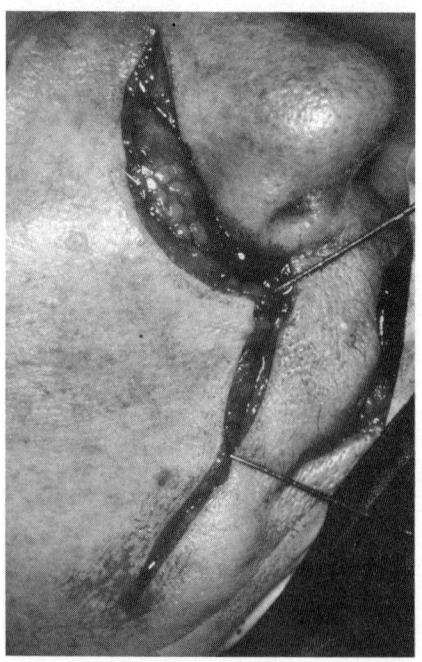

The cheek skin is undermined until enough advancement is obtained to close the defect with gentle traction on the flap edges using skin hooks.

CHAPTER 5
CHEEK RECONSTRUCTION

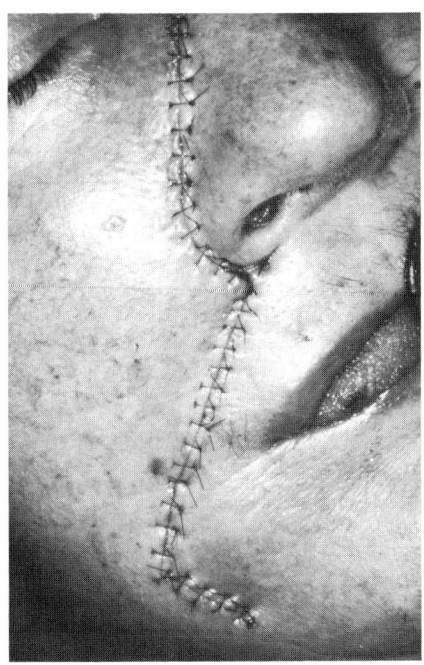

Suturing is begun superiorly. As the long lateral skin edge is approximated to the shorter medial skin edge, the cheek flap automatically advances, and the defect is closed. Minimal trimming is required.

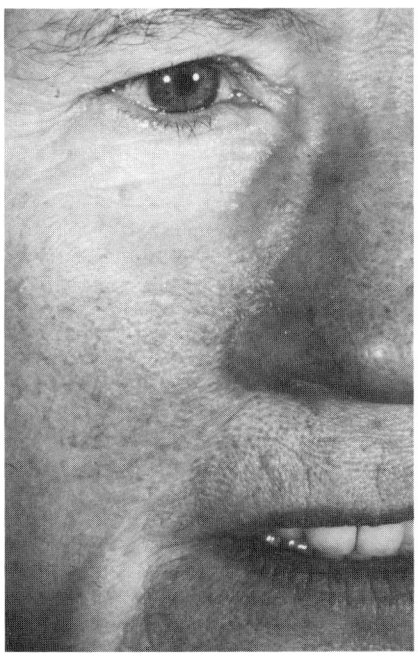

PROBLEMS

No problems have been encountered with this clever procedure. The scar line is long, but it falls into the natural line of the nose-cheek junction above and the nasolabial line below; thus it is rarely, if ever, a problem. The alar base–cheek relationship is beautifully preserved.

In some patients a slight flattening of the nasolabial fold will occur, leading to a very small degree of asymmetry. The perialar crescentic advancement flap can be used in younger patients to produce a very satisfactory cosmetic result.

SURGICAL TECHNIQUE OF CHOICE

Both methods described here have a place in reconstruction of the nasolabial region. A small defect in this area can be adequately dealt with by the triangular advancement flap. The scarring is complex but usually blends in well; some pincushioning may occur.

The ingenious perialar crescentic advancement flap is a pleasure to perform because large defects can be closed with minimal cosmetic deformity. Once the important principle of flap design underlying this method is understood, it can be applied elsewhere.

☐ Lateral to Alar Base Reconstruction

This region can be somewhat difficult to reconstruct because most methods—such as rhomboid, bilobed, rotation, and transposition flaps—tend to produce donor scars across the lines of minimal relaxed tension. As a result, the scars may appear very obvious.

INFERIOR ADVANCEMENT FLAP

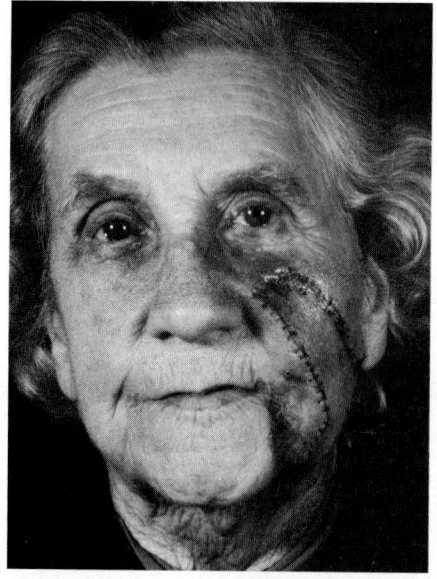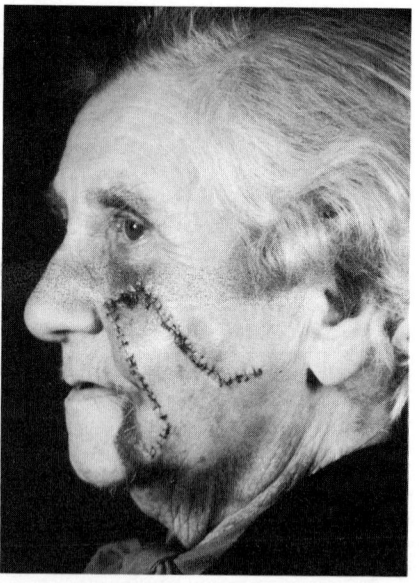

The inferior advancement flap will close fairly large defects.

This technique, which is identical to the one used for the patient shown on pp. 229 to 231, is recommended for reconstructing defects in the lateral to alar base region.

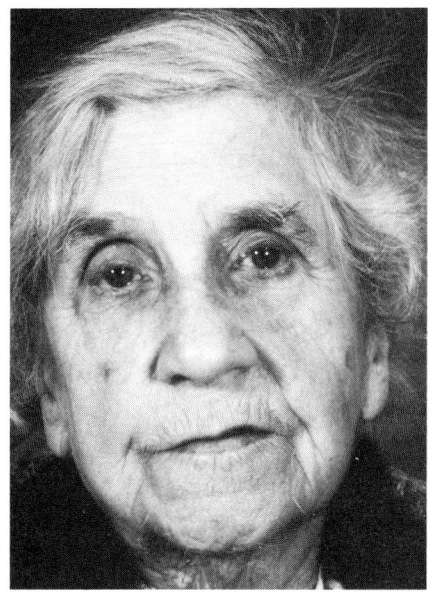
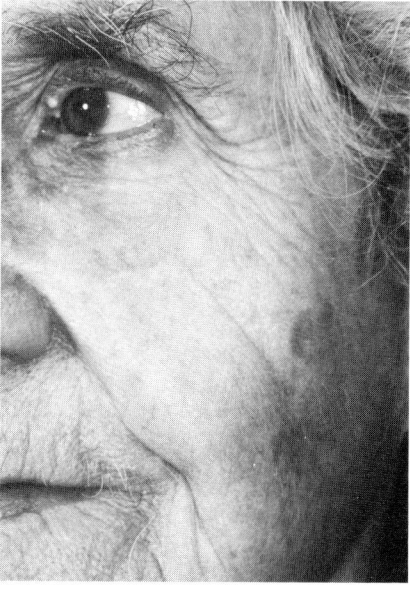

PROBLEMS

Apart from a slight deepening of the nasolabial fold, this method of reconstruction has been without problems.

REFERENCES

1. Mitz, V., and Peyronie, M.: Superficial musculo-aponeurotic system (SMAS) in the parotid and cheek area, Plast. Reconstr. Surg. **58:**80, 1976.
2. Webster, J.P.: Crescentic peri-alar cheek excision for upper lip flap advancement with a short history of upper lip repair, **16:**434, 1944.

CHAPTER 6

EAR RECONSTRUCTION

>That ruby which you wear
>hung from the tip of your soft ear
>
>ROBERT HERRICK
>*Hesperides*
>
>Elected Silence, sing to me
>and beat upon my whorled ear.
>
>GERARD MANLEY HOPKINS
>*The Habit of Perfection*

The ear is often taken for granted and is usually associated with function rather than with appearance. Yet an ear deformity is not often overlooked. In Western society prominent ears are a source of ridicule, and deformed, partial, or missing ears are obvious to everyone. Cup ears look strange, cauliflower ears denote pugilism, and pointed ears are suggestive of elves. Because of this awareness of the aesthetics of ear size, shape, and position, the artistic closure of ear defects is an important consideration for the surgeon in planning reconstruction.

■ ANATOMY

Ear skin is thin, pale, and shiny. It adheres closely to the underlying cartilage on the anterior aspect until the helical rim is reached. In this area the skin is pink, soft, and often matt in texture. From superior to inferior aspect along the rim, the amount of subcutaneous tissue (and consequently the excess skin) in relation to cartilage increases, culminating in an earlobe composed totally of skin and subcutaneous tissue. The earlobe is often red, matt, and soft; the skin in this region is fairly thick. On the posterior aspect of the ear the skin is thicker. More subcutaneous tissue is present and blood vessels are abundant. The skin is much less adherent to the cartilage. In the mastoid area the skin is pale and thick.

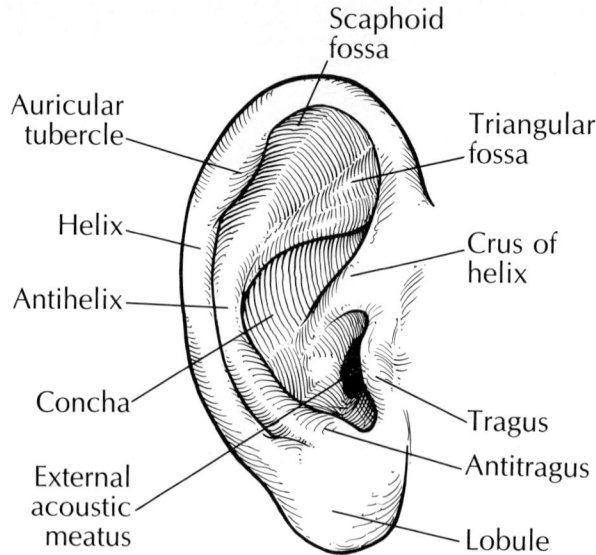

Configuration of the external ear is complicated and merits careful study.

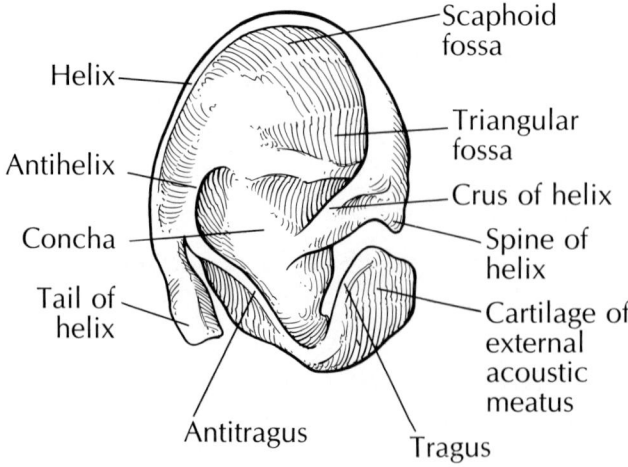

The structure of auricular cartilage is equally complex.

☐ Musculature

EXTRINSIC MUSCLES

Auricularis anterior: Arises from the lateral edge of the epicranial aponeurosis and is inserted into the spine of the helix.

Auricularis superior: Originates from the epicranial aponeurosis and is inserted into the upper part of the cranial surface of the auricle by a thin, flat tendon.

Auricularis posterior: Arises from the mastoid portion of the temporal bone and is inserted into the conchal eminence.

INTRINSIC MUSCLES

Helicis major: Lies upon the anterior margin of the helix. It arises from the helical spine and is inserted into the anterior border of the helix.

Helicis minor: Covers the crus helicis.

Tragicus: Lies on the lateral surface of the tragus.

Antitragicus: Arises from the outer part of the antitragus and is inserted into the tail of the helix and antihelix.

Transversus auriculae: Lies on the back of the ear over the conchal eminence.

Obliquus auriculae: Lies on the back of the ear and over the conchal eminence; it extends to the triangular eminence.

Both groups of muscles have little or no function in humans.

☐ Nerve Supply

MOTOR NERVES

Extrinsic muscles: The auricularis anterior and superior muscles are supplied by temporal branches of the facial nerve. The auricularis posterior muscle is supplied by the posterior auricular branch of the facial artery.

Intrinsic muscles: Those muscles of the lateral aspect are supplied by the temporal branches of the facial nerve. The ones on the posterior aspect are supplied by the posterior auricular branch of the facial nerve.

SENSORY NERVES

Sensation is supplied by the greater auricular and lesser occipital nerves from the cervical plexus, the auriculotemporal branch of the mandibular nerve, and the auricular branch of the vagus nerve.

☐ Blood Supply

The arteries include (a) the posterior auricular branches of the external carotid artery, which supply the posterior surface with some small branches extending to the lateral aspect; (b) the anterior auricular branches of the superficial temporal artery, which supply the lateral surface; and (c) a branch from the occipital artery, which adds to the supply to the posterior surface. The veins accompany the arteries.

☐ Lymphatic Drainage

The upper half of the cranial surface, the whole margin of the ear, and the posterior wall of the external auditory meatus drain to the upper deep cervical nodes and the mastoid lymph nodes. These nodes lie superficial to the mastoid insertion of the sternomastoid muscle.

The lobule of the ear and the floor of the external meatus drain to the superficial cervical lymph nodes; these nodes are situated along the external jugular vein superficial to the sternomastoid muscle. The middle ear drains to the deep parotid lymph nodes.

■ AESTHETICS

Because the ear protrudes from the side of the head, it is a prominent feature and any change in it is easily noticed. Alteration of one ear allows comparison with the other for symmetry.

■ PLACEMENT OF INCISIONS

The irregularities of the ear surface necessitate careful placement of incisions. If possible, incisions should not be taken across concavities; any scar contracture in this situation will cause obvious deformity. It is preferable to place the incisions within folds, where they are hidden from view.

■ AREAS OF TISSUE AVAILABILITY

There are limited options for flaps in ear reconstruction, and the indication for each of the available flaps is clear. If a resection is large, it is difficult to effect a very satisfactory result. Extra skin is available along the rim of the ear and in the postauricular area. For many reconstructions it is necessary to import skin from nonhairbearing areas around the ear.

Many ear lesions are handled either by elliptic excision and direct closure or by wedge resection. Posterior defects can almost always be closed directly. Large tumors may require either partial or total ear amputation. Superficial lesions, if extensive, may require excision and grafting. With a situation such as this, there is little call for local flaps. These flaps must be planned carefully to avoid ischemia or secondary ear deformity resulting from the flap donor site. Occasionally, small kite flaps, rim advancement flaps, or postauricular transposition flaps may be used on the rim of the ear.

■ AREAS TO BE RECONSTRUCTED

The area to be reconstructed may vary from part to all of the ear. A partial defect may consist of skin, skin and cartilage, or it may be full thickness. The ear, a cartilaginous appendage covered by skin, is a frequent site for cutaneous malignancy because of its prominence and resulting exposure to the sun and other elements. The convolutions of the ear are complex as becomes clear when a total ear reconstruction is being undertaken. Not only are there multiple convexities and concavities but the cartilage shows areas of varying thickness.

☐ Rim Defects

If there is a rim defect and wedge resection with direct closure, or if small triangular kite flaps moved along the rim from above and below the defect have been judged unsuitable, an advancement of the rim may be performed.

RIM ADVANCEMENT

Although rim advancement may seem somewhat hazardous, it is a perfectly reliable method of reconstruction. This procedure makes use of the excess of soft tissue available around the edge of the ear.

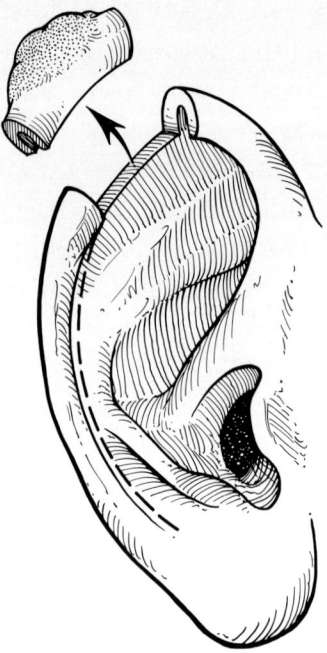

A lesion present on the rim is excised, with the full thickness of the rim being taken. This leaves an unsightly defect if closed directly; thus the reconstructive method of choice in this situation is a rim advancement flap.

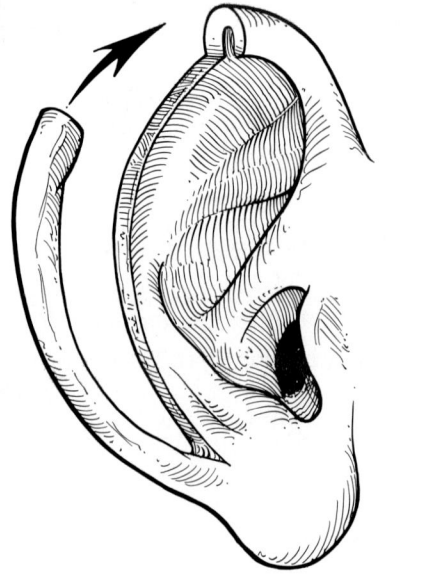 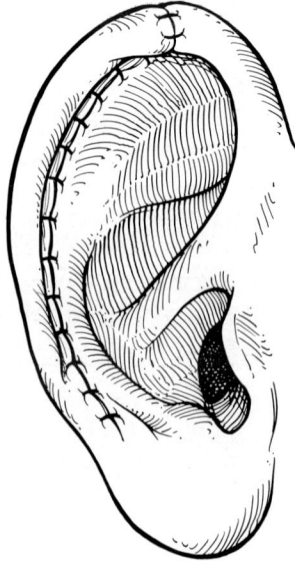

From the inferior portion of the defect, the rim is incised to the upper part of the lobule. The latter is soft, mobile, and extensile. These factors allow the rim to be advanced and the defect to be closed.

PROBLEMS

Distal necrosis of the flap may occur, but it is very unusual and would be minimal. Some distortion and shortening of the lobule may occur, and, if both lobules are closely inspected, asymmetry may be noted. This is not a significant problem.

☐ Anterior Conchal Defect

Lesions arising on the thin anterior skin of the concha involve the perichondrium, and thus adequate excision usually requires the removal of underlying conchal cartilage. The defect may be closed with a skin graft, but a local flap is quicker and gives better results in skin color, lack of contraction, and reestablishment of contour. The postauricular "revolving door" flap is ideally suited for this repair.

POSTAURICULAR "REVOLVING DOOR" ISLAND FLAP

Described by Masson,[2] the postauricular "revolving door" island flap is one of the most elegant reconstructive procedures in head and neck surgery. It is ideal for defects of the conchal area; the larger the defect the better, since this then allows a larger pedicle, a more secure flap, and total conchal replacement with flap skin.

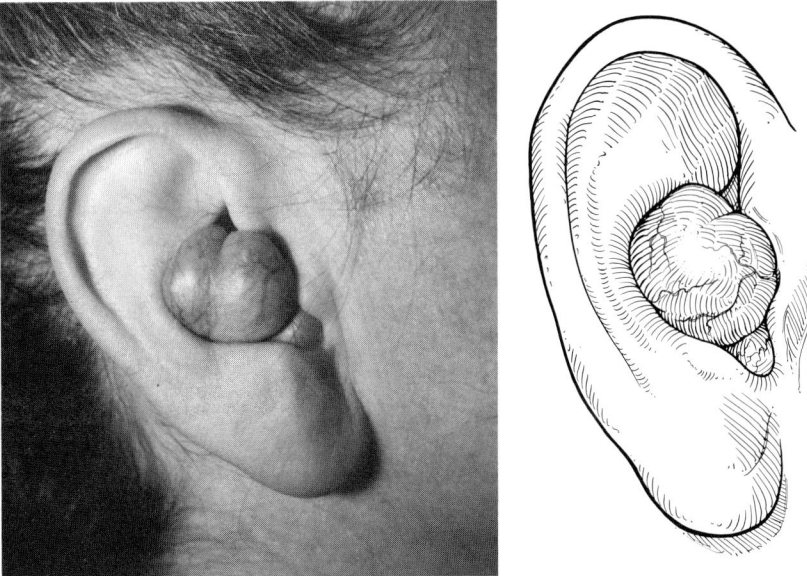

This illustration shows a neurofibroma of the concha of the right ear.

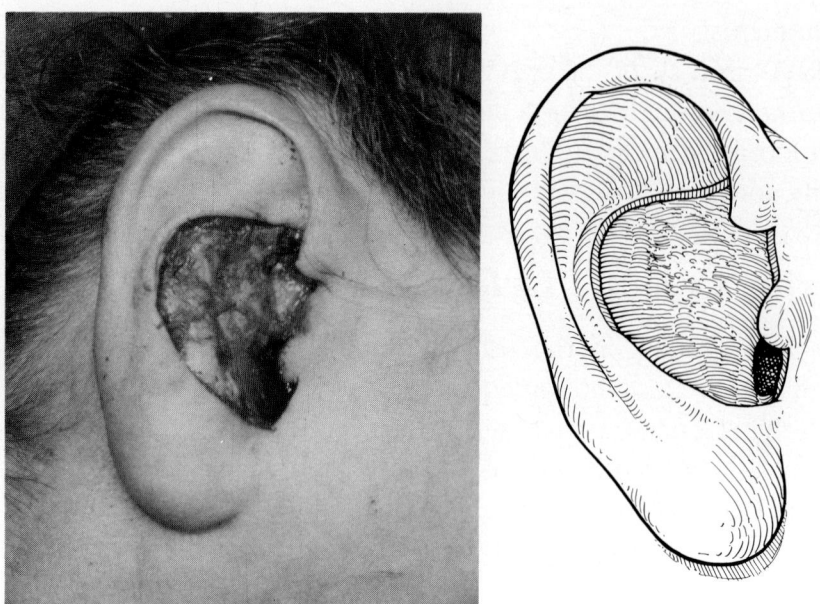

The neurofibroma was excised together with the underlying conchal cartilage.

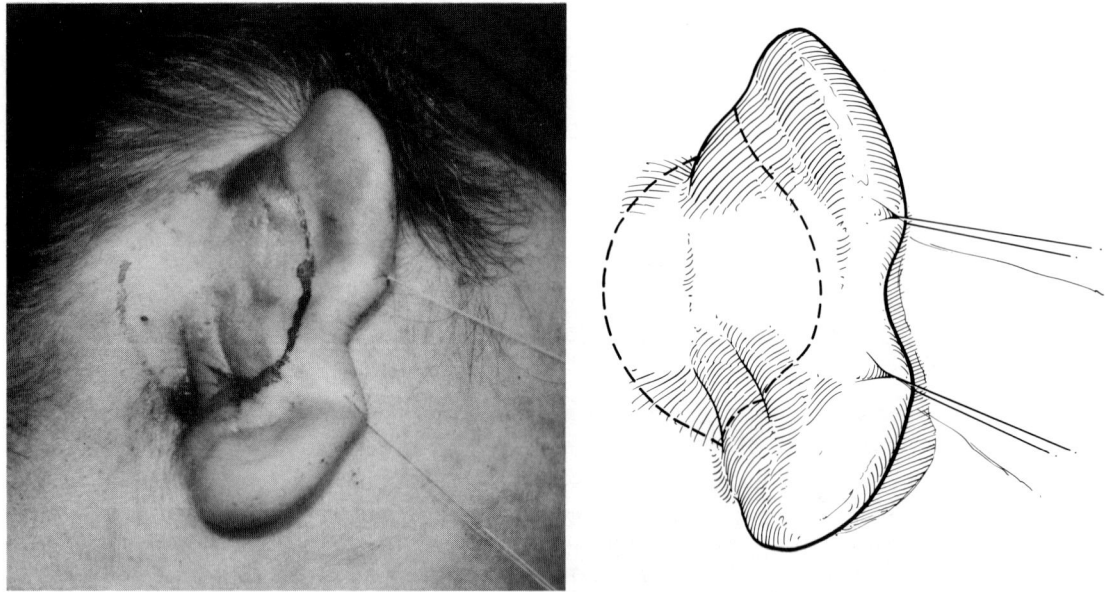

The ear is then pulled forward, and an island of skin is outlined, partly on the mastoid area and partly on the postauricular region.

CHAPTER 6
EAR RECONSTRUCTION

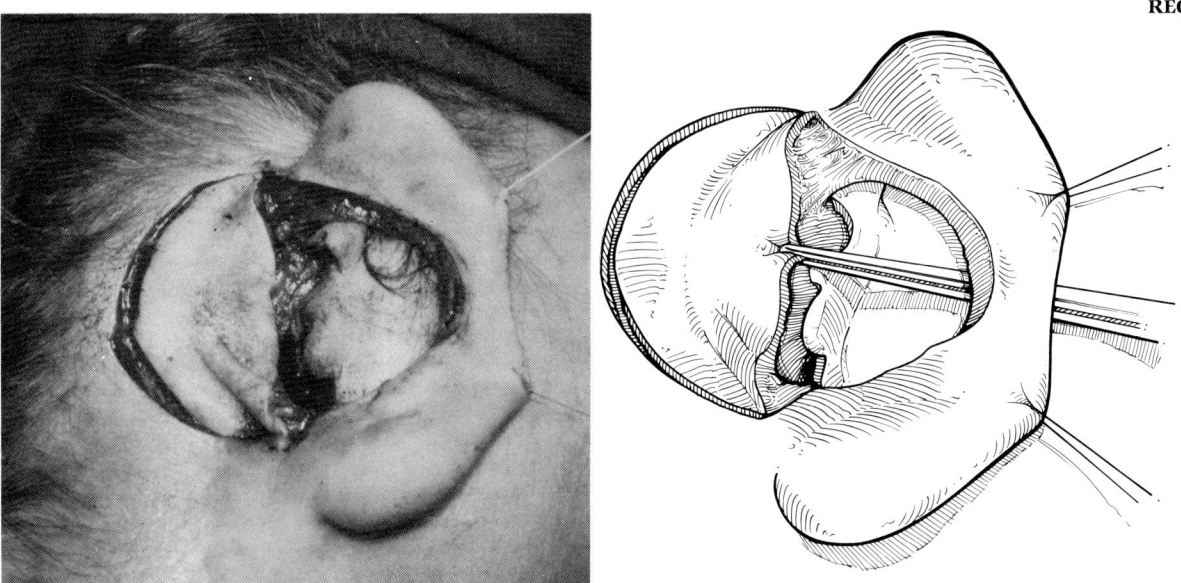

An incision is made around this island, and the flap is raised posteriorly and anteriorly. The skin is incised through to the anterior surface of the ear; the posterior skin elevation stops at the ear-mastoid groove. This vertical attachment becomes the pedicle, the hinge of the revolving door. The island is freed a little superiorly and inferiorly.

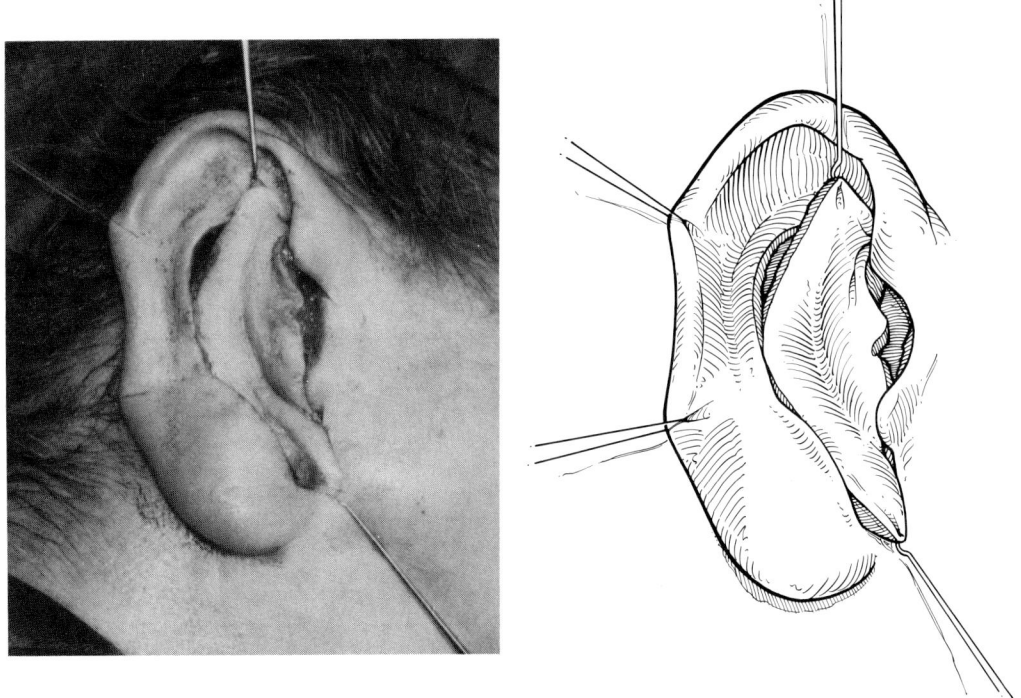

This posterior island can then be rotated like a revolving door, and the conchal defect is reconstructed.

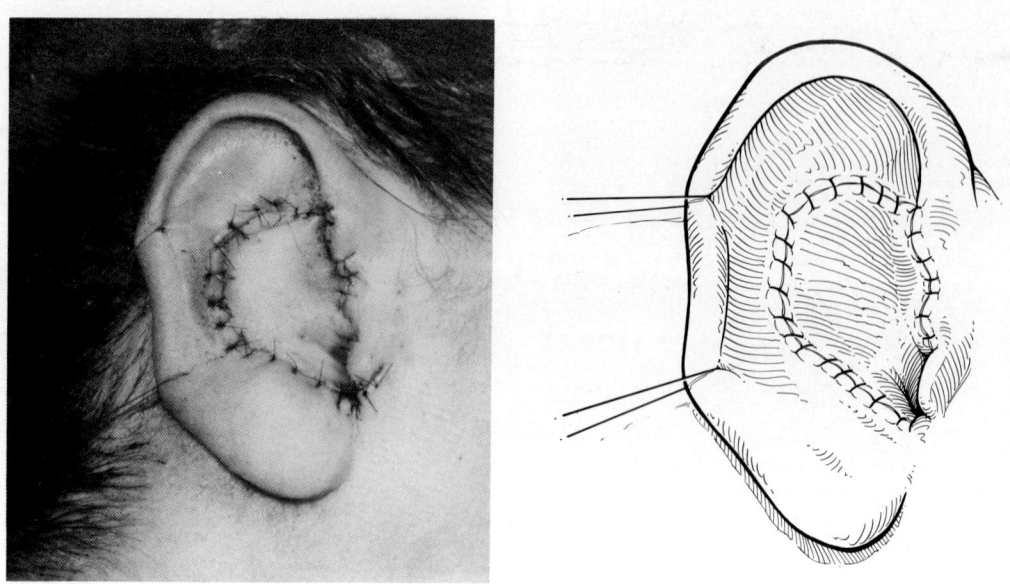

The postauricular defect is closed directly.

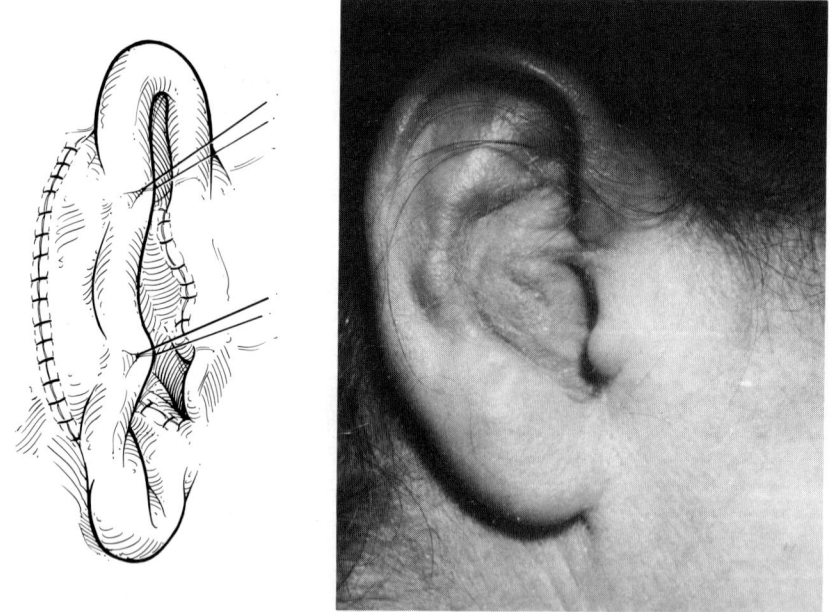

After this technique the ear looks almost completely normal.

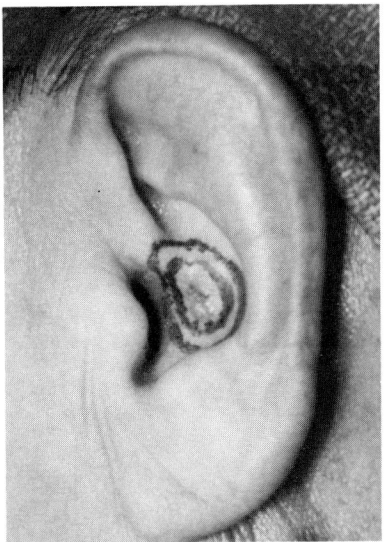 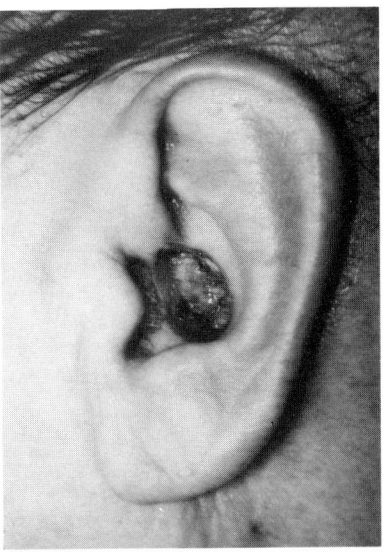 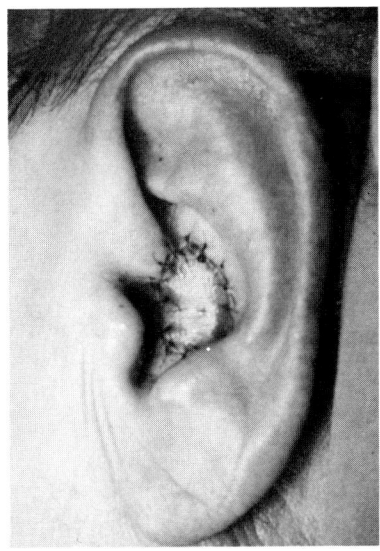

The use of this flap is also suitable for closing a smaller conchal defect following excision of a basal cell carcinoma.

PROBLEMS

Only two main problems may be encountered with this technique: flap necrosis, which may occur when small defects are being reconstructed, and infection. Although necrosis has not been encountered with this type of flap, if it occurred, it would be handled by frequent dressings and debridement or by wedge excision. Infection requires antibiotics. If chondritis occurs, it can be painful, may require debridement, and takes some time to eliminate. Occasionally hematoma may occur. If it does, the sutures are removed and the hematoma is expressed. These complications are rare.

☐ Partial Ear Defect

Trauma or tumor excision are the primary causes of partial ear loss; this usually occurs in the middle ear area. In the older patient a partial ear defect might be treated by a wedge resection, with approximation of the edges of the ear. In the younger person, however, the cupping of the ear resulting from this approach would be aesthetically unacceptable, and thus a more complete reconstruction is performed. If the patient has a full-thickness loss of rim, antehelical fold, and a variable amount of concha, this can be reconstructed only by a flap. The postauricular flap is the best solution for this problem.

■ POSTAURICULAR FLAP

The postauricular flap is a two-stage procedure, yet it is a rapid method of reconstructing a difficult defect. The bulk of the flap allows total reconstruction without the necessity for a cartilage graft.

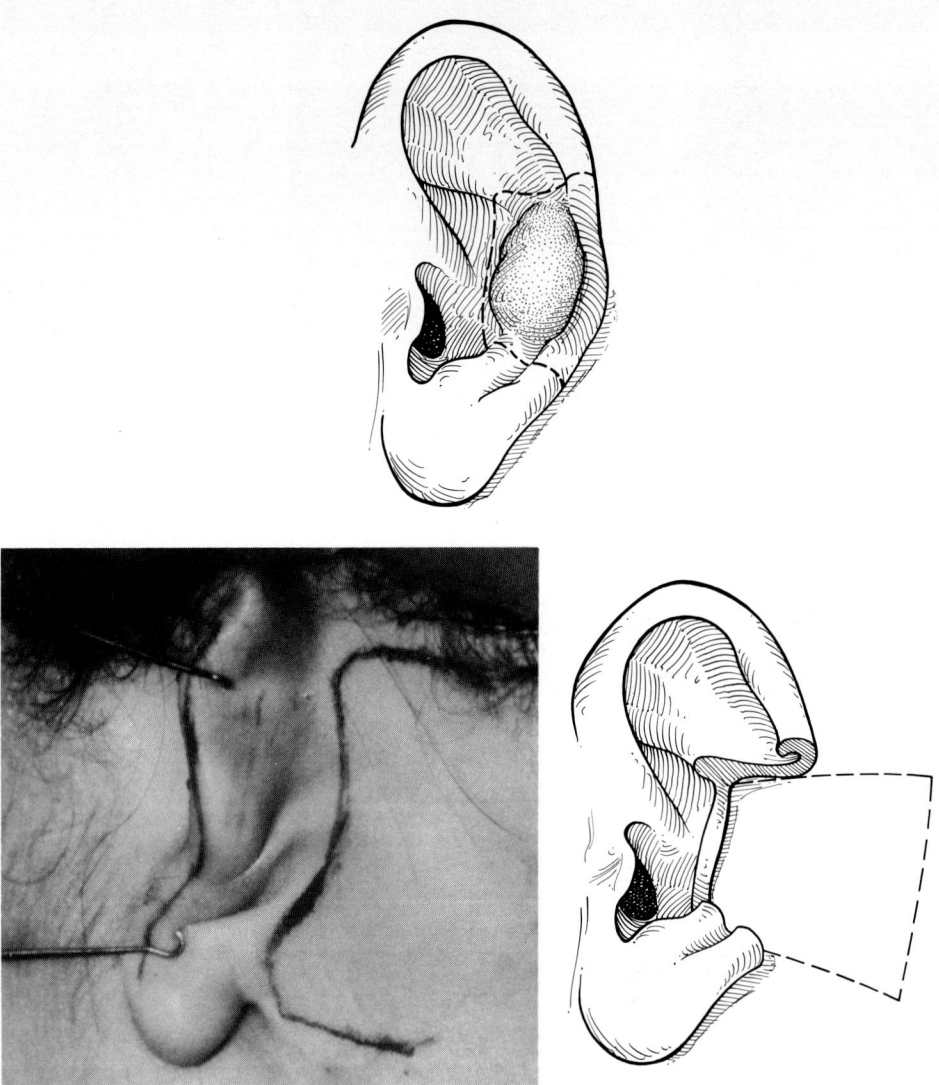

After creation of the defect, a flap is planned, based on the edge of the hairline. The breadth of the flap is equal to that of the defect; the length is such that it will reconstruct the anterior surface, the rim, and posterior surface.

CHAPTER 6
EAR RECONSTRUCTION

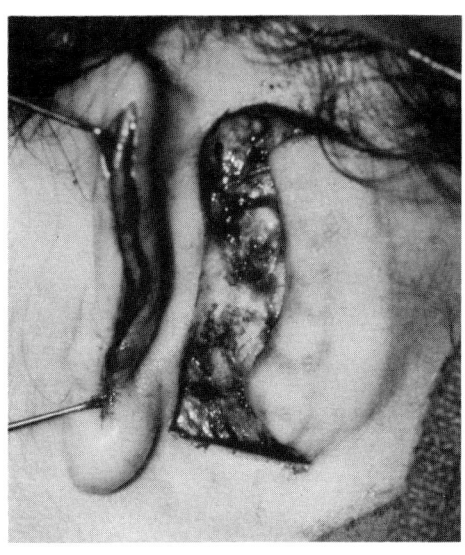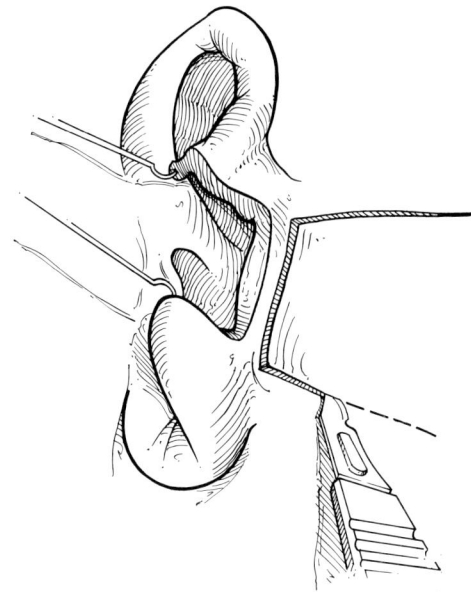

The flap is raised completely down to the postauricular fascia.

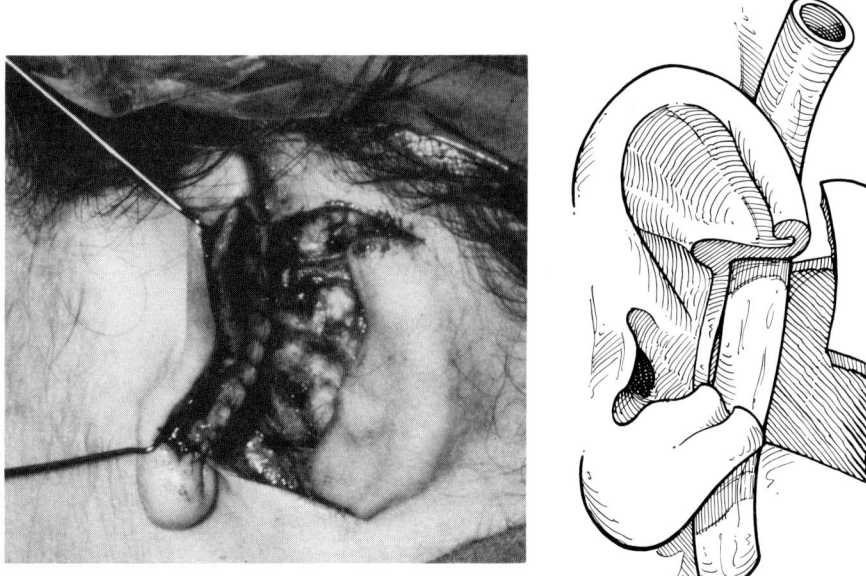

If sufficient skin is left anterior to the flap in the postauricular area, the free edge of this skin is sutured to the posterior edge of the ear defect over a portion of rubber or silicone tubing. If this is not possible, the tube is simply placed under the flap after it has been attached to the ear skin.

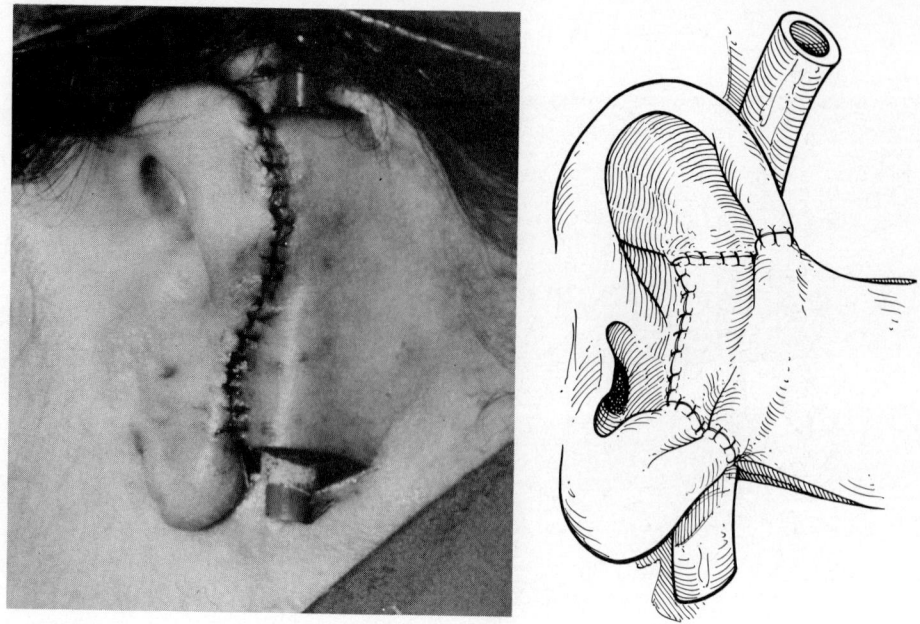

The free margin of the postauricular flap is sutured to the anterior free skin edge of the ear defect.

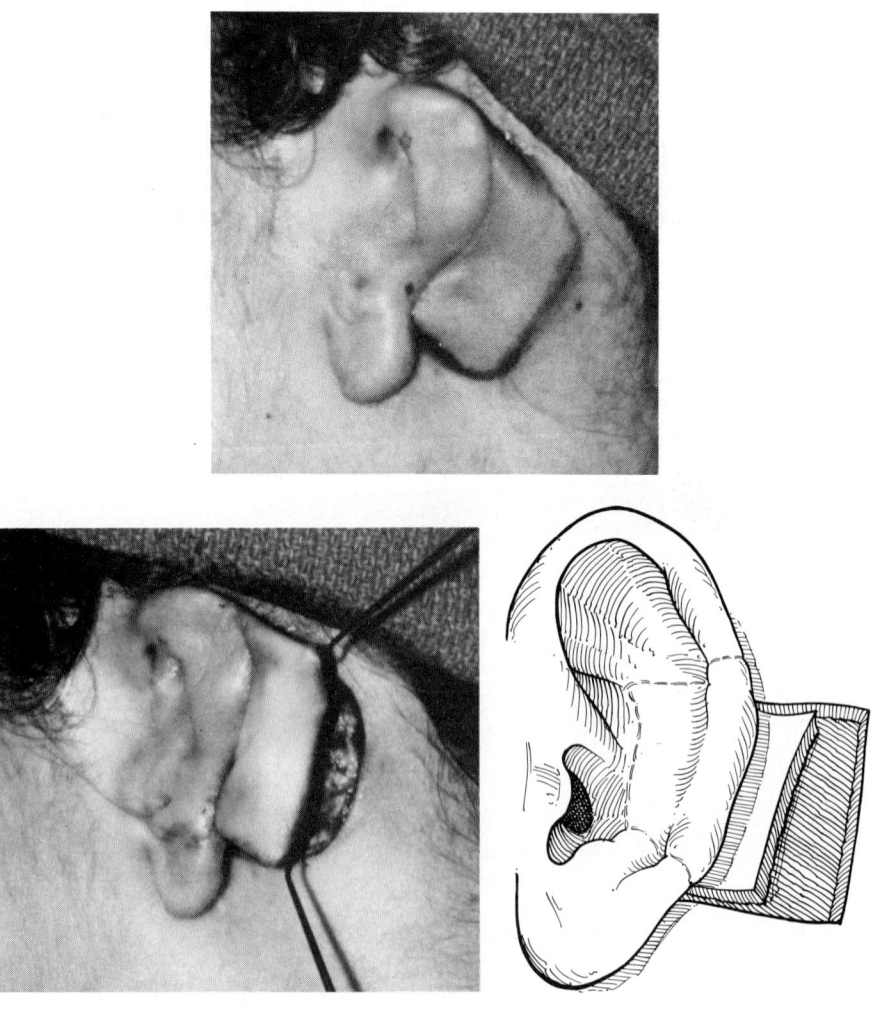

In 10 days the base of the flap is divided, and the remainder of the flap is used to resurface the posterior part of the ear.

CHAPTER 6
EAR RECONSTRUCTION

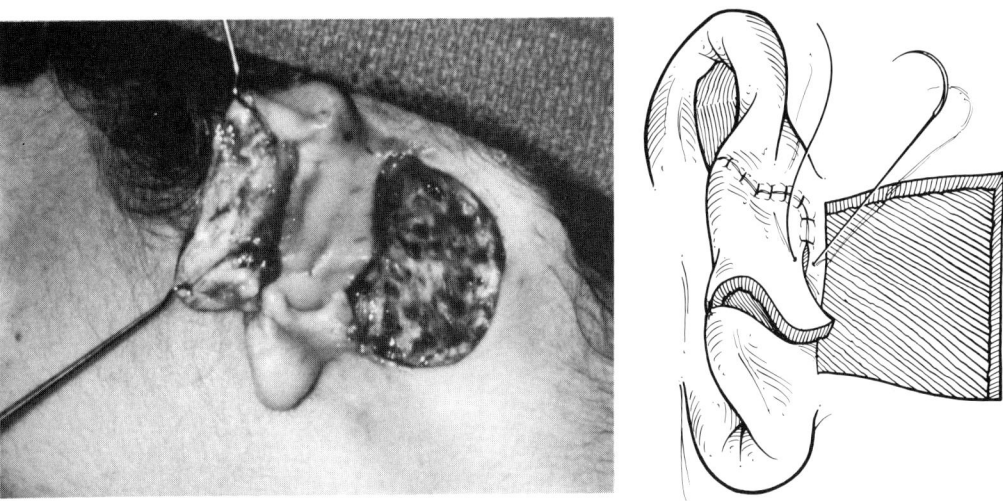

The ear defect is totally reconstructed by the flap being sutured to the posterior surface of the ear. A postauricular raw area results from division of the flap.

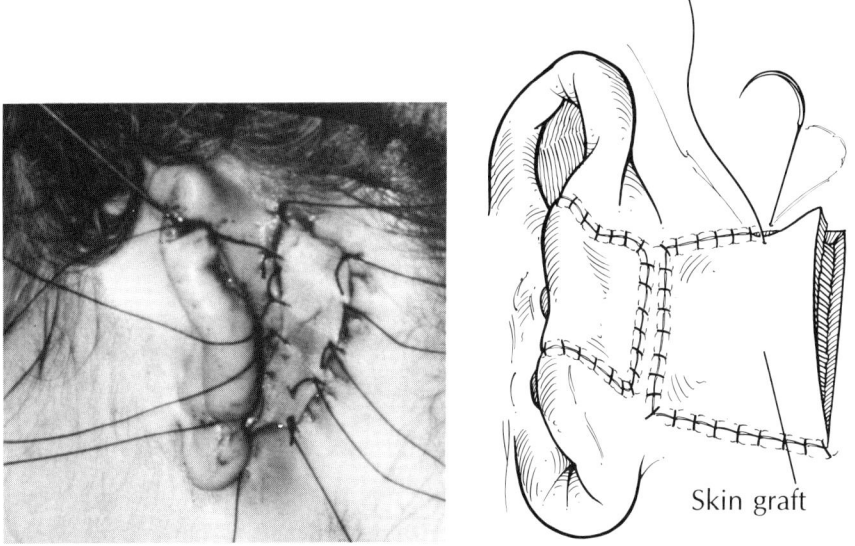

In some patients it is necessary to cover the raw donor area with skin graft. If the defect is small, it will heal spontaneously.

265

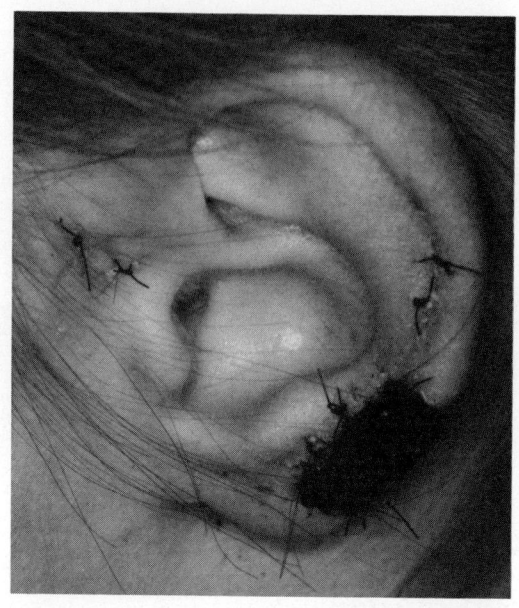

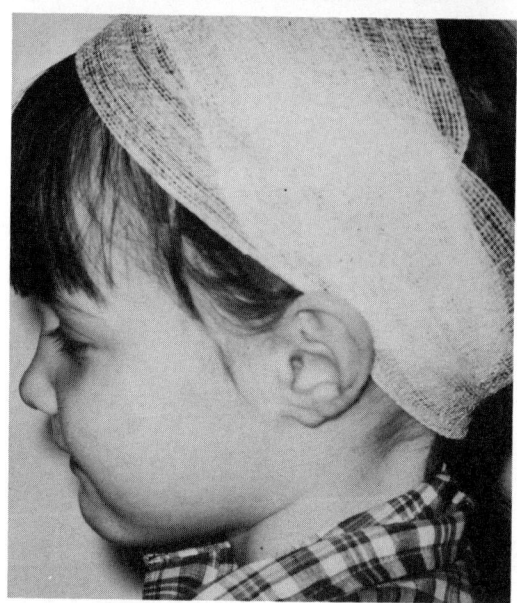

This patient lost a portion of the lower helical rim because of trauma. The treatment used was the postauricular flap reconstruction technique.

PROBLEMS

If the edge of the hairline comes close to the conchal mastoid groove, the flap may be short and a skin graft may need to be added to the posterior reconstruction. A further procedure involving flap defatting may be necessary to have an optimal aesthetic result, with a smooth helical rim. Flap loss from ischemia may occur, but this has not been observed. This is a safe and satisfactory method of reconstructing the defect.

CHAPTER 6
EAR RECONSTRUCTION

☐ Total Ear Resurfacing

A discussion of total ear reconstruction is not within the scope of this book. It is reasonable, however, to address the significant problem of skin cover when the total ear cartilage is exposed. An eventuality such as this is rare, but when it occurs, ingenuity is required. Any cover must be thin and must preserve ear contours; local skin flaps cannot fulfill these criteria. In such a situation the temporalis fascia flap may be used to advantage.

TEMPORALIS FASCIA FLAP[1]

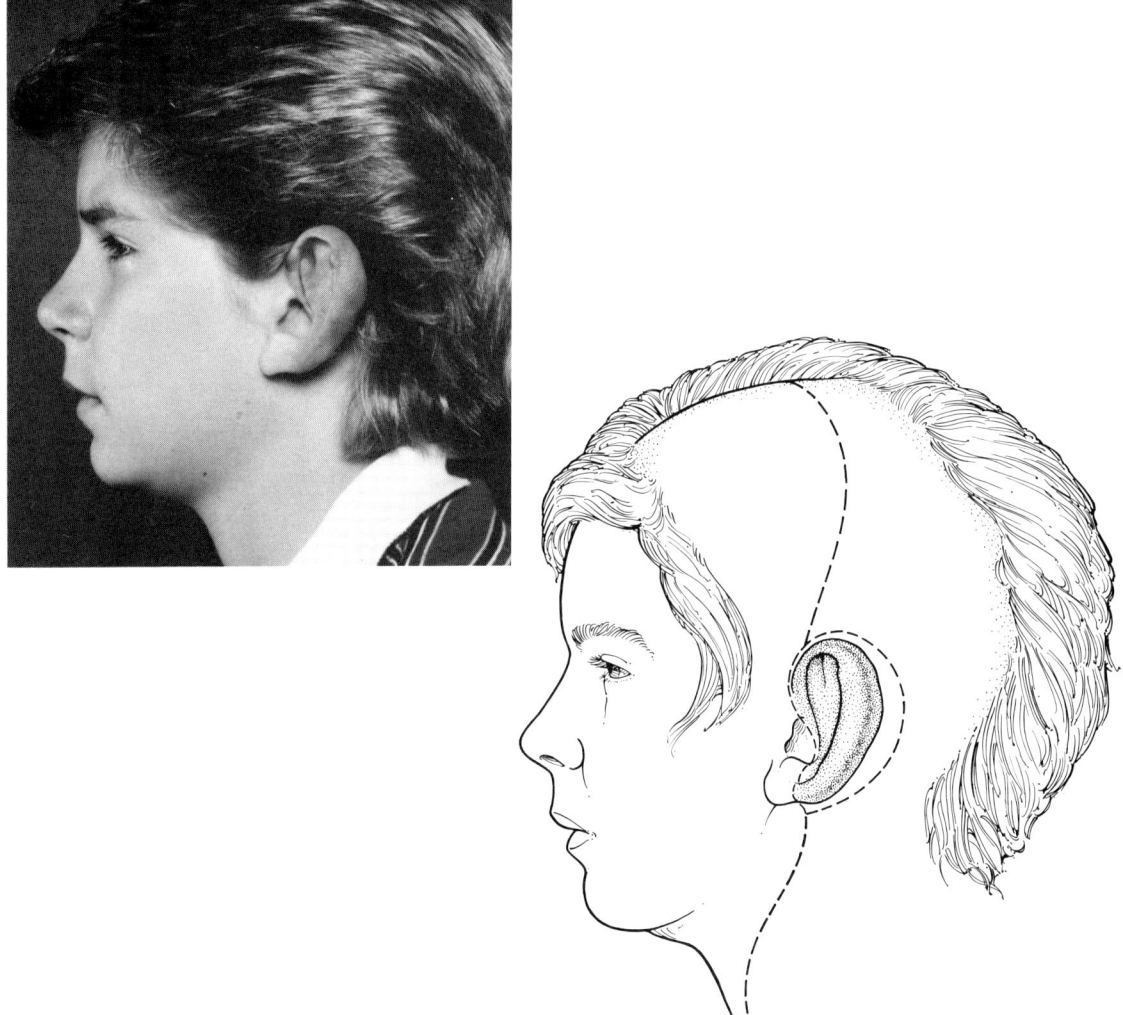

This boy has an arteriovenous malformation of the ear and postauricular area. It is a high flow, high shunt lesion that requires resection.

267

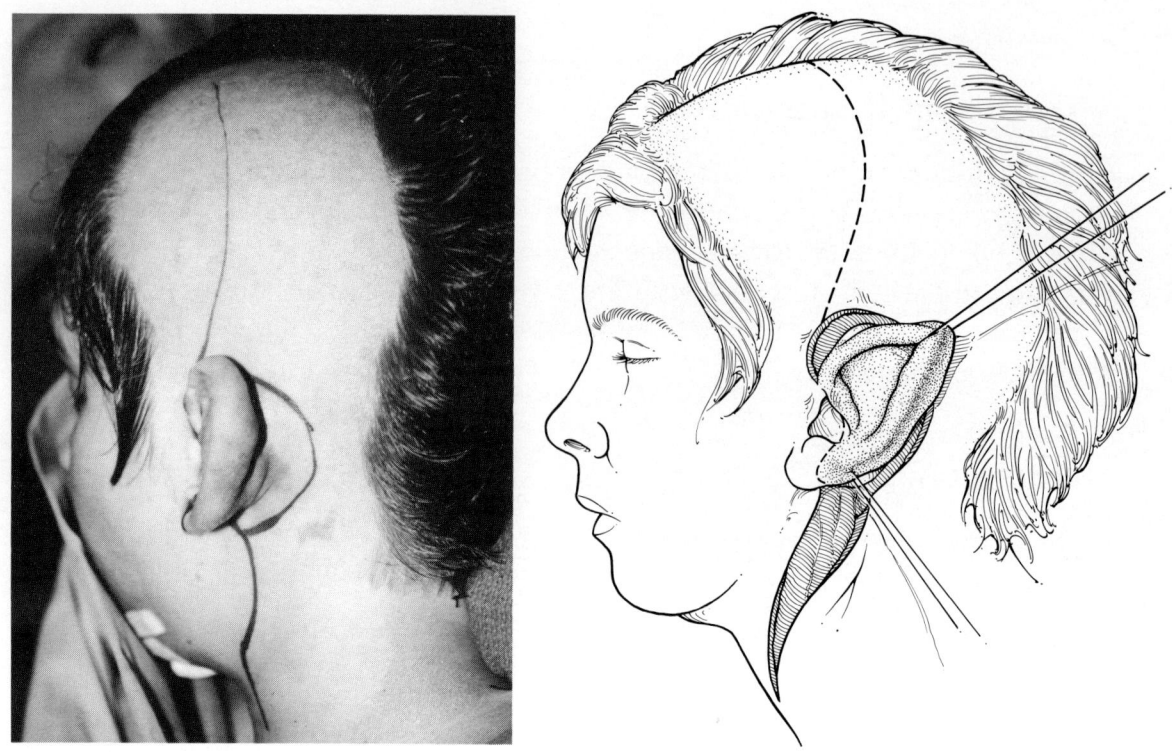

It was planned that a total resection of the lesion would be performed; the auricular cartilage would be retained and covered with an inferiorly based temporalis fascia flap.

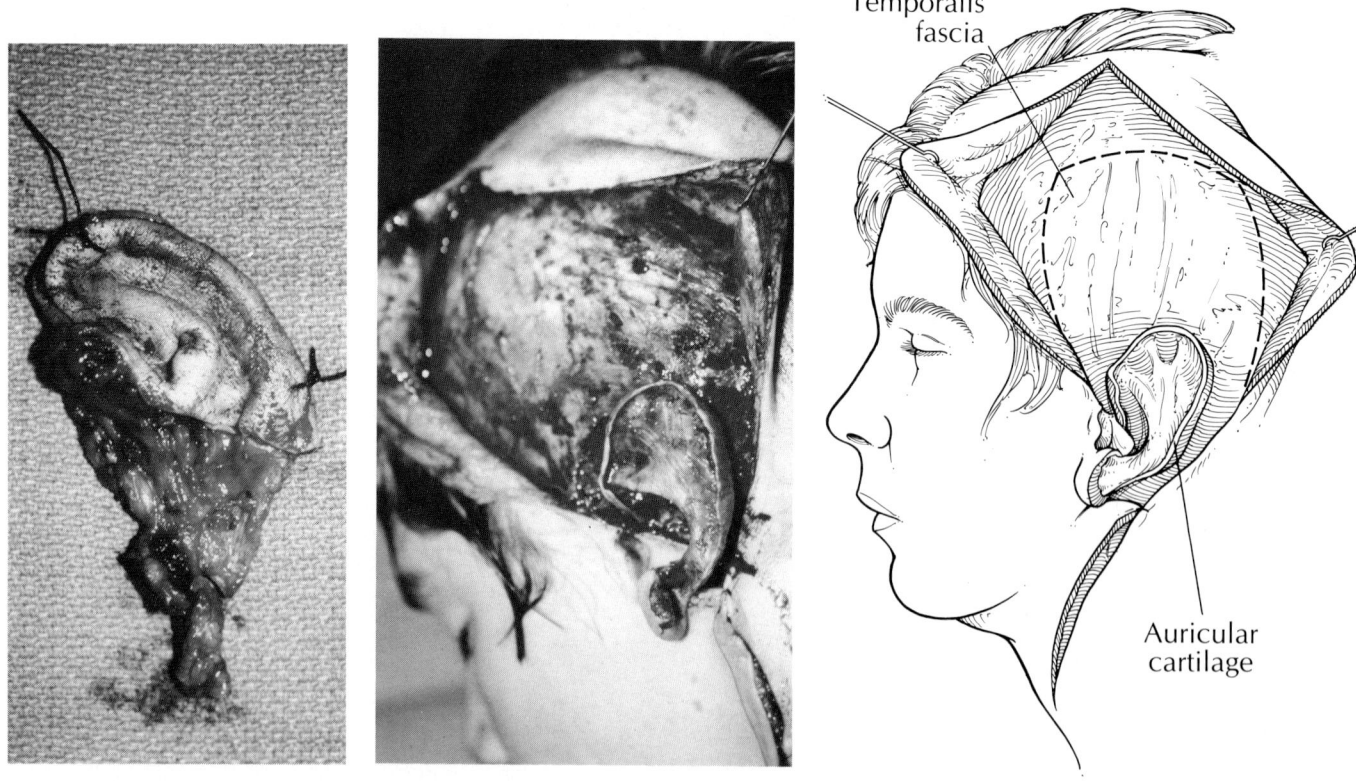

After control of the main arterial input has been gained in the neck, complete excision is carried out, and the auricular cartilage is left without perichondrium on its anterior and posterior surfaces.

CHAPTER 6
EAR RECONSTRUCTION

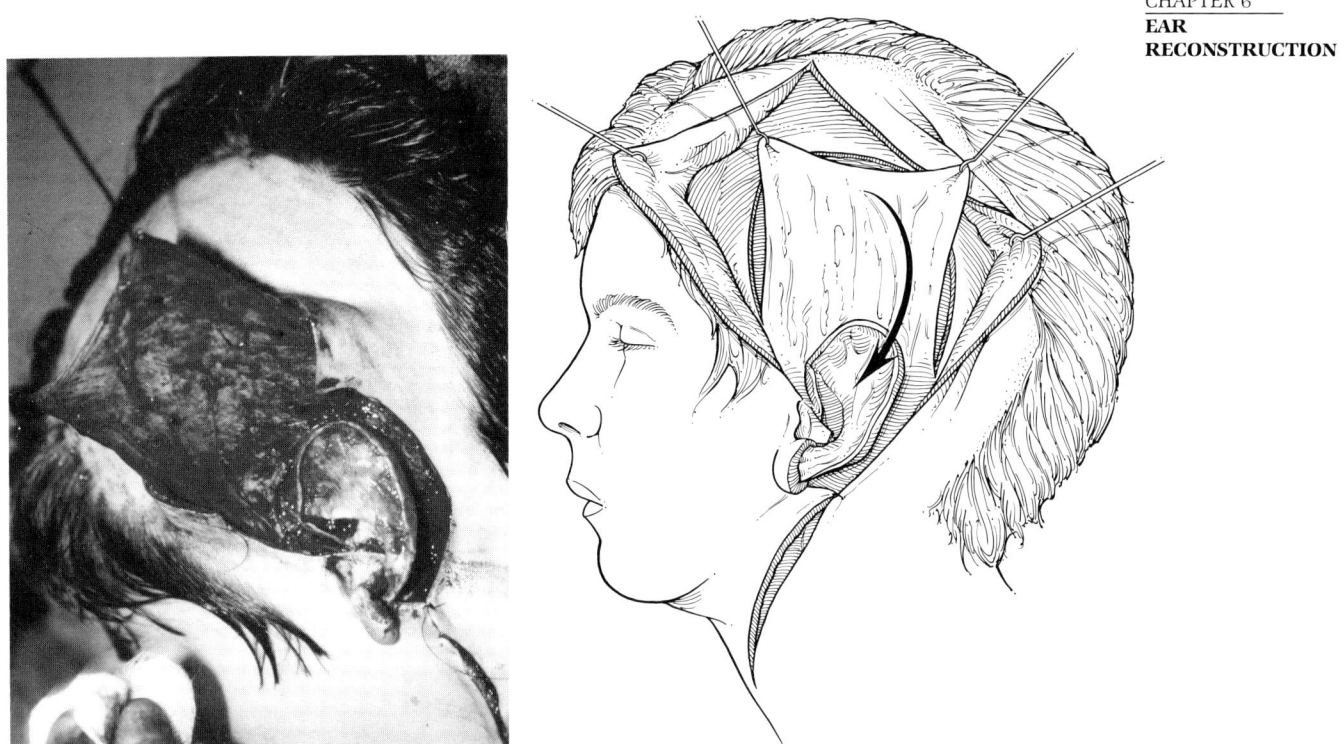

A vertical incision is made upward from the ear in the temporal area and the skin is elevated widely. The temporalis fascia is exposed, and a flap, based inferiorly, is lifted. The dimensions are those that will allow the ear to be covered completely anteriorly and posteriorly.

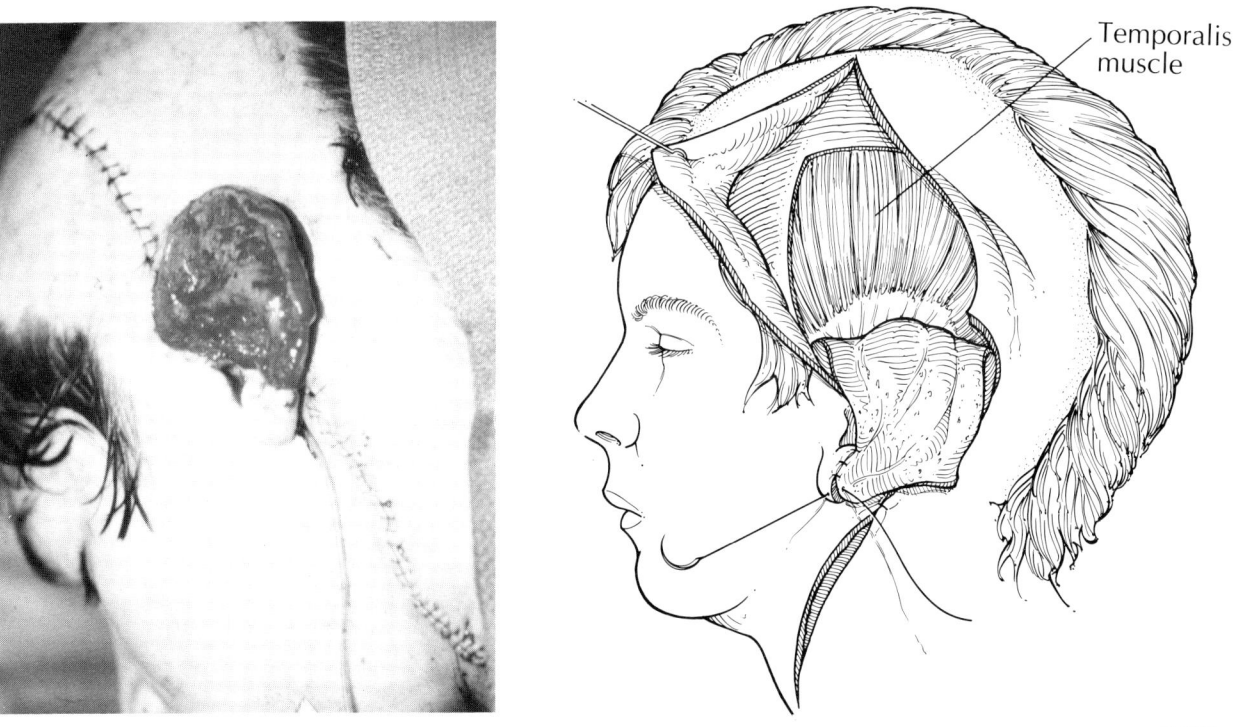

The fascia is turned down and sutured around the edges of the defect.

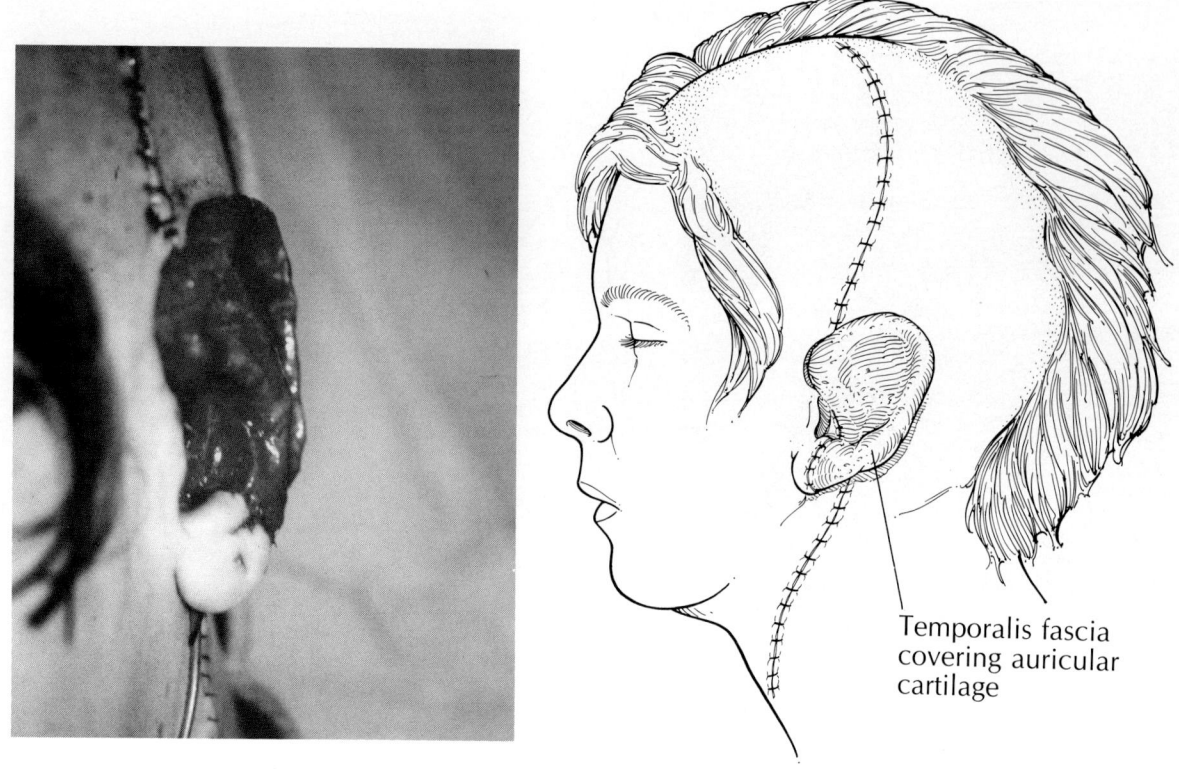

The area under the fascia is drained, since hematoma will result in flap failure. Once the fascia has ceased oozing, it is covered with a full-thickness skin graft.

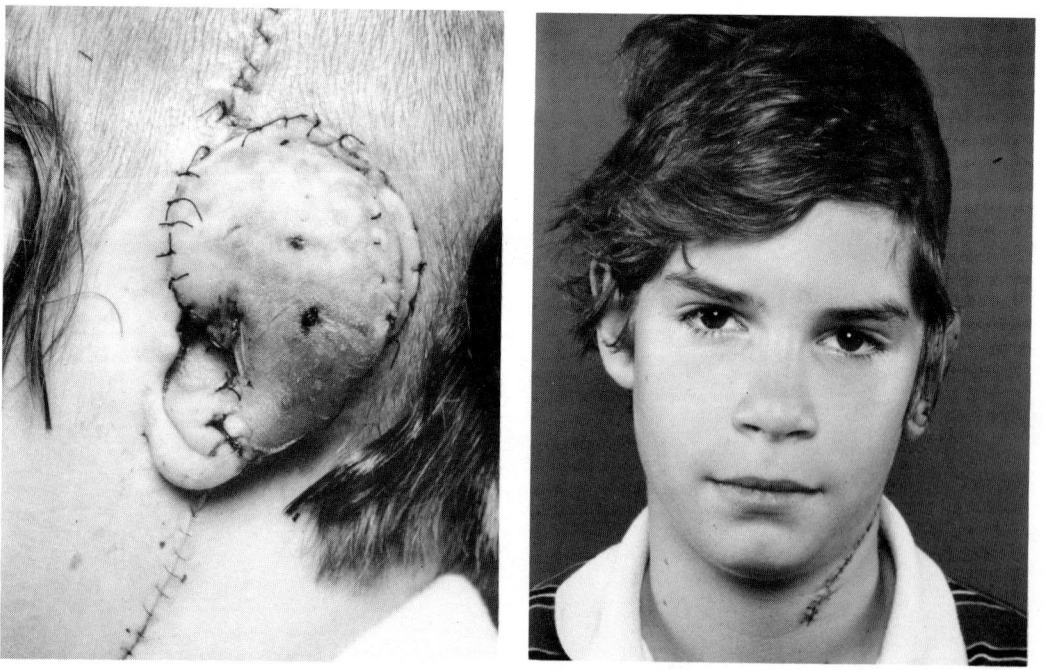

This approach gives a reasonably good ear contour.

PROBLEMS

Potential problems resulting from this method of reconstruction include loss of fascia, loss of skin graft, hematoma under the graft, and failure of the graft to take. (The delayed method of grafting largely obviates the last complication.) It takes almost 1 year for the reconstruction to settle and for the swelling to go down. In some cases a further procedure will be required to effect elevation of the ear from the side of the head. This is a good reconstructive method, since the only alternative is total resection and the fitting of a prosthetic ear.

☐ Lobule

The lobule can be reconstructed from small neck flaps or postauricular flaps. The former are preferable, but they produce more obvious scarring. If possible, trimming of the contralateral lobule for symmetry is the method of choice.

☐ Tube Pedicles

Small neck tube pedicles can be used for rim reconstruction. This method is becoming less popular for these reasons: it is time consuming, since the tubes must be moved over a considerable distance; and the procedure produces fairly extensive neck scarring. Occasionally, the result is satisfactory, but in most instances the skin color and the contours of the reconstruction do not resemble those of a normal ear. In severely burned patients this may be the only technique available.

REFERENCES

1. Brent, B., and Byrd, H.S.: Secondary ear reconstruction with cartilage grafts covered by axial, random and free flaps of temporoparietal fascia, Plast. Reconstr. Surg. **72:**141, 1983.
2. Masson, J.K.: A simple island flap for reconstruction of concha-helix defects, Br. J. Plast. Surg. **25:**399, 1972.

CHAPTER 7

EYELID AND CANTHAL REGION RECONSTRUCTION

*Let thy love in kisses rain
On my lips and eyelids pale*

PERCY BYSSHE SHELLEY
The Indian Serenade

*With fingers weary and worn
With eyelids heavy and red*

THOMAS HOOD
The Song of the Shirt

The eyelids are distinctive facial features that contribute to an individual's facial expressions. They may indicate tiredness, coquetry, or doubt. The primary importance of the eyelids is functional; they protect the cornea and contribute to tear drainage. In this respect the upper lid is vital. Absence of this lid exposes the cornea, resulting in ulceration, scarring, and blindness. Absence of the lower lid causes epiphora and conjunctivitis but little else apart from the gross aesthetic defect. During waking the upper lid closes over the cornea on blinking. During sleep Bell's reflex comes into play. The globe rotates upward and the cornea is protected under the upper lid.

ANATOMY
Skin

The eyelid skin is thin and usually pale; the upper lids are paler than the lower. With age, transverse wrinkles develop, indicating an excess of skin vertically. The subcutaneous layer is thin, and immediately under this lies the orbicularis oculi muscle layer. Deep to this muscle lie the tarsal plates—thin, elongated plates of connective tissue that are approximately 2.5 cm long. The tarsal plate of the upper eyelid is ovoid and larger than that of the lower lid; its maximal height is 10 mm. The levator palpebrae superioris is attached to its superior margin. The tarsal plate of the lower eyelid is smaller, its maximal height being approximately 5 mm. The orbital septum extends from the orbital margin to the tarsal plates. The ends of the tarsal plates are attached to the medial lateral orbital margins by the medial and lateral palpebral ligaments.

The conjunctiva lines the lids and the fornices and runs over the sclera to the cornea; the conjunctiva joins the cornea at the limbus.

Musculature

The orbicularis oculi muscles close the upper and lower lids. The levator palpebrae superioris muscle and Müller's muscle elevate the upper lid.

Nerve Supply

The upper half of the conjunctiva is supplied by the ophthalmic division of the trigeminal nerve (CN V) and the lower half by the maxillary division.

The orbicularis oculi is supplied by the facial nerve (CN VII).

The levator palpebrae superioris receives its nerve supply from the oculomotor nerve (CN III).

Blood Supply

The blood supply comes from the medial palpebral branches of the ophthalmic artery and the lateral palpebral branches of the lacrimal artery.

☐ Lymphatic Drainage

The lateral portion of the eyelids and the lateral canthus drain to the superficial and deep parotid nodes. The medial portion of the lids and the medial canthal area drain to the submandibular lymph nodes.

☐ Canthal Regions

MEDIAL CANTHUS

The skin around the medial canthus is very thin; a fine layer of subcutaneous tissue lies between it and the nasal bones. The canthus itself is complex and contains the caruncle and the puncti for the upper and lower canaliculi. Injury of these structures frequently results in stenosis of varying severity with resulting epiphora and at times conjunctivitis. The medial canthal ligament is attached to the nasal bones and secures the medial canthus in position; it is composed of a superficial layer and a deep layer. The lacrimal duct and sac lie medial and caudal to the canaliculus, behind the infraorbital rim.

LATERAL CANTHUS

The lateral canthus is less complex. Its ligament is a two-layered condensation of periorbitum that is attached to the lateral orbital rim and holds the lateral canthus in place. The periorbitum connecting the medial and lateral canthus inferiorly forms a sling for the orbital contents. This sling is referred to as Lockwood's suspensory ligament.

■ AESTHETICS

The palpebral openings are symmetric. Their shape, which is usually oval, is aesthetically pleasing. Any disturbance of the palpebral anatomy can cause a less satisfactory shape and result in facial asymmetry. The canthal areas are attractive and vary with racial characteristics. Again, these regions are symmetric, and therefore any variation in them is noticeable and aesthetically displeasing. Eyebrows and eyelashes are positive features that enhance one's appearance. If the eyebrows or the lash line are harmed in any way or displaced, the result may be disastrous both aesthetically and functionally; if displacement should occur, a functional problem may result. These aspects of this complex area must be kept in mind when reconstruction is planned.

■ FUNCTION

The eyelids have two basic functions: eye protection and tear drainage. Normally the lids are open during the day and closed at night. The cornea is protected by the upward rotation of the eye (Bell's reflex). During waking the orbicularis is usually relaxed and the levator keeps the lids open; during sleep the reverse occurs.

Tears are drained into the puncta by a dynamic lacrimal pump mechanism. During blinking negative pressure in the canaliculi draws the tears from the eye into the lacrimal system. This is largely the function of the lower canaliculus. In paralyzed or reconstructed lids this pump mechanism is damaged and epiphora results.

■ PLACEMENT OF INCISIONS

Ideally, incisions are made along the lid line transversely and in the crow's feet lines laterally. Vertical lid incisions may contract and deform the lid margin. Unfortunately, in lid reconstruction the position of the incisions is determined by the lesion to be excised.

In the medial canthal area horizontal incisions are better than vertical ones. Both types of incisions create problems, however, because the area is biconcave.

■ AREAS OF TISSUE AVAILABILITY

In older patients the upper eyelid skin is a good source of flaps for lower lid reconstruction because it is conveniently placed and offers good texture and color match. Forehead skin may be used, but only as a last resort; this skin is too thick and pale. Skin from the glabellar area is better; it is used frequently in the medial canthal region. Lower lid reconstruction is often accomplished with cheek or nasolabial skin.

■ AREAS TO BE RECONSTRUCTED

From a standpoint of reconstruction, the lower lid and the upper lid will be considered separately. Separate attention will also be directed to the problems of skin replacement and full-thickness reconstruction. The medial and lateral canthal areas will be examined individually, and the complexities of reconstruction in these regions will be defined.

CHAPTER 7
EYELID AND
CANTHAL REGION
RECONSTRUCTION

☐ Lower Eyelid Reconstruction

In lower eyelid reconstruction the aim is to form a lid of adequate height with a stable edge. Mucosa should not escape over the lid margin into the skin area.

Many techniques can be used to reconstruct the lower lid. This discussion, however, will be limited to examining those flaps that have produced consistently good aesthetic and functional results.

LOWER EYELID SKIN DEFECT RECONSTRUCTION

Although full-thickness skin grafts may be used to resurface full-thickness skin defects, the most uniformly secure method is to use a skin flap from the upper lid.[5]

Unilateral Tripier Flap

A skin defect on the lower lid can be conveniently reconstructed with this upper lid flap. Its proximity and security make it an attractive reconstructive choice.

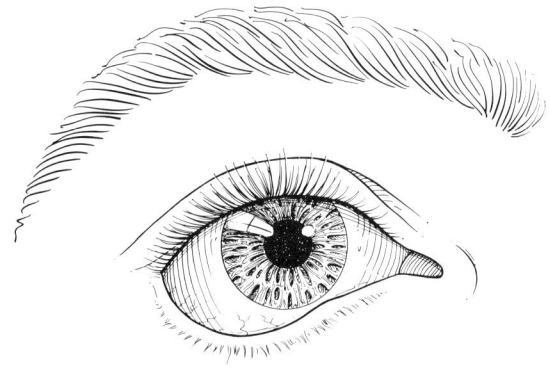

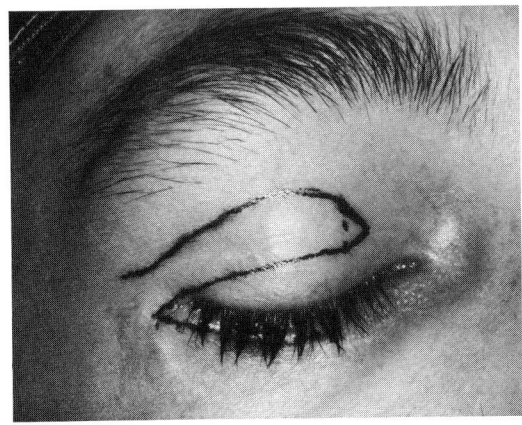

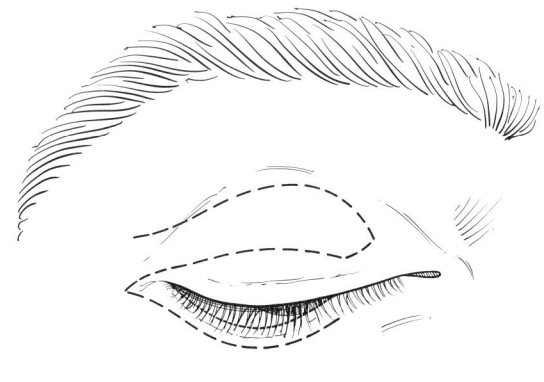

The unilateral tripier flap was used to repair the ectropion in this patient with Treacher Collins' syndrome.

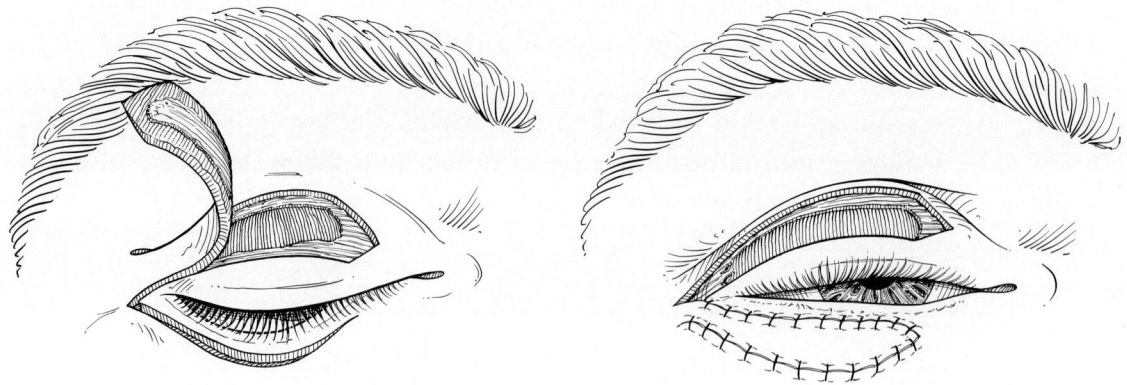

The defect in the lower lid is created, and a flap of corresponding dimensions is outlined on the upper lid. If two thirds of the length of the upper lid is required to perform the reconstruction, a single pedicle is sufficient. The flap is lifted with the underlying orbicularis muscle until it can be transposed easily down into the lower lid. The inclusion of the muscle on the flap ensures that vascularity is maintained.

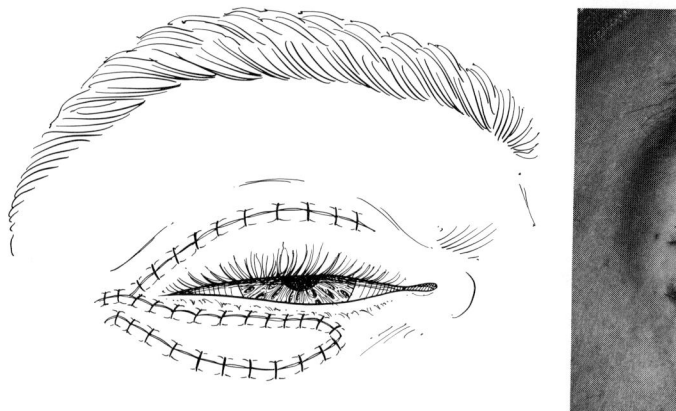 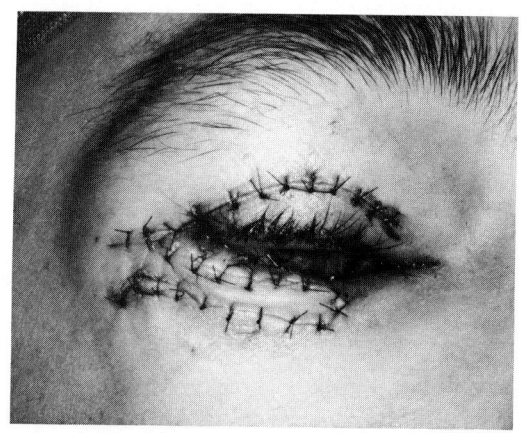

In some instances in which the lateral canthus is to be elevated, the lower lid incision joins the lower incision of the pedicle and the flap is directly inset. In this way the canthus is slightly elevated, a desirable effect for this patient because it combats the anti-mongoloid slant that is part of the syndrome. Some experts recommend the use of a tie over dressing. This technique is unnecessary when the orbicularis has been incorporated in the flap. When the pedicle is not directly inset, it must be divided and trimmed 10 to 14 days after the initial procedure.

Bilateral Tripier Flap

CHAPTER 7
EYELID AND
CANTHAL REGION
RECONSTRUCTION

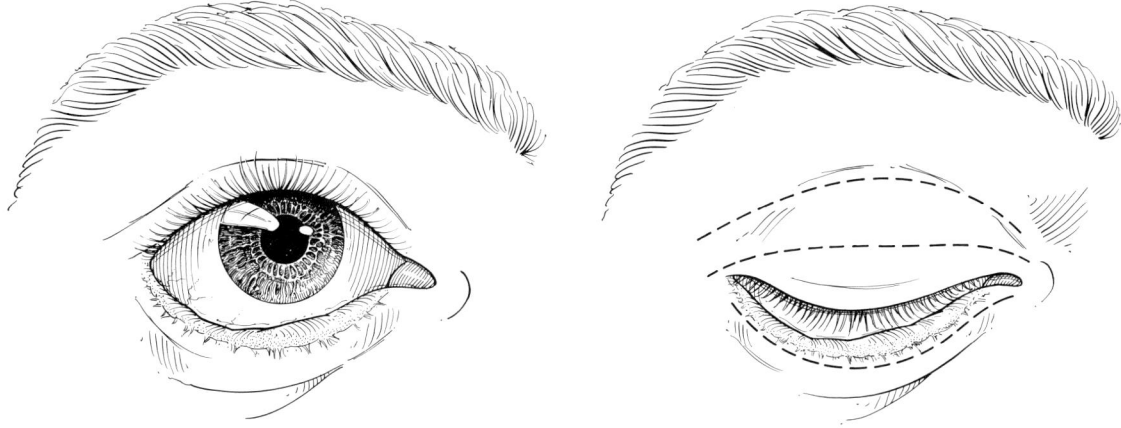

When the whole lower lid is to be resurfaced, a bilateral Tripier flap is used.

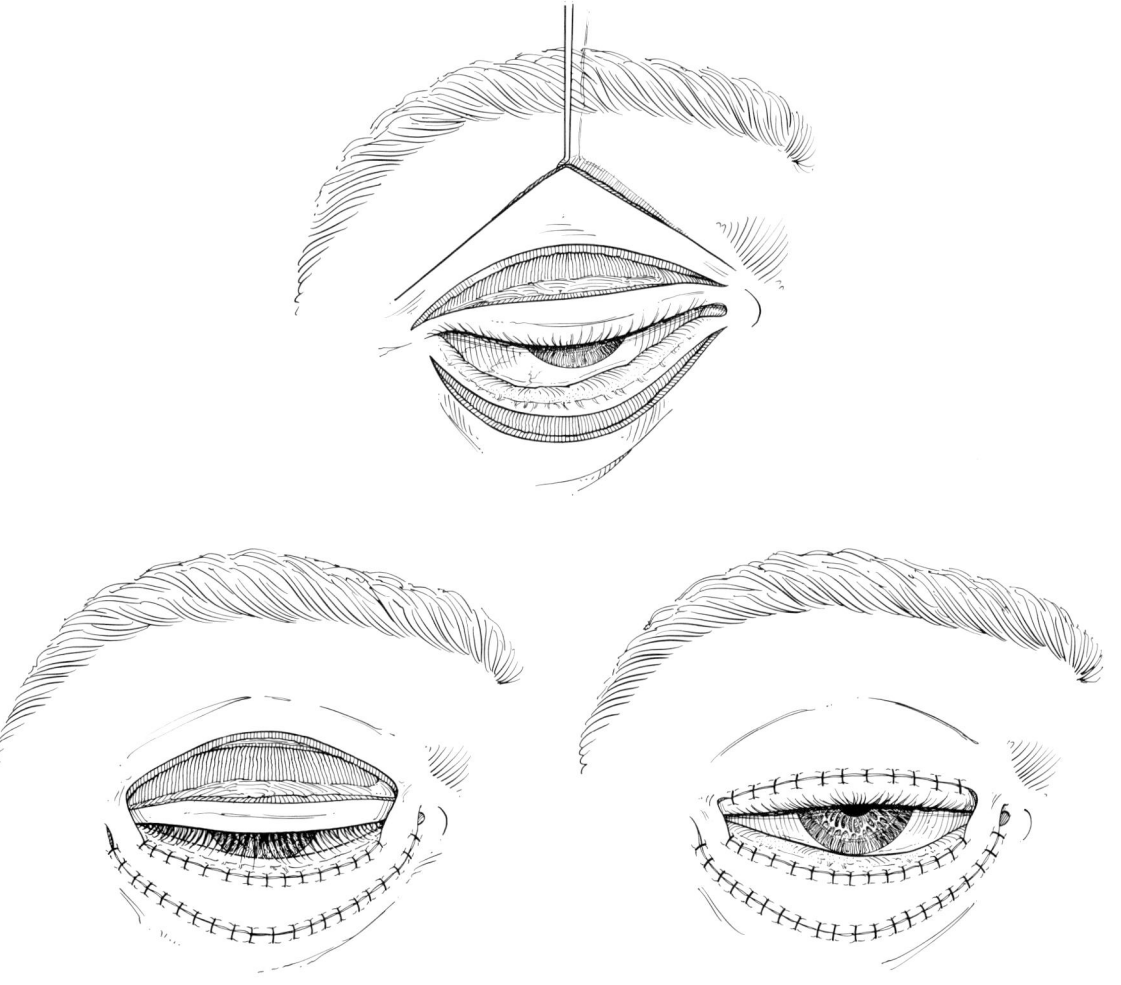

The flap is raised in exactly the same manner as the unilateral flap. The pedicles are left intact; in 10 to 14 days they are divided and trimmed.

PROBLEMS

Flap failure resulting from ischemia is a rare occurence. This has happened only when the orbicularis muscle has not been included in the flap. It is difficult to imagine anything more than a partial necrosis occurring in a myocutaneous flap. Slight pincushioning may occur, making the reconstruction obvious. When this flap is used for paralytic ectropion, the bilateral pedicles may be left undivided to act as a sling for supporting the lax lower lid.

☐ Partial Eyelid Reconstruction

In reconstructing part of a lid, a stable edge should be produced and the height of the lid should be preserved. The shape of the palpebral fissure and the lateral canthus should not be altered if at all possible.

CHEEK ROTATION FLAP

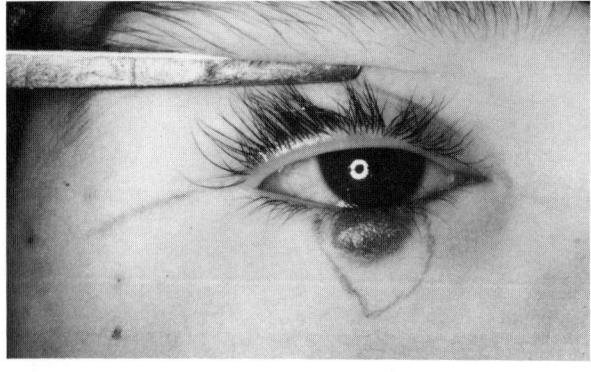

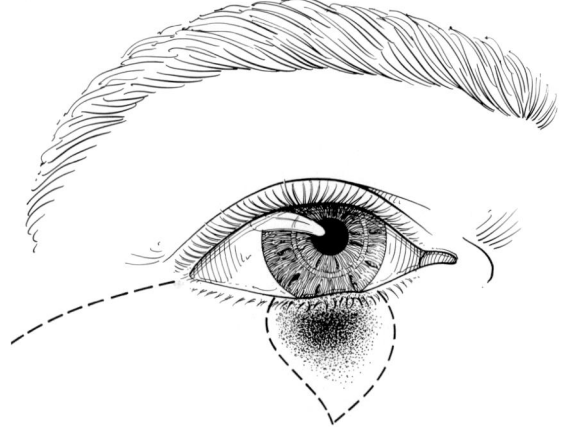

When the defect is subtotal, a rotation flap from the cheek produces the simplest and quickest reconstruction.

CHAPTER 7
EYELID AND CANTHAL REGION RECONSTRUCTION

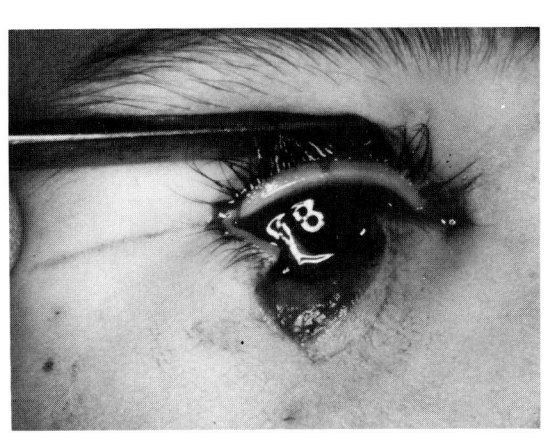 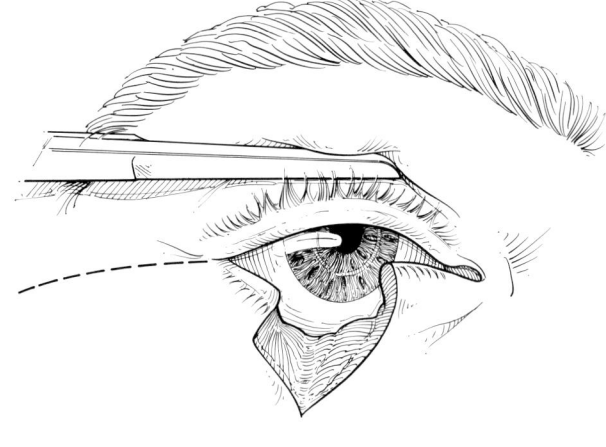

After the defect has been produced, an incision is taken out from the lateral canthus horizontally; it should be inclined in a cranial direction to prevent any pulling down of the lid and resulting ectropion. Initially the length of the incision is limited, and the lateral canthal division (described below) is performed.

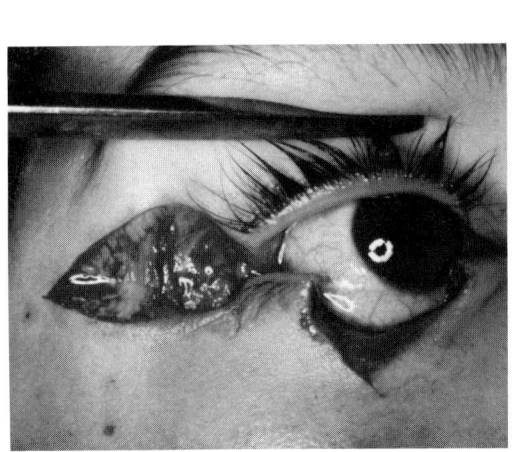 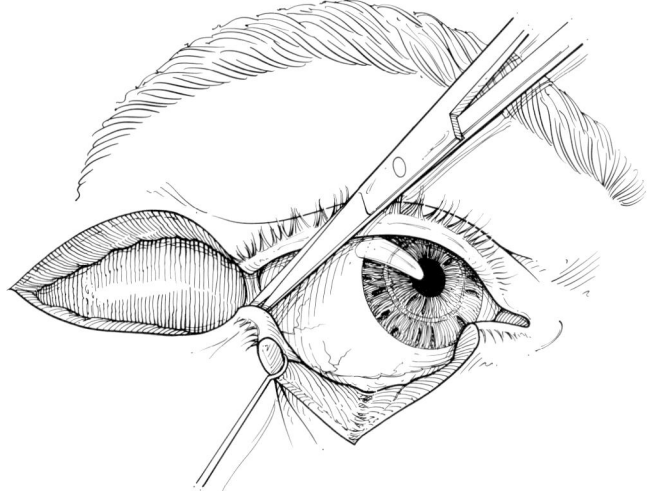

The incision is extended further laterally if additional length is required for closure. Long lateral incisions are rarely necessary. The skin is undermined at the suborbicularis level, onto the temporal area. At this point advancement is limited; in order to obtain the required skin shift, the lower limb of the lateral canthal ligament and the orbital septum are divided with sharply pointed scissors.

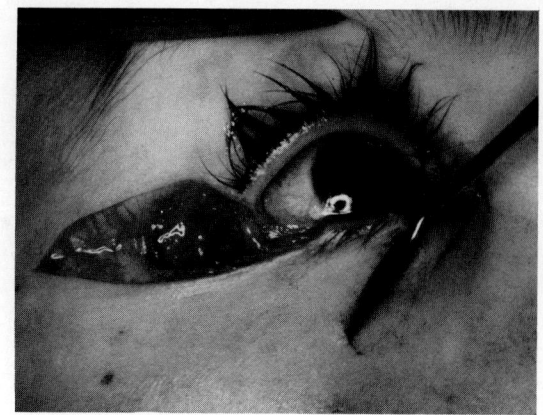

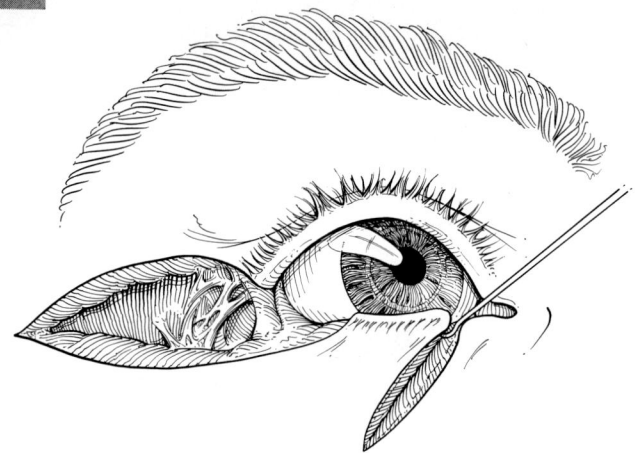

After this division it is easy to move the whole lid medially to close the defect.

A decision is now made about lining. If the defect is extensive or if it lies in the lateral half of the lid, lining will probably be necessary. Although buccal mucosa will provide good conjunctival replacement, the best cover *and* support is provided by the chondromucosal graft from the nasal septum, as described by Mustarde.[4] The technique for taking this graft is similar to the method used for a submucosal resection of the nasal septum. The low incision, however, is made through nasal mucosa and cartilage. The septal submucosal dissection is performed on the contralateral side of the cartilage. When the required extent of the dissection has been completed, further incisions are made through the mucosa and cartilage to provide a graft of adequate size. If a large chondromucosal graft is required, an incision is made around the alar base. Retraction of the base will give better exposure of the septum. The graft is then sutured to the raw area on the inner aspect of the flap.

CHAPTER 7
EYELID AND CANTHAL REGION RECONSTRUCTION

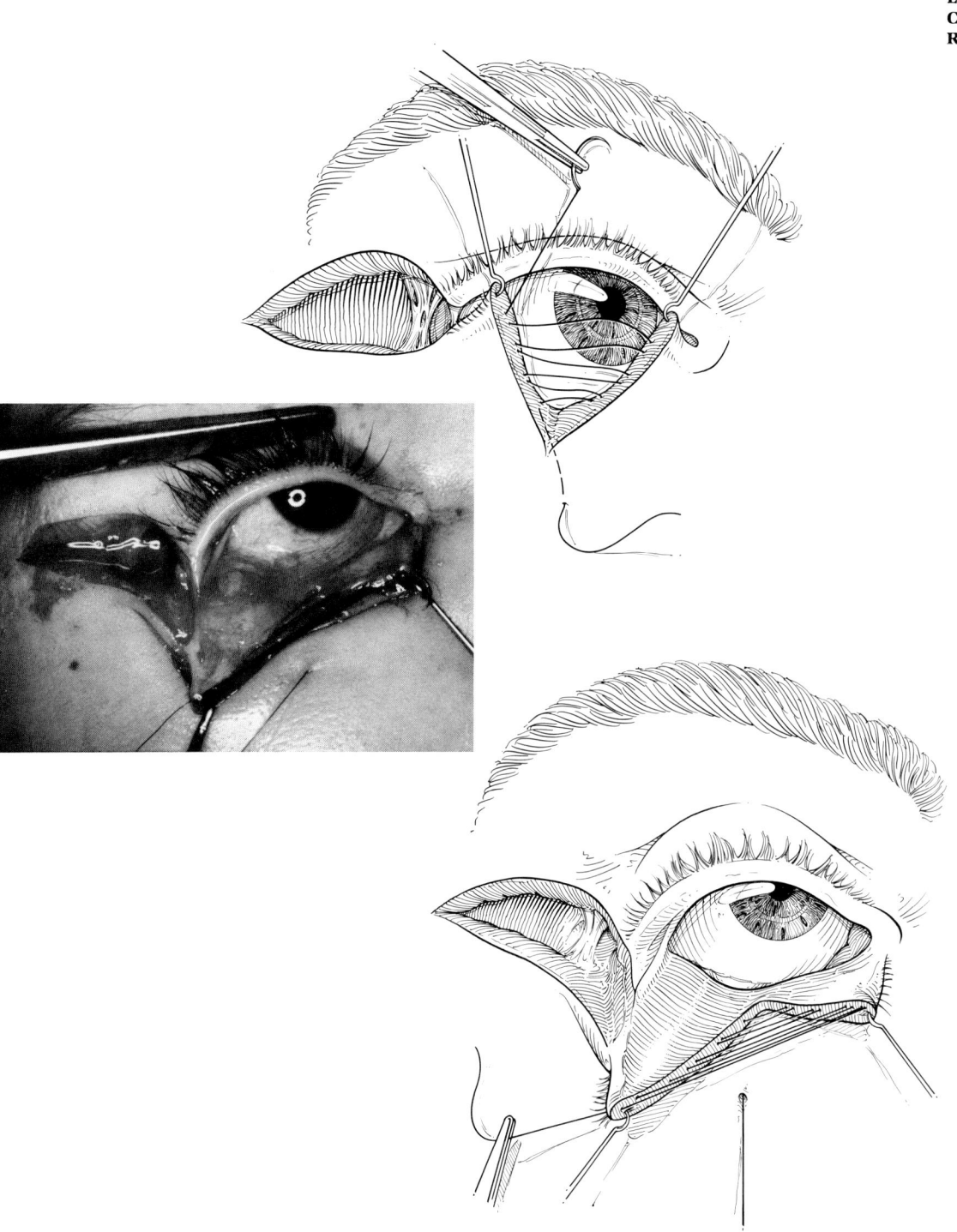

Vertical suturing of the eyelid is performed in layers, with 6-0 plain catgut used for the conjunctival and subconjunctival layers, 4-0 chromic catgut for the tarsal layer, and fine monofilament nylon for the skin.

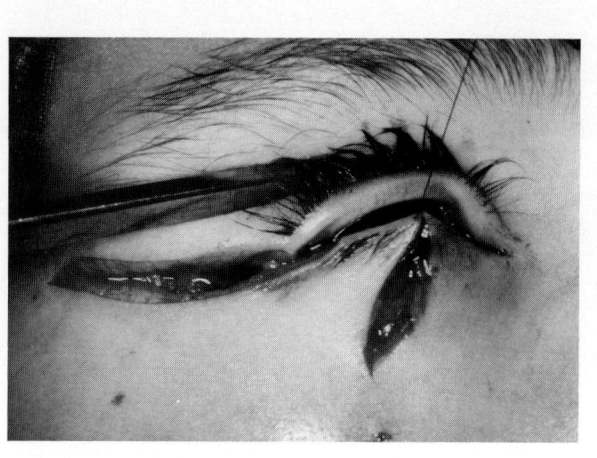
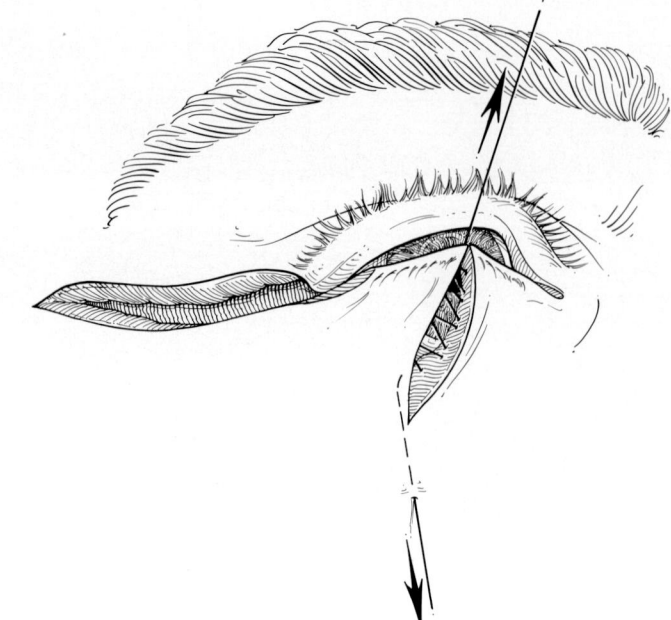

Care is taken to align the eyelid margin accurately, matching the gray line and the lash line on both sides of the incision.

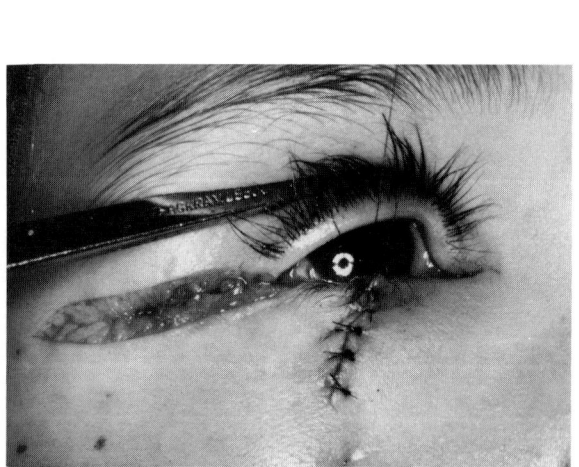
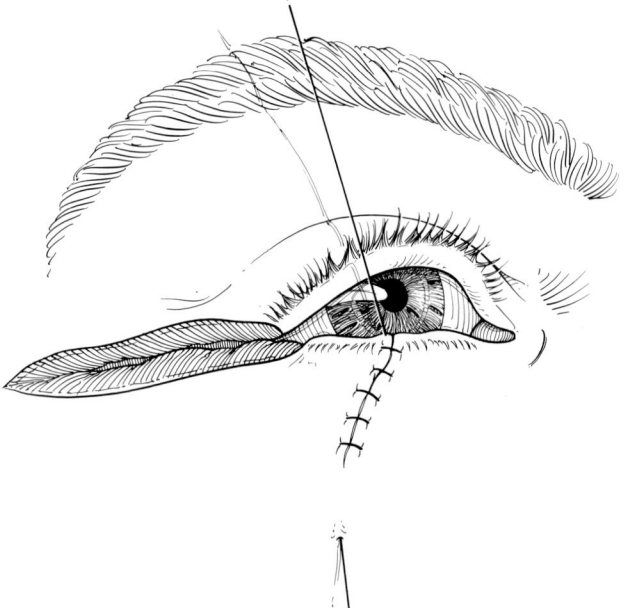

Closure of the defect and medial movement of the flap can be achieved without tension.

CHAPTER 7
EYELID AND CANTHAL REGION RECONSTRUCTION

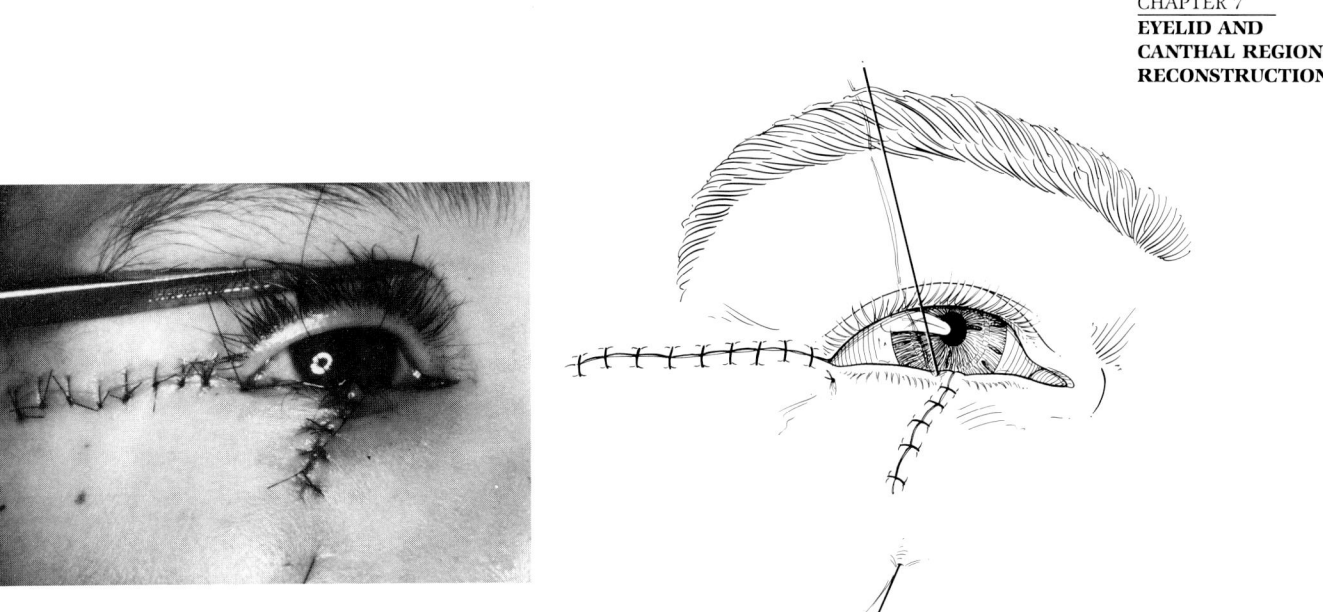

A Z-plasty at the outer end of the temporal incision has been described by McGregor[3] to relax the flap. This maneuver is never indicated for this particular reason. The real indication for this approach is to equalize the excess skin buildup above the lateral canthal incision as the cheek flap advances medially.

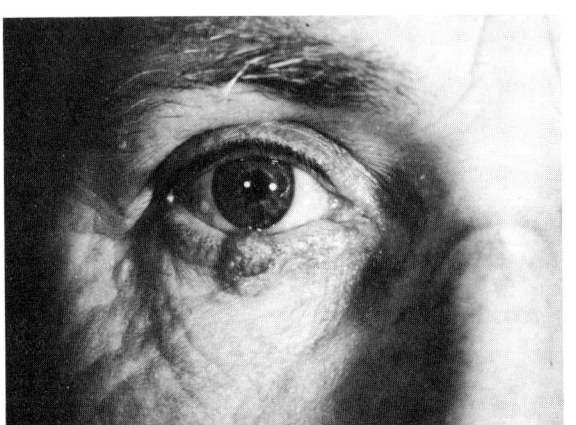
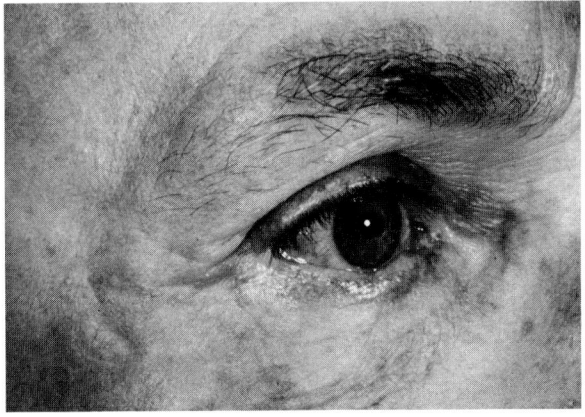

When used for this purpose, the Z-plasty works well and improves the aesthetic result, as can be seen after wedge excision of this basal cell carcinoma of the lower lid.

It is interesting to note that by dividing the inferior limb of the lateral canthal ligament some large defects in the middle eyelid region may be closed without any significant lateral canthal skin incision.

PROBLEMS

It is rare to encounter problems of any kind with this eyelid reconstruction. Occasionally, there may be slight notching of the lid margin, but it can usually be avoided by accurate suturing in this region. Slight sagging of the lateral portion of the reconstructed lid also may result. This sagging can occur for a number of reasons. The lining of the flap may have shrunk, or perhaps lining was not used and should have been. The lateral incision may have been directed caudally rather than cranially. This action and a failure to anchor the undersurface of the flap can cause a dragging force on the lid with resulting lateral ectopion. If this deformity occurs, it can be released and a skin graft or small Tripier flap inserted.

☐ Total Lower Eyelid Reconstruction

The requirements presented in the previous section for a partial lower lid reconstruction apply even more forcibly in total lower lid surgery. The surgeon must aim for correct height and a stable lid margin. There should be a deep conjunctival fornix. Good canthal positioning is important. A lid that conforms to the curvature of the globe is ideal.

Several methods can be employed for total eyelid reconstruction using the upper lid, the forehead skin, the nasolabial skin, or the skin over the cheek area as a rotation flap. Unless the surgeon has had extensive experience in eyelid surgery, it is best to select an approach that does not interfere with the upper lid. Significant disturbance of upper lid anatomy may cause serious functional problems that can ultimately result in corneal exposure or abrasion with the attendant complications. For this reason the method of cheek rotation flap and chondromucosal graft described here is recommended.

FOREHEAD FLAP

In the elderly patient, particularly when prolonged anesthesia is considered inadvisable, when there is some worry about the possibility of hematoma, when there has been irradiation to the cheek, or when the cheek and neck skin is tight, the surgeon may opt simply to use the forehead to reconstruct the lower lid in a two-stage procedure known as the Fricke flap.[1] A total excision of the lower eyelid is performed. Reconstruction of the tarso-conjunctival lining and support system is carried out with a composite chondromucosal graft from the nose, as shown here. Because of the thickness of the forehead skin, a buccal mucosal graft may be quite satisfactory.

CHAPTER 7
EYELID AND CANTHAL REGION RECONSTRUCTION

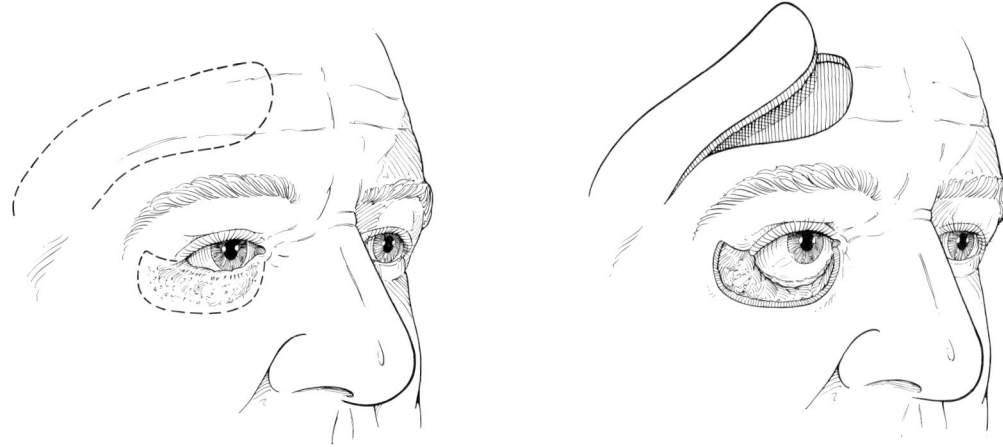

After the graft has been carefully sutured in place, a supraeyebrow forehead flap is raised; this flap has the correct dimensions for resurfacing the lower lid. The flap should be raised only at skin level, without frontalis, to obtain as thin a flap as possible.

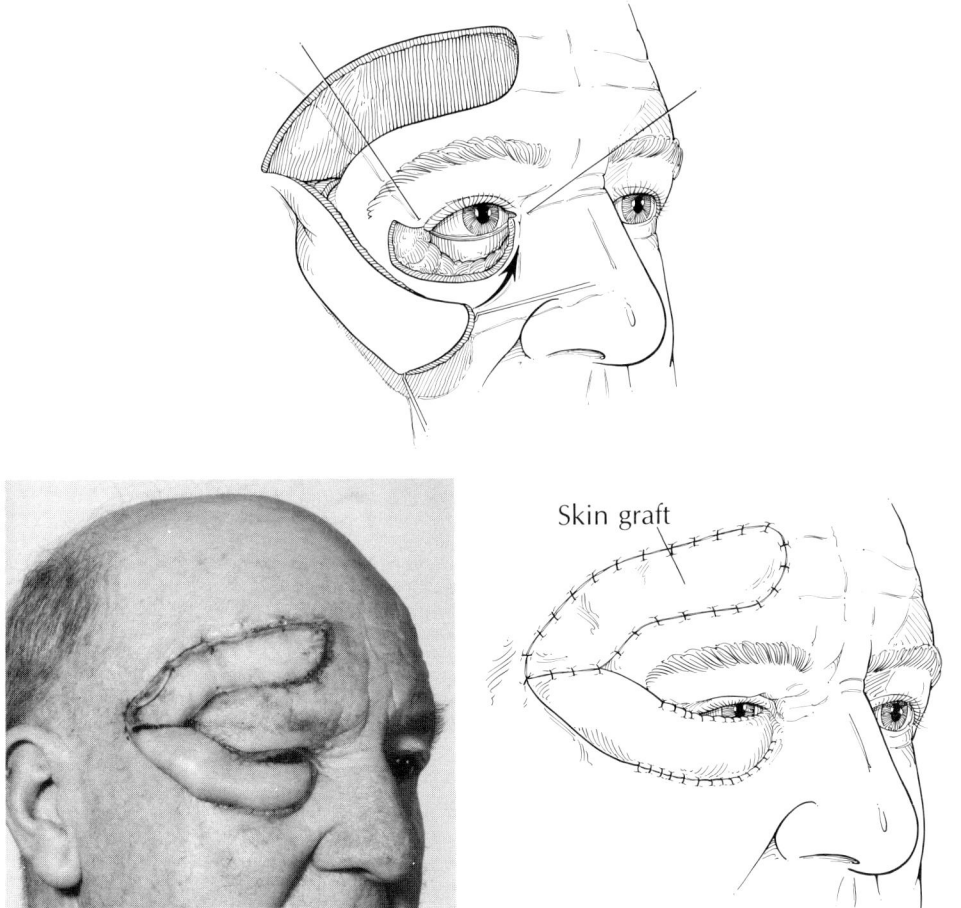

The flap is taken down and sutured into position to effect a skin reconstruction of the lid. The pedicle is left untubed, and a split-thickness skin graft is placed on the raw area of the forehead.

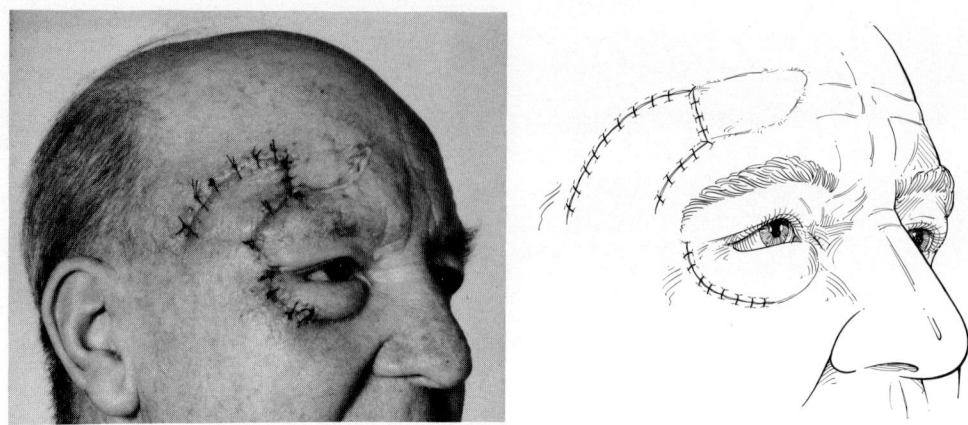

In 10 to 14 days the pedicle is divided and returned to the forehead area. The remainder of the lid reconstruction then is performed.

PROBLEMS

The skin of the forehead is much thicker than that of the lower eyelid, and the color tends to be lighter. Even after attempted thinning and Z-plasties around the edge of the flap, pincushioning of the flap occurs in almost every case.

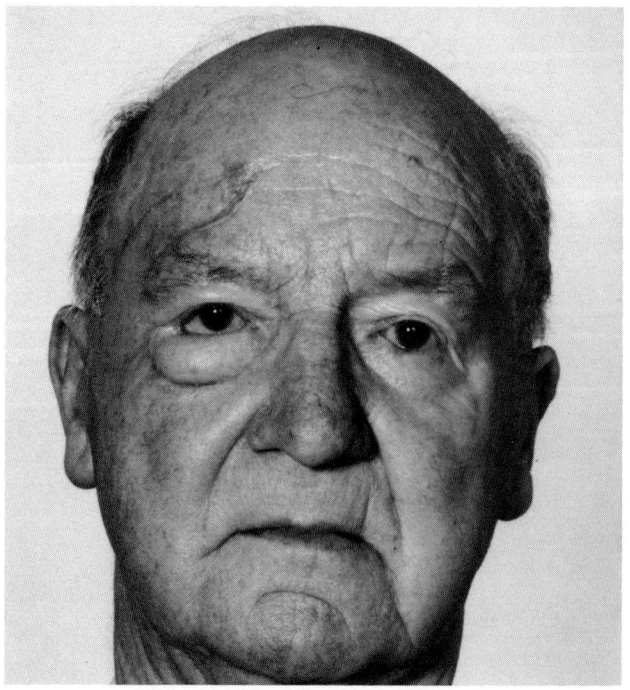

This can be clearly seen in the postoperative illustration.

CHAPTER 7
EYELID AND
CANTHAL REGION
RECONSTRUCTION

The pincushioning may also have the effect of turning skin in toward the cornea and causing some abrasion. This possible effect must be looked for very carefully at postoperative visits. The forehead flap does have the virtue of being a rapid and relatively atraumatic procedure that can be done under local anesthesia if necessary.

CHEEK ROTATION FLAP AND CHONDROMUCOSAL GRAFT

Three necessary components contribute to a total lower lid reconstruction: skin, support tissue, and lining. Undoubtedly, in our experience with all the available techniques of total lower eyelid reconstruction, the simplest and most consistently successful method is a cheek rotation flap for cover and a chondromucosal graft for support and lining. With careful planning and execution, few problems are encountered.

Most patients requiring this type of surgery are older and have a laxity of cheek skin. The amount of skin available for rotation is judged by using the fingers to push the skin from the malar area toward the nose. If the skin is tight, an alternative method of surgery should be considered.

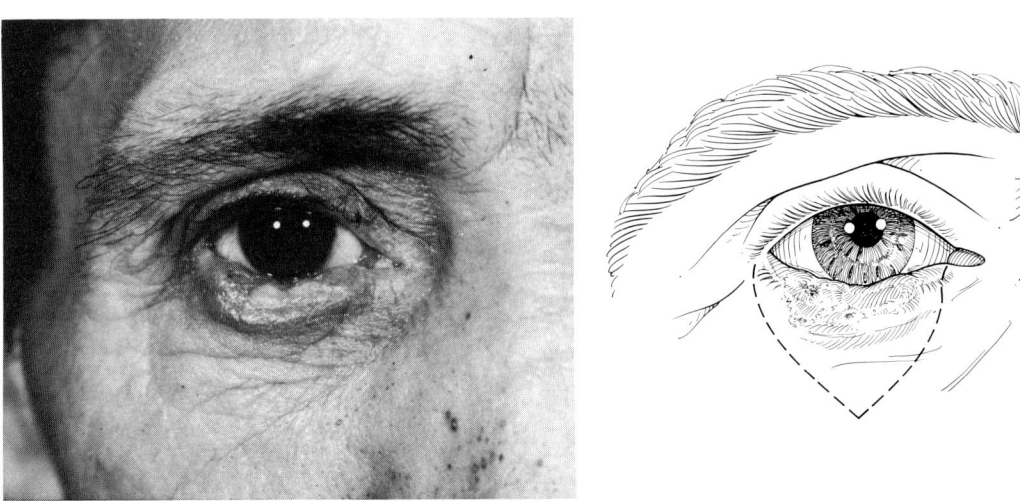

This patient with a basal cell carcinoma involving the whole rim of the right lower eyelid requires a total lid resection.

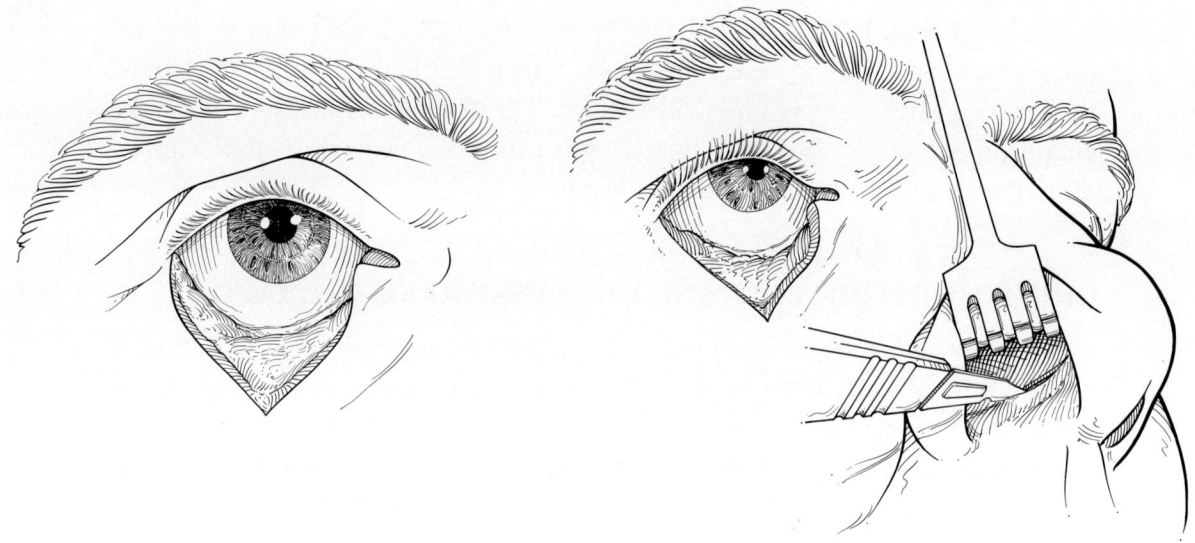

Once the eyelid has been resected, the chondromucosal graft is harvested. The graft must be large (it can be trimmed as necessary), but there is a tendency to underestimate its size. In order to obtain a large enough graft, it is wise to incise around the alar base to get good exposure of the septum. The graft is taken by means of a low incision in the septum through the mucosa and the septal cartilage.

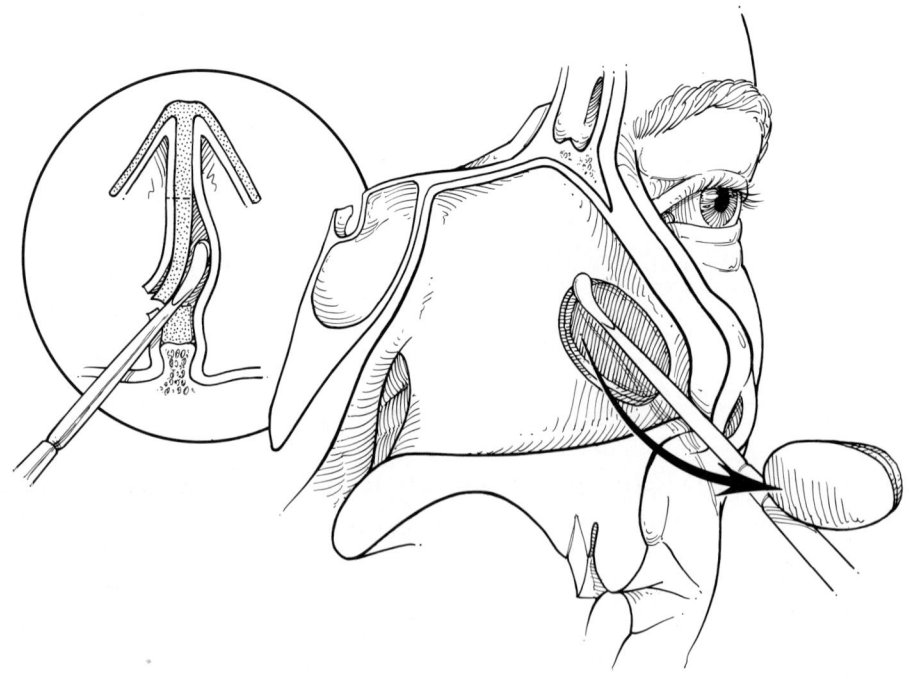

The mucosa on the other side is extensively raised, and a large composite graft is provided by incising through the mucosa and septum.

CHAPTER 7
EYELID AND CANTHAL REGION RECONSTRUCTION

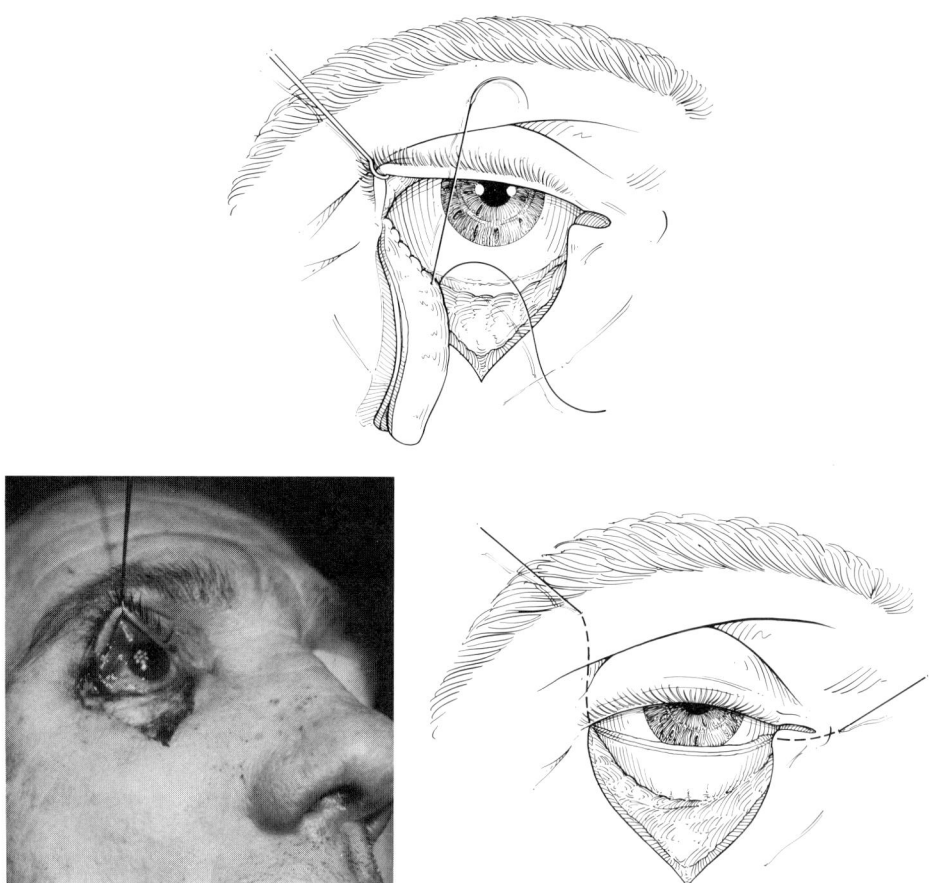

After the graft is taken, the septal cartilage is trimmed to leave a fringe of mucosa surrounding the central island of cartilage. The cartilage is thinned. This thinning may make the graft slightly convex on the cartilage side, providing it with a better contour for lid reconstruction. The graft is sutured to the conjunctiva with 6-0 plain catgut.

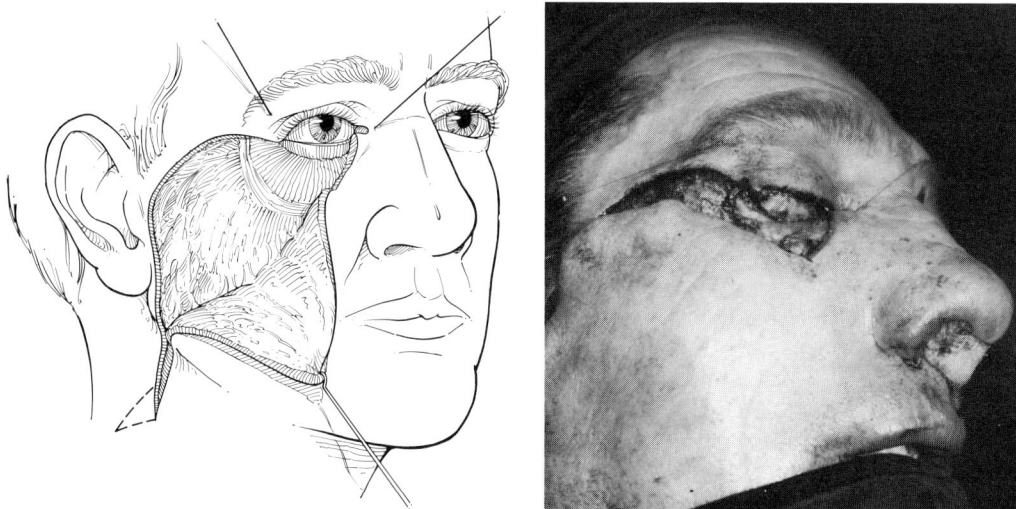

The cheek flap is designed. The incision goes laterally and upward; it then runs vertically in front of the ear into the neck as required. The flap is next raised at the face-lift level. Elevation extends down into the neck to maximally utilize the skin laxity in this area. Hemostasis is established.

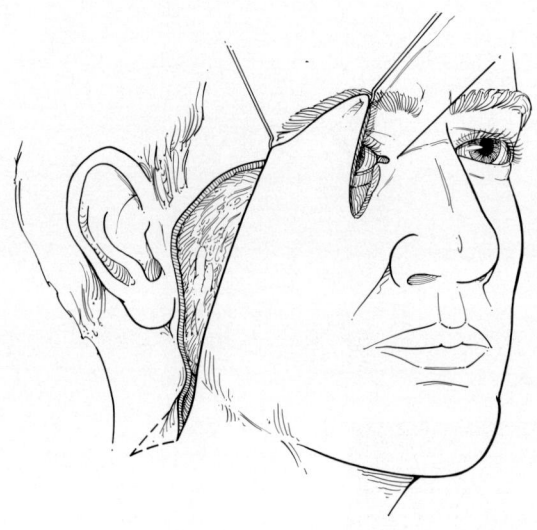

With the use of a hook the flap is gently pulled medially; it should not be forcibly dragged into position. If the flap is tight and defect closure is difficult, the incision is carried further into the neck and more extensive undermining is performed. The incision length and undermining is sufficient when the flap can be rotated effortlessly. Failure to check for pull on the flap may result in suturing under tension, with ischemia of the flap tip and loss of the reconstructed lid as possible consequences.

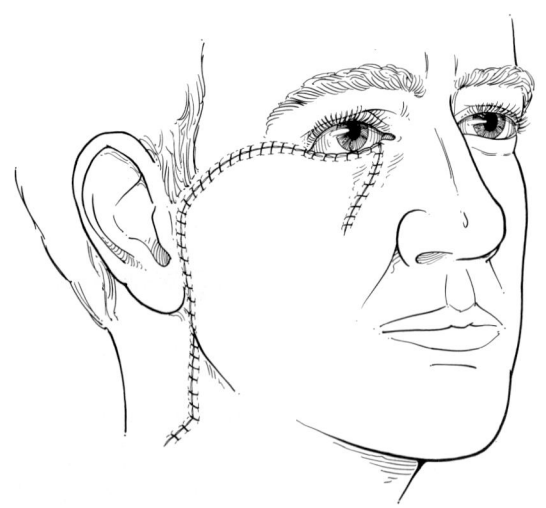

The flap is now rotated into position. It is sutured to the upper edge of the graft with running 6-0 plain catgut. The undersurface of the flap is anchored to the periosteum and soft tissue over the zygoma with nonabsorbable sutures. Anchoring prevents ptosis of the flap and subsequent ectropion.

Excess skin will remain in two areas: at the base of the vertical cheek suture line (because closure of the V defect leaves an inferior standing cone) and in the neck at the inferior posterior edge of the incision. Both of these areas must be trimmed. Suction drainage and pressure are important in order to prevent hematoma.

PROBLEMS

The most serious complication is flap loss because of ischemia, resulting from poor flap design, tension in closure, and hematoma. Infection is rare unless flap necrosis has occurred. Once necrosis is present, reconstruction is difficult. A bilateral Tripier flap or a nasolabial transposition flap offers the best solution.

Ectropion may occur if the flap is too tight in a vertical direction or because of skin laxity or a lack of flap stabilization to the zygomatic region.

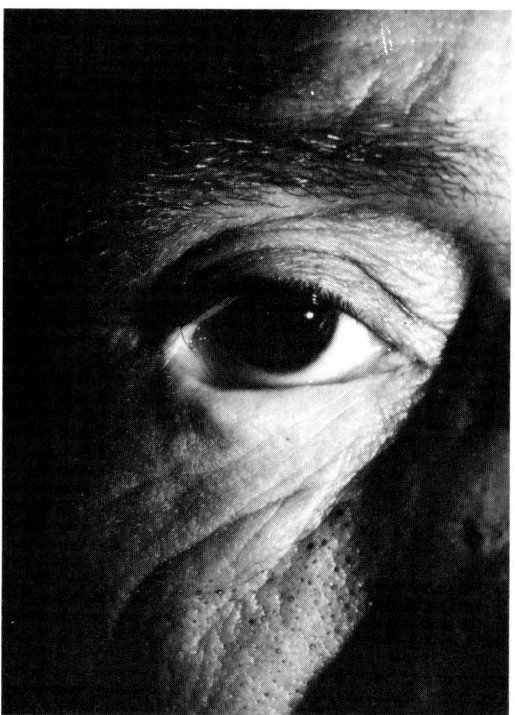

These conditions all result in a downward pull, as shown to a small extent in this illustration. Another quite different cause for ectropion is partial composite graft take, with resulting fibrosis and vertical contracture of the new lid. For a similar reason there may be entropion, or turning in of the skin, which may cause irritation and abrasion of the cornea. These problems require addition of tissue, either skin or mucosa.

SURGICAL TECHNIQUE OF CHOICE

The rotation flap is most satisfactory for partial or complete lower lid reconstruction. The flap is simple to design, and the skin color and texture are a good match for the normal lower lid skin. With good planning, correct execution, and efficient hemostasis, few complications should arise.

☐ Upper Eyelid Reconstruction

Because the skin of the upper eyelid is thin and supple, satisfactory replacement can be obtained from only a few areas. A flap from the forehead is too thick and the color is unsatisfactory. Skin defects only are best managed with full-thickness skin grafts from the other upper lid or from the retroauricular area. Split-thickness grafts should never be used unless no full-thickness donor sites are available. These grafts contract; in addition, they are pale in color, have a matte texture, and appear as obvious patches of foreign skin. After full-thickness resections it is necessary only to reconstruct a lid of three quarters the original length. The lid must never be short vertically; any significant defect of closure may cause corneal drying and ulceration.

PARTIAL UPPER LID RECONSTRUCTION

In partial upper lid reconstruction the lid should not be tight. Its height should be adequate to ensure closure of the palpebral tissue. There should be no notching of the free margin. This margin should be stable, with mucosa being contained within the inner surface of the lid.

Lid Switch Flap

If the edges of the lid defect cannot be brought together for primary closure, tissue must be imported. One method of doing this is the lid switch flap.

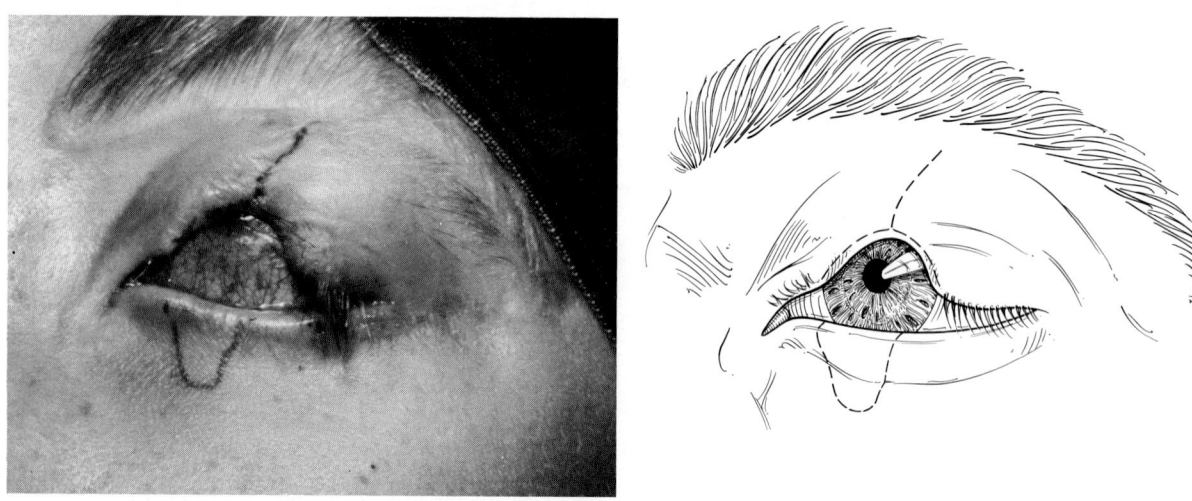

In this technique one quarter of the lower lid is used to reconstruct the upper lid defect. The lower lid is closed directly. The width of the upper lid defect is measured; a pentagonal wedge flap of half that width is drawn out on the lower lid.

CHAPTER 7
EYELID AND CANTHAL REGION RECONSTRUCTION

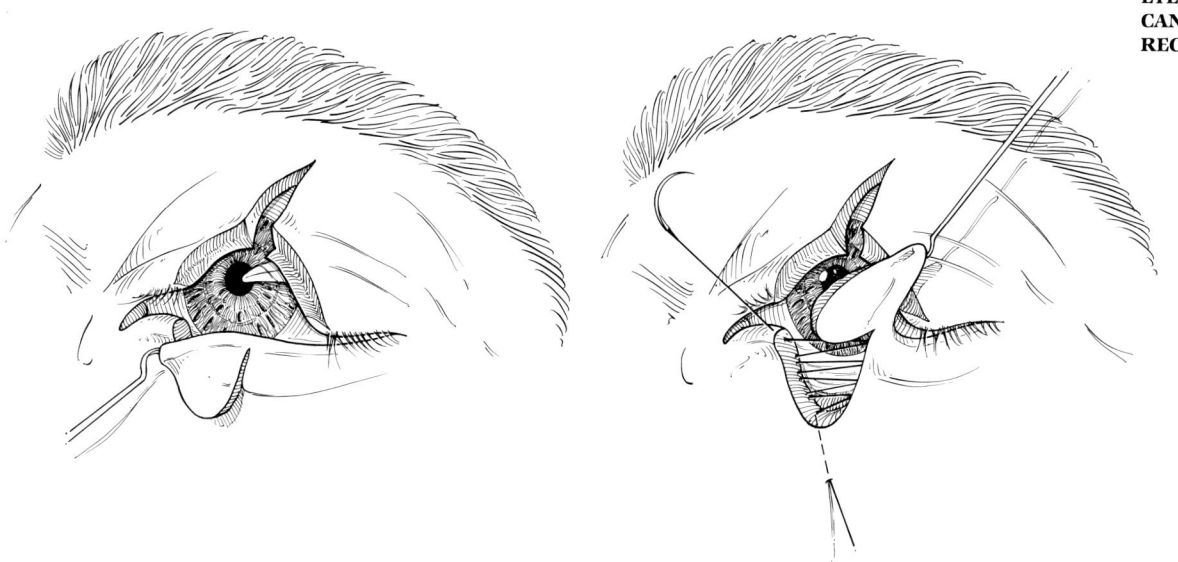

With the eye protected with a teaspoon or a specialized eye shield, and the lid margin held with hooks, the medial edge of the wedge is cut with straight iris scissors. Using a hook to keep the flap under tension, beginning at the apex of the wedge, the surgeon cuts through the lateral edge with a scalpel. The incision stops approximately 5 mm from the lid margin to prevent injury to the marginal vessels, which lie 3 mm from the free margin of the lid. The flap can be rotated on its pedicle to close the upper lid defect.

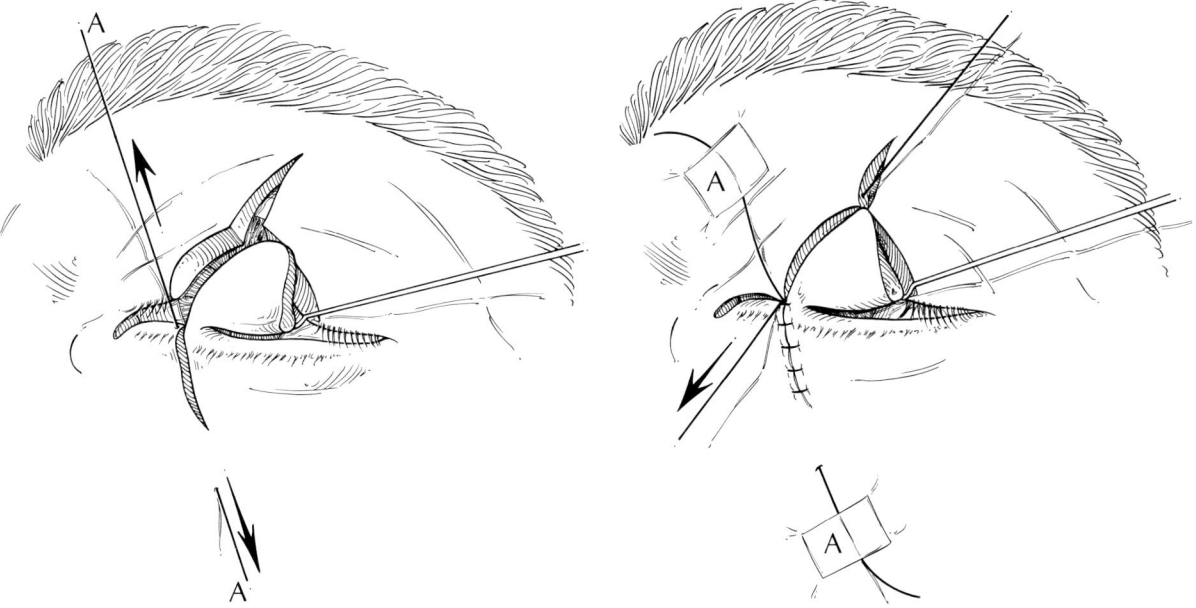

The lower lid is closed directly. Suturing of the flap into the upper lid and closure of the lower lid are performed in layers.

295

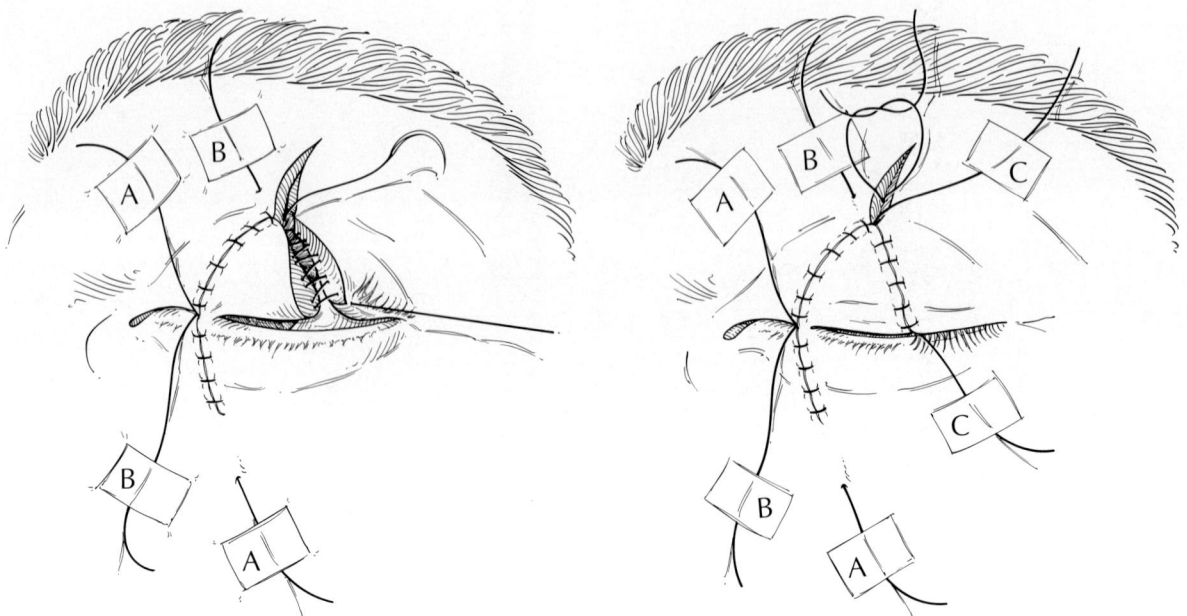

If nonabsorbable prolene or nylon subconjunctival sutures have been used for deep closure, the ends of the sutures should be covered with tape identifying which end is which. This makes for easy identification at the time of suture removal.

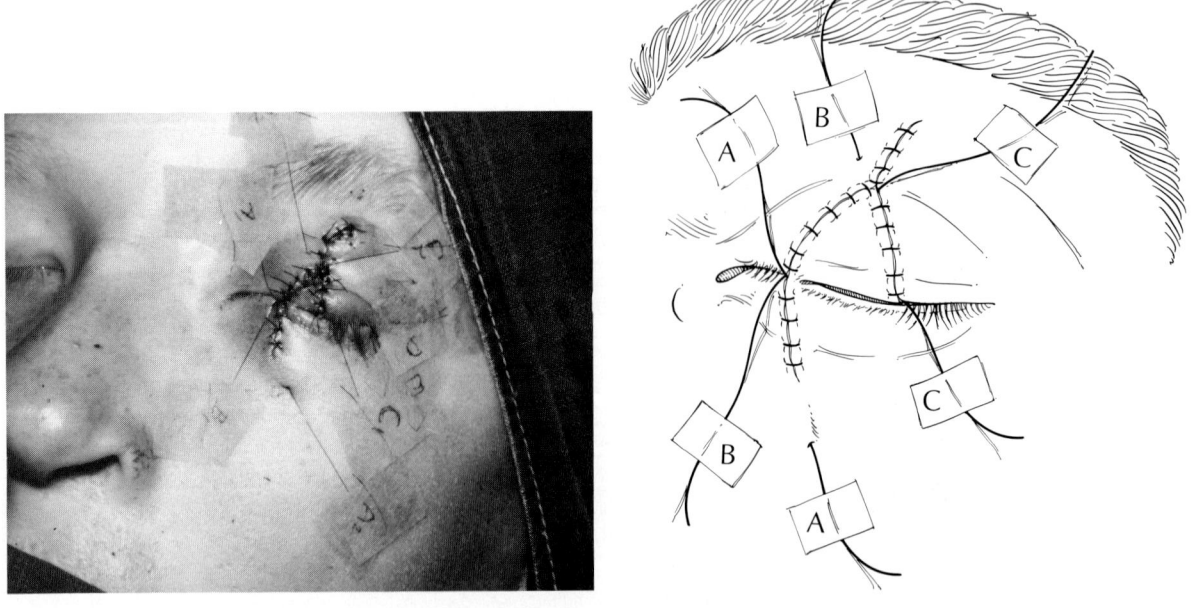

A Frost suture may be used to splint and protect the pedicle for 2 to 3 days. In 10 to 14 days the little vascular pedicle is divided.

CHAPTER 7
**EYELID AND
CANTHAL REGION
RECONSTRUCTION**

The lid switch flap also may be used for larger defects. In such cases the flap is correspondingly larger and is based on a small cheek rotation flap fashioned in the standard way by a lateral canthal incision. The rotation flap closes the lower lid defect. This procedure will be discussed further in relation to total upper eyelid reconstruction.

PROBLEMS

Although the lid switch flap can provide excellent results in skin color, texture, lid anatomy and function, it is not a technique for the inexperienced.

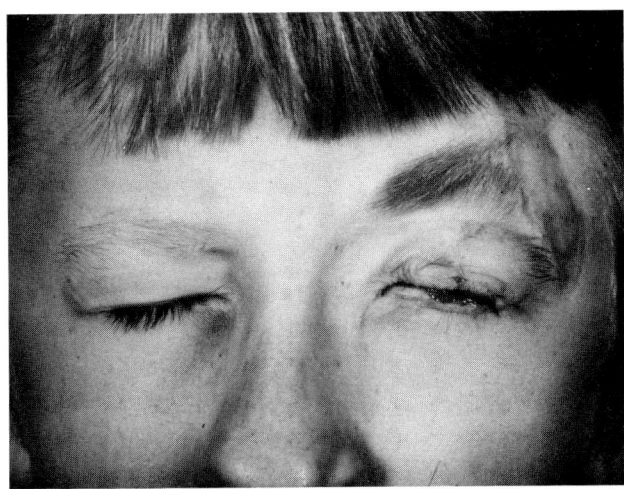

Inaccurate planning of the flap may result in too little tissue to adequately close the defect. Lack of care in approaching the lid margin may damage the blood supply and cause flap necrosis. Tight suturing around the pedicle at the margin of the lower lid can strangle the vessels in the pedicle, likewise leading to flap necrosis. Irregularities may occur at the rim of the upper lid with entropion or ectropion and corneal irritation from the eyelashes.

Upper Lid Rotation Flap

An alternative to the lid switch flap is the upper lid rotation flap. This technique is also used for defects ranging from one quarter to one half of the lid length. The best way to plan the procedure is to stand at the patient's head, look down, and consider the upper lid as the lower lid. In this way both the planning and the performance of the procedure are made much easier.

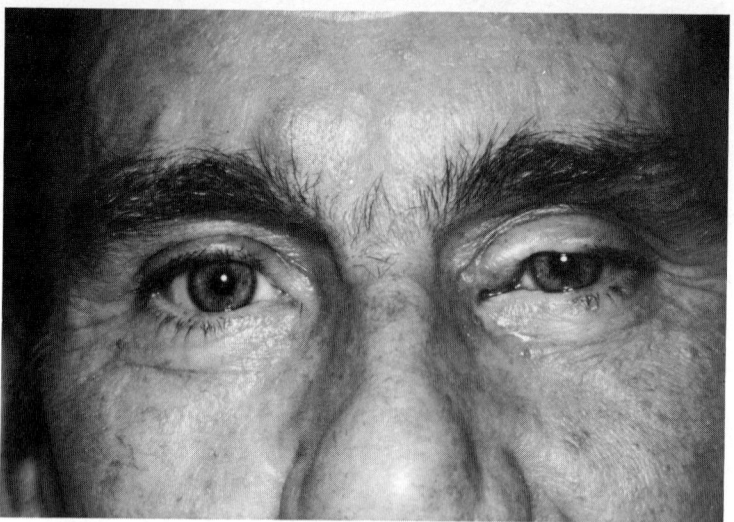

The patient shown here had a basal cell carcinoma involving the full thickness of the medial third of the left upper eyelid.

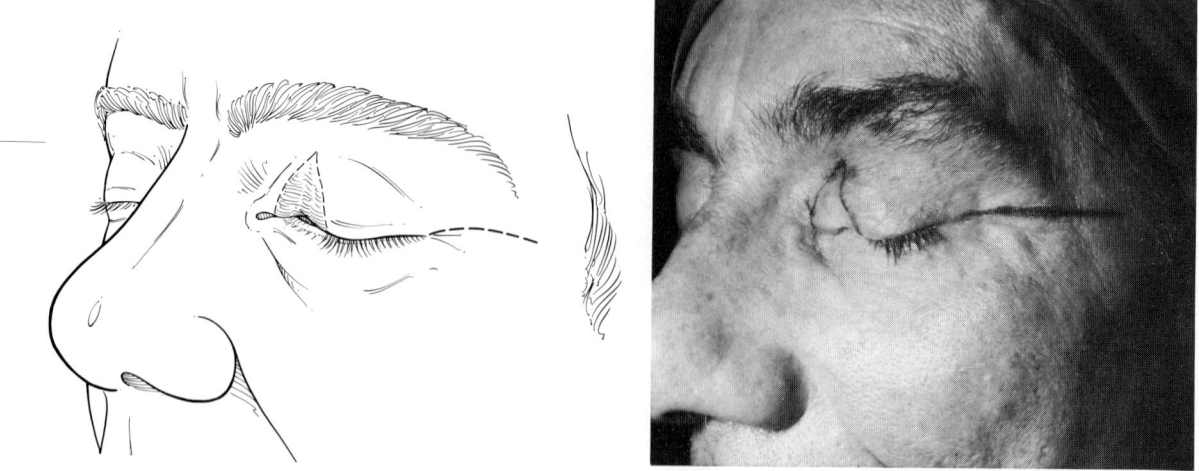

The projected resection is fashioned as a standard pentagonal wedge.

CHAPTER 7
**EYELID AND
CANTHAL REGION
RECONSTRUCTION**

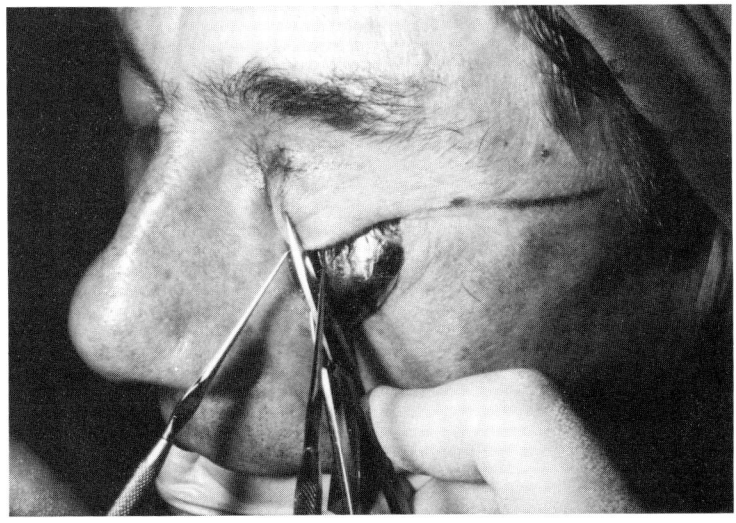

With the eye protected by means of a teaspoon, the upper lid is resected with straight iris scissors.

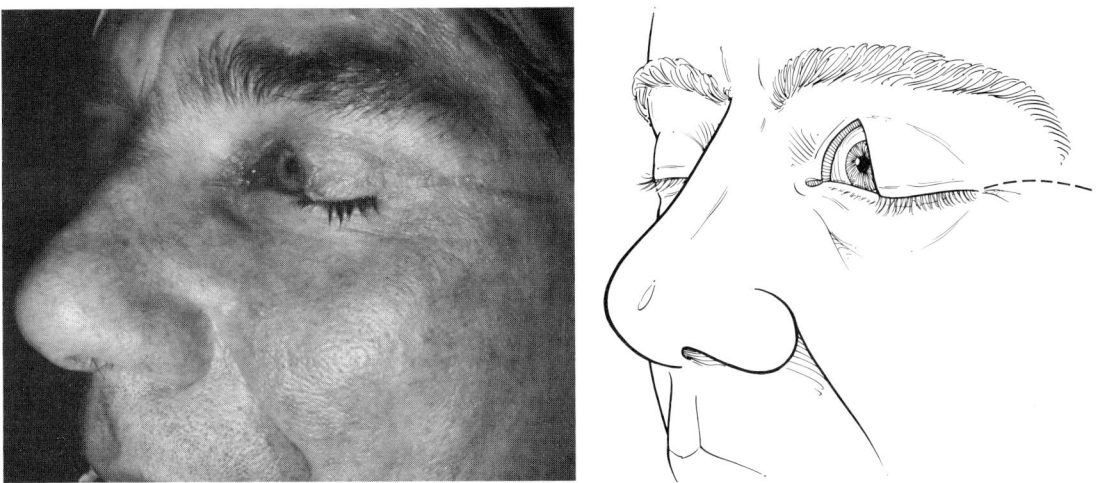

An incision is made through the lateral canthus extending out onto the temporal area.

299

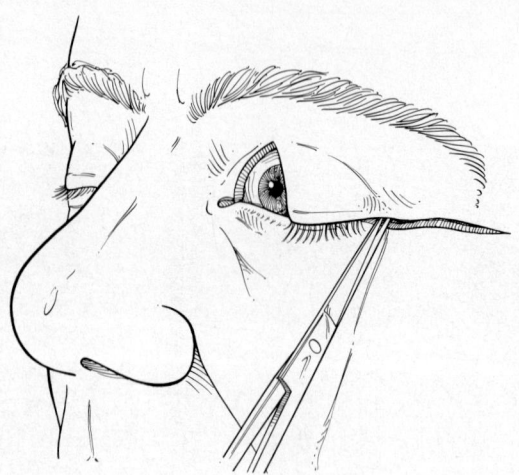

The upper limb of the lateral canthal ligament is divided with sharp pointed scissors.

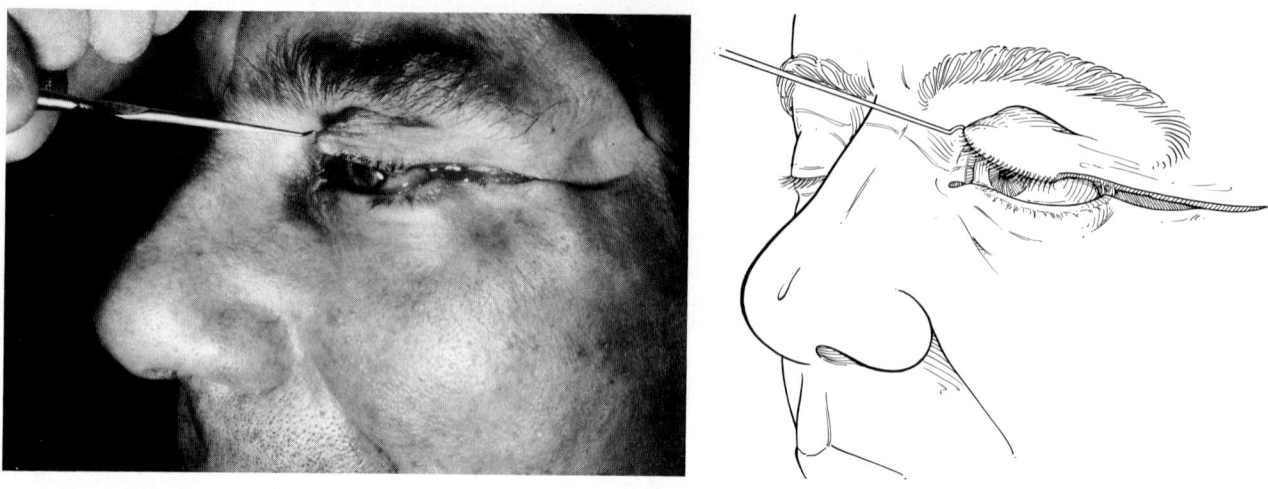

When this maneuver is performed, the lid can be moved medially to close the defect. If any tension is present, the lateral incision is extended. However, this incision rarely extends far into the temporal area.

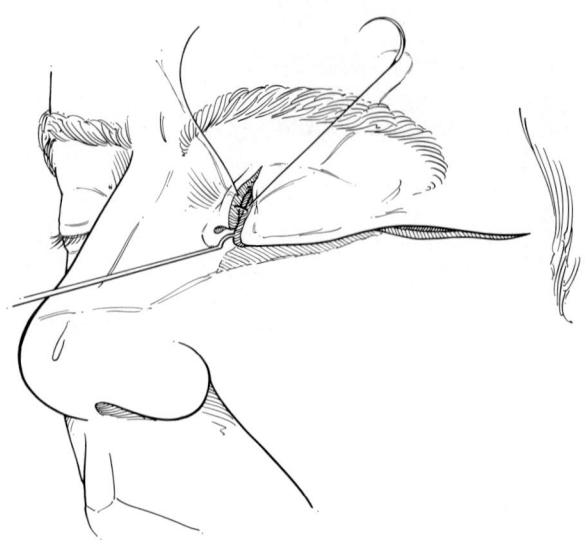

CHAPTER 7
EYELID AND CANTHAL REGION RECONSTRUCTION

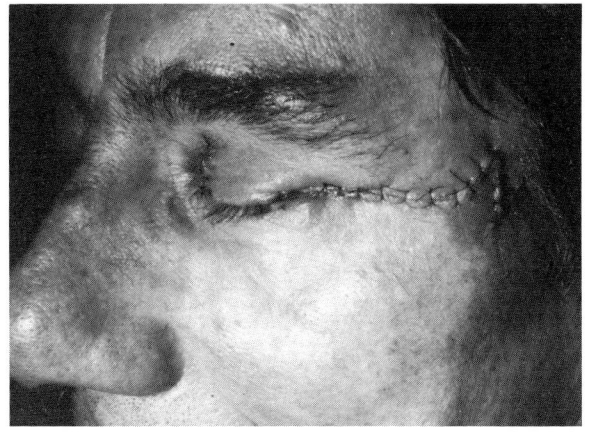

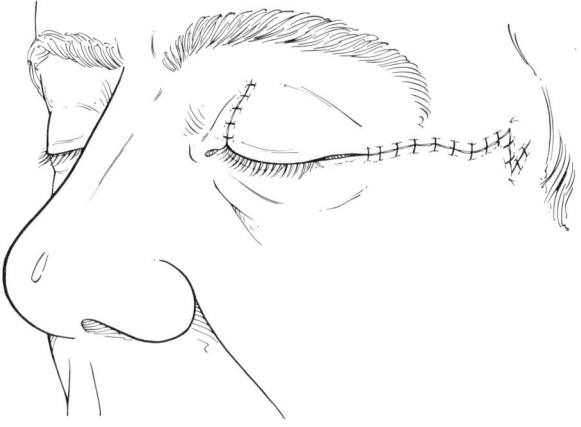

As with the rotation flap in lower lid reconstruction, a temporal Z-plasty can be done, but this is mainly for cosmetic reasons and adds little or nothing to the lid advancement. The edges of the defect are closed in layers.

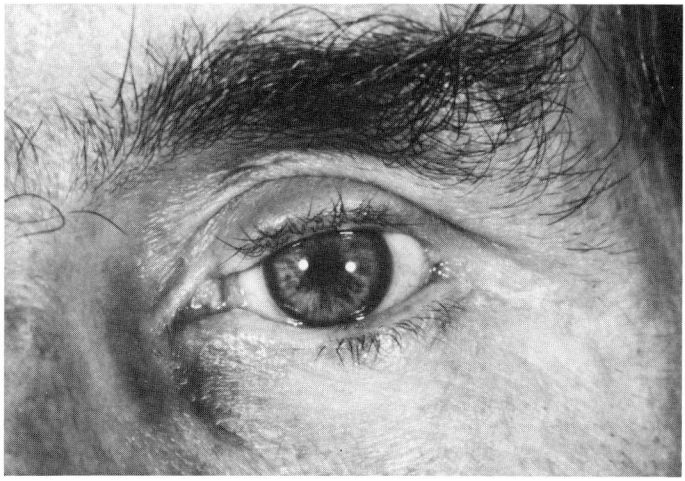

The result can be aesthetically excellent.

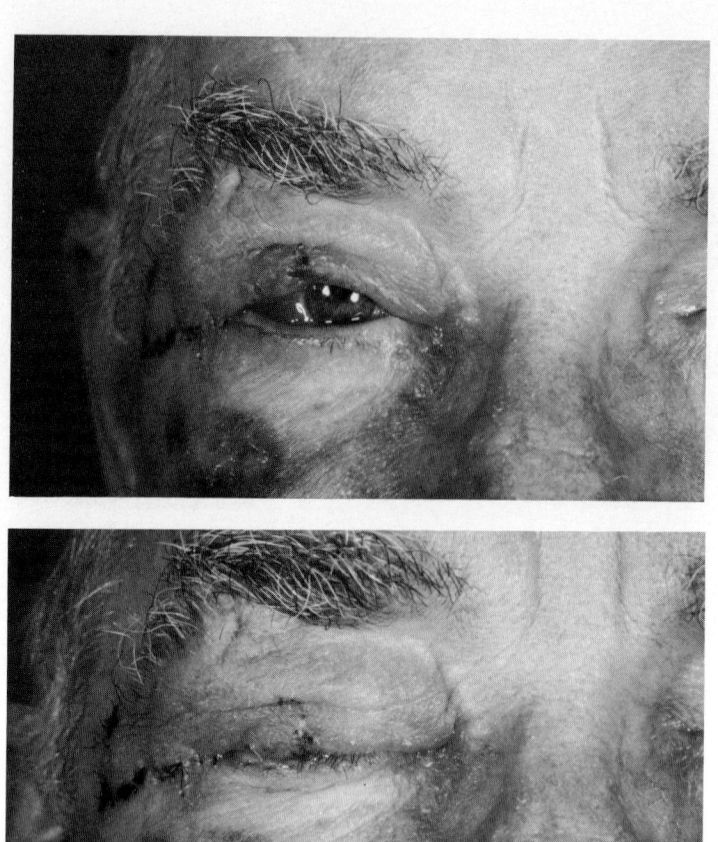

These illustrations show a patient with a recent upper lid reconstruction and preservation of full eyelid function.

PROBLEMS

Few problems are encountered with the upper lid rotation flap. However, some should be considered, at least in theory. If the defect is too large, the upper lid can be unduly tight. Fortunately, the flap will usually stretch with time. Entropion and corneal irritation may occur. Upper lid ptosis also may occur, but normally this is a temporary phenomenon.

Surgical Technique of Choice

Because the upper lid rotation flap is simple to design, uncomplicated to perform, and produces an excellent aesthetic and functional result, it is the reconstructive method of choice. The secret to performing this technique is in the planning process; the surgeon needs to consider the upper lid as though it were the lower lid and then plan the surgery accordingly.

TOTAL UPPER LID RECONSTRUCTION

The upper lid is of paramount importance, both aesthetically and functionally. This structure is essential for corneal protection, since without its cover the cornea dries and ulcerates and scarring and blindness result. Reconstruction of an upper lid is a matter of urgency. The other important attribute of the upper lid is its ability to open and close. If possible, this movement should be maintained. Since the lower lid is much less important functionally, it can be used as a source of reconstructive material.

Simultaneous Cheek Rotation and Total Lower Lid Switch Flap

As mentioned in the preceding discussion, the lower lid has a less important functional role than the upper lid. Therefore, when the total upper lid has been sacrificed, the lower lid can be used in its entirety to effect a satisfactory reconstruction.

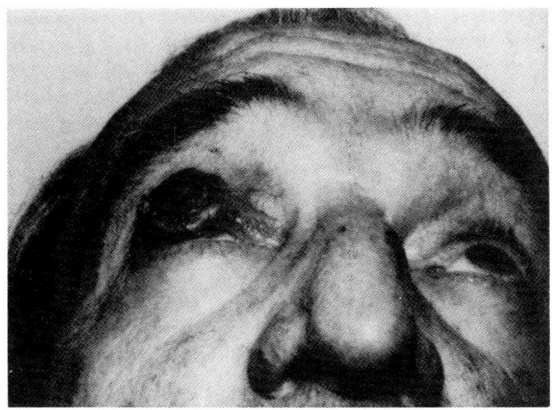 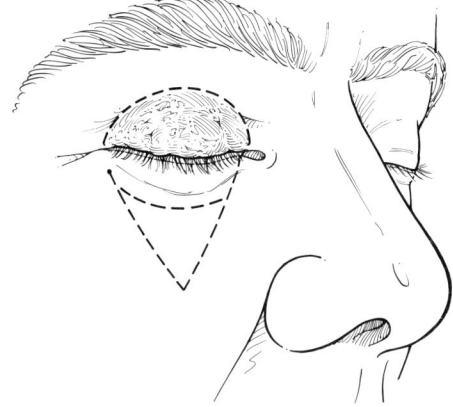

The patient presented here had a large squamous cell carcinoma of the upper lid.

After total upper lid resection has been performed, the operative plan is outlined on the lower lid and cheek. The whole of the lower lid will be taken, with the lower punctum and the medial canthal area left undisturbed.

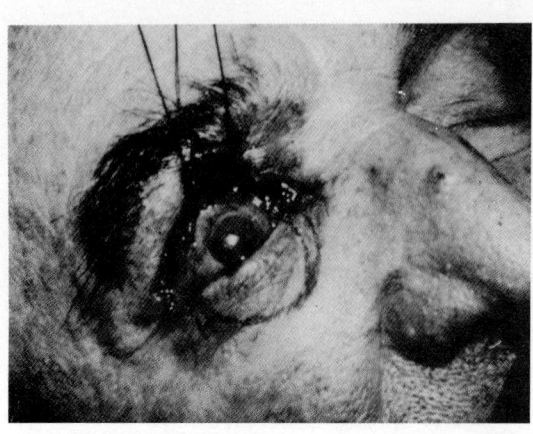 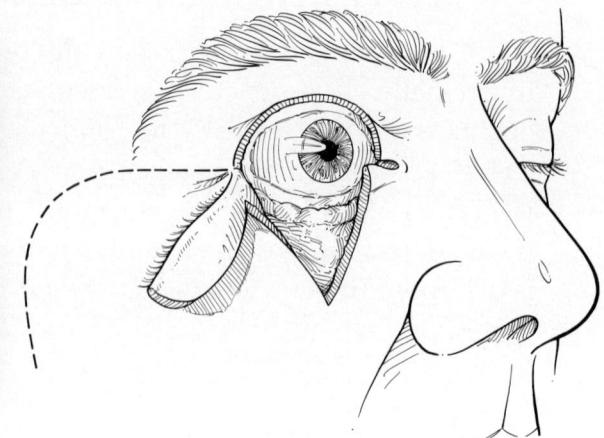

The required amount of skin is drawn out, and the lateral part of the incision is taken to within 5 to 7 mm from the lateral lid margin in the region of the lateral canthus. A standard cheek rotation flap is drawn out on the cheek. This flap must be planned to be large enough to reconstruct the lower lid.

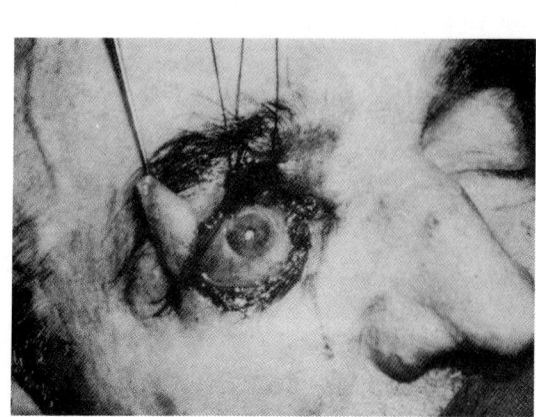 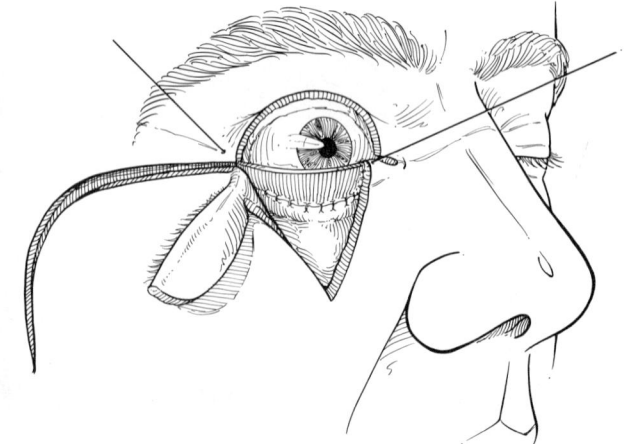

The lower lid flap is cut with straight iris scissors and scalpel, maintaining the lateral pedicle. The cheek flap is widely elevated, as described earlier. At this point the lid flap and the cheek flap are temporarily rotated into their final positions. This allows the excess cheek skin under the lower lid excision to be estimated. When this calculation has been made, the required wedge of skin is excised.

A composite chondromucosal graft is taken from the nasal septum. With the large amount of tissue required, it is usually necessary to incise around the alar base to give better exposure to the septum.

This graft is sutured in position, as described for lower lid reconstruction.

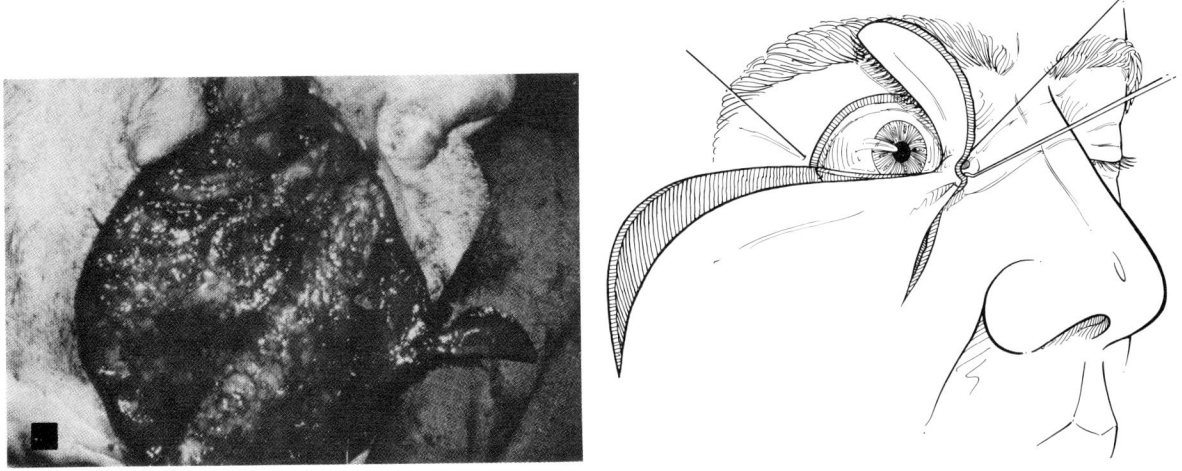

At this point the lid and cheek flap are temporarily rotated into their final positions. This allows the excess cheek skin under the lower lid excision to be estimated. When this has been done, the calculated wedge of skin is excised.

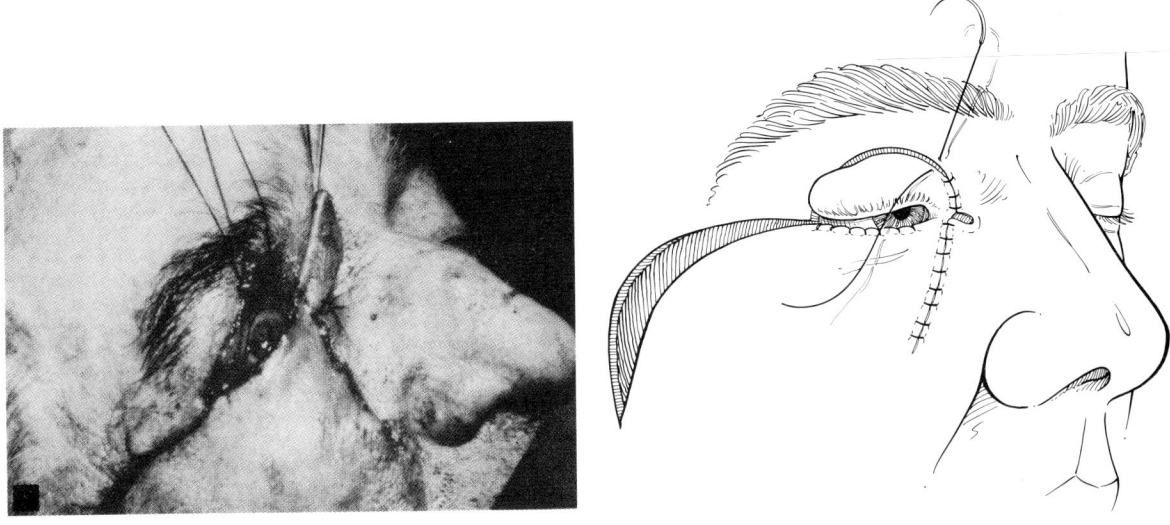

The lower lid is rotated to form the upper lid, with the medial end of the lower lid becoming the lateral end of the upper lid. The levator muscle is sutured to the orbicularis muscle.

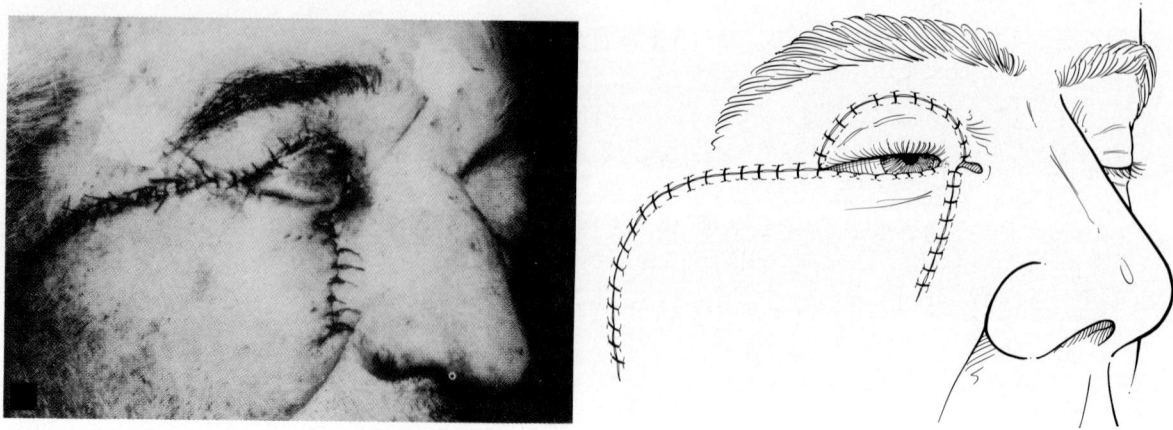

As this is done, the cheek flap rotates to close the cheek defect. Care should be taken to anchor the undersurface of the flap to the malar area and to prevent sagging of the reconstructed lower lid. The upper lid pedicle is left in situ for 2 to 3 weeks to ensure good vascularity of the lid; after this time the pedicle is severed.

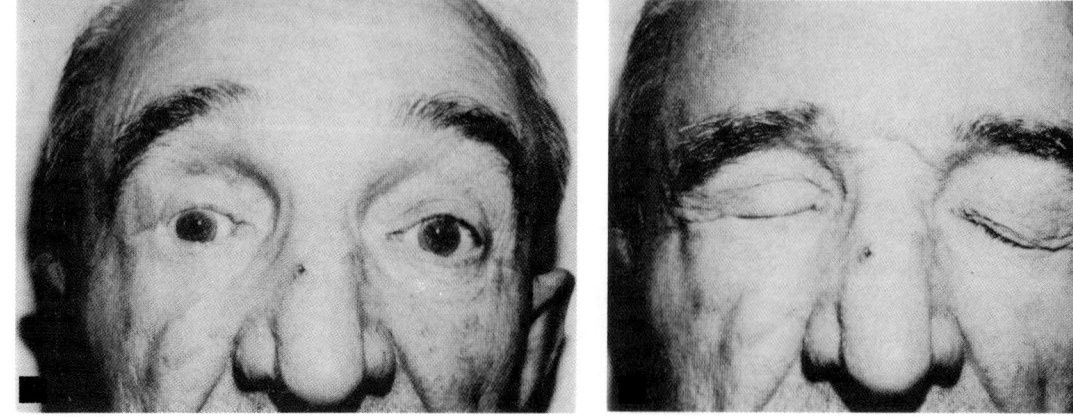

Excellent aesthetic and functional results can be achieved with this procedure.

PROBLEMS

The vascularity of the transferred lower lid may be a problem. If significant ischemia occurs, with necrosis of the new upper lid, further upper lid reconstruction becomes a matter of great urgency. Solutions to this problem are limited and unsatisfactory from both a functional and a cosmetic point of view. Concurrent loss of the cheek flap resulting in an eye without lids is another possibility. Immediate closure with a mucosa-lined forehead flap would be the solution to this horrifying complication. After healing had occurred, further procedures would be used to refine the lids.

Two-Stage Lower Lid Switch and Cheek Rotation Flap

The advantage of this technique of total upper eyelid reconstruction is its safety. Because the repair is done as a two-stage procedure, the vascularity is much less tenuous. In addition, the two stages allow for more trimming and more refined reconstruction.

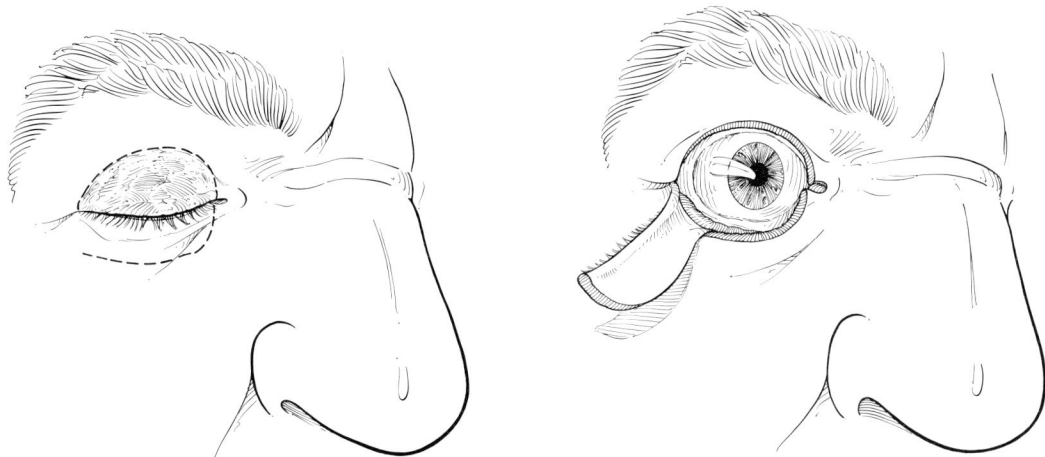

After resection of the upper lid, the lower lid is incised, either medially or laterally, until it can be swung up and sutured to the lateral half of the upper lid defect.

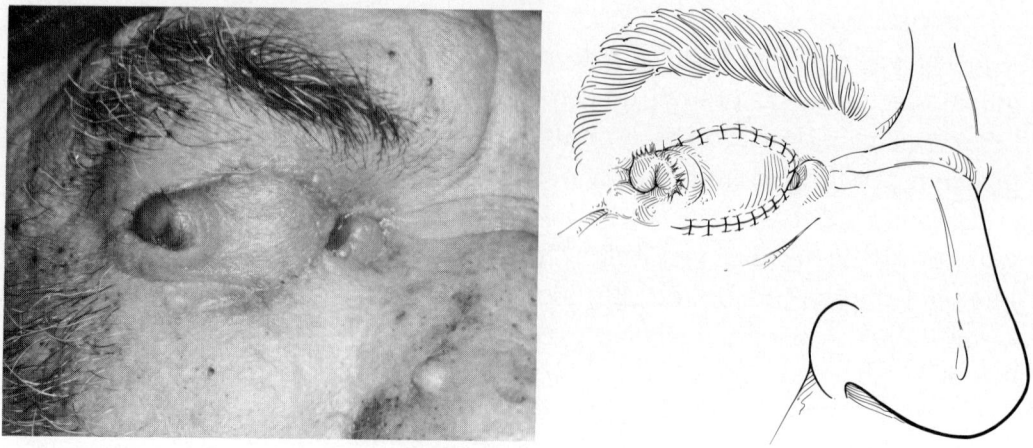

It is important to spare the punctum. In this way the lid is based on a much wider pedicle than with the conventional lid switch flap. The levator muscle is attached to the orbicularis muscle over as wide a distance as possible. The raw areas are closed by suturing the conjunctiva to the skin.

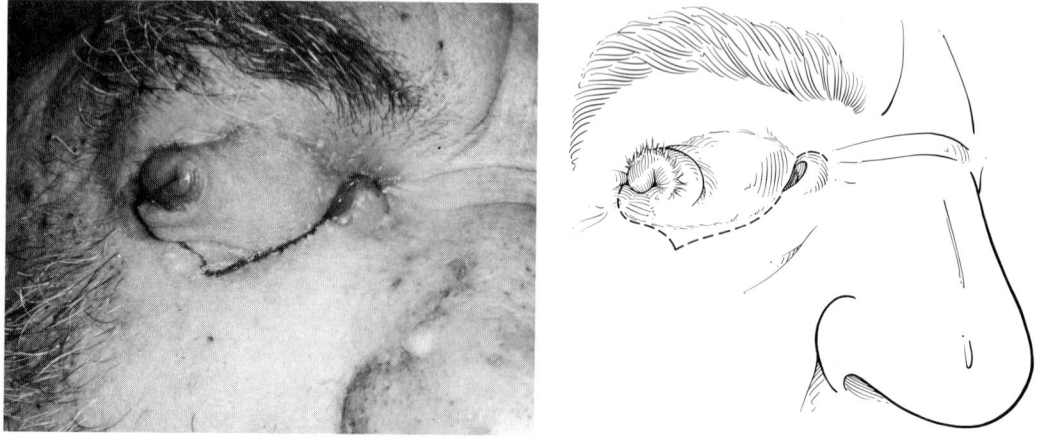

The position of the lid pedicle is such that it covers and protects the cornea during the 2 weeks it is left attached. At that time the amount of lower lid required to totally reconstruct the upper lid is marked on the lid.

CHAPTER 7
**EYELID AND
CANTHAL REGION
RECONSTRUCTION**

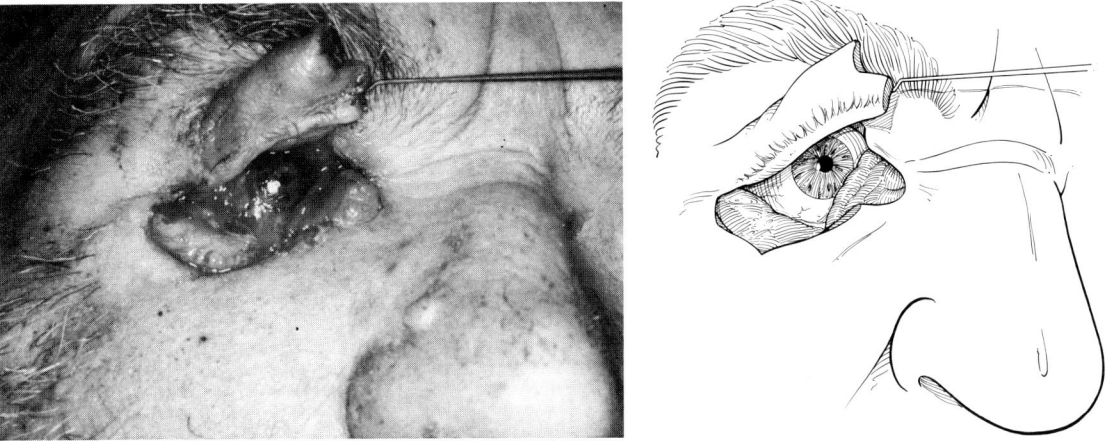

The base of the upper lid is divided, and the lower lid is swung up into the freshened area on the medial aspect of the upper lid defect.

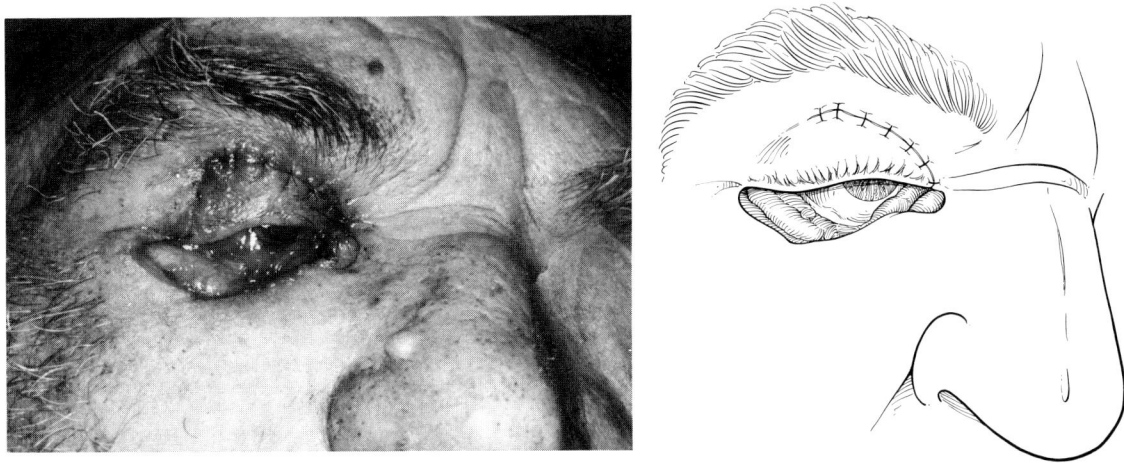

Thus upper lid reconstruction is completed. If possible, the levator is identified and sutured to the tarsal plate.

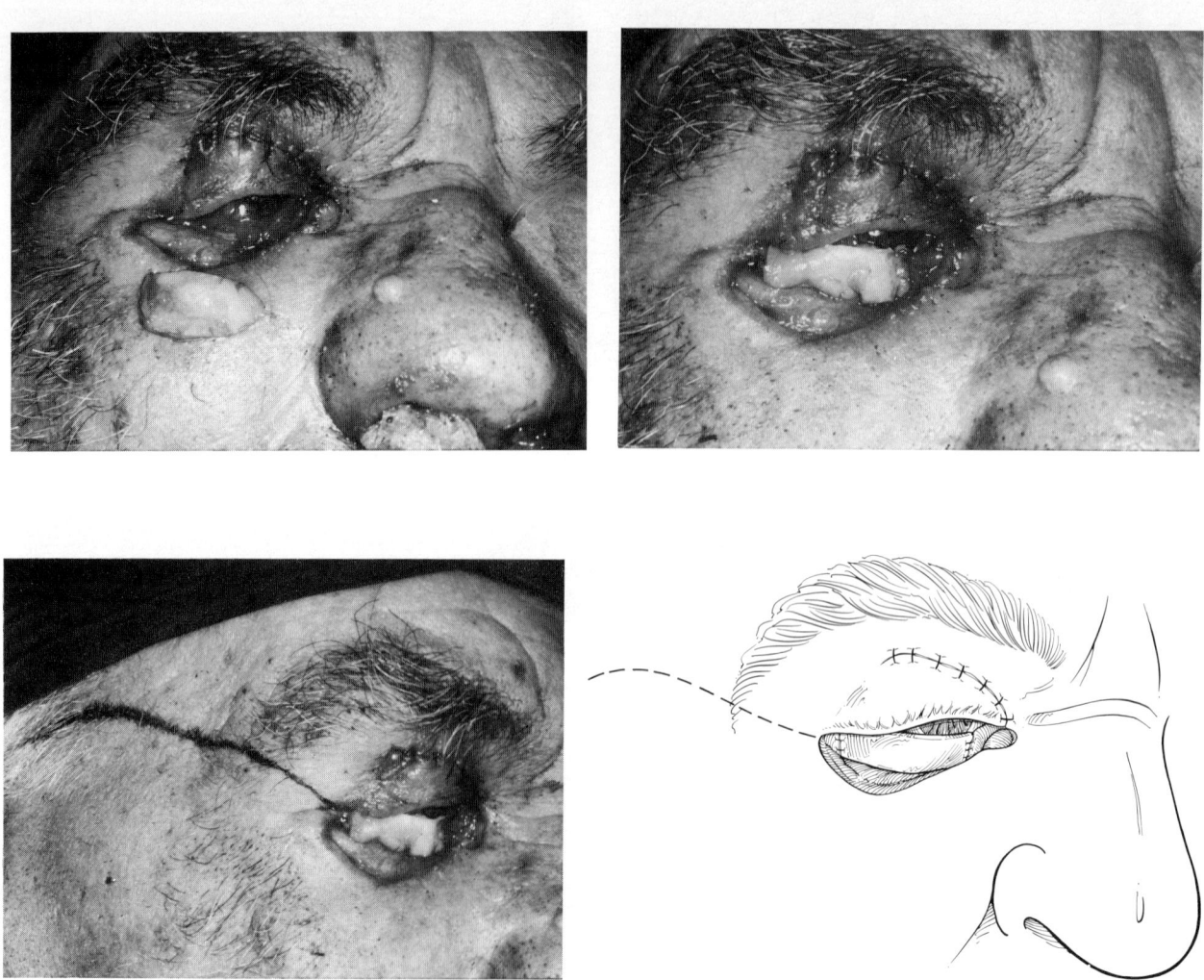

The lower lid is reconstructed by the conventional cheek rotation flap–chondromucosal graft method described earlier.

CHAPTER 7
**EYELID AND
CANTHAL REGION
RECONSTRUCTION**

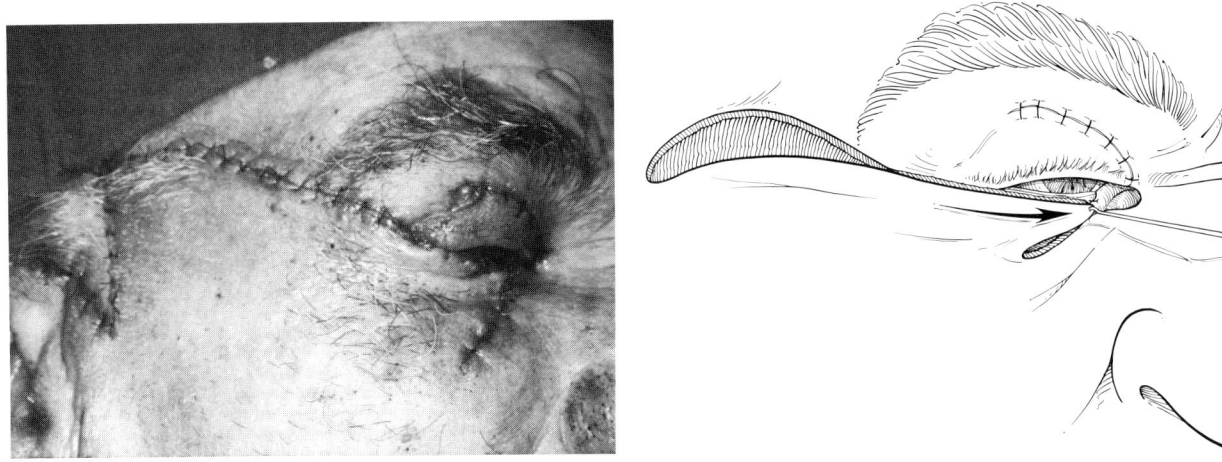

With an extended lateral canthal incision, the cheek flap is elevated at the face-lift plane and rotated medially to resurface the skin of the lower lid.

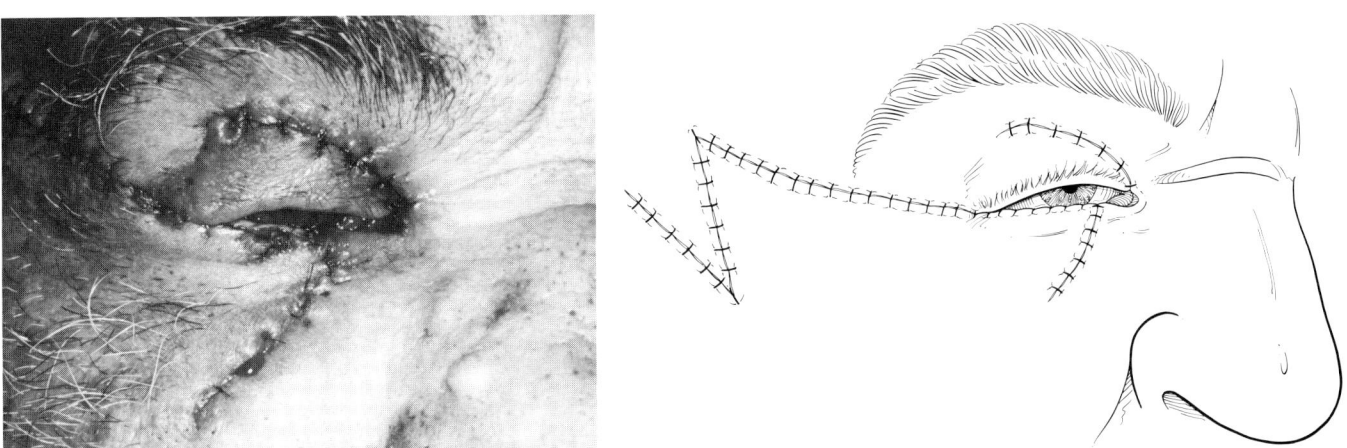

Excess skin at the base of the vertical incision on the cheek is removed as a dog ear.

PROBLEMS

Vascularity is not a problem for the upper lid reconstruction, but, as with all large cheek rotation flaps, ischemia can be a problem for the lower lid. If ischemia does occur, then the lower lid reconstruction will fail and a forehead or nasolabial flap with mucosal lining will be necessary for subsequent reconstruction.

311

Reconstruction of Choice

Only the two-stage method of reconstruction should be considered because of its secure vascularity. There is little likelihood of losing the upper lid reconstruction if the pedicle is kept wide. Even if the lower lid reconstruction is lost, the eye is protected with the new upper lid. The entire area can then be allowed to heal before reconstruction of the lower lid begins once more.

☐ Reconstruction of Medial Canthus

The medial canthal area has been included with the eyelids because excision in this region frequently extends to the lids, occasionally involving sacrifice of the full thickness of the lids, lacrimal puncta, and canaliculi. In the medial canthus incomplete excision of carcinoma can result in later extension of the cancer into the ethmoid sinuses, and from there to the cribriform area with resulting intracranial invasion. In removing superficial lesions, excision of periosteum is also recommended, particularly if there is any suggestion of subdermal involvement. If periosteal involvement is noted, underlying nasal bone should be resected. It is true that skin grafts allow early detection of recurrence, but their use may lead to initial inadequate tumor excision. The reason for this is that the surgeon will tend to leave a base of periosteum on which to place a skin graft, since without periosteum a graft will not take. It is more logical to resect down to bone or to include bone in order to get one layer ahead of the tumor; in this situation a skin graft cannot be used. The defect is reconstructed with a local flap.[2]

When the excision has been completed, the canthus must be reconstructed. It should be placed in the correct anatomic position and fixed to bone. Failure to do this leads to obvious asymmetry. At this stage it is probably unwise to perform a complicated lacrimal reconstruction. Such reconstruction may not be necessary because epiphora may not be a problem in the long term. The possibility of tumor recurrence exists. It is much better to adopt a wait and see policy. If all is well and reconstruction is indicated, it can be performed later.

SPLIT FINGER FLAP

The split finger flap may be used when the side of the nasal bridgeline, including the periosteum and sometimes bone, and the medial ends of both eyelids have been sacrificed.

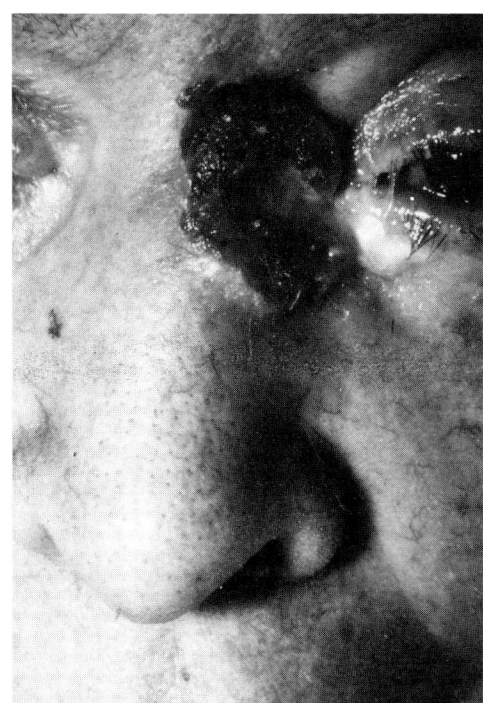

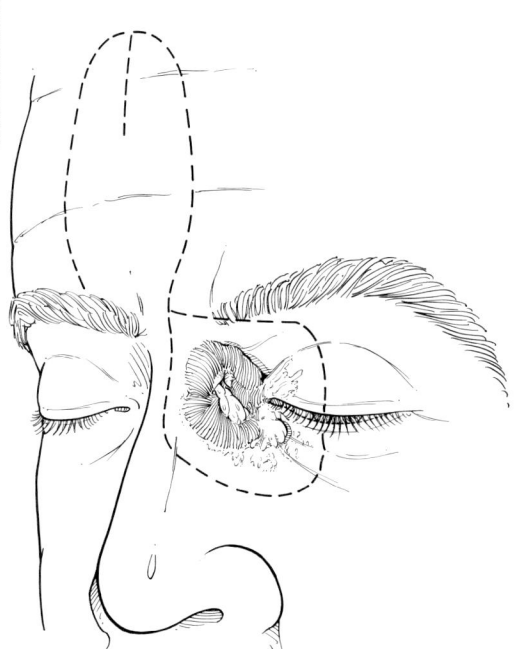

The patient shown here had a penetrating basal cell carcinoma of the medial canthal area. The planned excision and the split finger flap are outlined. The flap is planned slightly wider and larger than the standard finger flap.

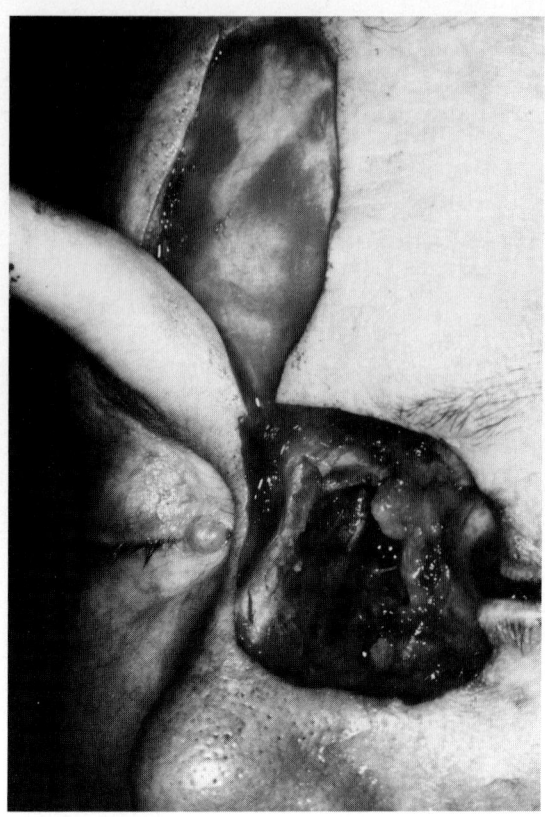
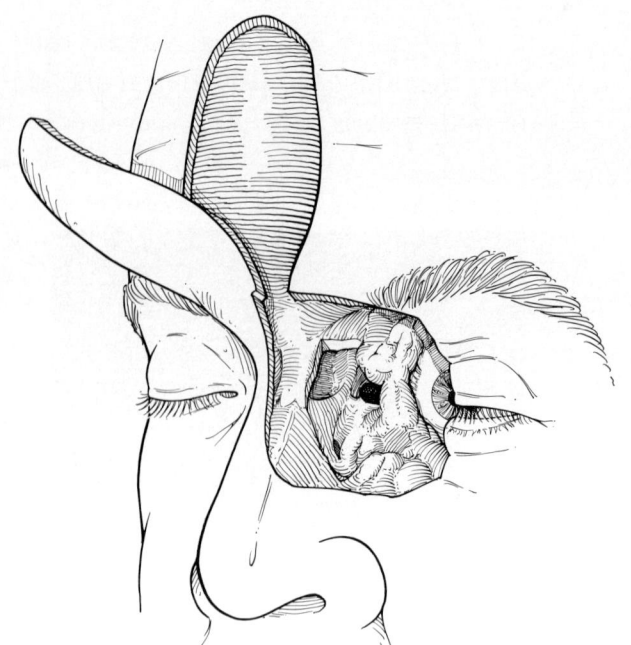

The tumor is resected with underlying bone and ethnoid sinuses. The whole medial canthus and the medial ends of the upper and lower lids are sacrificed. The medial conjunctival pocket is reconstructed by mobilization of the conjunctiva to the limbus, if necessary. The conjunctiva is sutured horizontally and provides lid lining.

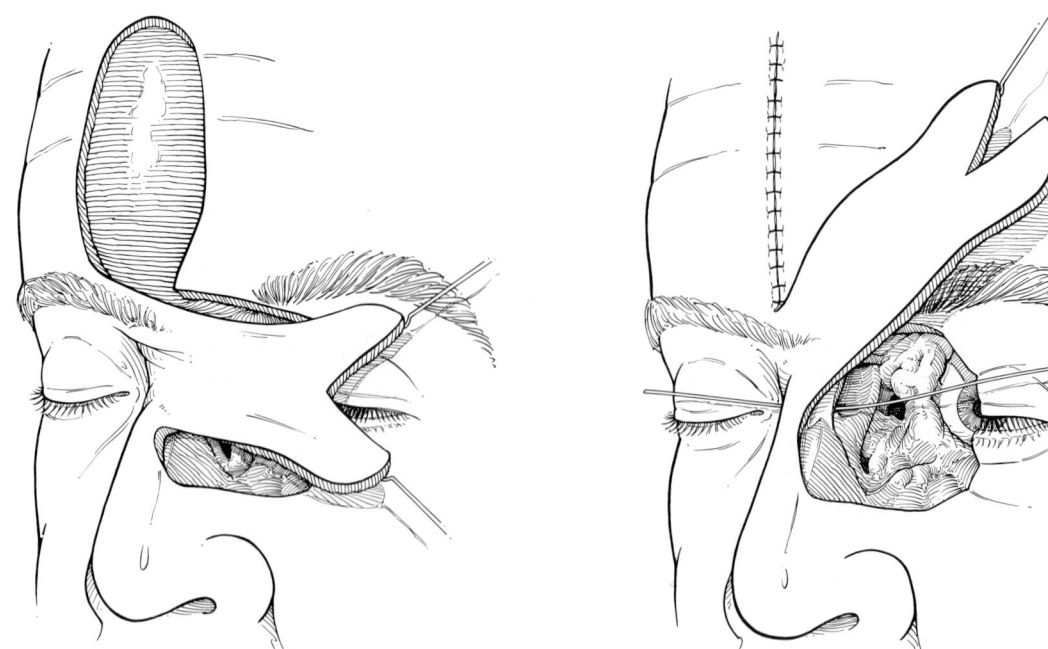

The flap is then rotated into the defect and split at its free end until the correct position for the new medial canthus is obtained. The forehead defect is closed directly.

CHAPTER 7
EYELID AND CANTHAL REGION RECONSTRUCTION

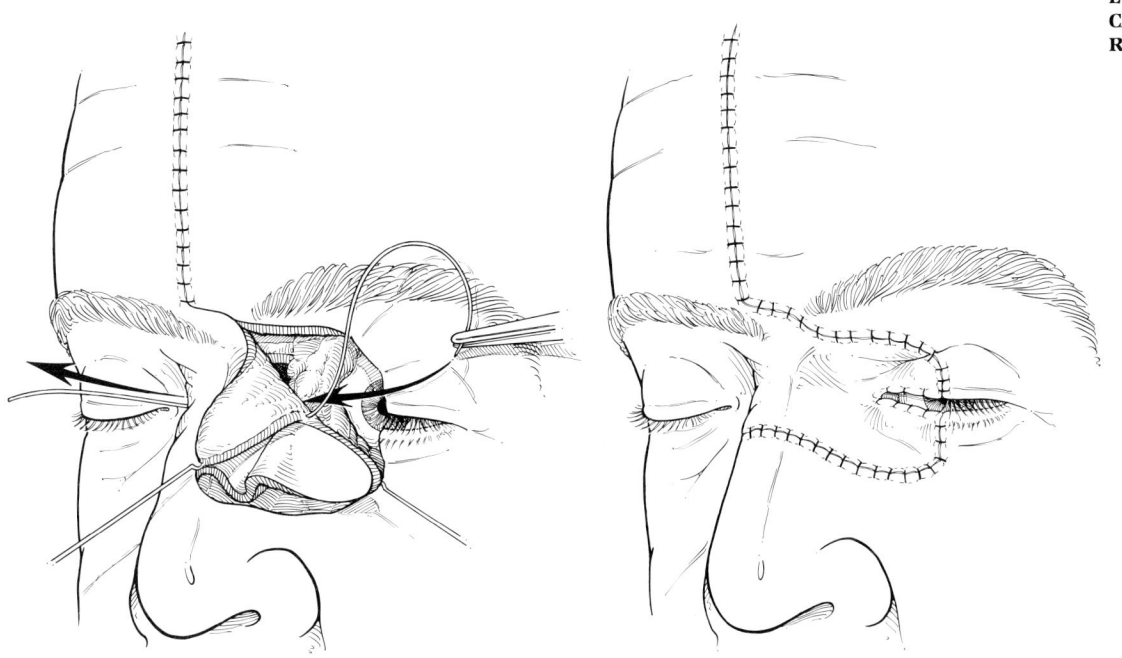

Using an incision on the other side of the nose, the surgeon exposes the noninvolved nasal bone. Two drillholes are made in this area, and a wire is passed through to the area of the medial canthus. Here the wire is threaded through the deep layer of the flap and taken back out the second of the two holes. Gentle tightening of the wire brings the new canthus securely into its correct position and ensures the correct biconcave contour in this area. The flap is then sutured onto the eyelid defects. Some trimming is necessary to deal with the potential dog ear on the nose.

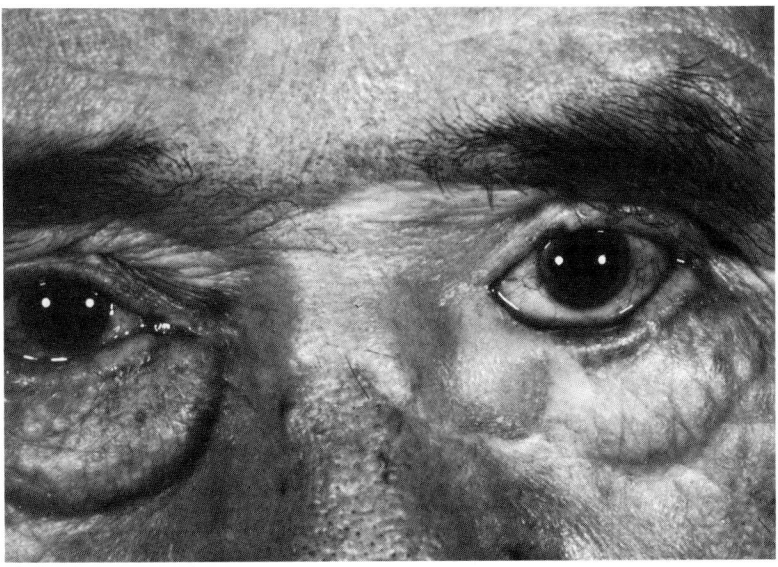

Rarely is any secondary contouring surgery necessary.

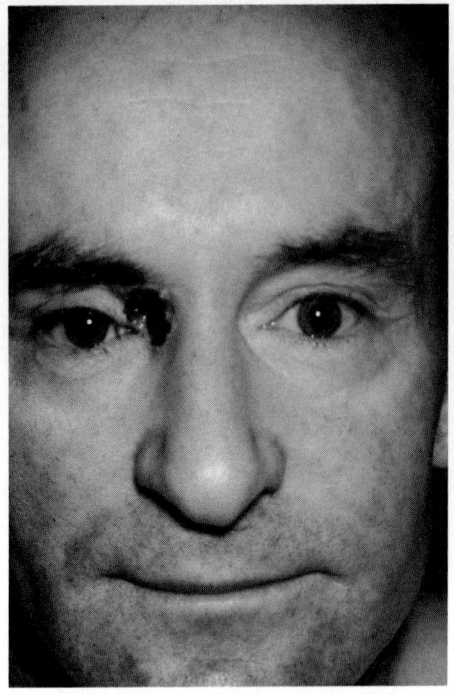 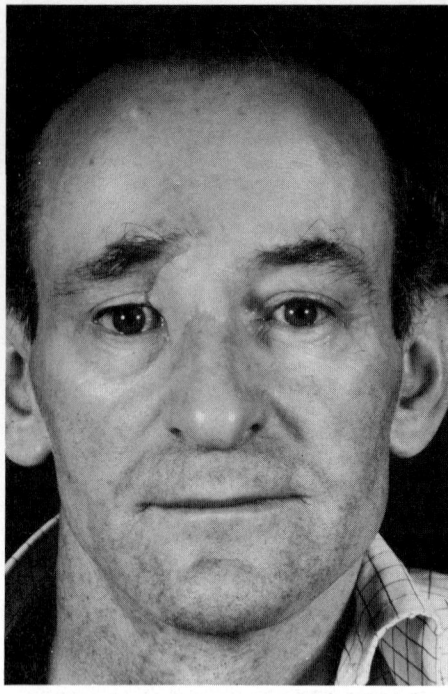

These illustrations show the recommended resection for a penetrating basal cell carcinoma in the medial canthal region. Again, the nasal bones and ethnoid sinuses are sacrificed. The defect is covered with a diagonal forehead flap. It should be noted that the thick forehead flap fits snugly into the bony defect and thus the potential contour deficiency is well filled.

PROBLEMS

The flap may be bulky and require later thinning, but this problem is unusual. Displacement of the medial canthal attachment can occur and reattachment may be necessary.

☐ Complex Reconstruction

Frequently tumor resection will result in a defect that requires medial canthal reconstruction together with full-thickness lid reconstruction. The lower lid is involved more frequently than the upper lid. This situation calls for a combination of flaps. Again, the lacrimal drainage system is sacrificed. The medial canthal ligament also may be resected and may require reconstruction.

FOREHEAD FLAP AND CHEEK ROTATION FLAP

A defect such as the one just described will require a complex reconstruction using combinations of techniques. The cheek and the forehead bear the brunt of these reconstructive efforts.

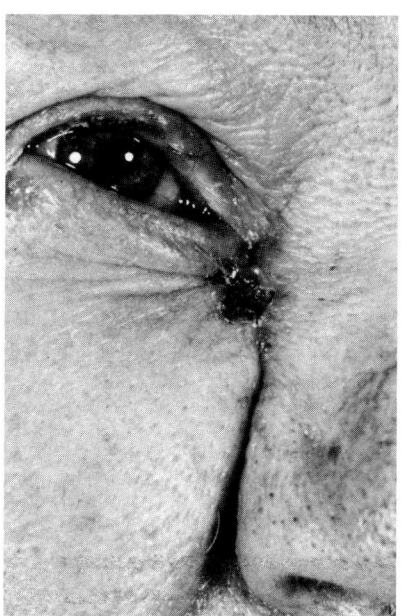

The patient illustrated here had an extensive postradiation therapy medial canthal basal cell carcinoma.

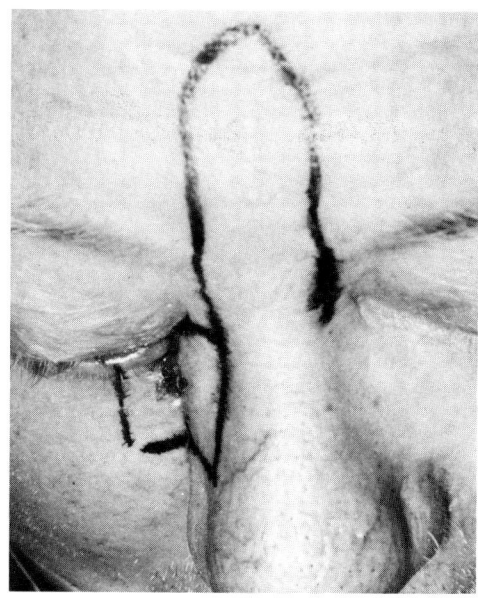
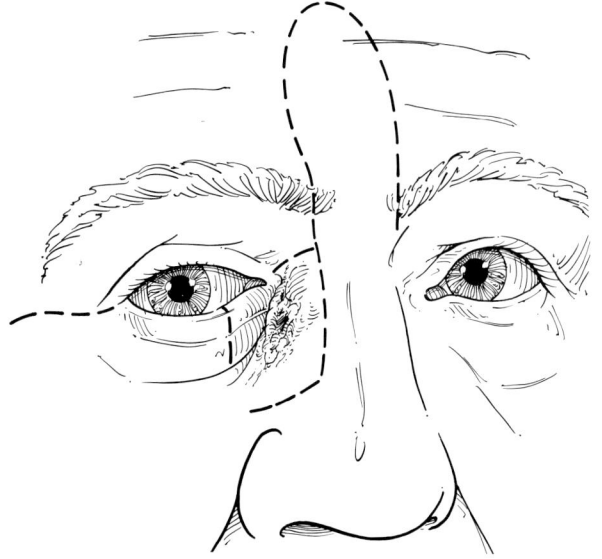

The planned skin excision—together with underlying nasal bone, infraorbital rim, lacrimal apparatus, and ethmoid sinuses—is drawn. Medial cover will be with a forehead flap.

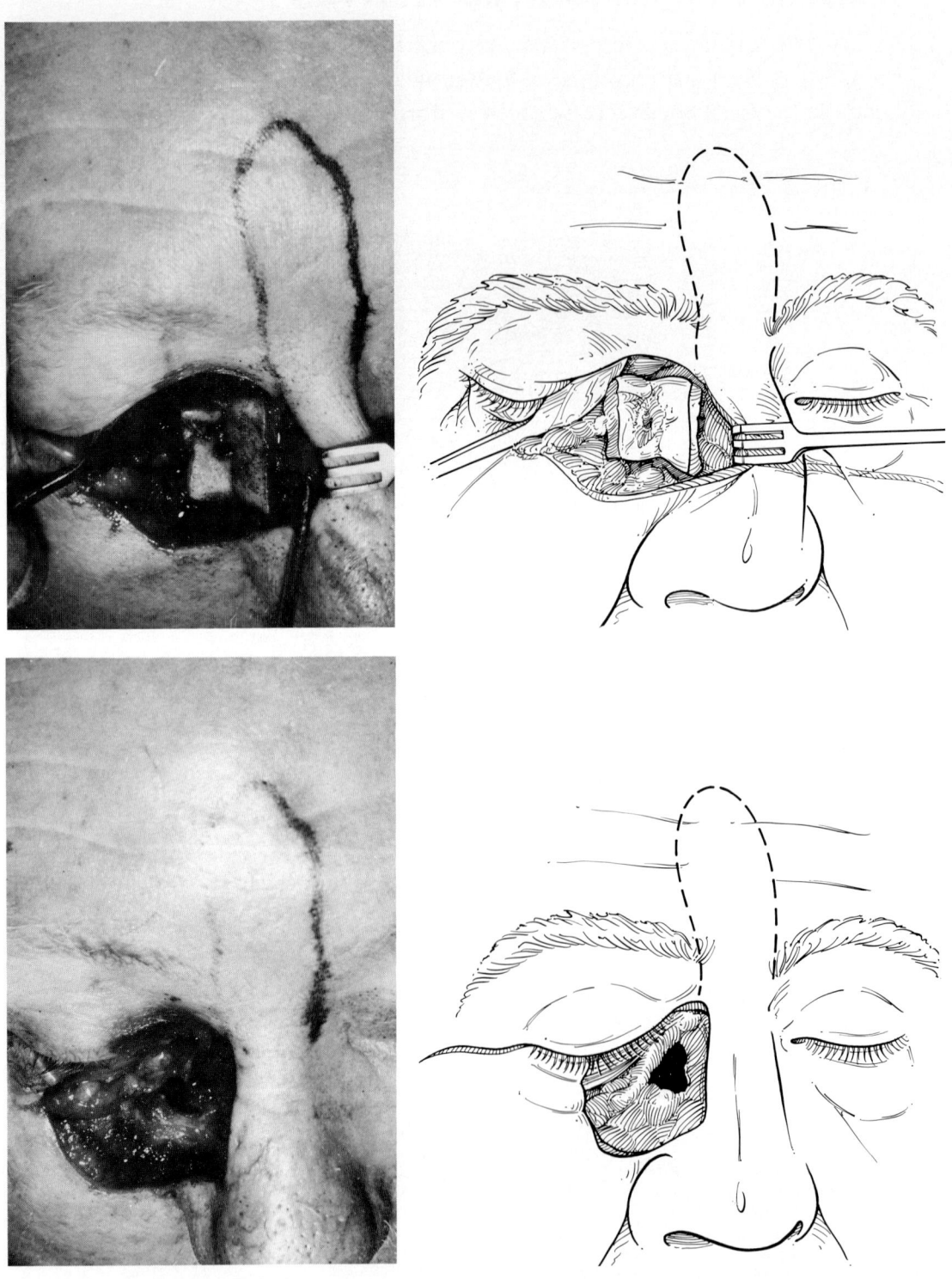

The excision is completed, with the expected defect left for reconstruction.

CHAPTER 7
EYELID AND CANTHAL REGION RECONSTRUCTION

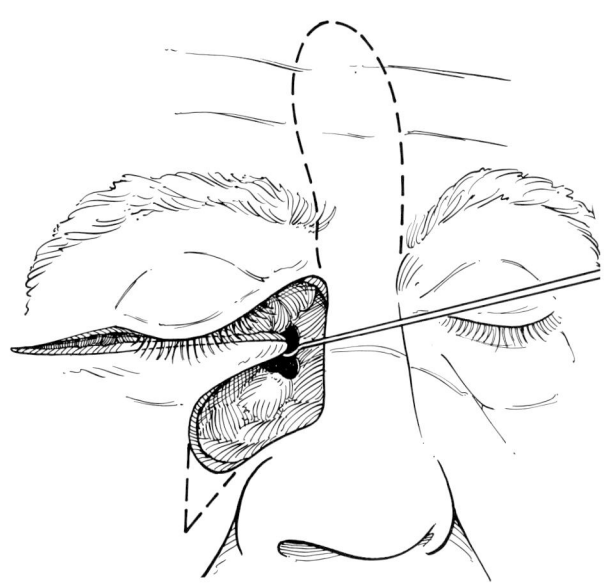

A lateral canthal cheek incision is made with division of the lower limb of the lateral canthal ligament; this allows the cheek and the lower eyelid to advance medially.

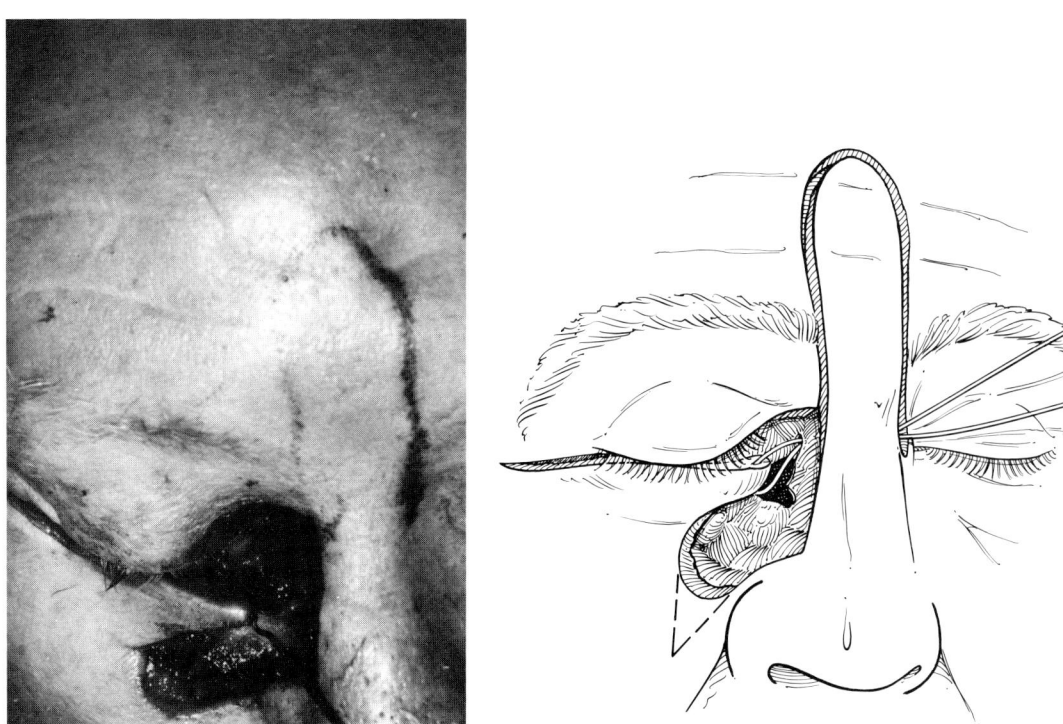

A transnasal canthopexy is performed as described earlier. The medial end of the lower lid is fixed in its correct position by the transnasal wire.

319

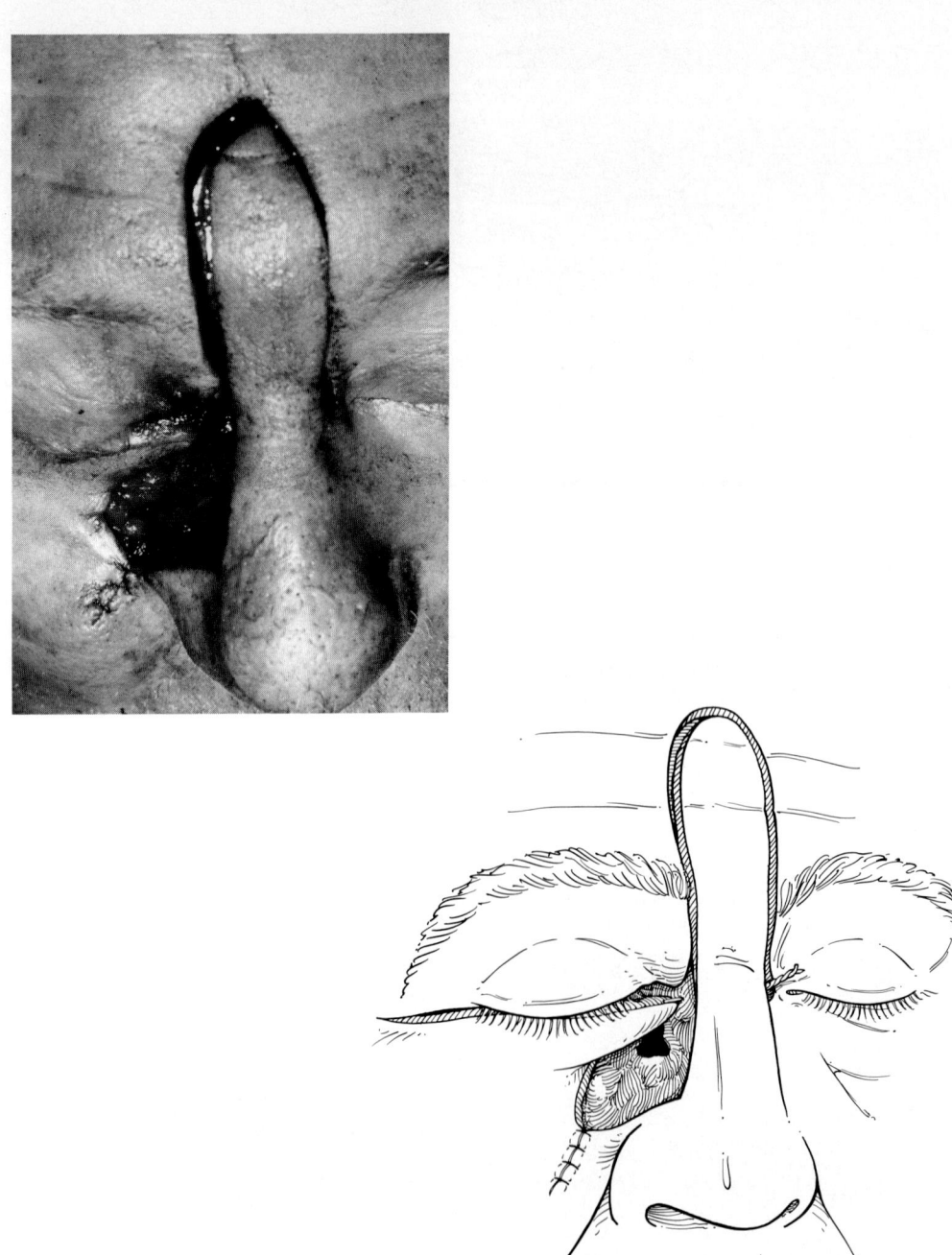

A small excess of cheek under the defect, caused by the cheek rotation, is excised.

CHAPTER 7
EYELID AND CANTHAL REGION RECONSTRUCTION

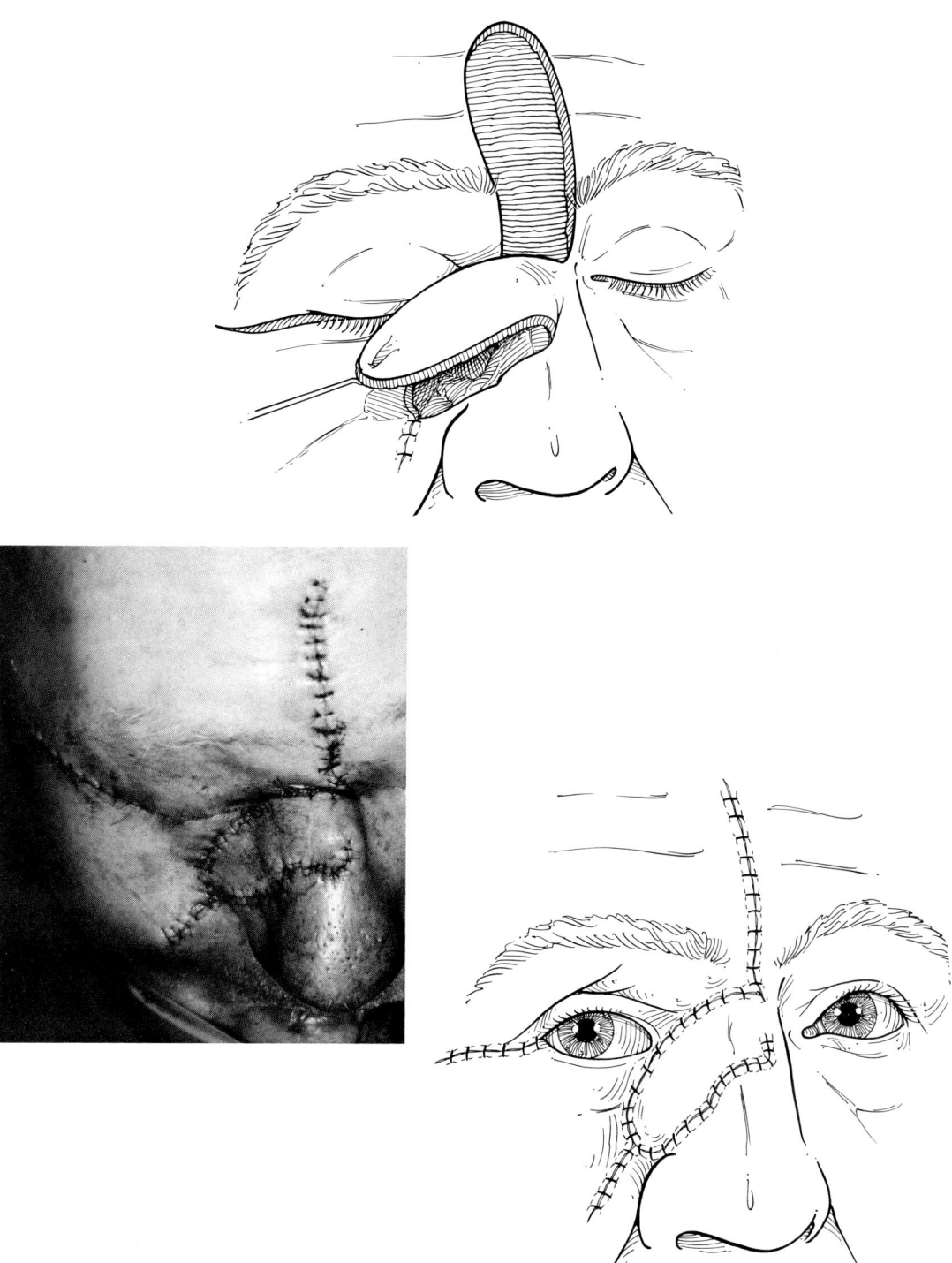

The forehead flap is swung down and sutured into position. Alternatives to this procedure would be the glabellar flap or an island flap from the forehead in the midline. These procedures are performed exactly as described earlier.

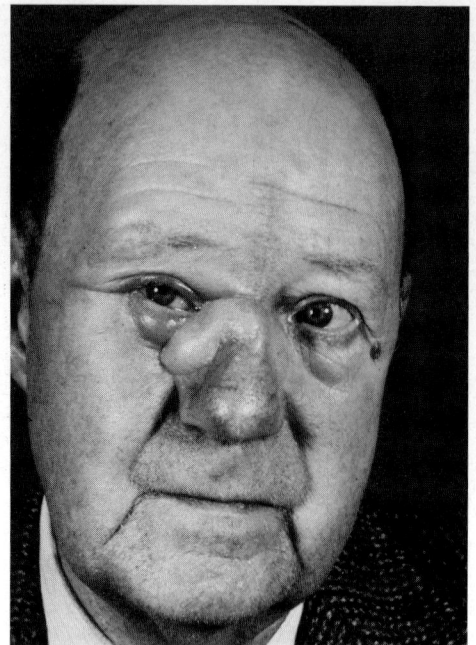 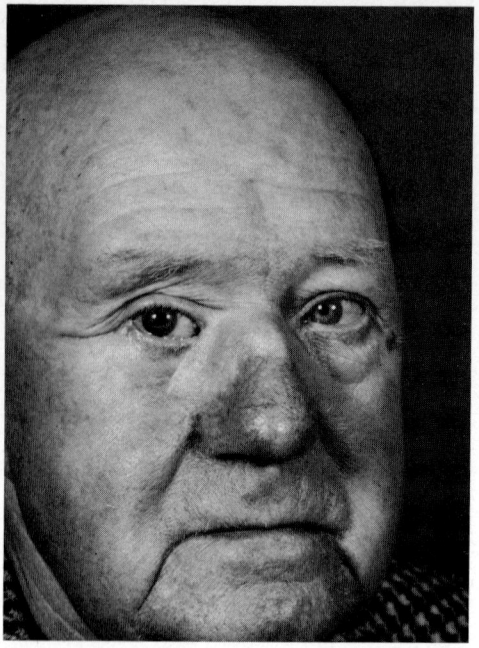

Initially lower lid edema is present, and the forehead finger flap is very bulky. With time all areas settle in a satisfactory fashion. It has not been necessary to perform any secondary surgery.

PROBLEMS

Epiphora may occur because of sacrifice of the canaliculus, but this complication is uncommon. Therefore the surgeon should not strive unduly to obtain primary lacrimal drainage. It is rarely successful and should be left for a future date, when the area has settled and the risk of tumor recurrence has receded. It is more important to establish the correct medial canthal position. Unless a secure canthopexy is achieved, it may be displaced later and give an unsightly telecanthus, which will require a secondary correction. Such a procedure is more difficult than a primary medial canthopexy. Pincushioning of the forehead may occur, and thinning may be necessary.

Reconstruction of Lateral Canthus

In the lateral canthal area the correct topography of the region is a basic consideration in planning reconstruction. The lateral canthal position needs to be reestablished, both vertically and horizontally.

Lateral canthal defects rarely occur. However, when they do, they pose a significant reconstructive problem because of the absence of local flap donor sites possessing the same type of skin as the lateral canthal and lid regions. If possible, a full-thickness skin graft is used. If bone is exposed, it is necessary to use a local flap. If only the lower portion of the lateral canthal area needs to be reconstructed, a standard cheek rotation flap or a rhomboid flap gives a good result. (See pp. 218 to 220 and pp. 210 to 213 for further description.)

FOREHEAD (FRICKE) FLAP

The forehead, or Fricke,[1] flap is easily planned and rapidly executed. It can replace the lateral canthal area, or it may be split to form the canthus and a portion of the lids.

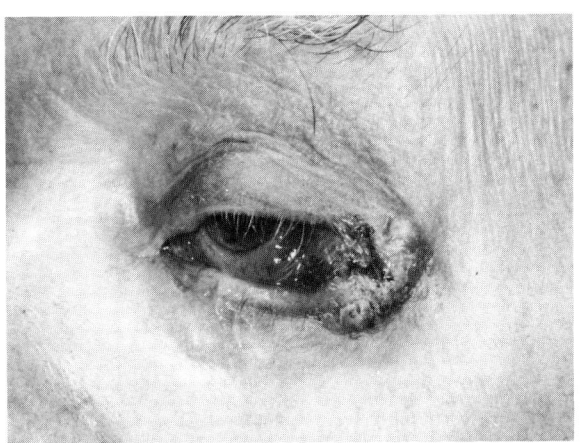
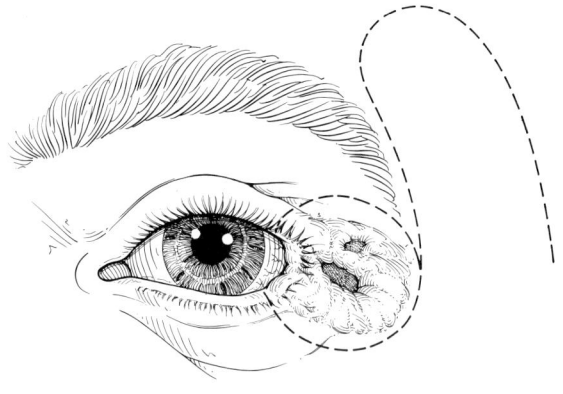

The elderly patient illustrated here had an extensive basal cell carcinoma of the lateral canthal area. The flap is based laterally and consists of skin lateral to and above the eyebrow. Occasionally, it may be a one-stage procedure, but more often it is performed in two stages.

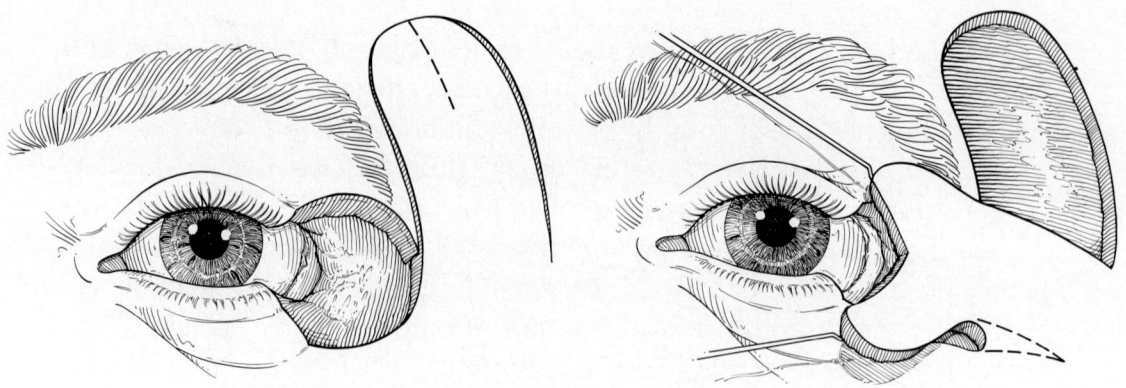

The flap is elevated, its length being that required to give a satisfactory canthal and lid reconstruction. The flap is split at the end to allow a more normal canthus to be formed.

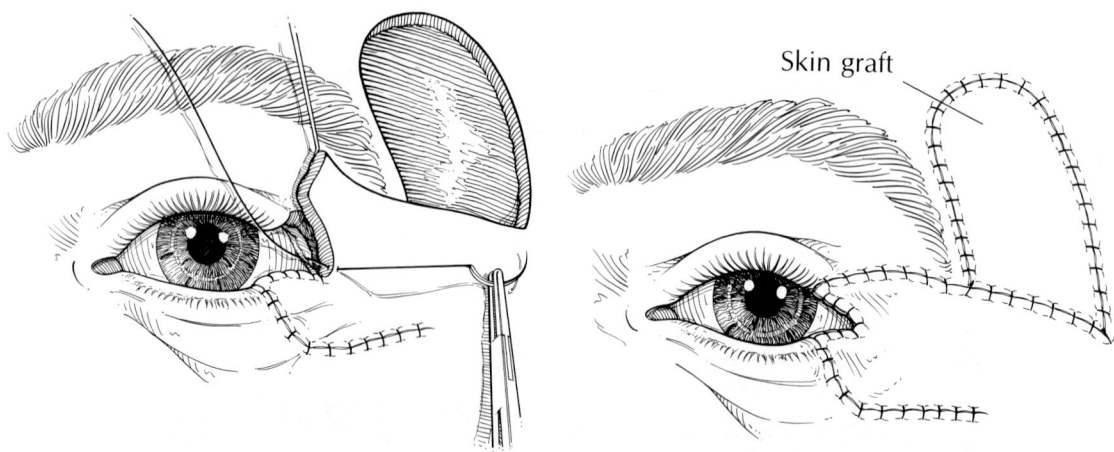

It is usually possible to mobilize enough conjunctiva to resurface the inner aspect of the flap. If this is not possible, then a free buccal or nasal mucosal graft is used. With such a thick flap, support of a chondromucosal graft is not necessary. The flap (and if necessary the graft) is sutured in position. The donor site can rarely be closed directly. This would distort the eyebrow, and the raw area would then need to be covered with a skin graft.

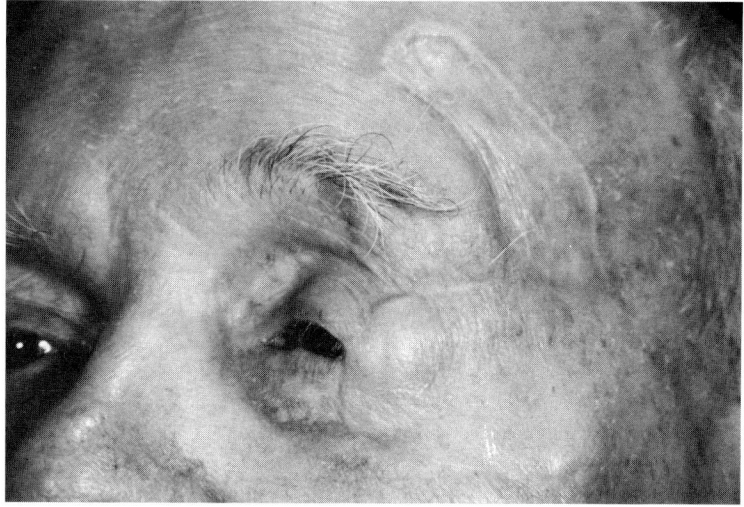

In many cases the flap is inset directly and no further procedure is required. In other cases, when a pedicle remains, this is divided in 10 to 14 days, and the unused portion of the flap is returned to the forehead.

PROBLEMS

The skin of the forehead, which is thick, obviates the necessity for lid support but produces a very obvious, bulky reconstruction. In many individuals the forehead skin is paler than that of the lids, a further reason for a poor reconstruction. The donor site is unsatisfactory; if this site is closed directly, the eyebrow position and shape are distorted. If grafted, the pale, mat, depressed skin graft causes a very obvious cosmetic defect.

SURGICAL TECHNIQUE OF CHOICE

In summary, lateral canthal reconstruction is not very satisfactory when both lids are involved. Fortunately, this is not an area that frequently requires reconstruction. Lower defects are closed with local cheek flaps. For more extensive areas the forehead flap should be considered.

REFERENCES

1. Fricke, J.C.G.: Die Bildung der Augenlider (Blepheroplastik) nach Zerstörungen und. dadurch hervorgebrachten Auswärtswendungen derselben, Hamburg, 1829, Perthes & Besser.
2. Jackson, I.T., Laws, E.R., Jr., and Martin, R.D.: A craniofacial approach to advanced recurrent cancer of the central face, Head Neck Surg. **5:**474, 1983.
3. McGregor, I.: Eyelid reconstruction following subtotal resection of upper or lower lid, Br. J. Plast. Surg. **26:**346, 1973.
4. Mustardé, J.C.: Repair and reconstruction in the orbital region, Edinburgh, 1980, Churchill Livingstone.
5. Tripier, L.: Du lambeau musculocutané en forme de pont appliqué à la restauration des paupières, Rev. Chir. **4,** 1890.

CHAPTER 8

LIP RECONSTRUCTION

But the loveliest things of beauty God ever has showed to me are her voice, and her hair, and eyes and the dear red curve of her lips

JOHN MASEFIELD
Beauty

A man had given all other bliss and all lies worldly warmth for this to make his whole heart in one kiss upon her perfect lips

ALFRED LORD TENNYSON
Sir Lancelot and Queen Guinevere

 The lips are particularly expressive facial features, conveying emotional and sexual connotations. Their thinness, thickness, and general contours add to or detract from the overall beauty of the face. Lips vary considerably among different ethnic groups. What is considered attractive in one group may be far from that in another. The lip deformities created by certain African tribes in the quest for beauty would merit reconstructive surgery in the Western world.

■ ANATOMY

The skin of the lip is soft and pink; the lower lip skin has a higher content of yellow pigment in it. The mucosa varies from individual to individual, but it is identical on the upper and lower lips.

☐ Musculature

The basic muscle of the lip is the orbicularis oris. The surprising complexity of its anatomy has been revealed in recent studies.[3,6-10,17]

The muscle decussates in the midline of the upper and lower lip, but it also has a decussation at the commissures. In addition, there are bands of muscle fibers in the lip margins that decussate only at the commissures. These fibers are more prominent in young children. In the philtral area vertically oriented muscle fibers can be seen in relation to the philtral columns.

Other muscles act on the lips. These are the buccinator, levator anguli oris, depressor anguli oris, levator labii superioris, depressor labii superioris, and zygomaticus major and minor. The risorius is a narrow bundle of muscle fibers that arises from the parotid fascia and is inserted into the skin of the angle of the mouth. It retracts the angle of the mouth to give a somewhat unpleasant grin.

☐ Nerve Supply

The sensory nerve supply is from the infraorbital nerve, the second division of the trigeminal nerve.

The motor nerve supply to the muscles is provided by the lower buccal and mandibular branches of the facial nerve.

☐ Blood Supply

The arterial supply is from the superior and inferior labial arteries, which arise from the facial artery.

The venous drainage is through the superior and inferior labial veins, which drain into the anterior facial vein.

☐ Lymphatic Drainage

The lymphatic drainage is to the submental nodes and to those nodes around the vessels at the edge of the body of the mandible.

The upper lip and the lateral segments of the lower lip drain to the submandibular and facial lymph nodes. The central portion of the lower lip drains to the submental nodes. These nodes lie on the surface of the mylohyoid muscle between the anterior bellies of the two digastric muscles.

■ AESTHETICS

The lips are normally symmetric in form and function, with the philtrum and the Cupid's bow contributing to this delicate symmetry. The mucosa is not sharply divided from the skin but is separated by the white roll area that is highlighted along the mucocutaneous junction. In the male the upper lip and the central portion of the lower lip are hairbearing. This is not so in the female, although many females have very fine silky hairs on the upper lip.

■ PLACEMENT OF INCISIONS

If possible, all lip incisions should be vertical. At the commissure, scars extending horizontally toward the cheek are acceptable.

■ AREAS OF TISSUE AVAILABILITY

The lips can be reconstructed with cheek tissue obtained by advancement or by transposition from the nasolabial folds. The neck has been used as a rotation flap, and distant flaps from the scalp, forehead, and cheek have been employed frequently.

■ AREAS TO BE RECONSTRUCTED

In discussing lip reconstruction, defects of the mucosa and the skin will be considered first; then methods used to reconstruct full-thickness defects of varying sizes in the upper and lower lips will be discussed. The commissure will be considered separately in view of its complexity; it poses considerable difficulties because there is a contralateral *normal* commissure for comparison.

☐ Reconstruction of Lip Mucosa

The vermilion tends to be a neglected area. Defects in this area may be reconstructed with flaps or grafts. Mucosal grafts do not always take well and tend to lack the necessary bulk when the defect is of a significant depth. Mucosal flaps, on the other hand, frequently contract to produce areas of excess mucosa. Mucosal repairs must be handled with care and accuracy.

ROTATION FLAPS

Small to moderate defects, which cannot be closed directly without causing deformity, must be reconstructed with neighboring mucosa used as a flap. The defect is triangulated and mucosa can be rotated in to close the raw area (as in the standard rotation flap method described in Chapter 1). There is no secondary defect; mucosa is plentiful and can be stretched.

PROBLEMS

Pincushioning may occur because of contracture along the suture line. This contracture causes lip deformity and makes further correction necessary; the prominent area is excised or thinned.

V-Y ADVANCEMENT FLAP

The V-Y advancement technique is used to fill small lip deficiencies, especially in the secondary cleft lip deformity. The area to be augmented is marked out; from this, a long V is drawn with its apex toward the buccal sulcus. The lines are incised and the mucosa within the V is elevated at a deep submucosal level. The V is closed as a Y until the defect is well filled by the resulting mucosal advancement. It is advisable to overdo this advancement to allow for later reduction in the bulk of the flap. If this is not done, there may be partial recurrence of the initial deformity.

PROBLEMS

It is not uncommon for this flap to be made too small in terms of the length of the V. If this is the case, inadequate advancement is obtained and the defect is not filled out. Similarly, if the defect is not overcorrected, the result will be inadequate with time. Contraction lines may occur on either side of the V with resulting labial notches.

TRIANGULAR ISLAND ADVANCEMENT FLAP

The triangular island advancement flap is particularly indicated when the defect extends to the mucocutaneous junction.

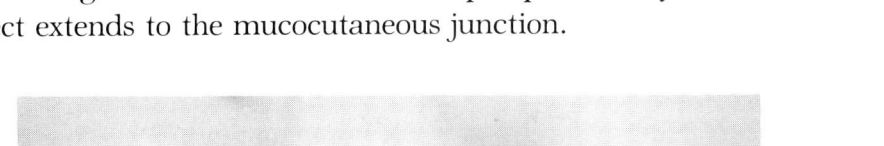

The patient illustrated has an electrical burn of the lower lip.

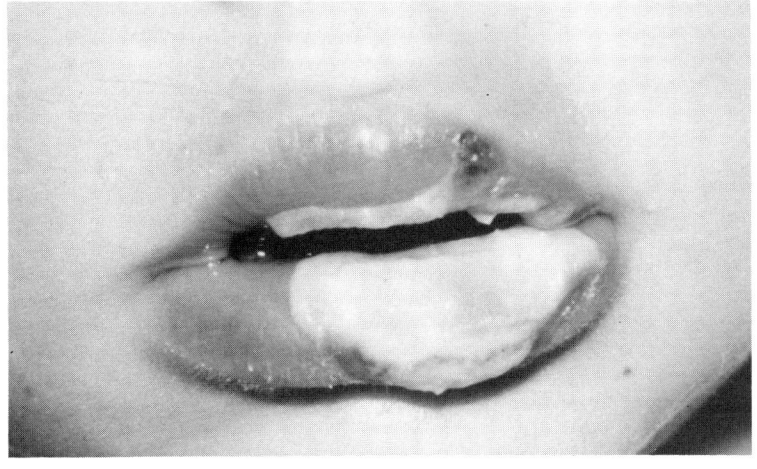

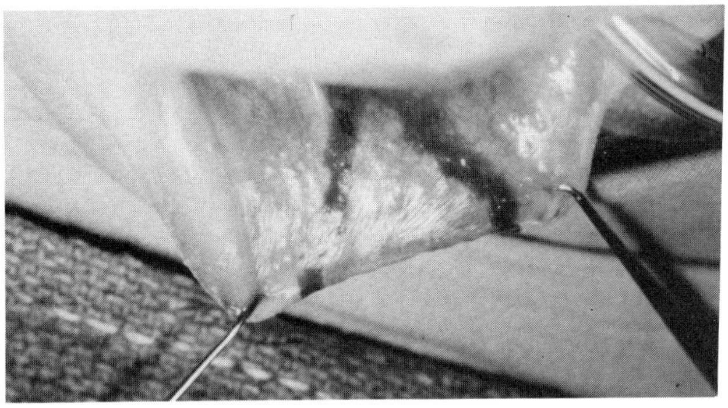

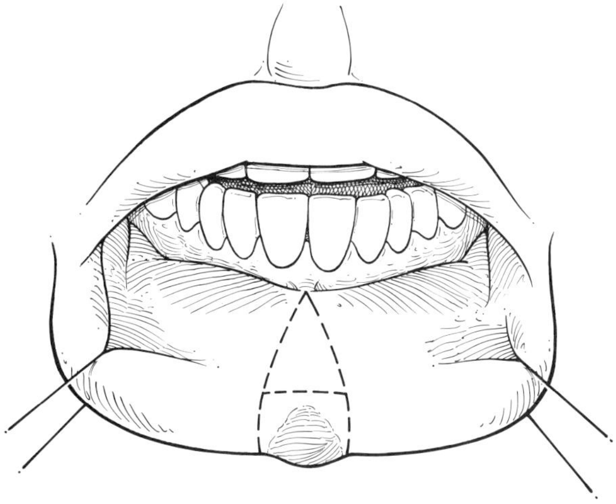

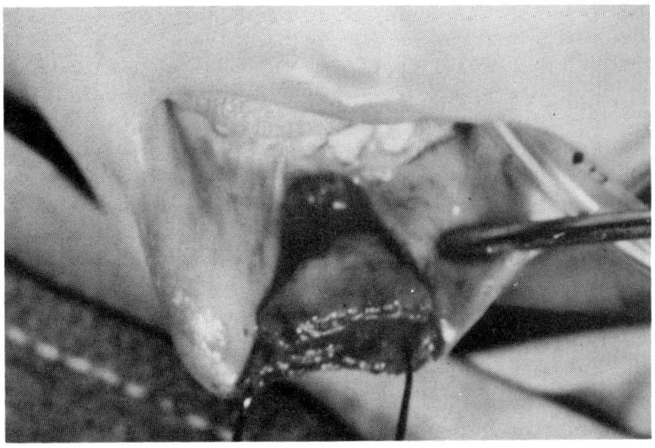

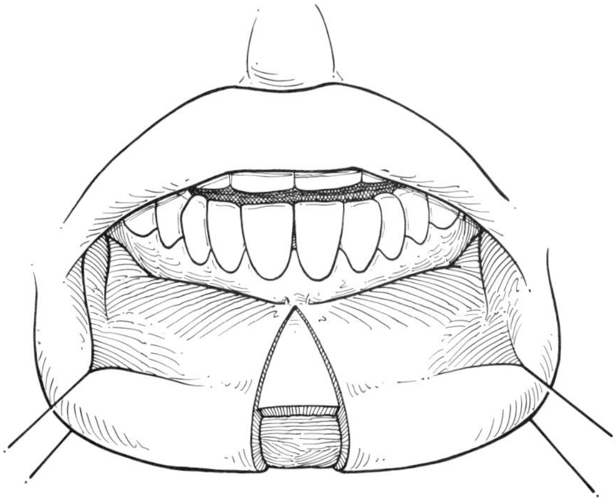

When the defect is square (for example, after resection of a small hemangioma), the oral edge of the square is made the base of a triangular island flap.

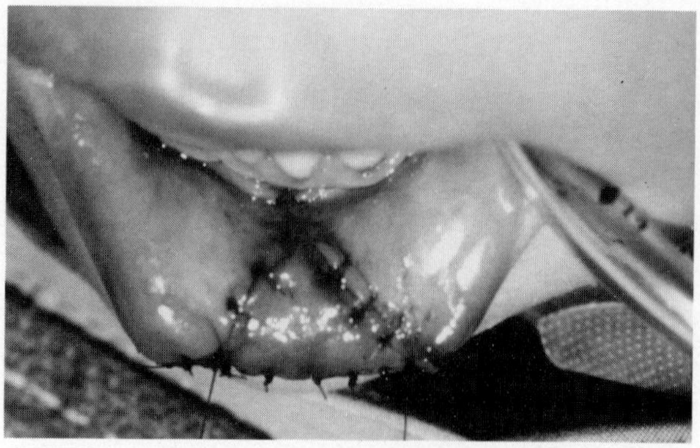

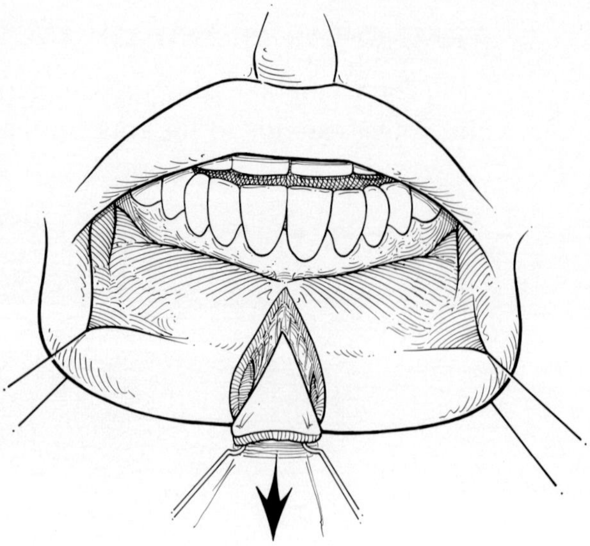

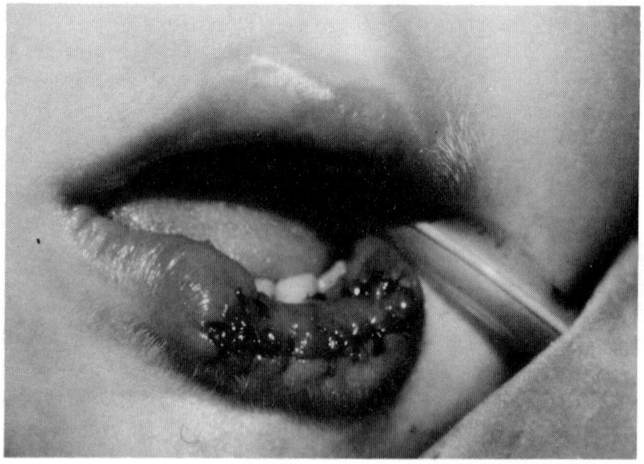

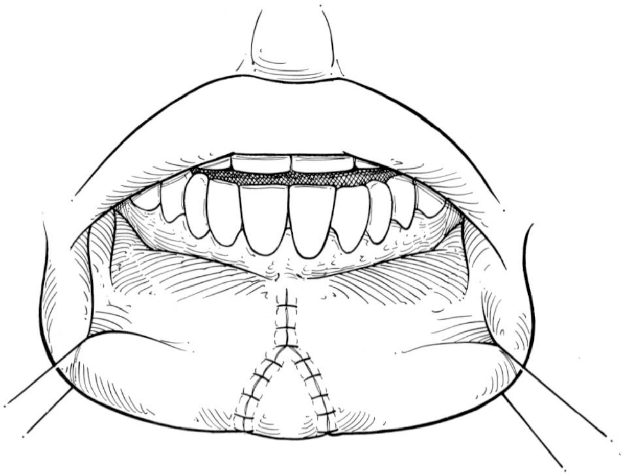

The island flap is raised on a submucosal pedicle and then advanced to close the defect. The donor area is closed in a V-Y fashion. This dissection need not be too extensive, since the submucosal tissues are extremely lax.

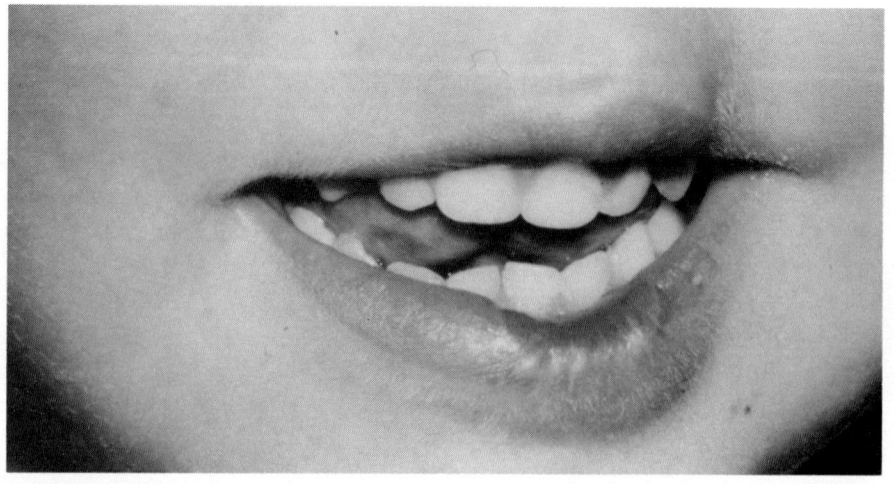

The result shows a slight deficiency of mucosa, which usually improves with time.

PROBLEMS

If the pedicle is made too narrow, ischemia of the flap with necrosis could occur. With proper planning this is not seen. There may be small grooves on the lip margin on either side of the flap because of scar contracture. These may be corrected by excision and small Z-plasties.

TRANSVERSE TRIANGULAR ISLAND ADVANCEMENT FLAPS

Transverse triangular island advancement flaps are designed using a principle introduced by Kapetansky,[15] who described "pendulum" island flaps based on the orbicularis muscle. These were used to fill the central lip deficiency in the bilateral cleft. When this problem is present to a small degree and a total rerepair of the lip is not being contemplated, island flaps, based on submucosal pedicles, can be designed. The technique is mainly applied to the upper lip because of its use in the cleft lip deformity. However, it can also be employed in the lower lip as a double or single advancement flap.

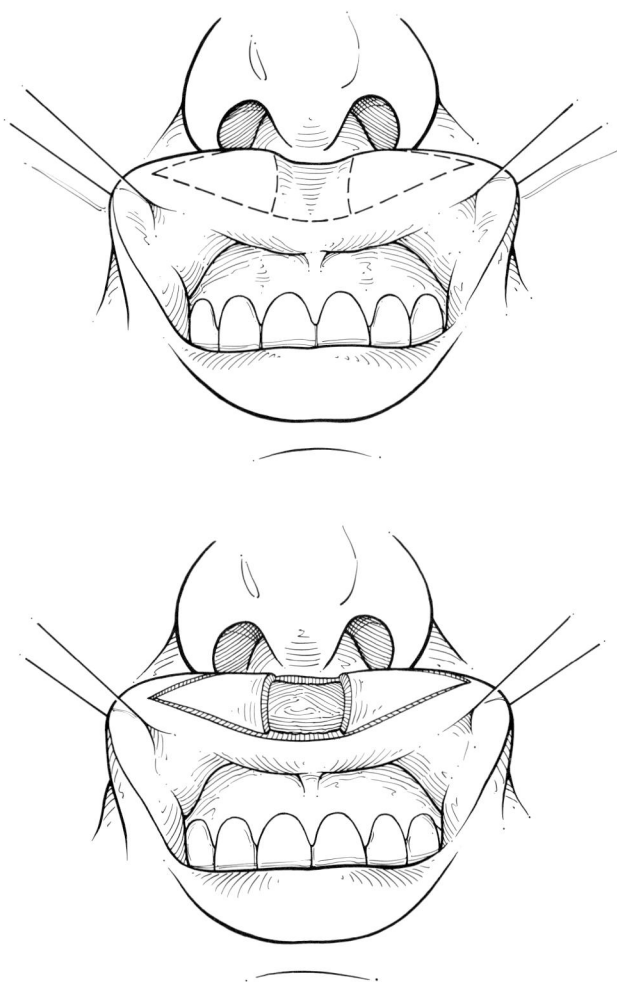

The flaps are raised on both sides of the deficient area, with the bases of the triangles facing each other. The area between the flaps is resected.

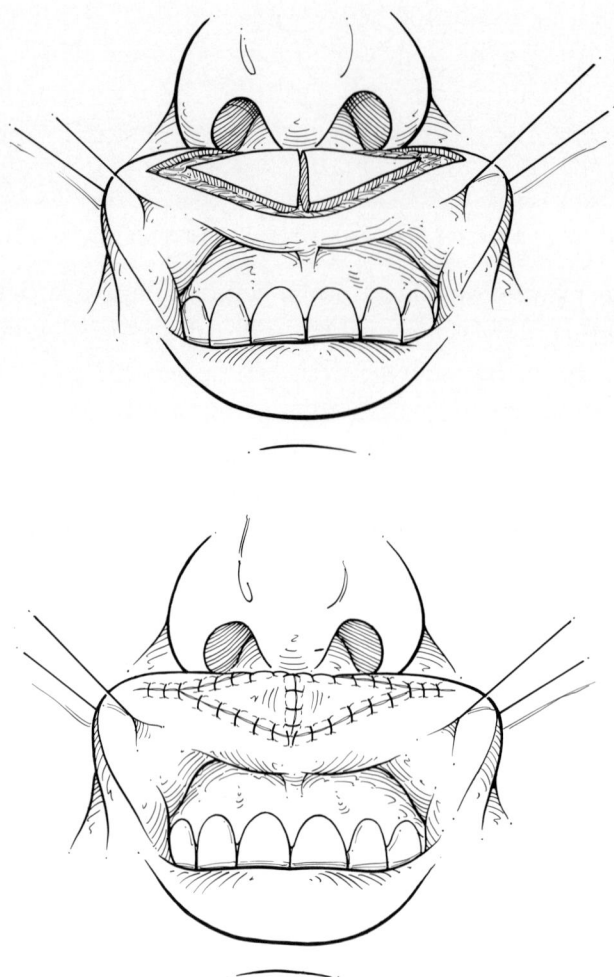

When the pedicles have been mobilized sufficiently, the triangles are moved together and the bases are sutured to each other. Laterally, there is a V-Y closure. This arrangement gives central bulk to the lip with lateral grooves. The resulting lip margin closely resembles the normal anatomic situation of a central tubercle with gentle valleys on either side.

PROBLEMS

Technical problems may result from making the flaps too small and thus having too little bulk for the central tubercle. If the pedicle is overmobilized, flap ischemia and necrosis may result. This unfortunate situation has not been encountered.

SURGICAL TECHNIQUE OF CHOICE

There is no single method of choice for localized lip mucosal reconstruction. Each technique has its individual merits and can be applied according to specific indications.

CHAPTER 8
LIP RECONSTRUCTION

☐ Extensive Lower Lip Mucosal Defect Reconstruction

FACTORS TO CONSIDER

If there is an extensive defect of the lower lip mucosa, it is usually advisable to excise the mucosa of the entire lower lip and then resurface it with intraoral mucosa or tongue. In this way lip cover is uniform in color and texture.

MUCOSAL ADVANCEMENT

Where only mucosa is to be supplied and bulk is not required, the mucosa is simply advanced, usually without undermining. The mucosa is sutured to the skin of the lip with a fine running absorbable suture.

PROBLEMS

The mucosa covering the lips is unique. When intraoral mucosa is transferred to the lips, it never becomes true lip mucosa. Thus drying, scaling, and flaking occur, and so the area must be kept lubricated with petroleum jelly or lanolin at all times.

TONGUE FLAP

When some muscle has been excised, a bulkier reconstruction is required. In such a situation the tongue flap is used.

The original tongue flap was described by Guerrero-Santos and others[12]; in this case the dorsum of the tongue was used to reconstruct the lip. This approach is contrary to the basic principles of reconstruction outlined earlier, which state that, if possible, like tissue should be used to replace like tissue. The color of dorsal tongue mucosa is not the same as that of the lip, and its texture is rough rather than smooth. In fact, an upper-surface tongue flap on the lip always looks like tongue; it does not change or improve with time. In order to overcome this problem, the undersurface of the tongue has been used.[13,14] The undersurface is smooth, without papillae, and its color is a more satisfactory match for the lip.

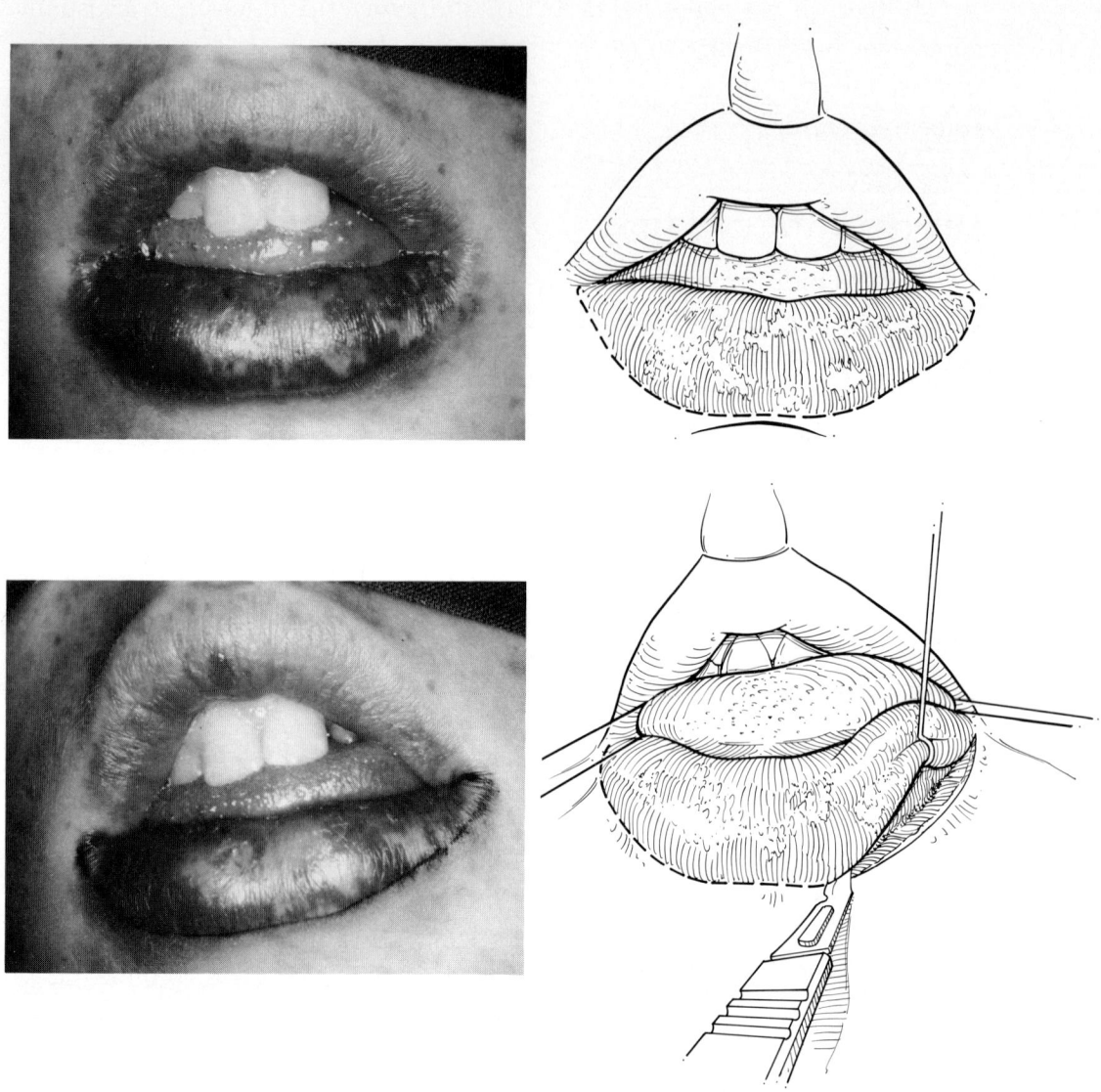

The patient illustrated above has a hemangioma of the lower lip that has caused color change and lip enlargement. The postexcisional defect may be part or all of the length of the lower lip. It consists of mucosa, submucosa, and often a layer of orbicularis.

CHAPTER 8
LIP RECONSTRUCTION

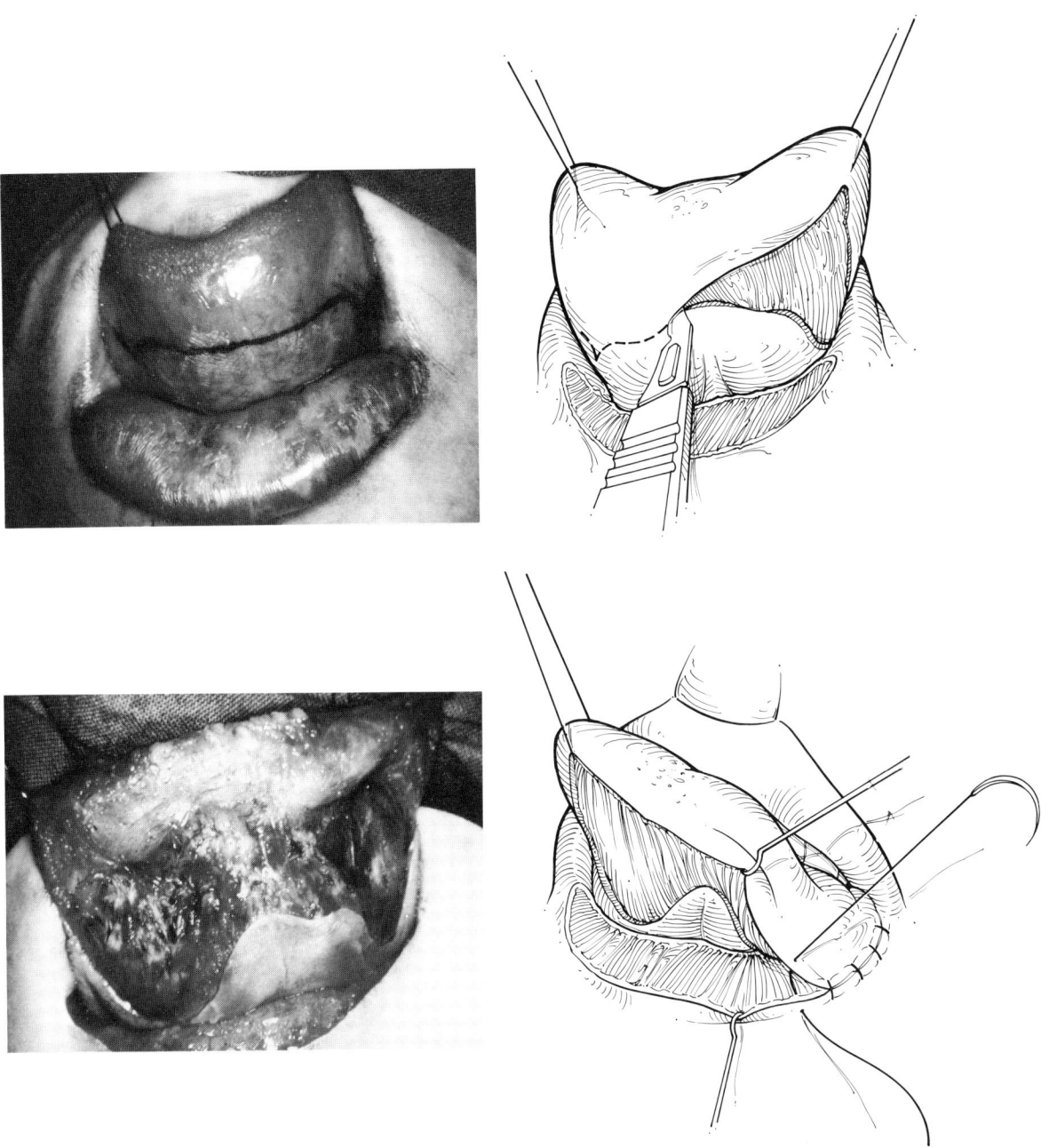

A suture is placed on either side of the tongue, and the required flap is outlined on the undersurface. A flap of the required size is elevated, based anteriorly. The thickness of the flap is that required to reconstruct the lip.

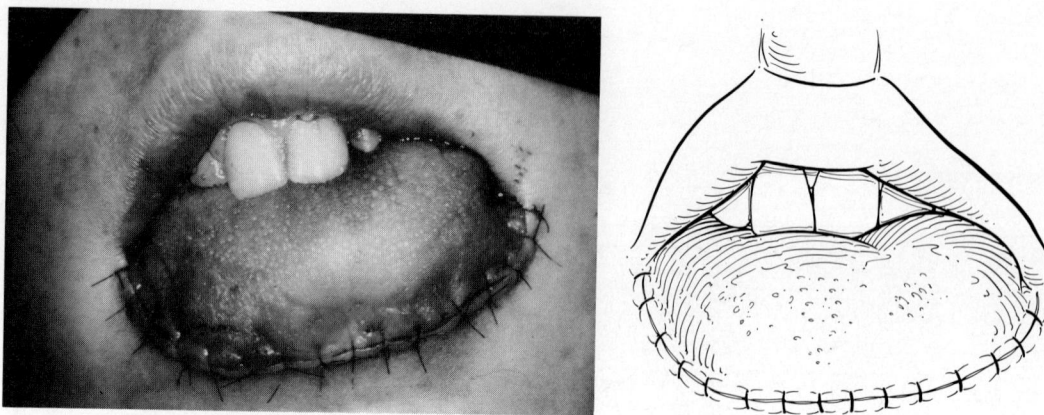

The posterior edge of the flap is then brought forward and sutured to the cutaneous border of the defect. It is also sutured laterally. The raw area on the undersurface of the tongue remains, with no attempt at closure being made.

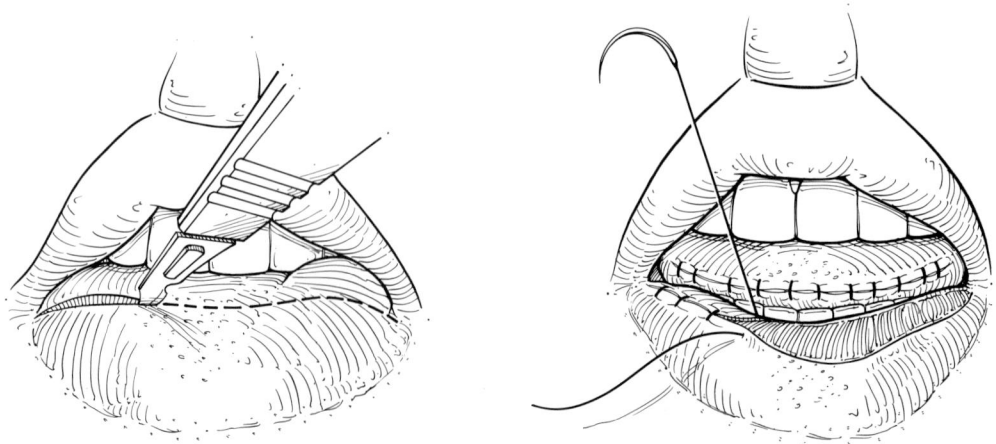

The tongue flap is left attached to the lip for 10 days and then is divided. At this point it is important to make sure that enough tongue mucosa is transferred to generously close the residual defect. In this way an adequate resurfacing is obtained. Failure to transfer sufficient mucosa will result in a thin pincushioned ridge of tongue mucosa.

The incision on the tongue is closed with a continuous absorbable suture. If there is significant induration, causing difficulty in closure, the defect may be left unsutured and will close spontaneously.

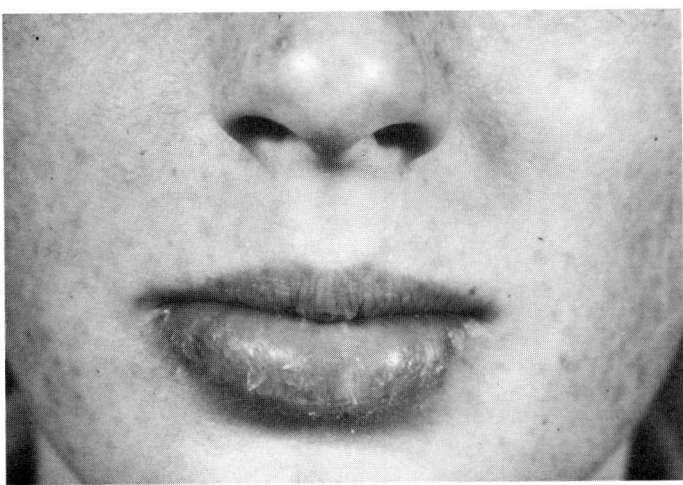

A reasonably normal-looking vermilion can be obtained. Scaling of the mucosa because of drying can be seen in this case.

PROBLEMS

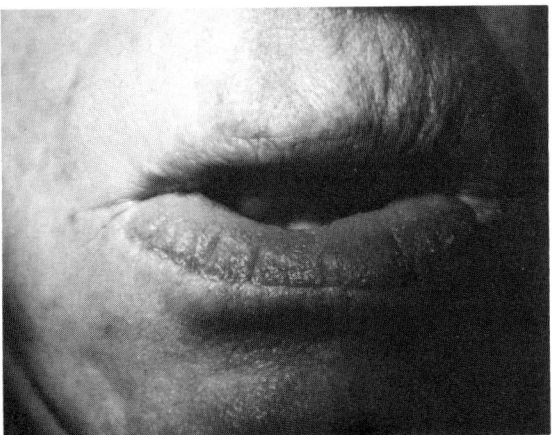

As long as the undersurface of the tongue is used, the color match and mucosal texture are good. The figure above illustrates the poor result obtained when the upper surface of the tongue is used. It is possible that the flap may be torn from the lip in the immediate postoperative phase, but this has never been encountered. The inferior surface flap actually lengthens the tongue and allows more movement of the tip.

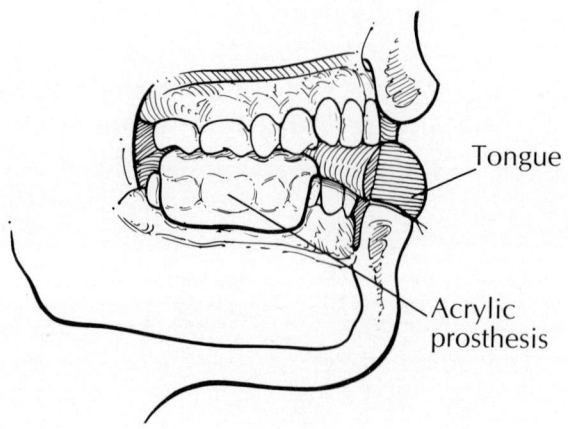

In the immediate postoperative phase a potential problem in the dentulous patient is biting through the flap with the incisors. This is prevented by using bilateral acrylic molar bite blocks, which ensure an anterior open bite sufficient to allow protection of the tongue flap pedicle. The blocks can be cemented onto the lower molar teeth before surgery.

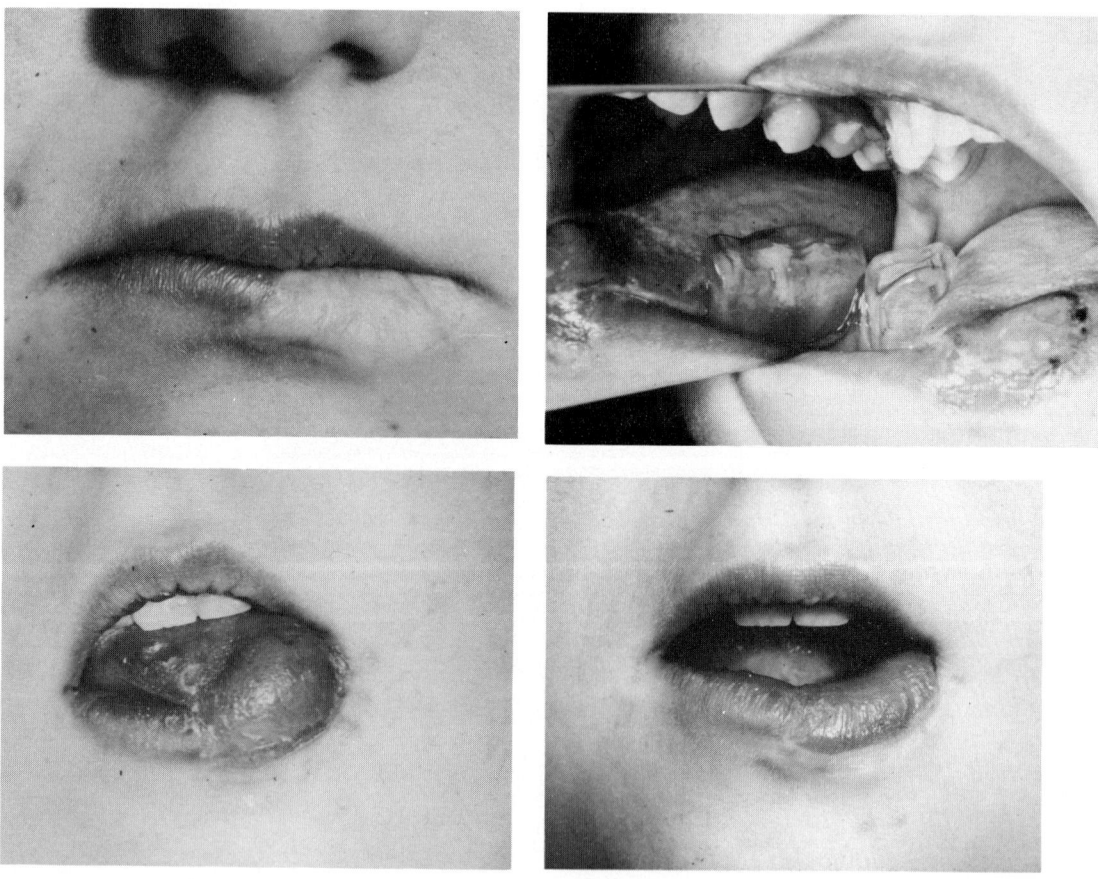

The use of this technique is illustrated above by a case in which half the lower lip mucosa has been replaced with a dorsal tongue flap following an electrical burn.

Extensive Upper Lip Mucosal Defect Reconstruction

FACTORS TO CONSIDER

Fortunately, it is rarely necessary to reconstruct a large mucosal defect on the upper lip. Since this area does not have the same exposure to weather conditions as the lower lip, premalignant and malignant change is uncommon. The reason for reconstruction is usually to complete a total lip reconstruction rather than resection of mucosal malignancy. Significant lip mucosal defects are very difficult to reconstruct. The amount of mucosa is limited, and advancement from the intraoral area onto the lip is not possible, since it would cause an ugly in-rolled deformity of the lip anterior. Tongue flaps tend to pull off readily because the tongue is in a less normal and less comfortable position when attached to the upper lip.

TONGUE FLAP

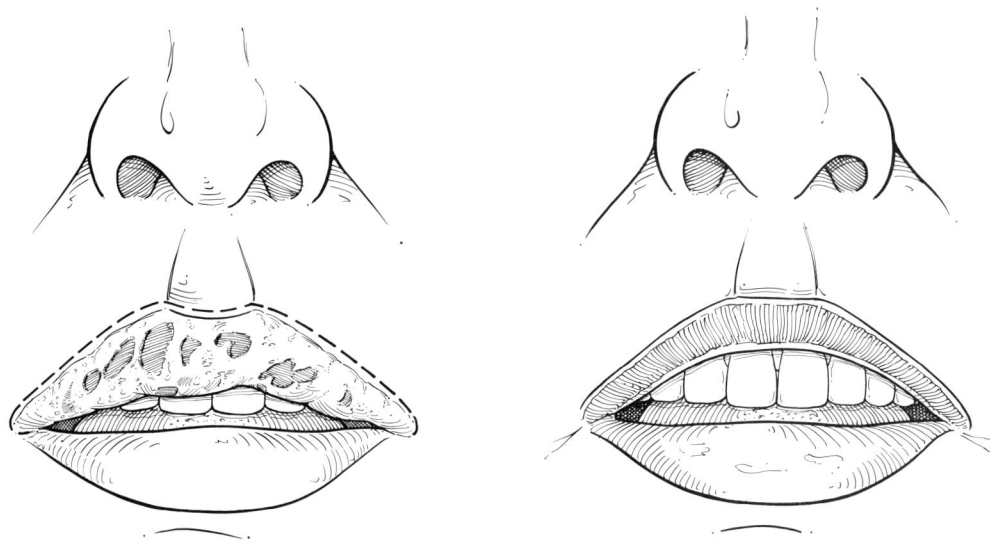

The mucosa of the upper lip can be reconstructed with tongue mucosa, but the standard undersurface flaps cannot be used in this situation.

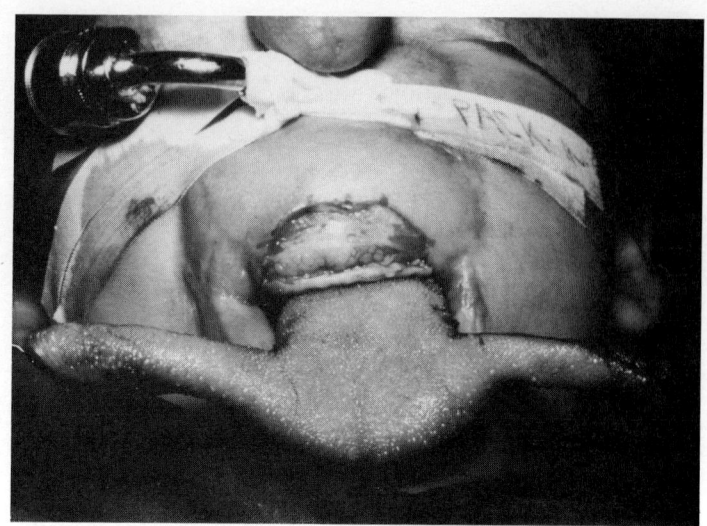 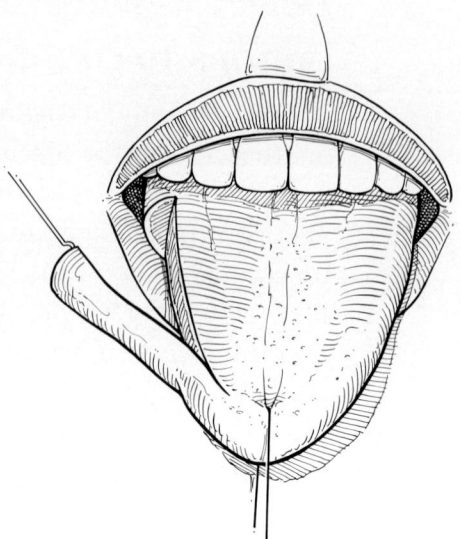

It is advisable to use anteriorly based lateral flaps. The thickness will vary with the depth of the defect.

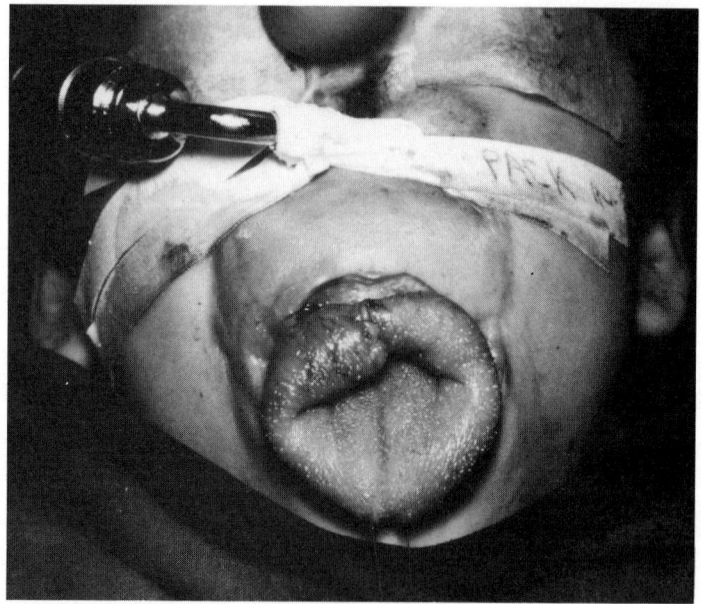 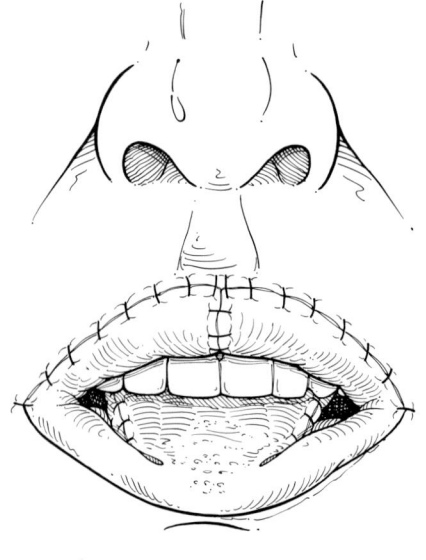

The flaps are swung up and initially sutured end to end. This mucosal bridge is then sutured to the lip margins anteriorly and posteriorly in order to reconstruct the defect. The tongue donor sites are closed directly.

CHAPTER 8
LIP RECONSTRUCTION

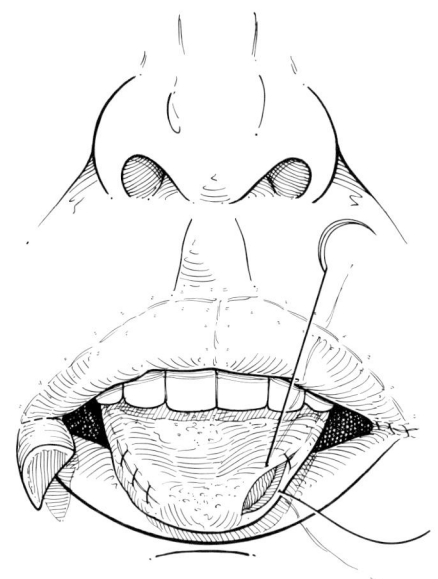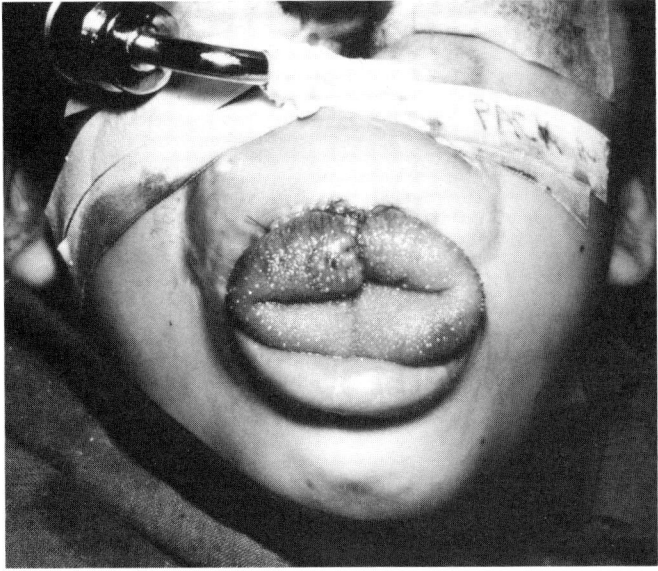

In 10 days the pedicles are divided, and the flaps are trimmed and inset into the lips. The small raw areas on the tongue are closed with a few sutures.

PROBLEMS

In upper lip reconstruction the tension on the tongue flap is much greater than the tension involved in lower lip resurfacing. Suturing the lateral edges of the tongue to the lip helps to stabilize the reconstruction and prevent separation of the flap. Usually some of the upper surface of the tongue is included in the reconstruction. Forming a Cupid's bow is a very difficult task. If the bow can be made, it suffers from the deficiency seen when this structure is created by skin mucosal contouring in a cleft lip patient. No white roll is present, and there is a very sharp and artificial-looking junction between the skin and the vermilion.

☐ Upper Lip Reconstruction

The upper lip has a complex symmetry that is difficult to reestablish after resection. In the male, hairbearing skin must be used. The alar base area and the nasolabial region should not be disturbed. The commissure position should not be altered. Any reconstruction should not cause lip shortening or tightness.

SKIN DEFECTS

Perialar Crescentic Advancement Flap

If the defect lies on the lateral third of the lip, it can be dealt with by means of the perialar crescentic advancement flap described by Webster.[20] This cleverly conceived advancement flap will close fairly large defects without causing deformity of the alar base, the lip, or the oral commissure. The defect should be triangulated with the base superiorly. However, the long axis should not be vertical; if this were so, any closure would tend to lengthen the lip. Instead, the long axis lies diagonally.

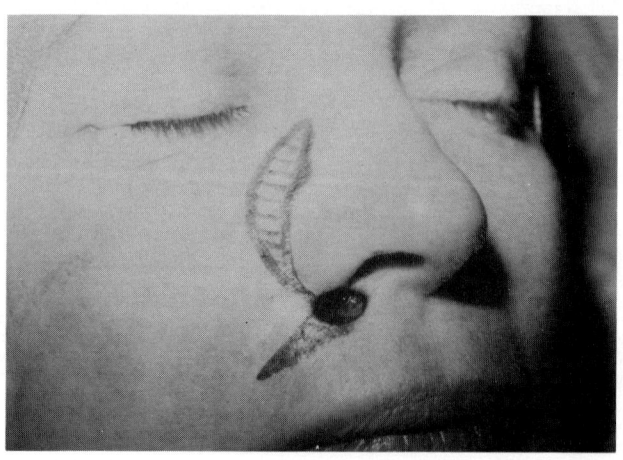 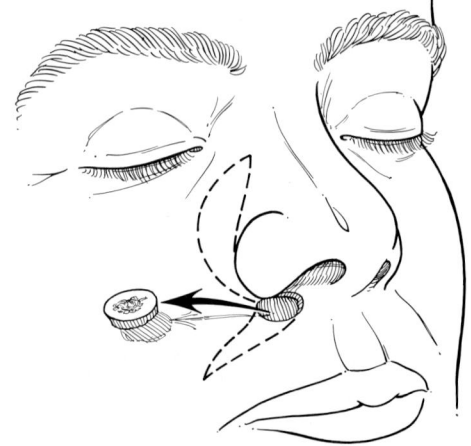

From the lateral end of the triangle base, an ellipse of skin is outlined on the paranasal area. If a large shift is required, excision of a wider ellipse is planned. As the ellipse is made wider, the outer edge of the flap becomes longer and more shift of cheek skin into the lip is obtained (see Chapter 1). Excision of the potential dog ear inferiorly on the lip at the apex of the triangular excision may be planned at this point.

CHAPTER 8
LIP RECONSTRUCTION

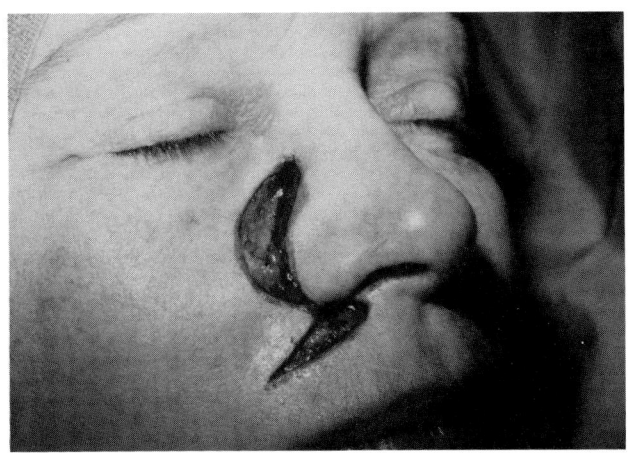 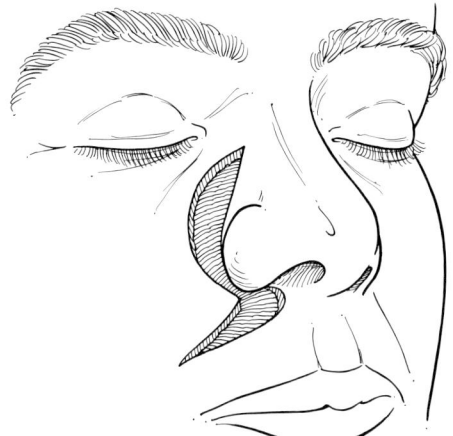

The planned amount of skin is now excised.

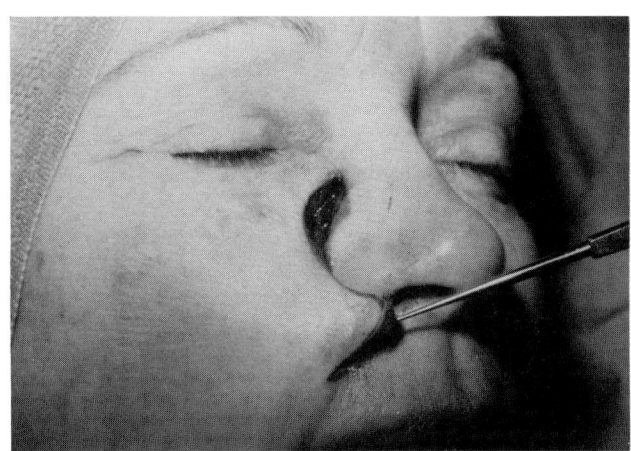 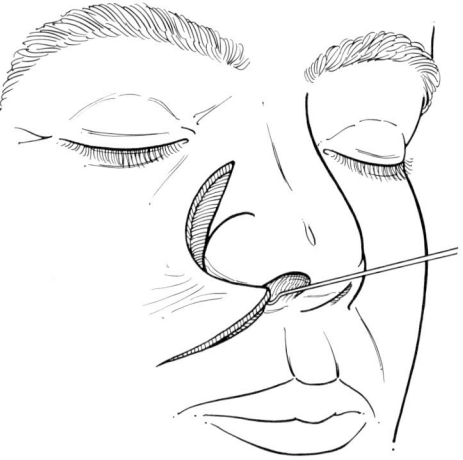

The cheek is undermined until the skin can be advanced comfortably with a hook to close the defect without tension.

345

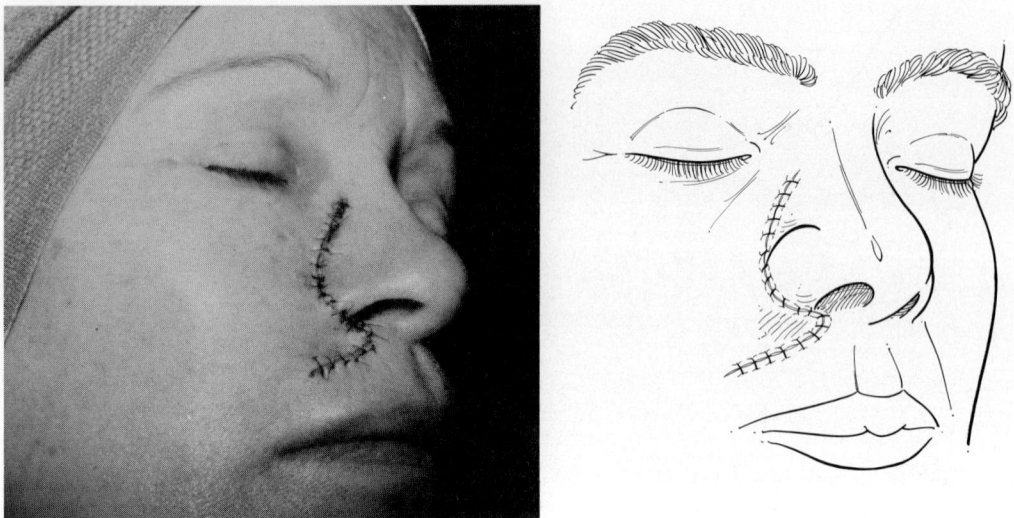

Suturing commences at the superior part of the ellipse; as the long outer line is joined to the shorter inner line, the cheek flap automatically advances. With this movement the triangular defect is closed. The suture line lies in a very satisfactory position on the nasal cheek line, below the alar base and at an angle on the lip.

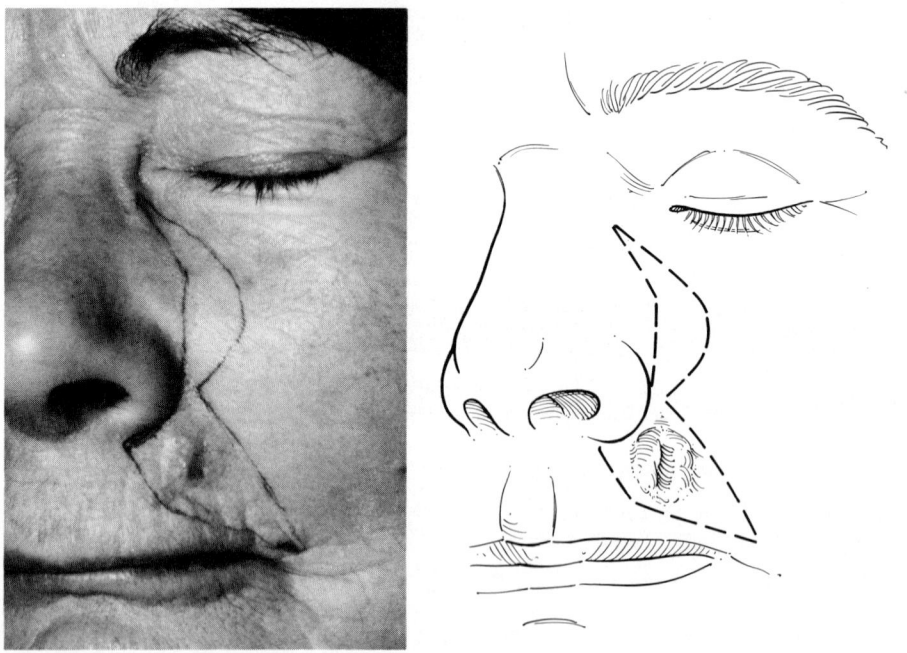

This method can also be used for lesions situated lower on the lip.

CHAPTER 8
LIP RECONSTRUCTION

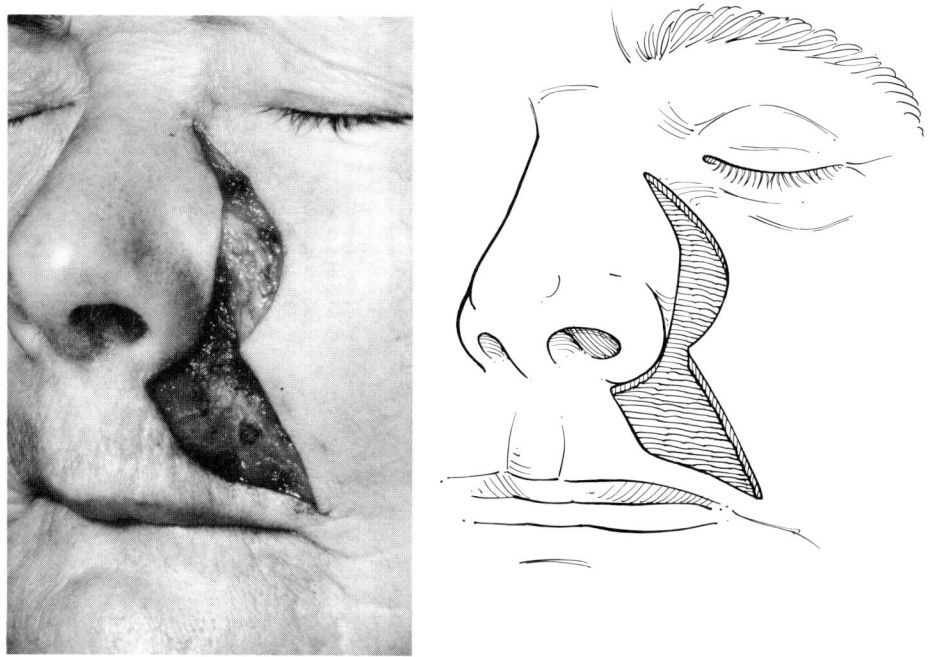

The position of the triangle chosen for excision should be noted. This permits closure of the defect without lengthening of the lip or distortion of the alar base area.

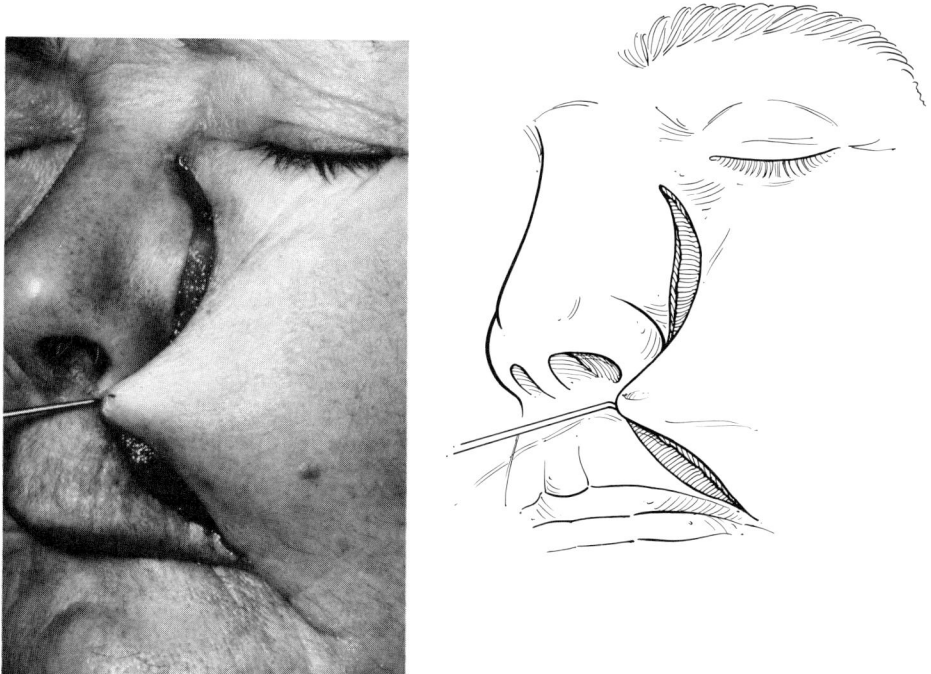

The cheek is undermined in the face-lift plane extensively enough to allow the flap to be advanced without tension; closure of the defect presents no problem.

347

MODIFICATION OF PERIALAR CRESCENTIC ADVANCEMENT FLAP

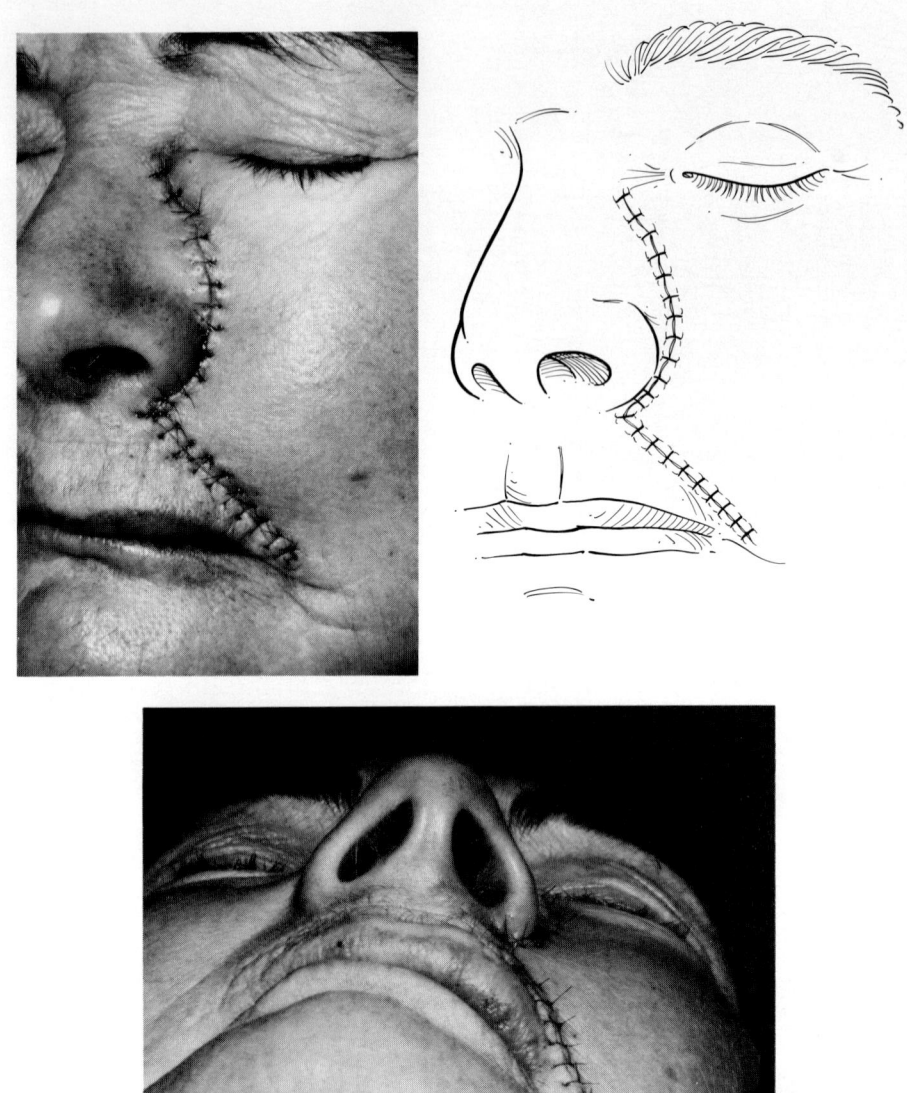

In some instances when the lesion lies close to the mucocutaneous junction, the technique needs to be modified, as seen after excision of the upper lip basal cell carcinoma shown on the opposite page.

CHAPTER 8
LIP RECONSTRUCTION

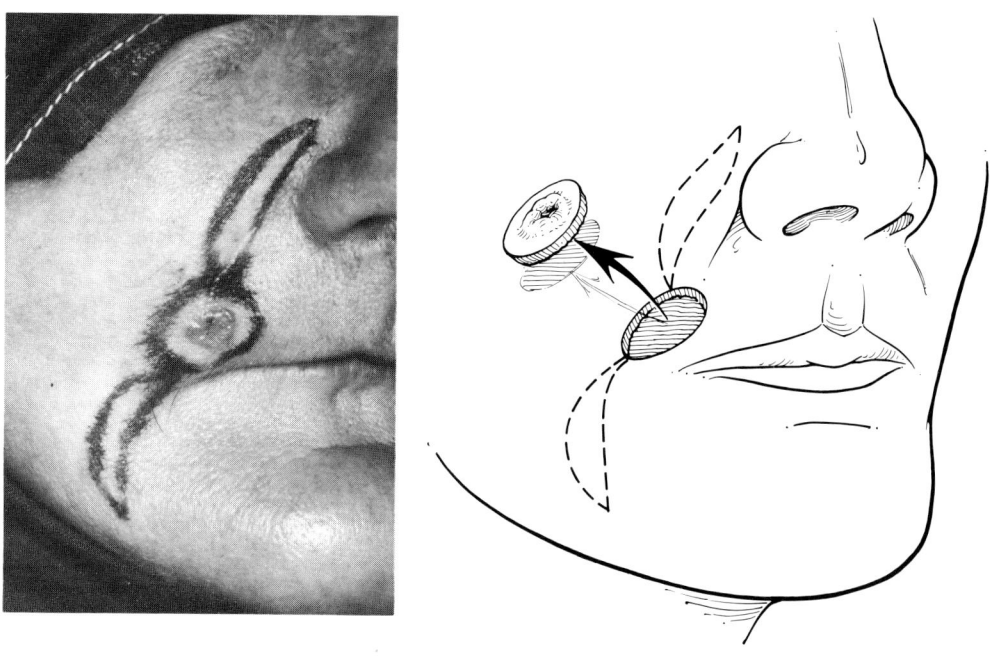

Both superior and inferior ellipses are planned; the latter is taken around the commissure.

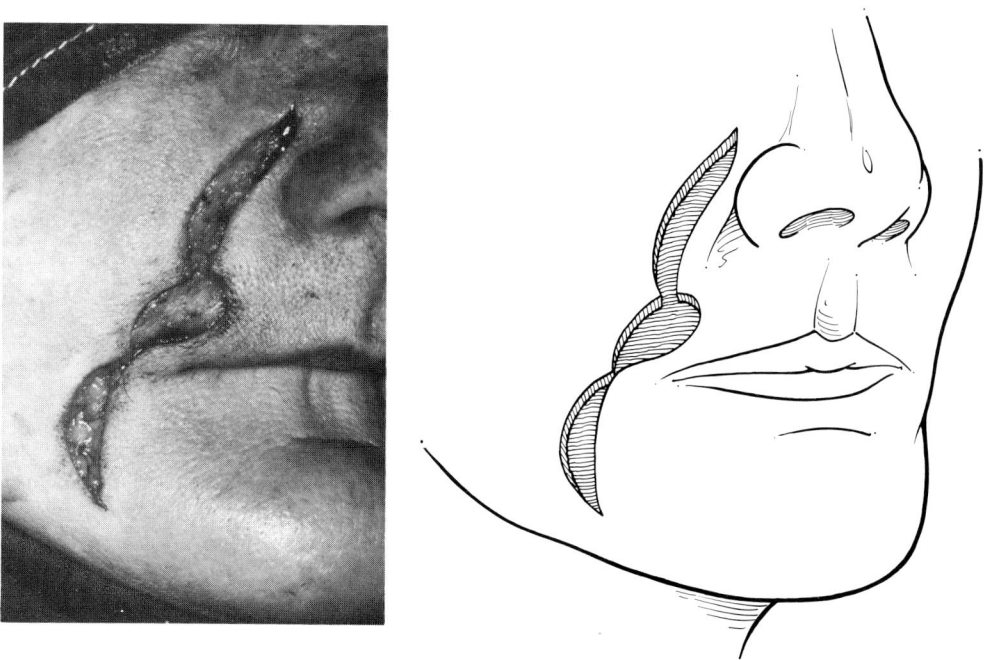

The lesion and the planned amount of normal skin are excised.

349

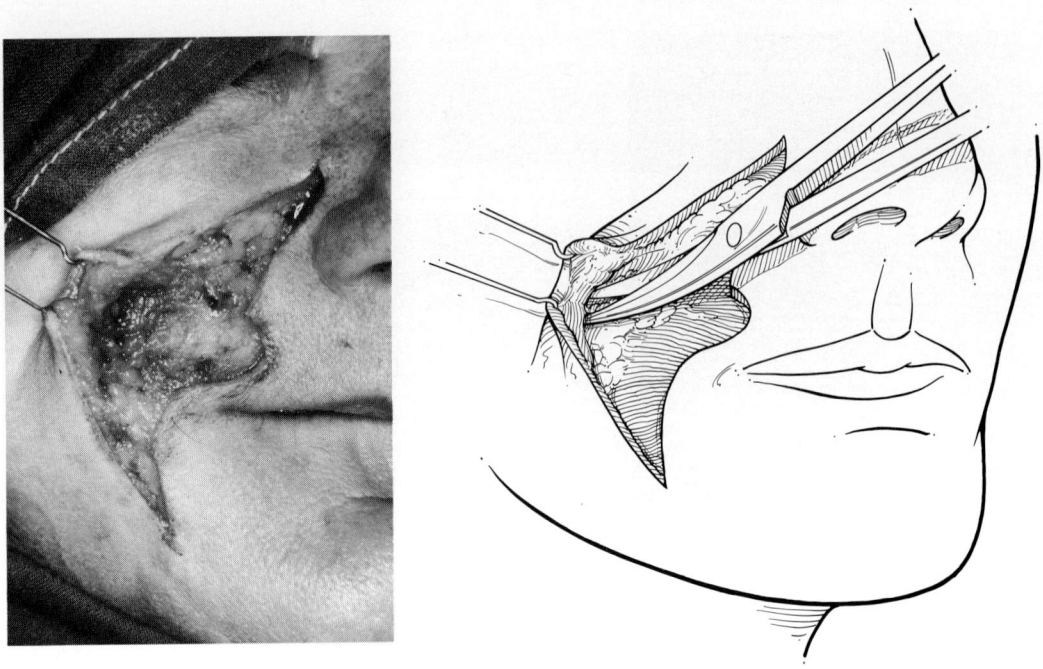

The cheek is undermined to a degree sufficient to allow closure.

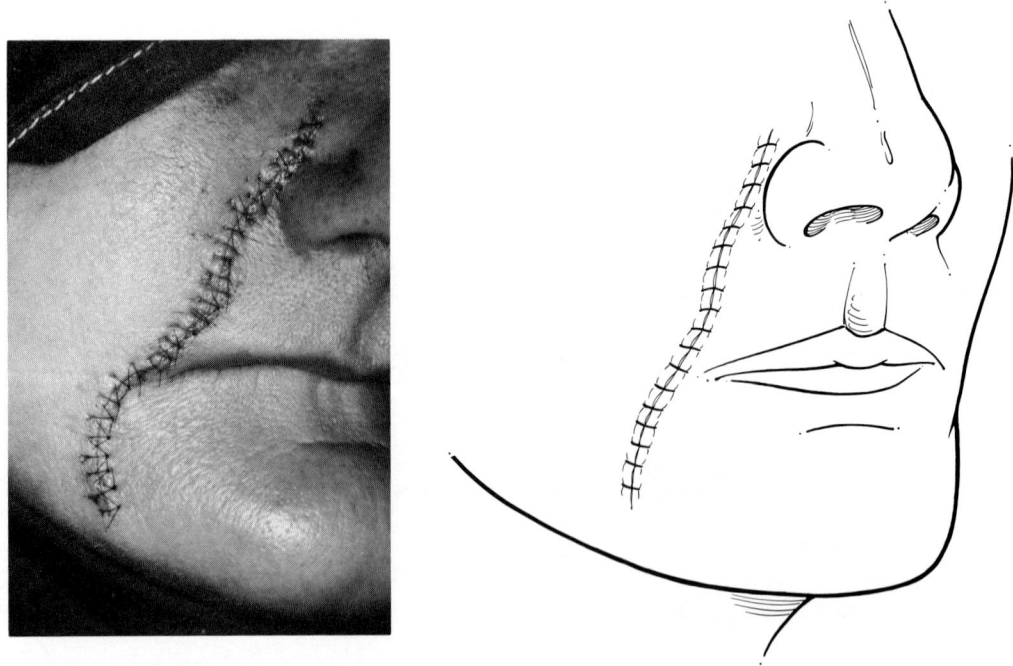

After satisfactory trimming of the skin, closure is obtained in the nasolabial line.

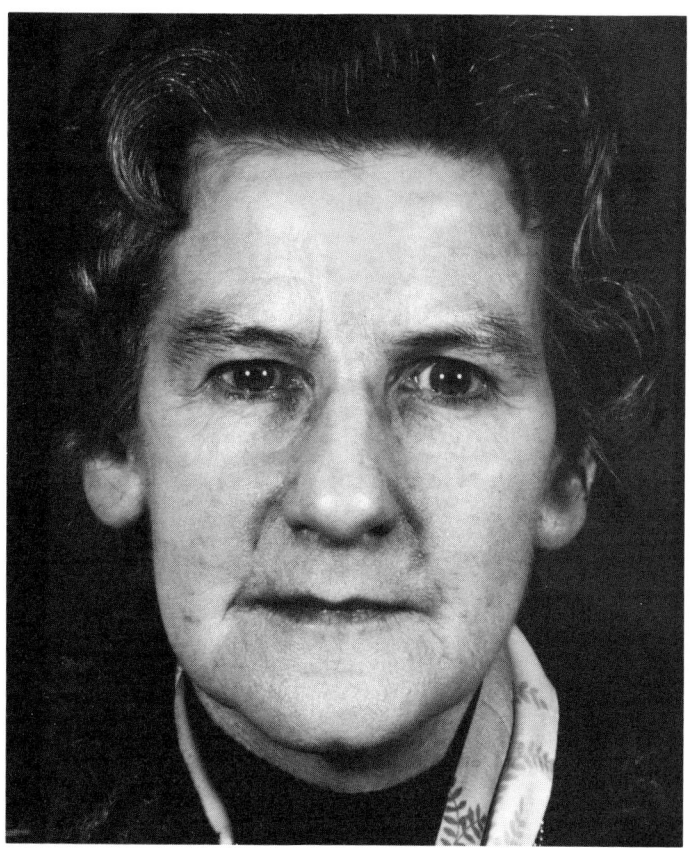

This gives a good result with little distortion of normal anatomy.

PROBLEMS

Few difficulties are associated with this elegant technique. Occasionally, when a relatively large defect is reconstructed, the nasolabial fold may be partially obliterated, but this does not cause problems and does not require correction. In some individuals the cheek skin is more highly colored and thicker than is usual; as a result, this skin may be obvious when advanced into the lip. For some males the advanced cheek area may not be hairbearing, and this may draw attention to the reconstruction.

Two-Stage Nasolabial Flap

The nasolabial area is a useful donor site for flaps used to reconstruct lip skin, especially for large defects. The skin is plentiful, and in the male it is hairbearing.

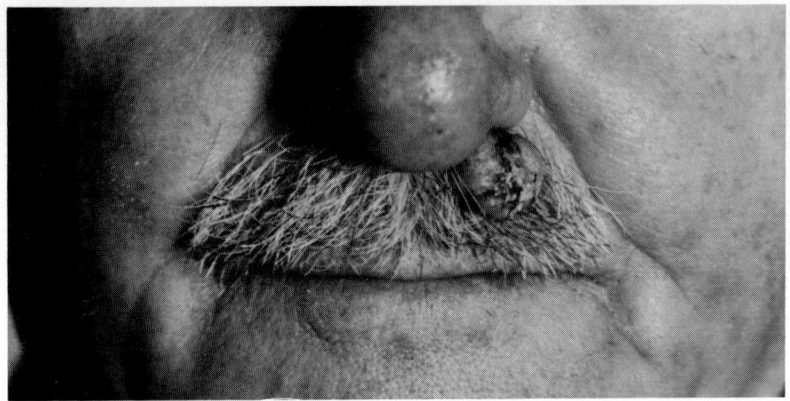

The two-stage nasolabial flap is ideally suited for reconstruction of the defect resulting from excision of the basal cell carcinoma of the upper lip illustrated here.

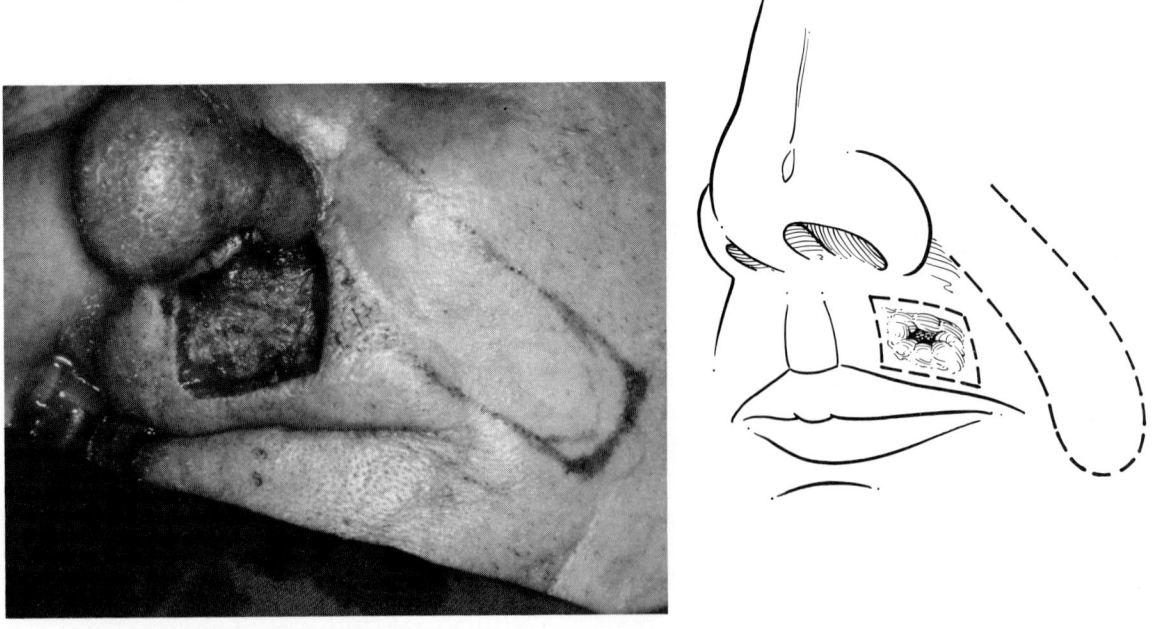

The flap is based superiorly and made long enough and wide enough to resurface the lip defect.

CHAPTER 8
LIP RECONSTRUCTION

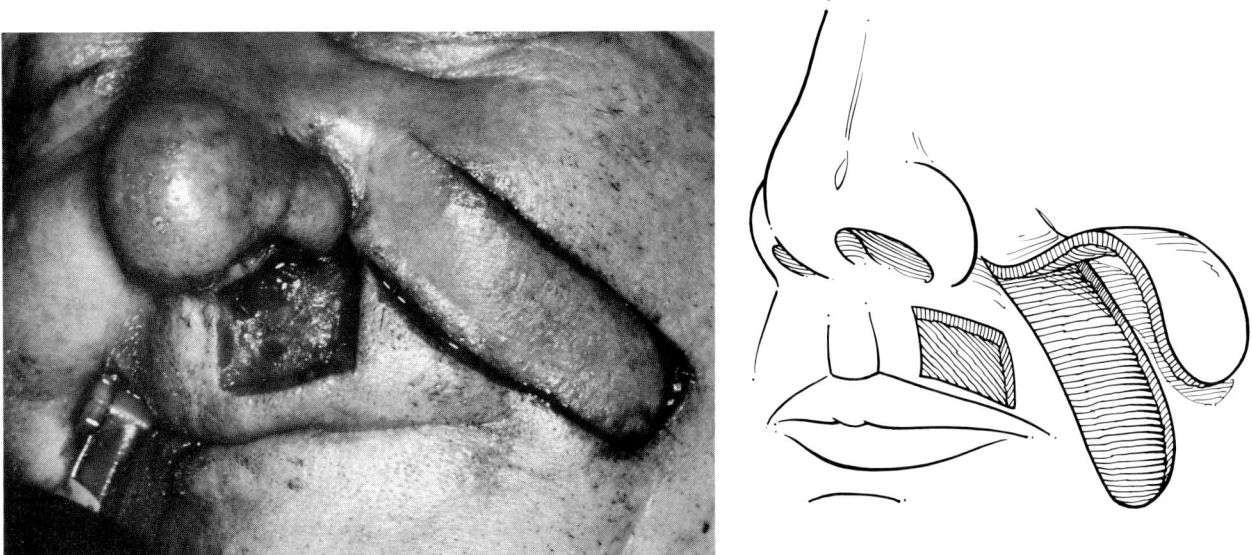

The flap is lifted just above the facial muscles. Deep dissection should be avoided in order to ensure that facial nerve branches are not divided.

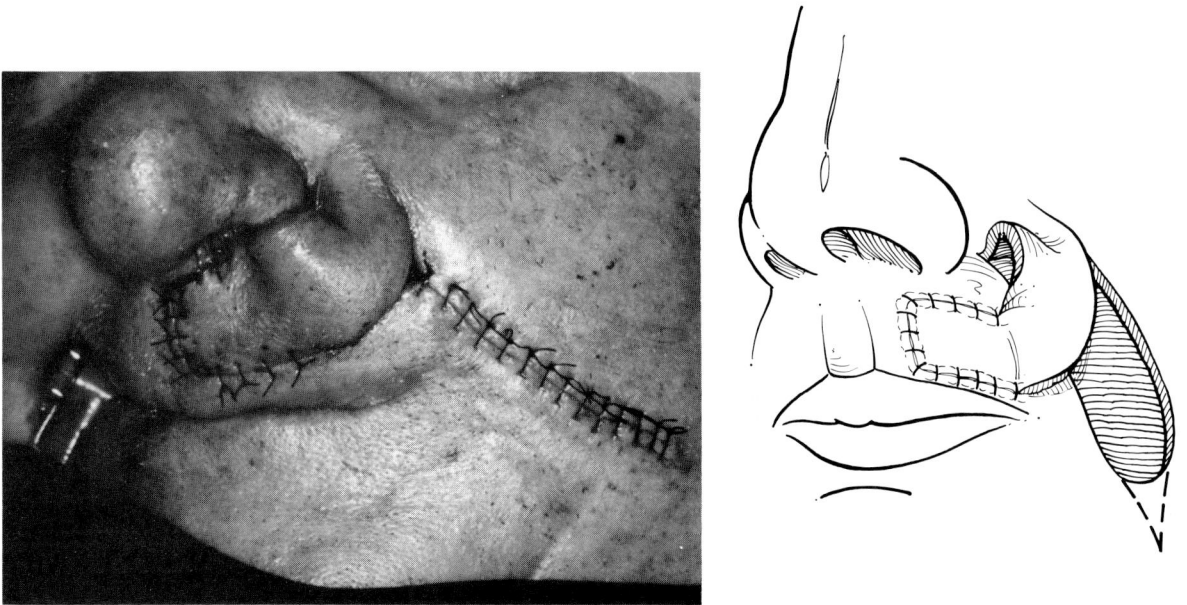

The flap is transposed medially to close the lip defect. The nasolabial defect is closed directly.

353

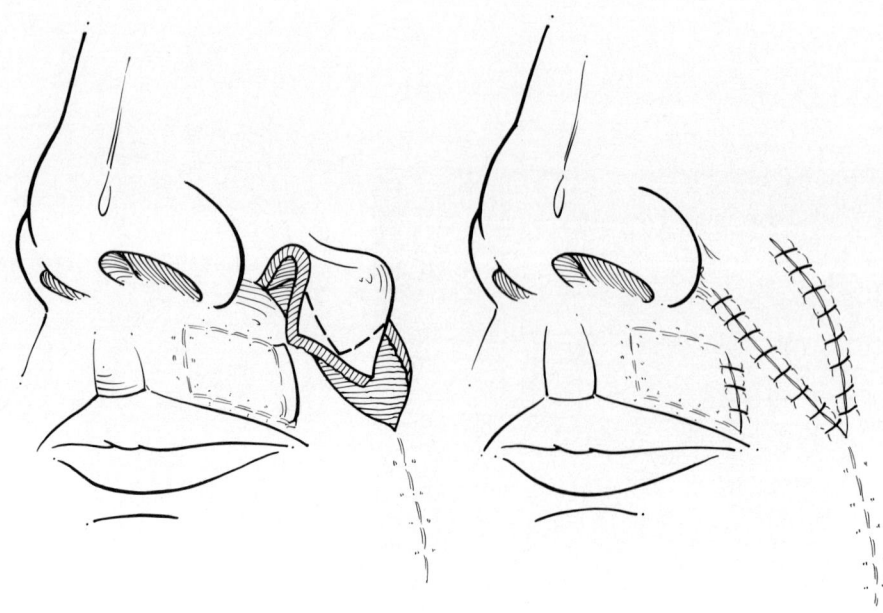

The flap is left in position for 10 to 14 days and then divided and inset. The unused portion of the flap pedicle is returned to the nasolabial area, trimmed and inset to restore normal contours.

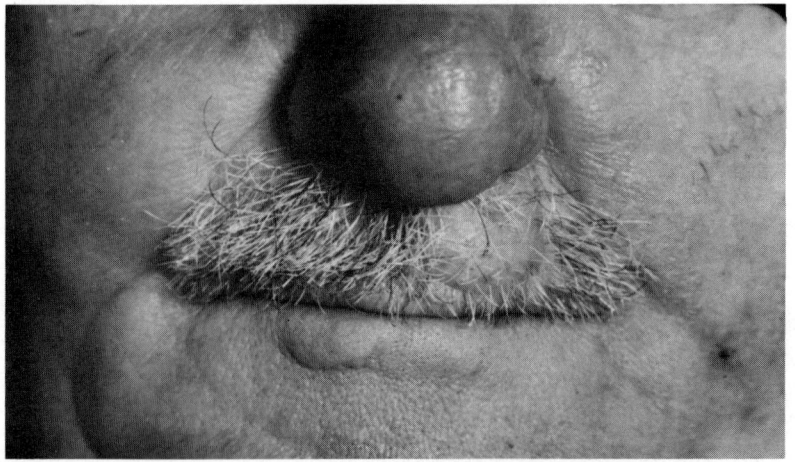

The illustration above shows how well this flap provides hairbearing skin for an individual who wears a mustache.

PROBLEMS

Few problems are encountered with the two-stage nasolabial flap. The flap may pincushion and require trimming. In a female patient there may be a color and texture difference between the reconstructed lip and the normal lip skin. Some asymmetry of the nasolabial areas may be noted. In most instances the scars are not a significant problem.

Surgical Technique of Choice

If the defect is small enough and in a convenient position, the perialar crescentic advancement flap is best. It is a one-stage procedure, and the scars lie in a good aesthetic position, directly in the line of minimal relaxed tension. When the defect is large, deep, and complex, the two-stage nasolabial flap is the method of choice. It is particularly appropriate when the defect is located toward the center of the lip, since cheek rotation to this area is not possible.

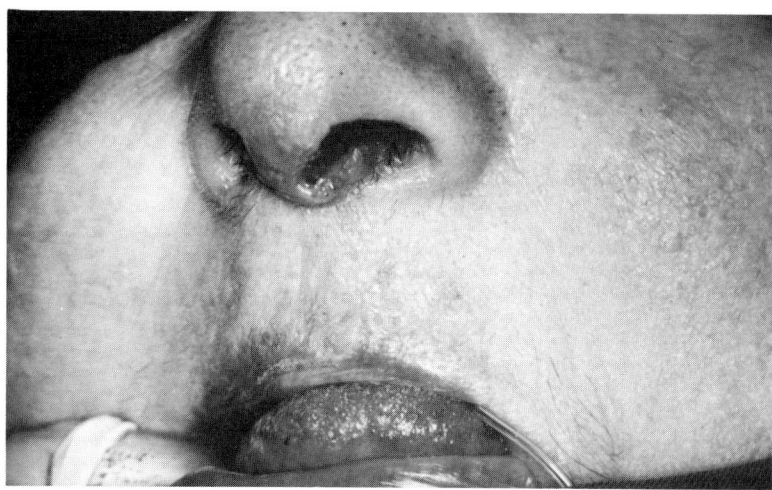

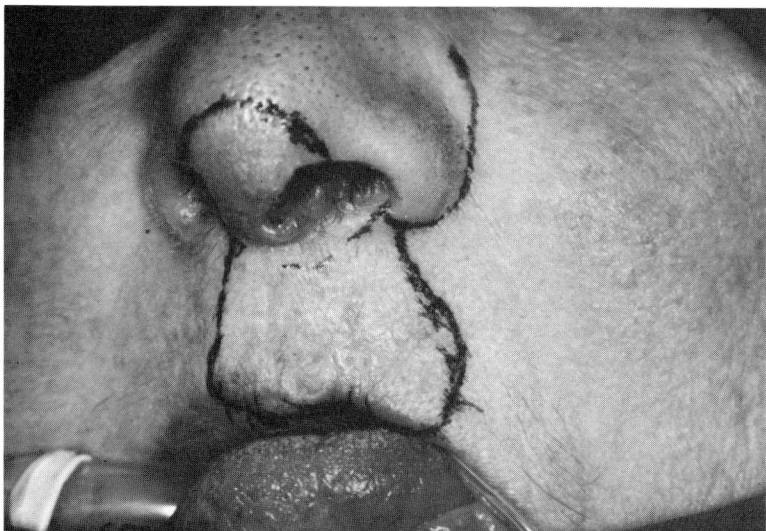

This is well illustrated above. In this patient with a squamous cell carcinoma of upper lip, columella, and membranous septum, a wide excision was necessary.

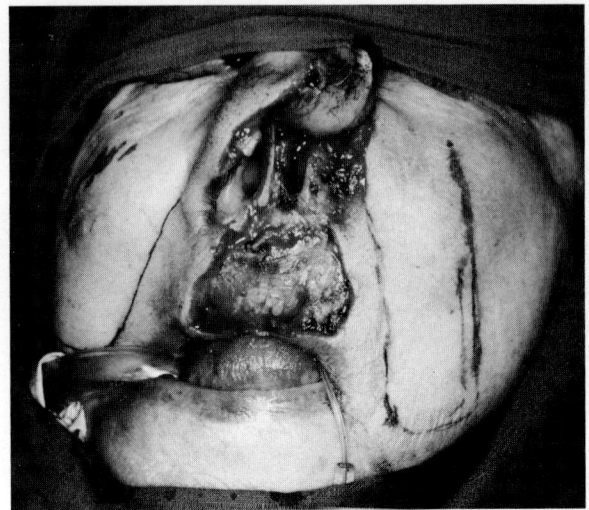 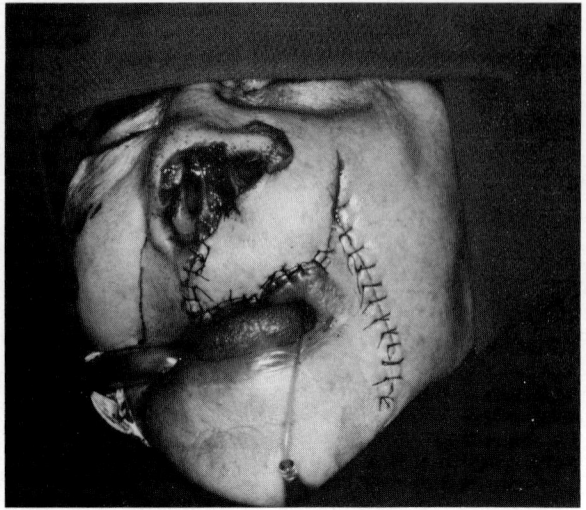

After resection long bilateral nasolabial flaps were used for the reconstruction. One flap was employed to reconstruct the defect in the upper lip.

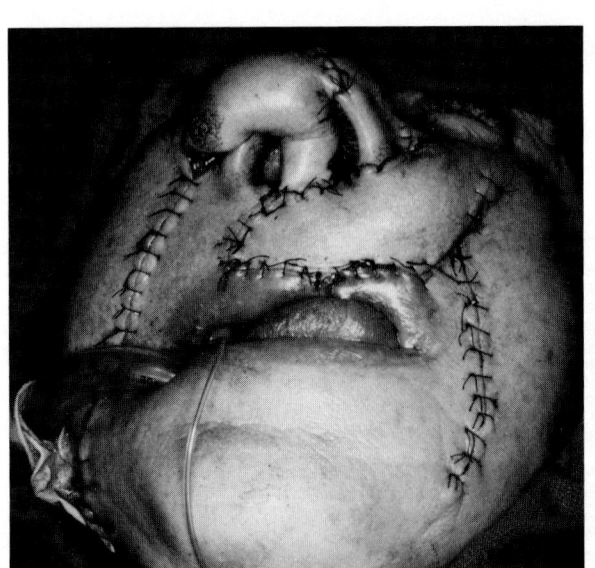 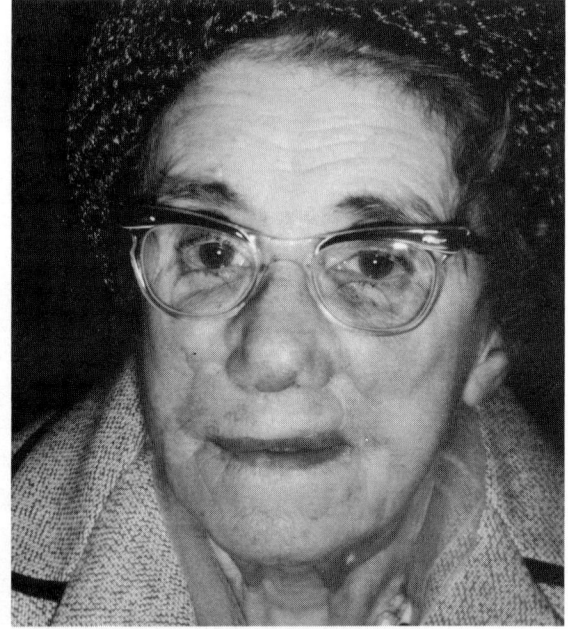

The other was elevated, folded, and sutured to the raw edges of the septum to form the columella. With this two-stage procedure a good result was obtained in reconstruction of this complex defect of columella and lip. No further surgery was necessary in this older patient.

FULL-THICKNESS DEFECTS OF UPPER LIP

As with replacement of skin, symmetry should be achieved with as little disturbance of the surrounding anatomic features as possible. In most individuals one quarter of the lip can be sacrificed and the defect can be closed directly without difficulty. In others, such as persons with lax lips, even larger defects may be closed in this fashion. If it is judged impossible to close the defects without causing lip distortion, then a flap is used.

Abbe Flap

The Abbe flap, or lip switch flap, was first described by Sabattini,[18] Stein,[19] Buck,[4] Estlander,[5] and later by Abbe.[1] However, as often happens, the originator's name was lost in antiquity. In spite of attempts to rename this the Stein flap, it has remained the Abbe flap. This flap can be used to reconstruct as much as one third of the upper lip.

The lower lip is always lax and can supply a flap of one quarter of its length to reconstruct defects of the upper lip. The Abbe flap offers immediate replacement of the total lip anatomy.

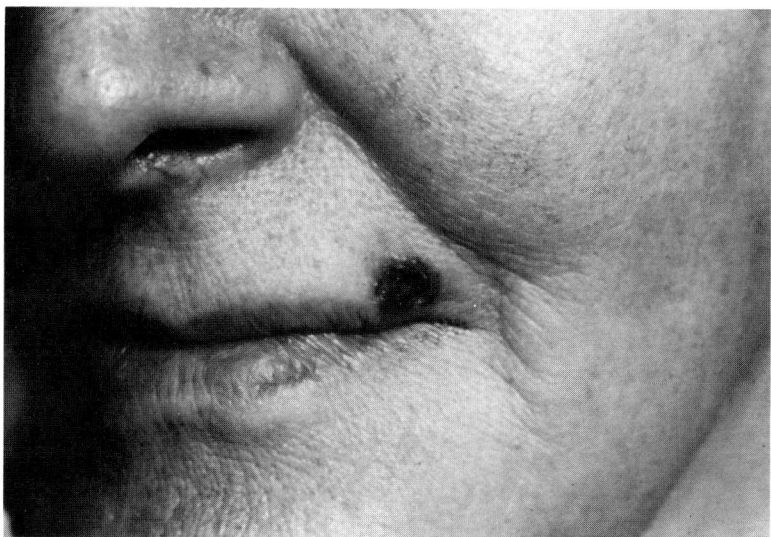

This technique was used after reconstruction of the squamous cell carcinoma of the upper lip illustrated here.

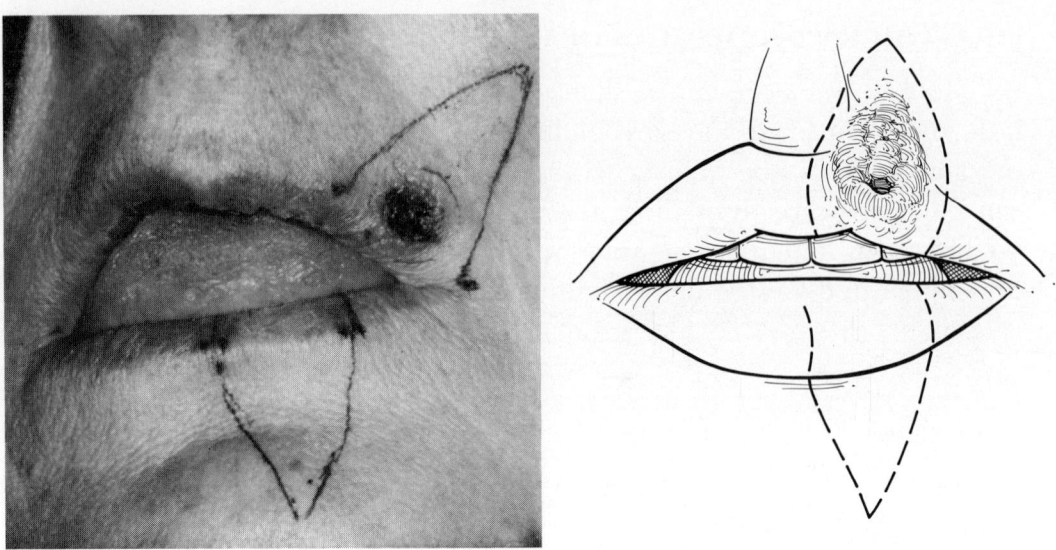

The projected upper lip defect is assessed, and a flap of sufficient dimensions to close this defect is drawn on the lower lip. The rotation point of the flap is chosen on the basis of convenience, usually in order to leave the largest oral opening during the period of lip adherence.

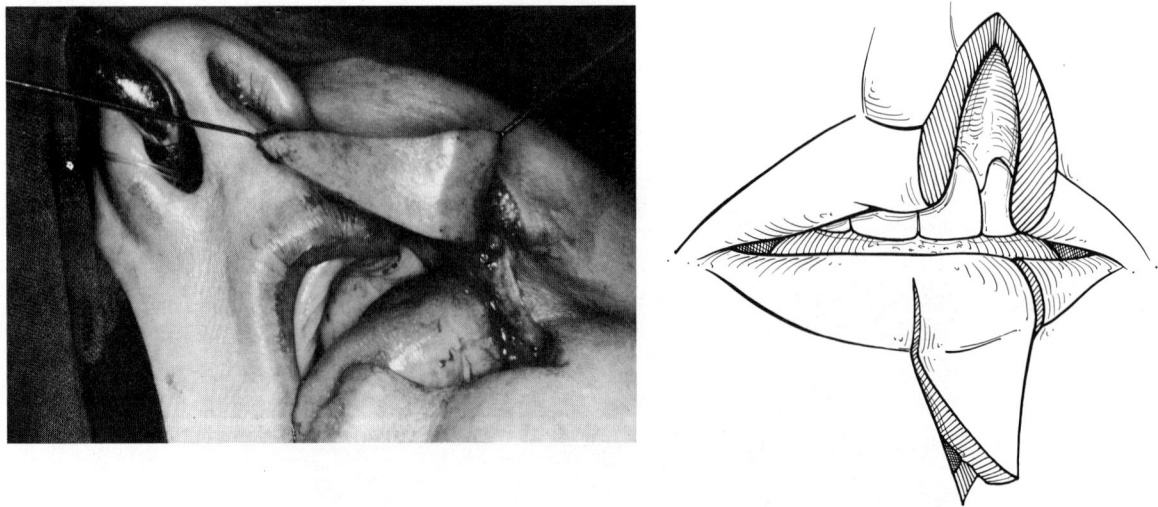

The upper lip resection is completed. The lower lip flap is totally incised on the side away from the pedicle, and the position of the labial artery is noted. On the other side the lip is incised until only a small cuff of subcutaneous tissue and muscle surrounds the vascular pedicle.

CHAPTER 8
LIP RECONSTRUCTION

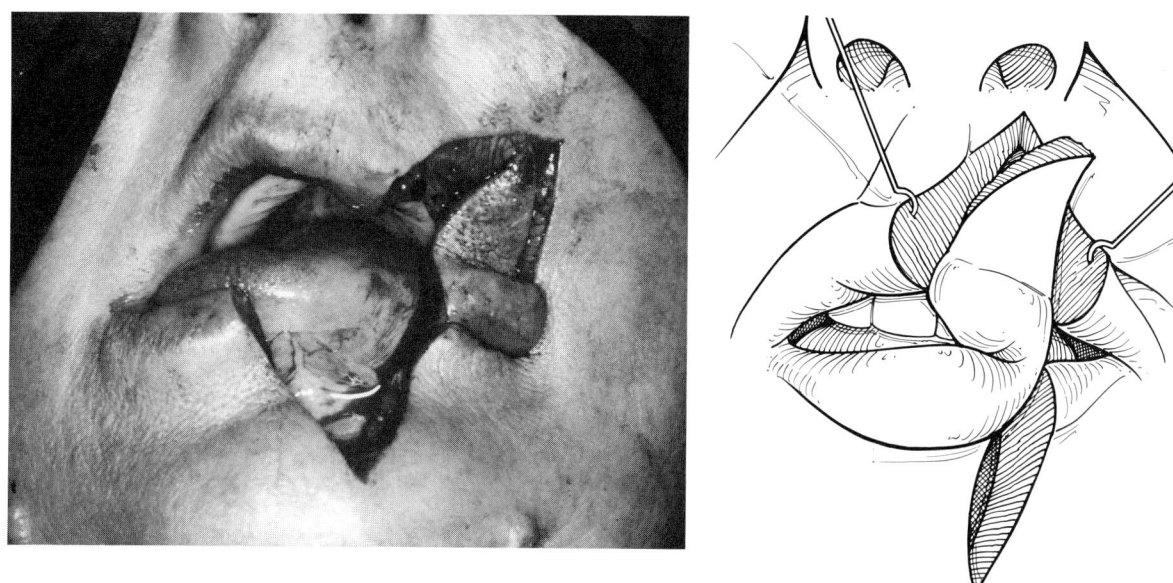

This makes for very easy rotation of the flap into the upper lip defect.

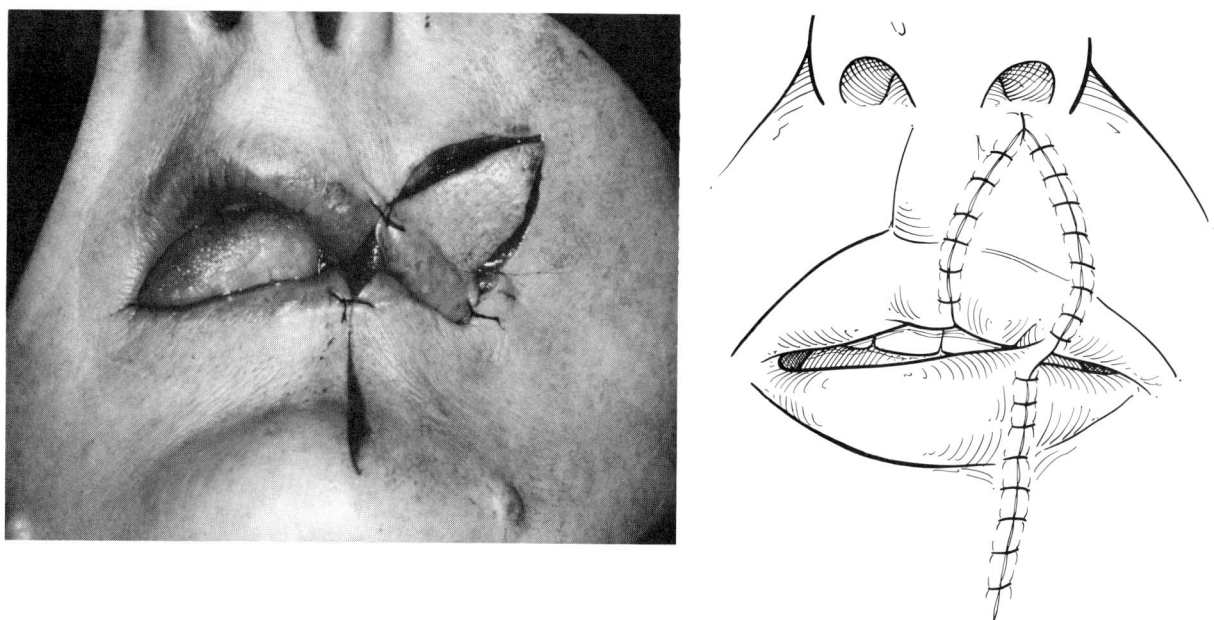

Closure is performed in layers. The mucosa of the upper and lower lip is closed with an absorbable suture, and this is followed by suturing of the muscle and the skin. Care must be taken in suturing around the pedicle, since blood flow may be compromised. Persistent cyanosis calls for mandatory suture removal in this area. Then the flap color should revert to normal.

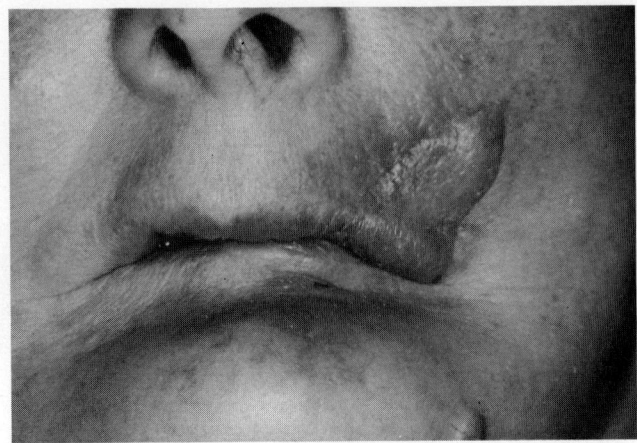

A wide adhesive tape is placed under the chin and run up to the cheeks to support the chin and keep the lips together.

The pedicle is divided after 10 to 14 days. Any necessary trimming is carried out at this time.

Abbe-Estlander Flap

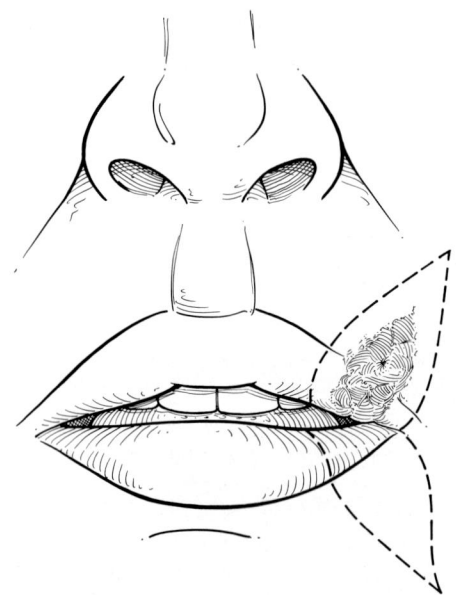

When the flap is being used to reconstruct a defect that requires partial commissure reconstruction, it is known as the Abbe-Estlander flap.

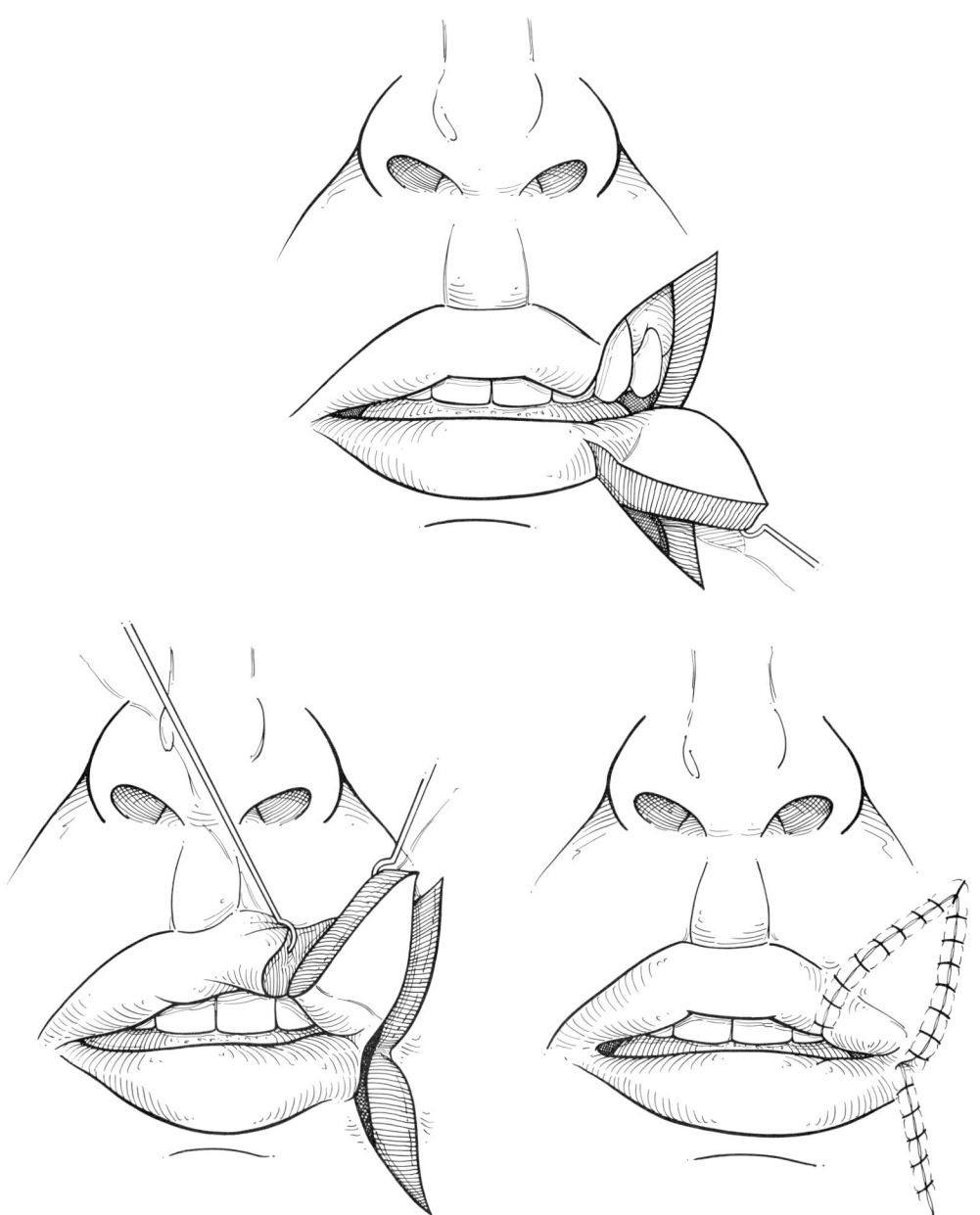

The method is essentially the same as described above, except that the medial pedicle becomes the commissure. Often immediate postoperative asymmetry is noted and later adjustment is necessary.

PROBLEMS

By incorrectly positioning sutures or by direct trauma to the vessels during cutting of the flap, it is possible to injure the pedicle of the flap and cause vascular occlusion. This will result in flap necrosis. If the surgeon has a clear understanding of the vascular anatomy, it is unlikely that the pedicle would be damaged in this fashion. As the flap is cut on the side opposite the pedicle, the exact position of the labial vessels can be noted. This allows safe incision of skin, muscle, and mucosa on the other side of the flap, with the formation of a very narrow but secure pedicle.

Perialar Crescentic Advancement Flap

The perialar crescentic advancement flap was described in detail earlier in this chapter and in Chapter 1. The patient illustrated here has an adenocystic carcinoma of the minor salivary glands in the left cheek–upper lip area.

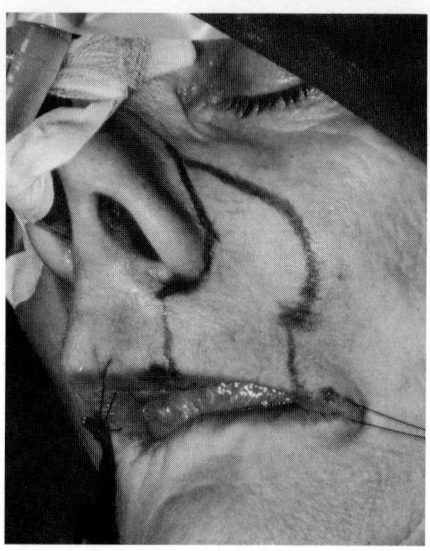 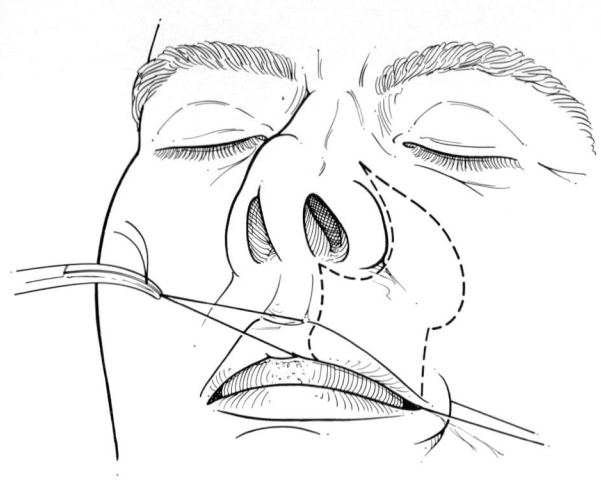

A wide excision is planned in the perialar crescentic fashion.

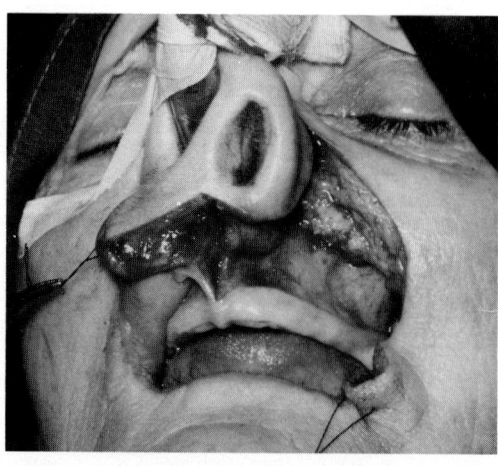 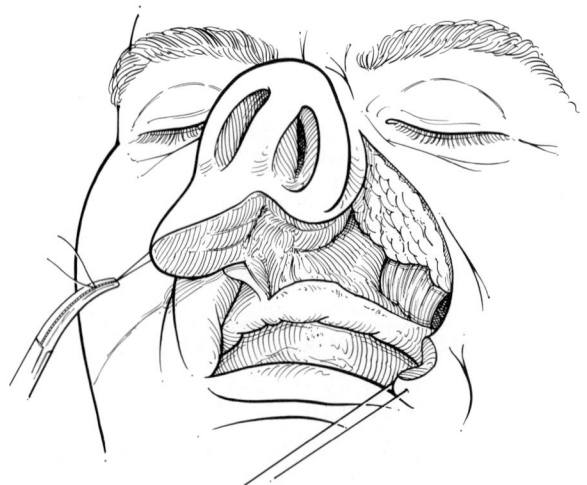

The full thickness of the lip and cheek is excised down to and including the maxillary periosteum.

CHAPTER 8
LIP RECONSTRUCTION

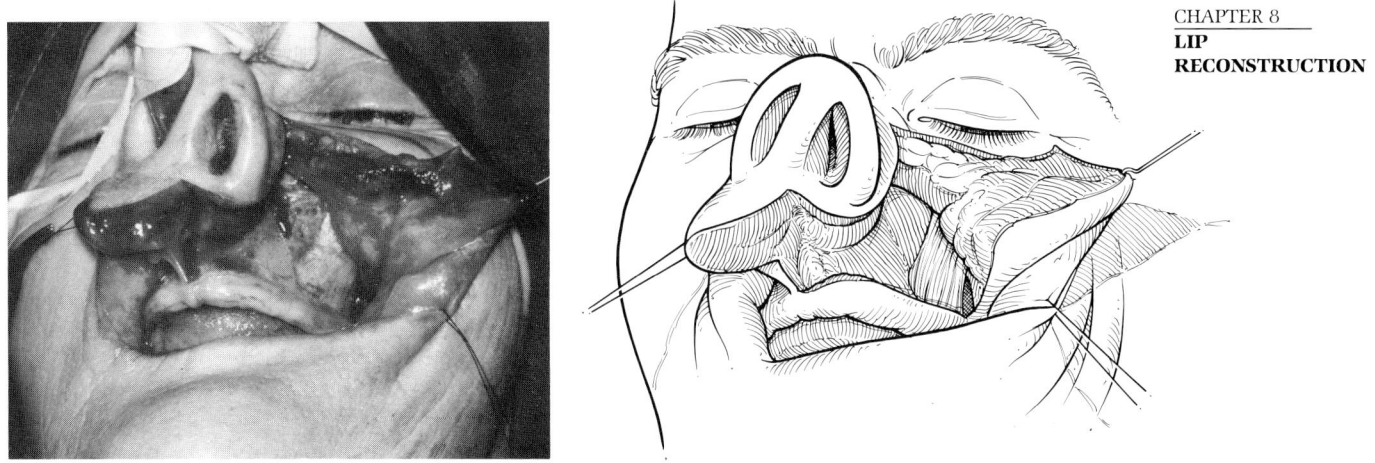

The mucosa in the apex of the upper buccal sulcus is incised, and the cheek is elevated further laterally.

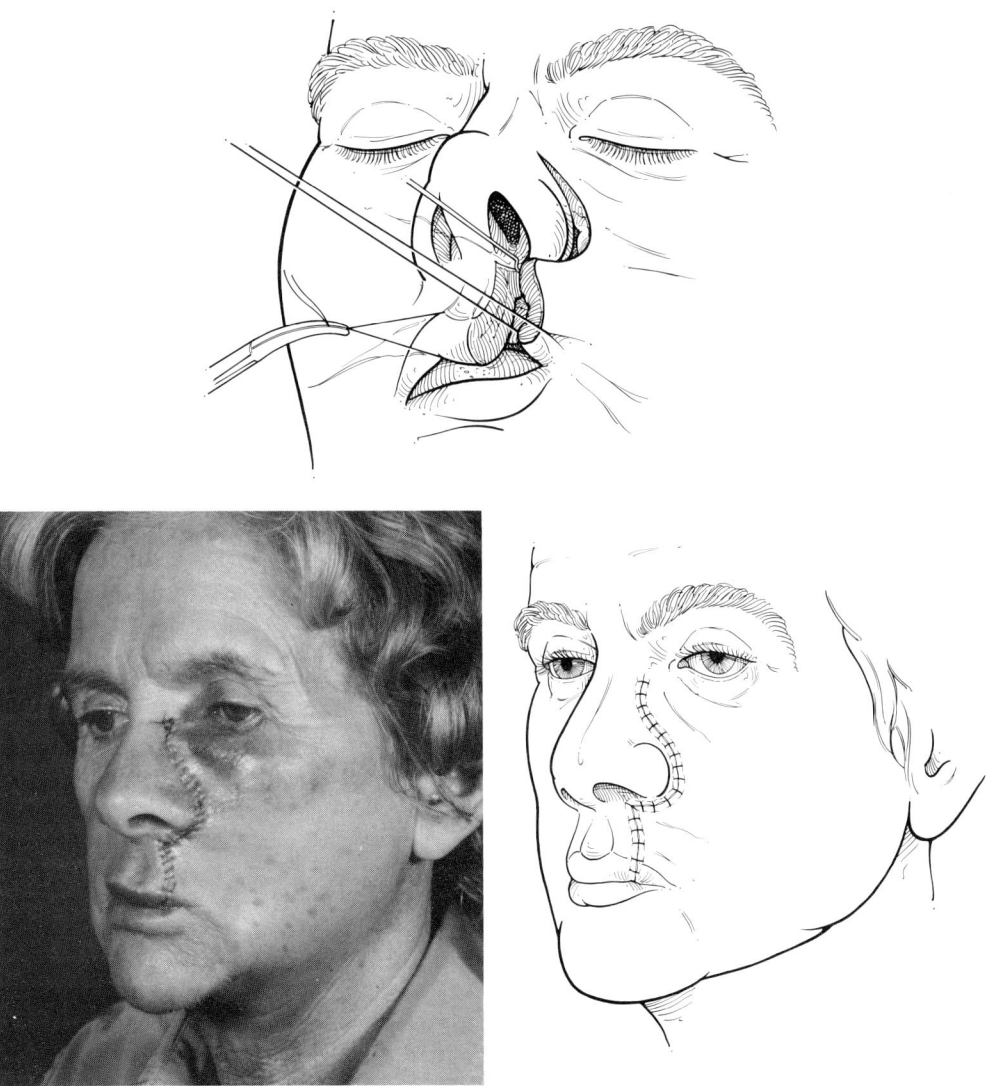

The remainder of the lip and cheek can now be advanced medially with ease in order to close the defect.

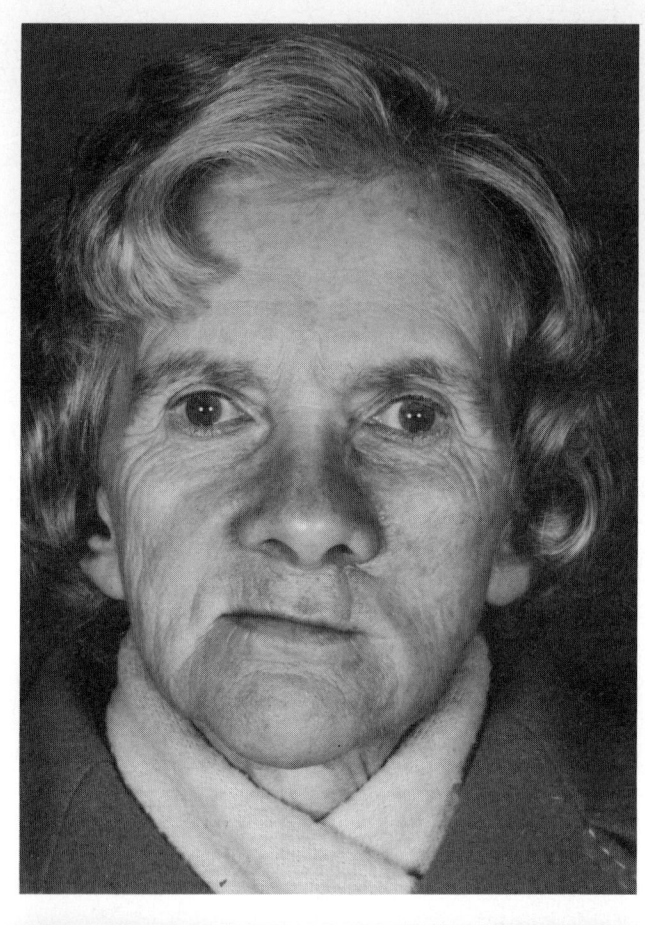

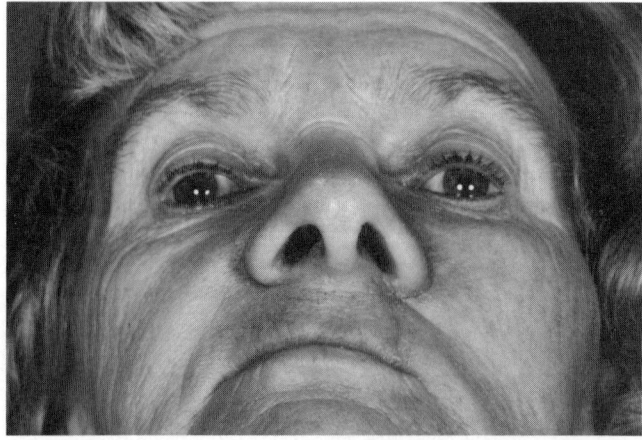

The result is good, without distortion of the lip, cheek, or nose.

Bilateral Perialar Crescentic Advancement Flaps

For a defect of one third of the lip length, a single flap may be used. If the defect is larger than one third, it can be reconstructed by means of a bilateral variation of the Webster principle, as demonstrated in this patient with a leiomyosarcoma of the upper lip.

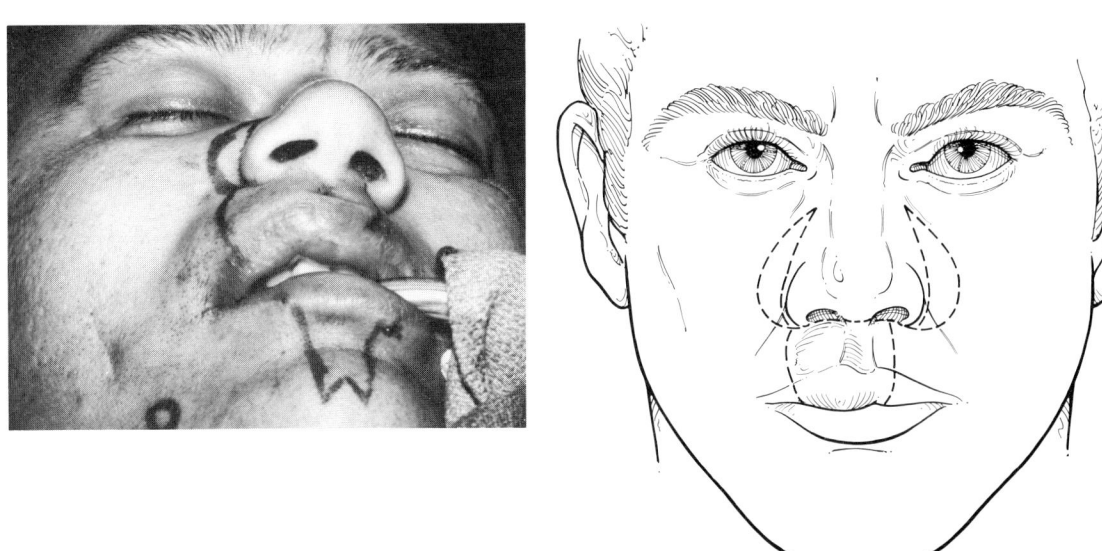

The Abbe flap design on the lower lip was an alternative reconstruction that was considered.

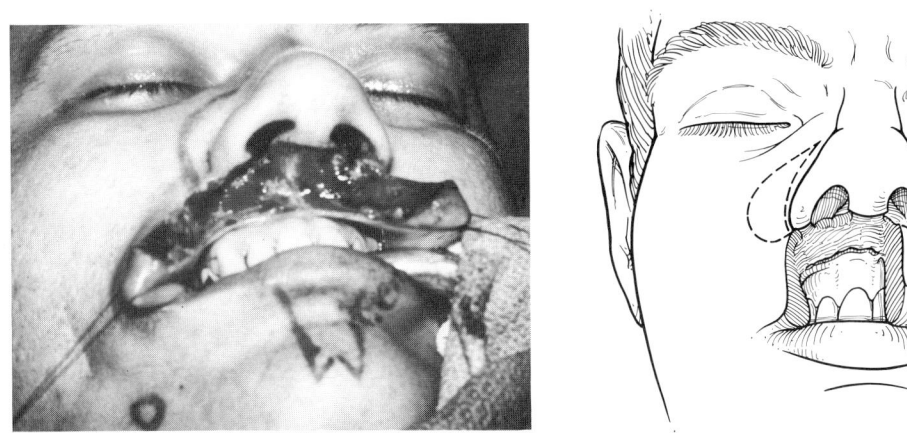

Just over one half of the lip is excised, along with portions of the alar bases, the nostril sills, and the base of the columella.

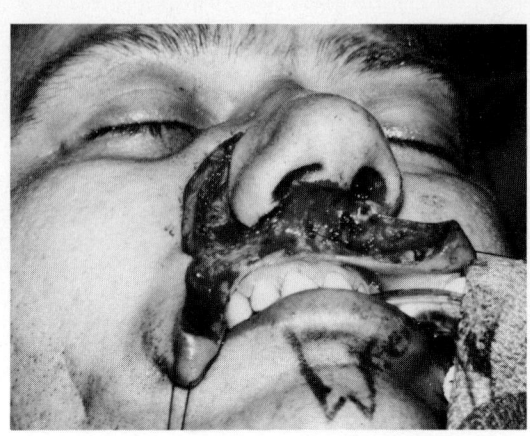
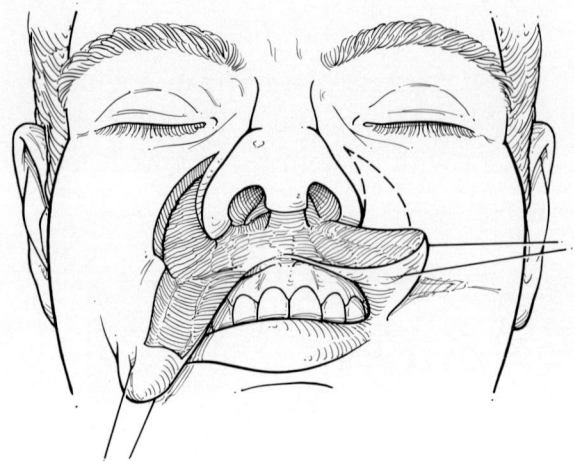

The crescentic excision is wider and lower in this case; it is taken around the alar base.

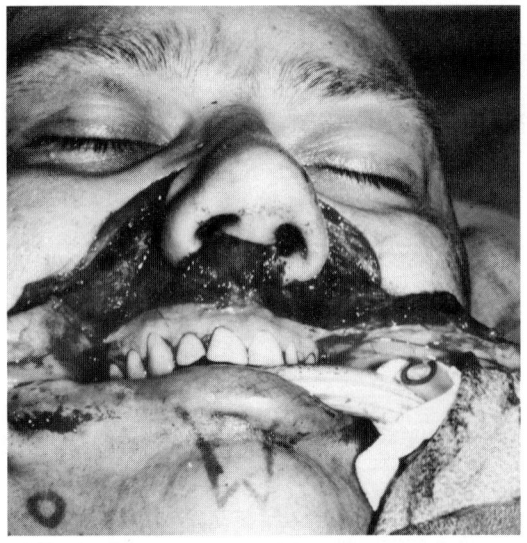
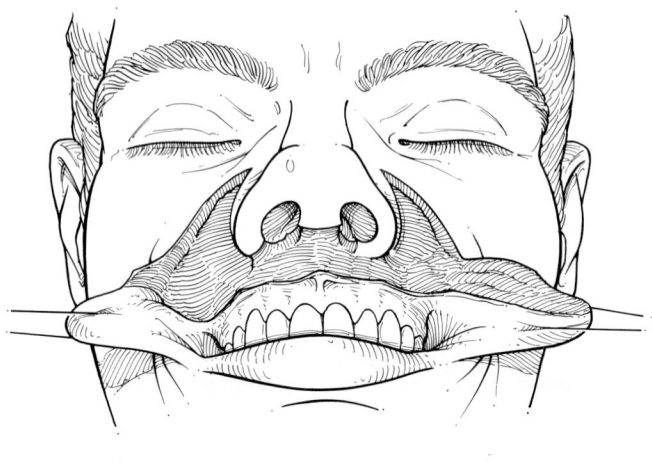

It may also be necessary to free the mucosa in the buccal sulcus and undermine the cheeks further. The result is a full-thickness cheek flap.

CHAPTER 8
LIP RECONSTRUCTION

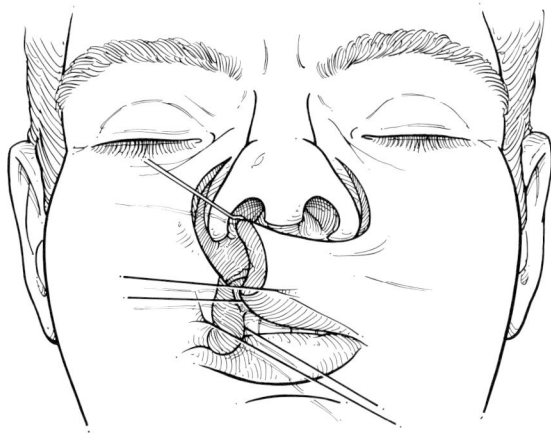

Following this maneuver the remnants of the lip are advanced to close the defect.

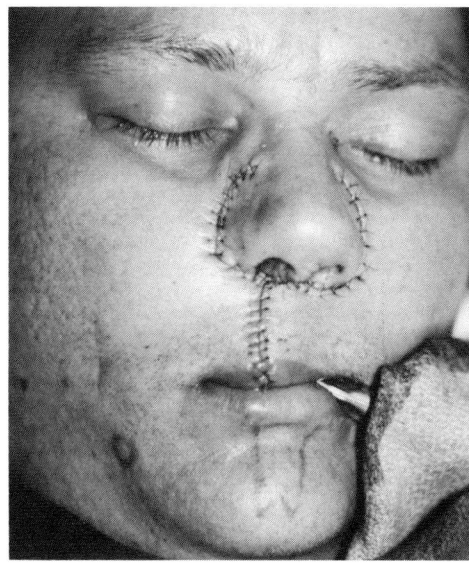
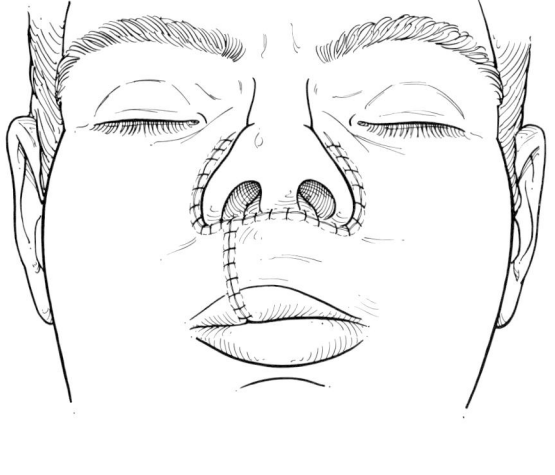

The lip is sutured in layers.

367

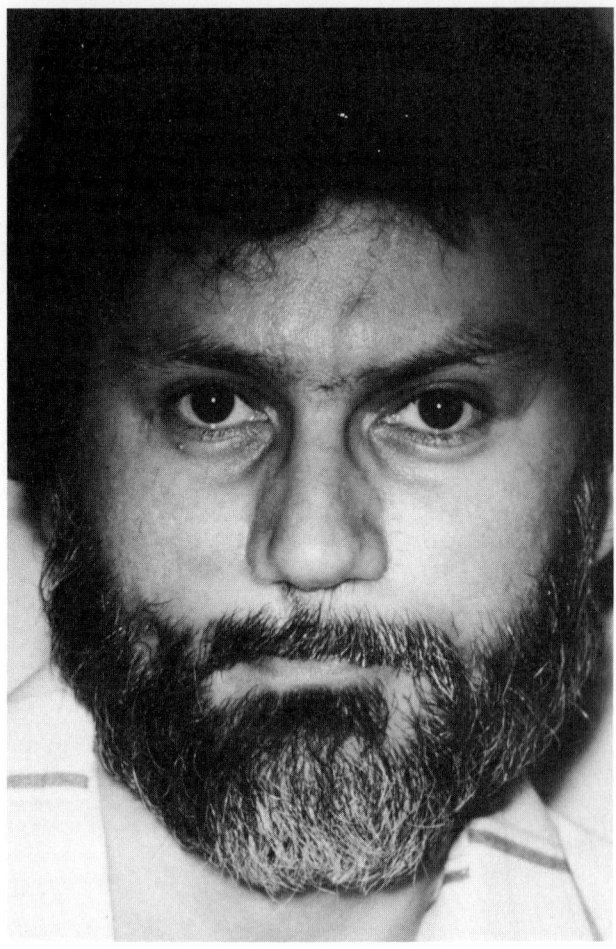
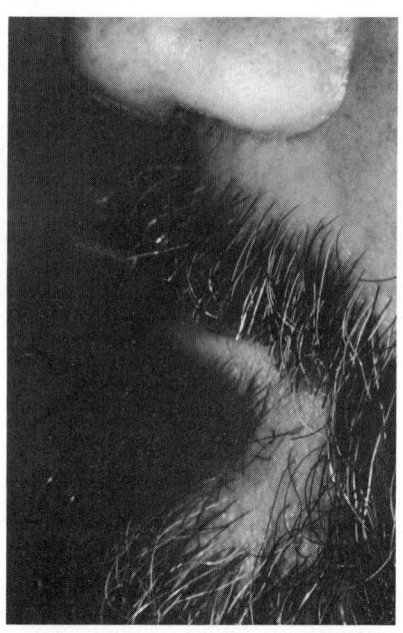

A slight tightness of the upper lip is noted in the result, but the lip relationship is reasonably satisfactory.

PROBLEMS

With the perialar crescentic advancement flap, the lip is not augmented and the position of the commissures is changed, which results in a smaller mouth opening. The diminished mouth size can be a significant problem for patients who wear dentures. In addition, an obvious tightness of the upper lip occurs, although this improves slightly with time.

Reversed Karapandzic Flap

For reconstructing large lip defects that exceed one third of the lip length, a lower lip sharing procedure may be used. This approach has the advantage of using like tissue for filling the defect. The repair is based on a principle published by Karapandzic in 1974.[16] With this technique incisions are made around both commissures to provide full-thickness flaps equal to the width of the lip. The initial incision is made through the skin. The muscles are divided by a mixture of blunt and sharp dissection with perservation of the nerve and vascular supply. Thus the segments advanced to form the lip are well vascularized and functional. In upper lip reconstruction, unlike reconstruction of the lower lip, the mucosa is incised along the buccal sulcus. It is now possible to advance the segments and reconstruct the lip. The reconstructed lip is usually somewhat tight. This method will be discussed in more detail in the section on lower lip reconstruction, where the results from this approach are much better.

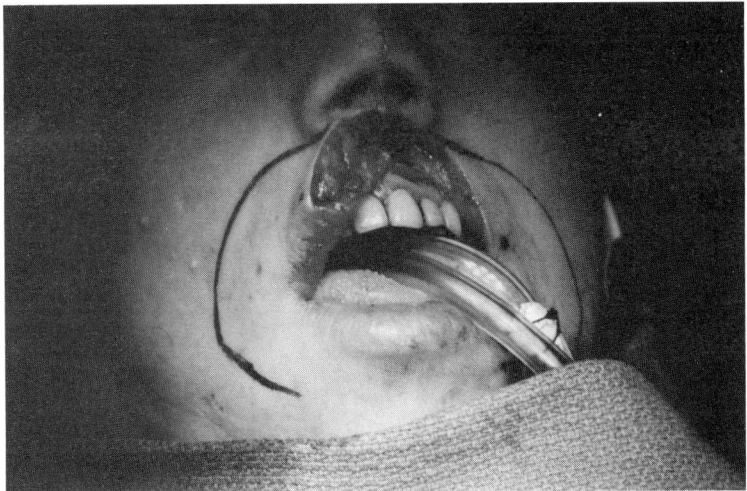

The reversed Karapandzic method was chosen for this patient, who had a Merkel's cell tumor excised from the upper lip and the columella.

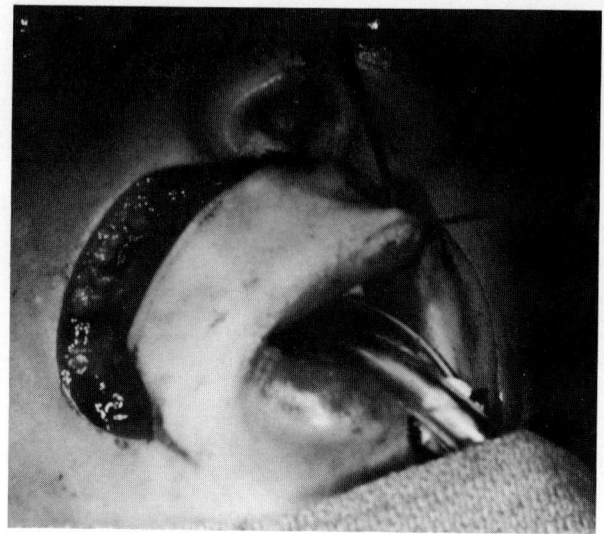 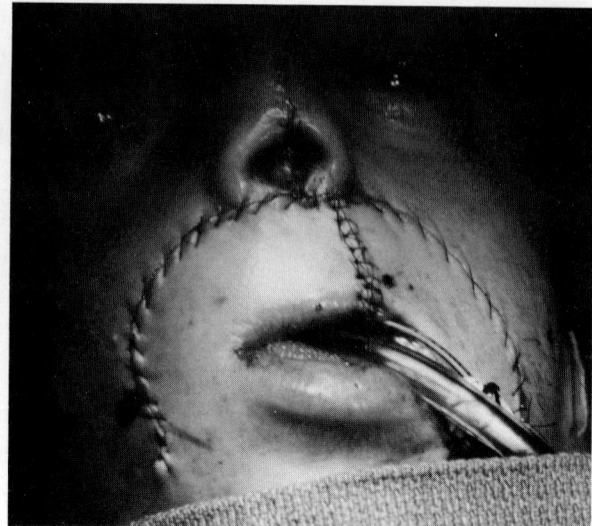

After this procedure the lip was reconstructed with bilateral Karapandzic flaps. The reconstruction was tight and not aesthetically satisfactory. Soon after the procedure the patient succumbed to distant metastases from this aggressive tumor.

PROBLEMS

Tightness of the upper lip and an inability to rotate the commissures adequately are the main problems associated with this approach. The lip tightness is combined with a small mouth aperature, which can cause problems for denture wearers. It may be necessary to perform a commissurotomy at a later date to widen the mouth.

Surgical Technique of Choice

Undoubtedly, the best results are obtained from the Webster method. The lip is not so tight as with other procedures, and the aesthetic result is superior. Moreover, the flap does not involve the lower lip, with the resulting ugly scar created by the Abbe flap donor site.

☐ Total Upper Lip Reconstruction

Total upper lip reconstruction is an extremely difficult problem with no truly satisfactory solution. The aesthetics of the reconstruction are suboptimal, as is the function. The tissue necessary to achieve symmetry and normal anatomy and function is not available.

Fortunately, total upper lip reconstruction is rarely required. Several methods are available, and all involve the use of nasolabial tissue. Simple nasolabial flaps based inferiorly or superiorly can be used, or more formal fan-type flaps (Gillies) can be employed.

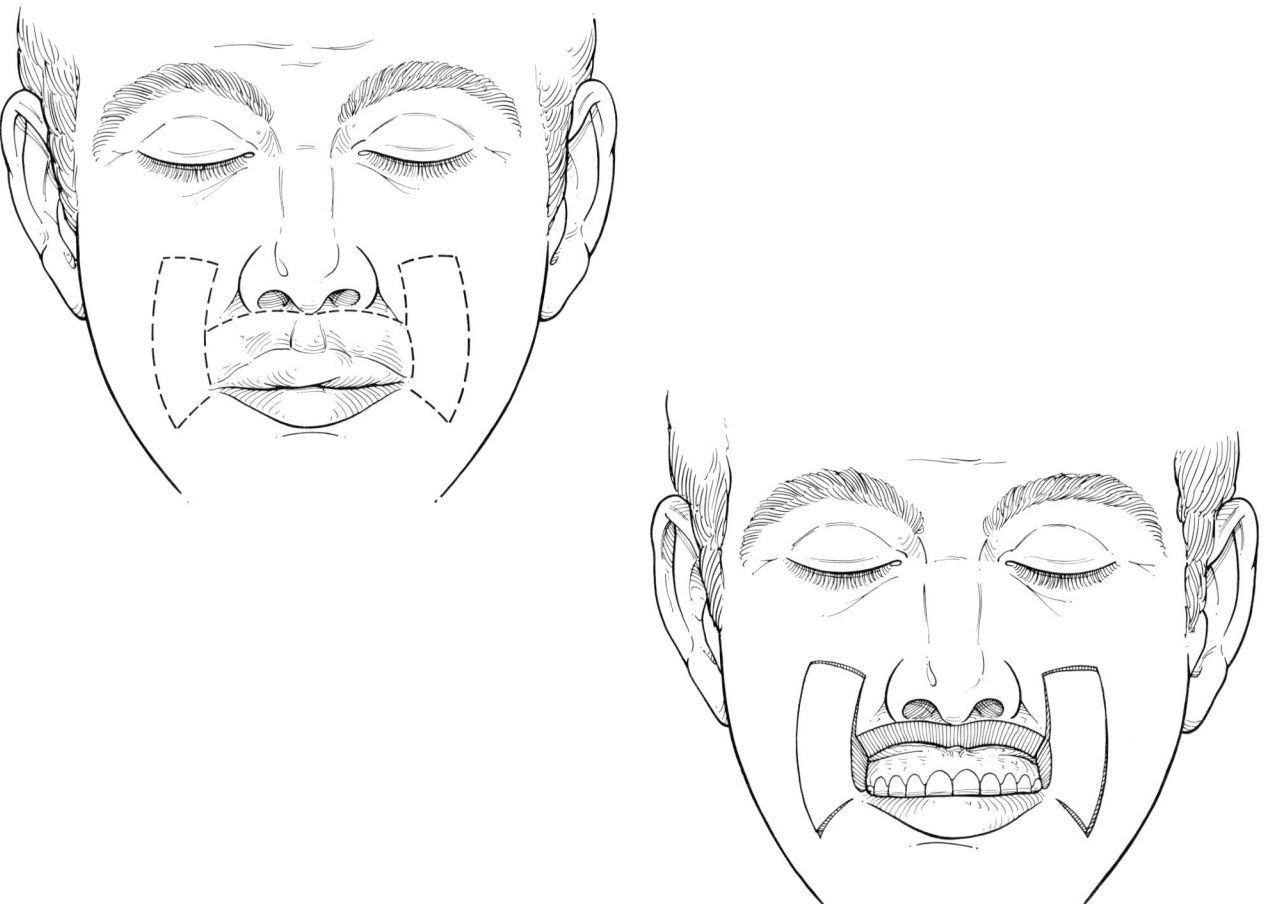

The flaps are based on an inferior medial pedicle; they are full-thickness cheek flaps that include the mucosa. Considerable care is taken at the pedicle area to avoid traumatizing the vessels around the commissures. A conscious effort is made to maintain a subcutaneous pedicle that is wider than the skin or mucosal pedicle.

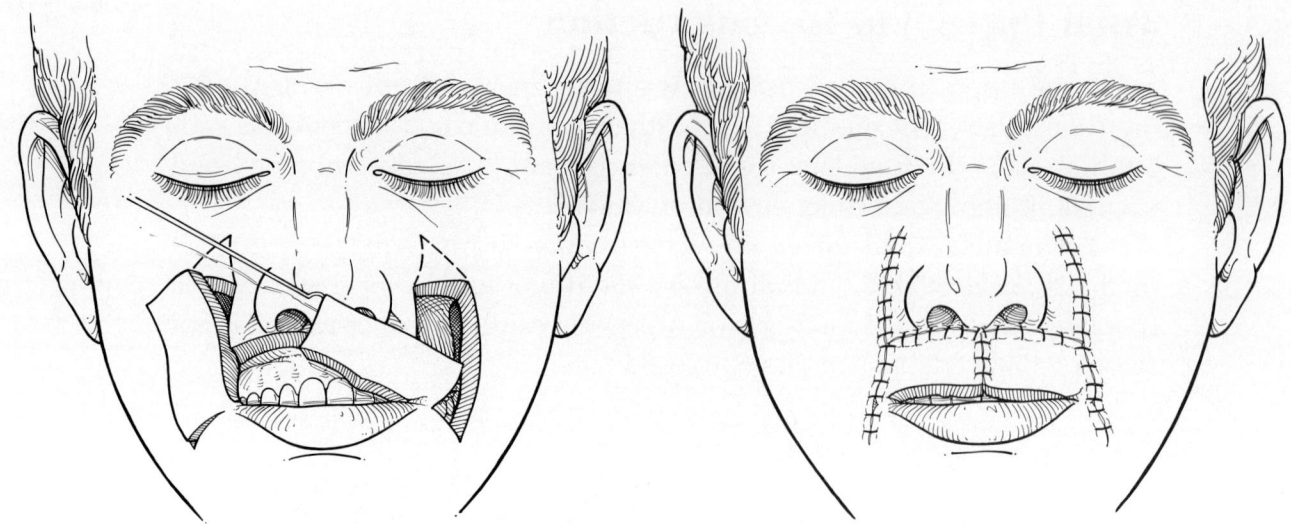

After the flaps have been incised, they are rotated medially to form the upper lip. The donor defect is closed directly after excision of superior dog ears of excess skin.

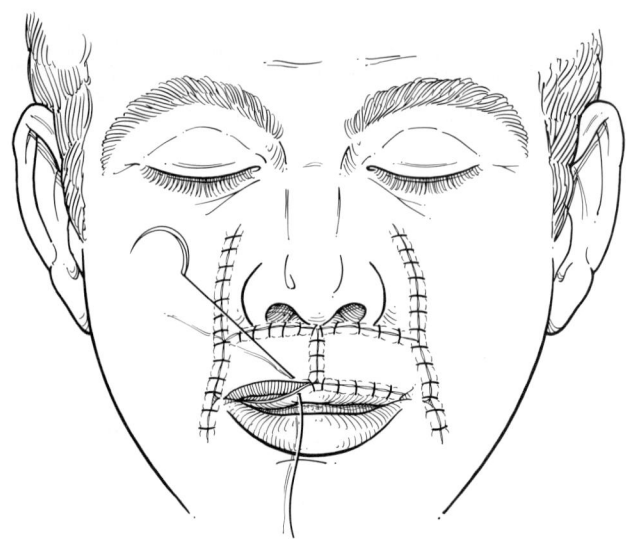

The mucosa is reconstructed by advancement. Use of a tongue flap is too hazardous in this situation; it would probably become detached.

Frequently, it is necessary to employ distant flaps, such as the deltopectoral flap, for adequate reconstruction. In the male, once the bulk of the lip has been supplied, skin cover can be exchanged for a narrow scalp flap, which provides hairbearing skin. From this, a moustache can be grown to disguise the reconstruction and make up for any discrepancy between the lips. Recently attempts have been made to supply function by tunneling flaps of vascularized and neurotomized platysma or frontalis into the lip. It is too early to assess the results of these procedures.

☐ Lower Lip Reconstruction

Symmetry, normal contours, and normal function are the goals in lower lip reconstruction. Poor lower lip function causes embarrassing drooling and can produce faulty vocal articulation.

SKIN DEFECTS

As with the upper lip, skin defects of the lower lip may be closed directly, skin grafted, or, if deep and extensive, reconstructed with an inferiorly based nasolabial flap or a rotation flap. The results of this approach are quite good, but there is a tendency for those flaps to pincushion and to defy revisional surgery for this problem.

Inferiorly Based Nasolabial Flap

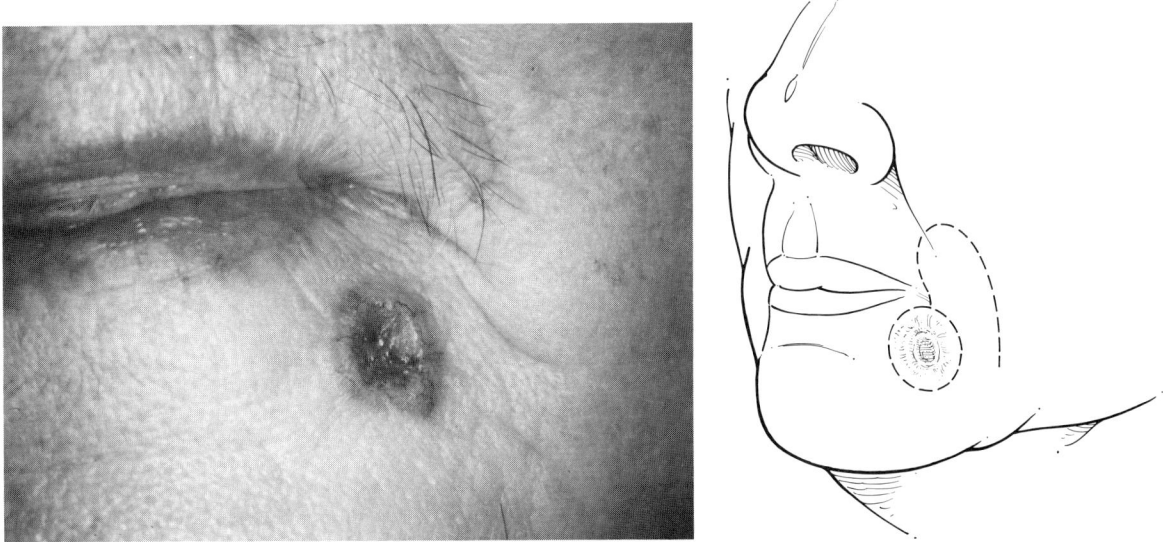

The patient illustrated here had a basal cell carcinoma of the lower lip. This is excised and reconstruction is planned with an inferiorly based nasolabial flap.

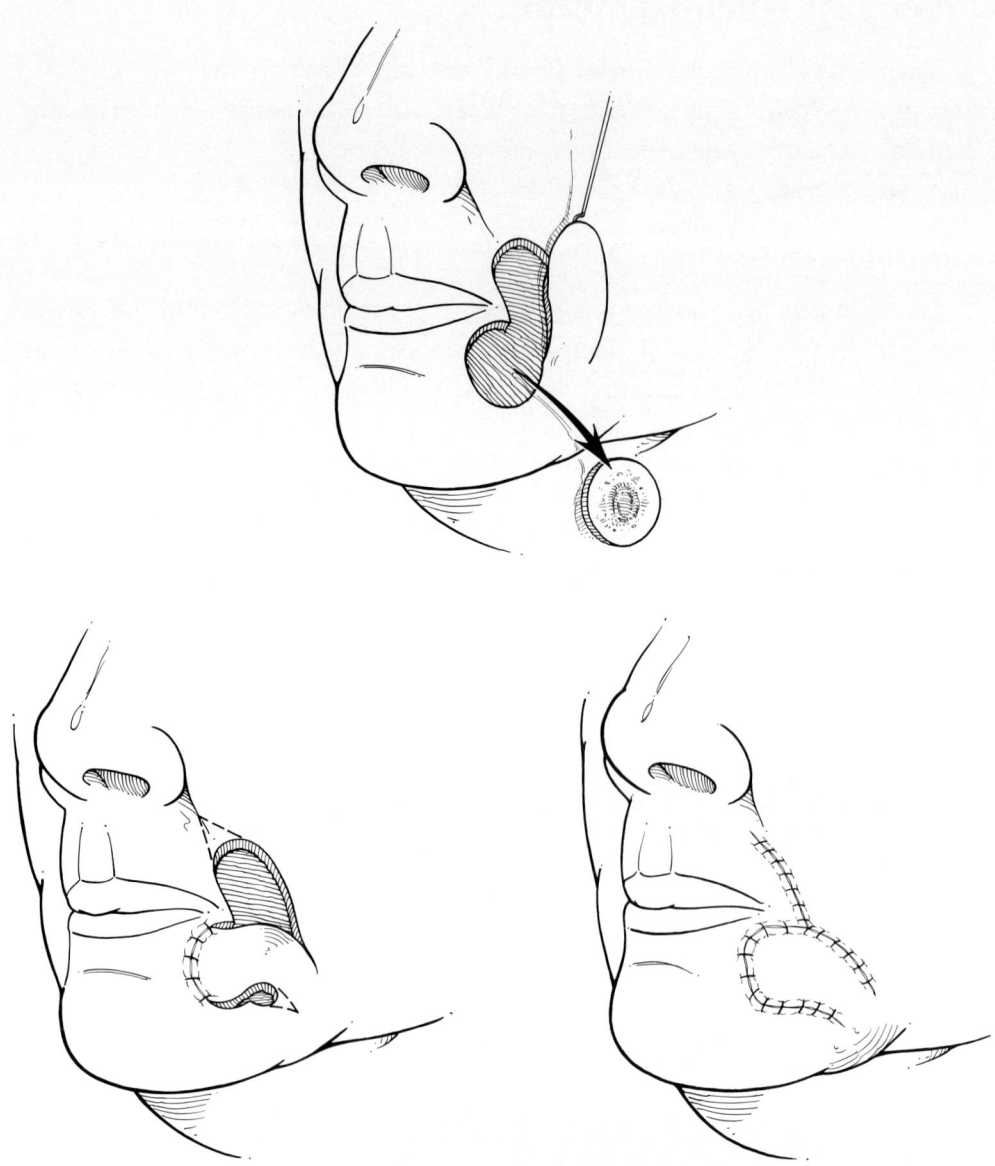

The flap is elevated (with care taken not to damage facial nerve branches), transposed to the lower lip, and sutured into position. The donor defect is closed directly.

CHAPTER 8
LIP RECONSTRUCTION

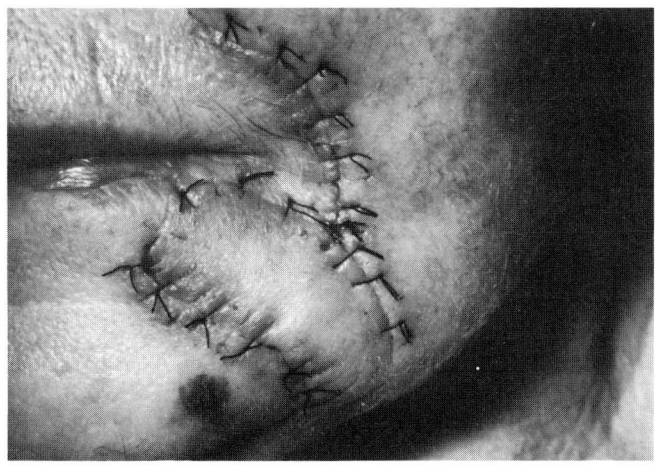

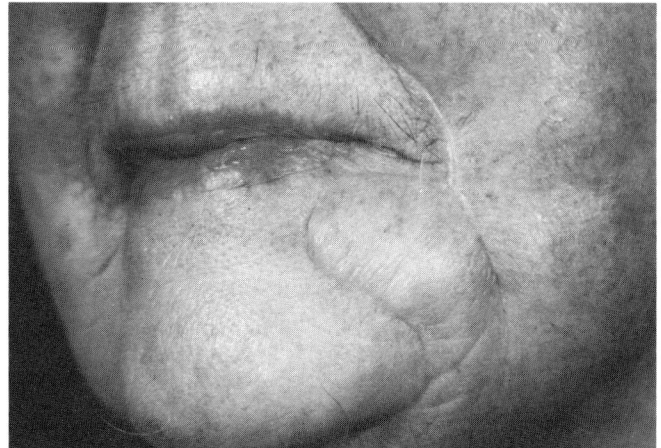

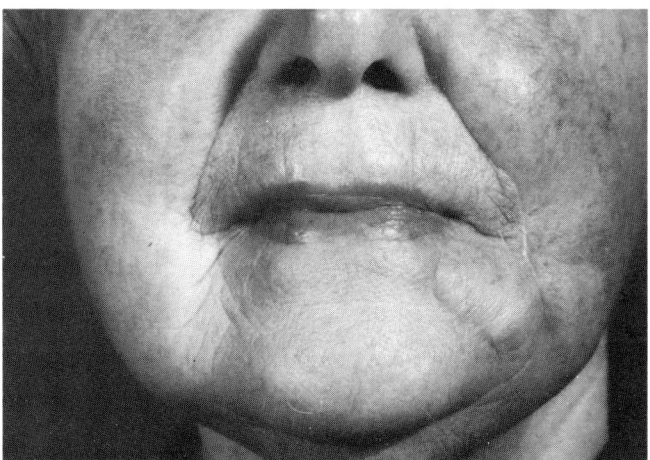

The result is good. The mouth is symmetric, the lip level is horizontal, and only slight pincushioning of the flap is present.

PROBLEMS

With the inferiorly based nasolabial flap, the main disadvantage is pincushioning. This makes the scars more obvious. However, the color match is reasonably good.

SMALL FULL-THICKNESS LIP DEFECTS

Small full-thickness defects of the lip are usually simple to reconstruct. The height of the lip must be maintained, and there should be no mucosal notching.

Direct Closure

If the defect is less extensive than one third of the lip, direct closure in layers is possible and will give an excellent result.

PROBLEMS

Occasionally a notch may occur in the free vermilion edge. In reconstructions for carcinoma this irregularity should be accepted and later corrected after the fear of recurrence has subsided. Complex scar lines should be avoided in cancer resections, since they make follow-up difficult. In nonmalignant conditions a Z-plasty is performed to lengthen the mucosa and thus maintain the anteroposterior lip convexity.

LARGE FULL-THICKNESS DEFECTS

In reconstructing large full-thickness defects, the surgeon should be careful not to make the lip too tight. The lower lip would then have a reversed relationship with the upper lip. The lip should be functional and of the correct height.

Reversed Abbe Flaps

Abbe flaps (see pp. 357 to 360 for a fuller description) can be taken from the upper lip to reconstruct lower lip defects. However, these flaps can be only one third of the upper lip and thus cannot fill large lower lip defects. If the lower lip defect is in the commissure area, a reversed Abbe-Estlander flap is used; again, the medial free margin of the upper lip flap is inserted into the lateral edge of the lower lip defect.

CHAPTER 8
LIP RECONSTRUCTION

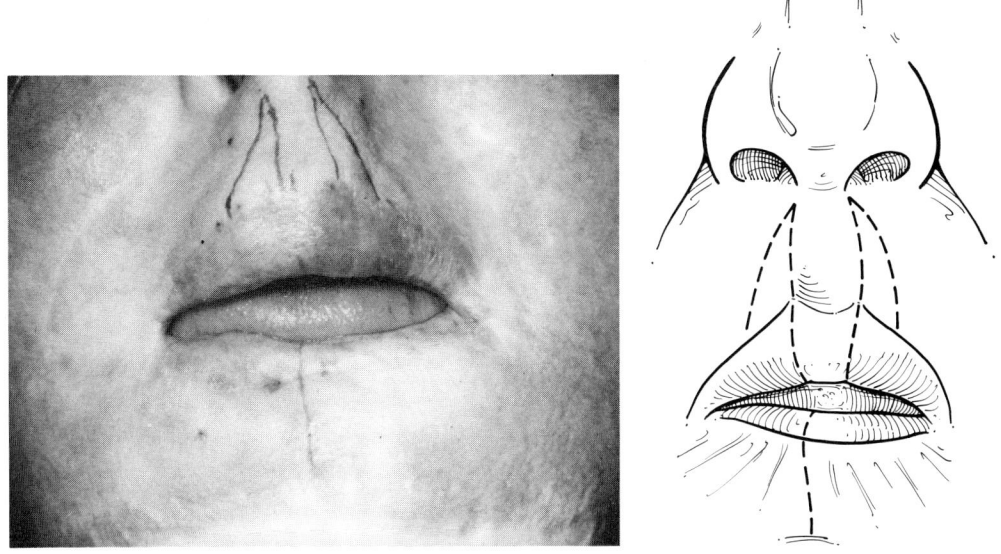

Bilateral Abbe flaps are planned to augment this total lower lip reconstruction after cancer resection.

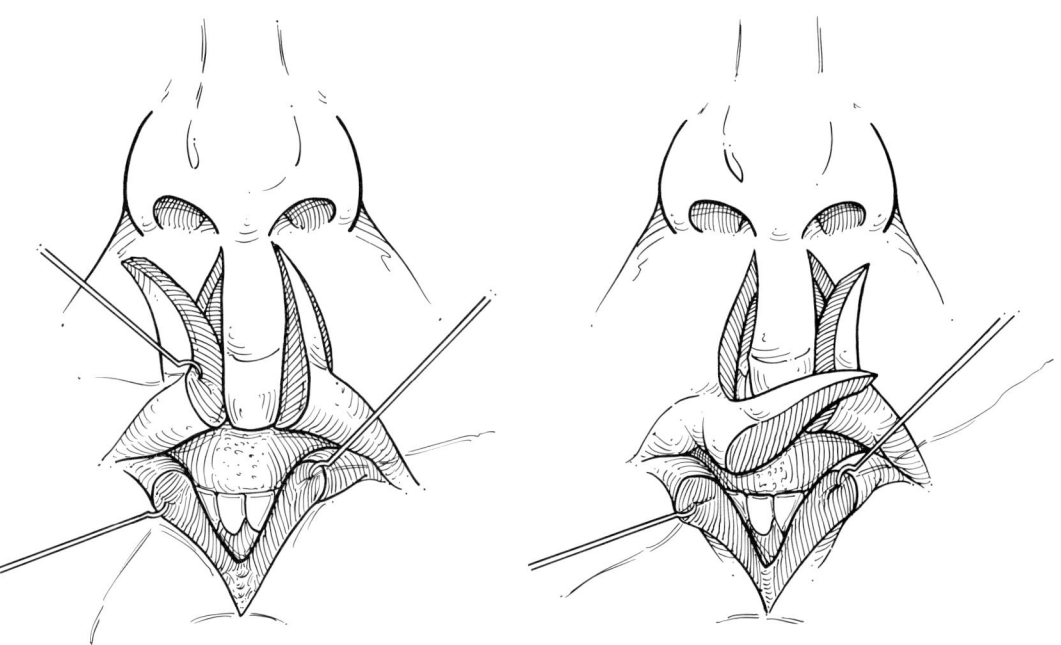

The flaps incorporate the philtral columns, and the vascular pedicles are located on the lateral edges of the flaps. The position of the vessels is noted on the medial incision, which completely divides the lip. This knowledge allows a narrow pedicle to be created laterally with complete security.

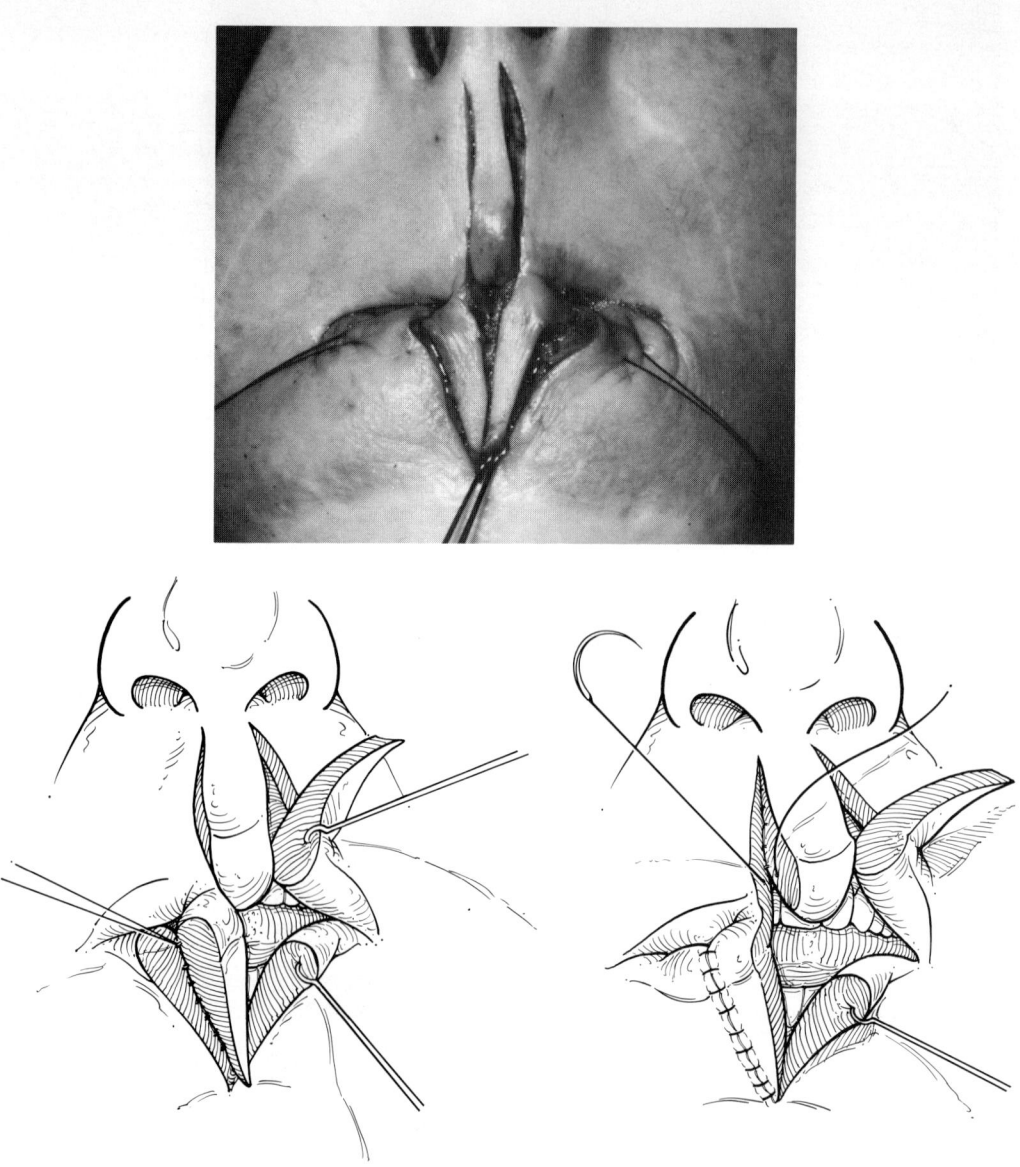

The narrow pedicle permits greater ease of rotation from upper to lower lip: as the flaps are rotated into the lower lip, the laterally placed pedicles move medially.

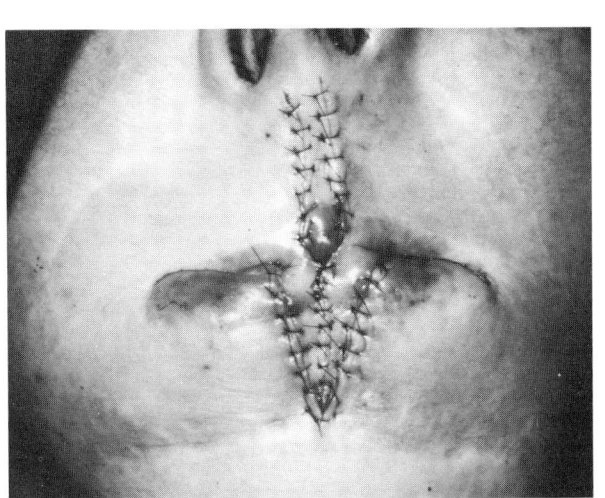 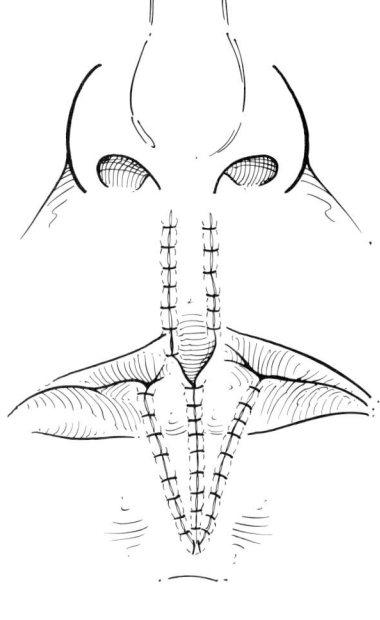

The lack of bulk makes the period between reconstruction and pedicle division more comfortable for the patient. All lip incisions are closed in layers.

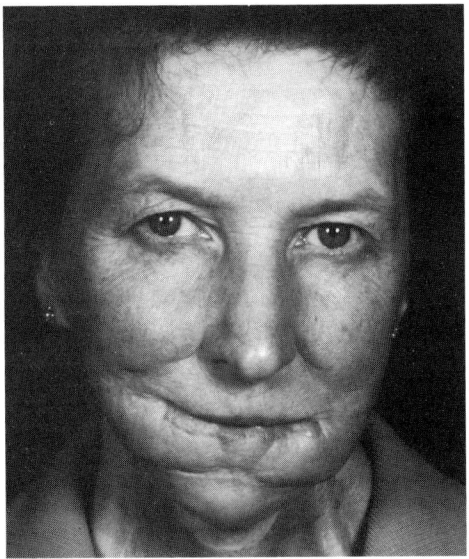

The pedicles are divided in 7 to 10 days. The donor site scars are remarkably inconspicious, and the upper lip distortion is minimal.

PROBLEMS

As with the conventional Abbe flap, problems may arise from pedicle compression. However, if planning and surgery are executed carefully, this has never been a problem with the reversed technique.

Karapandzic Technique

The Karapandzic technique can be used to reconstruct up to three quarters of the lower lip. It is simple, quick to perform, and results in a functional and aesthetically acceptable lip.

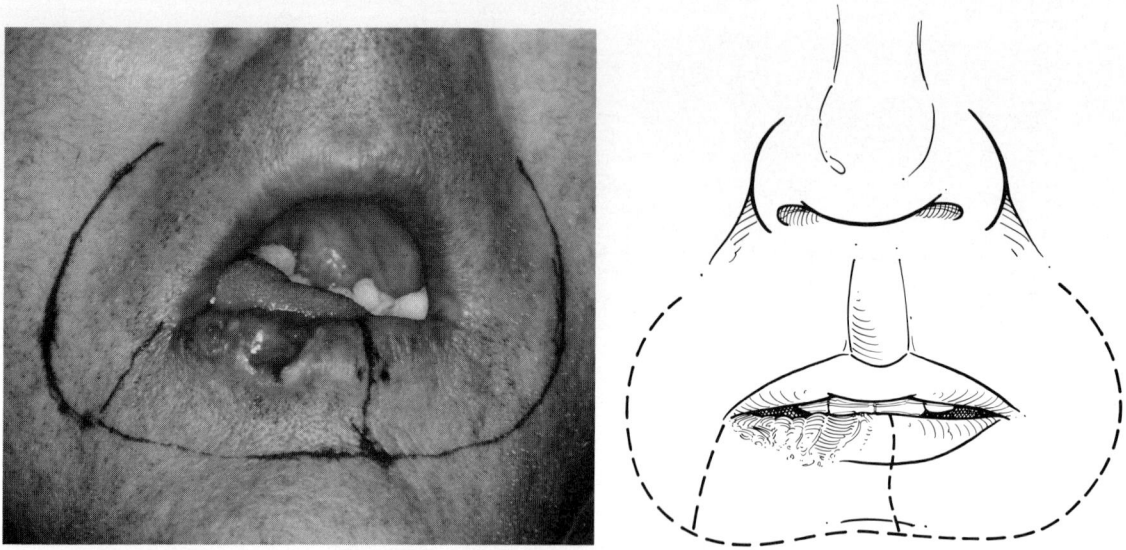

The plan for the procedure is outlined for this carcinoma of the lower lip.

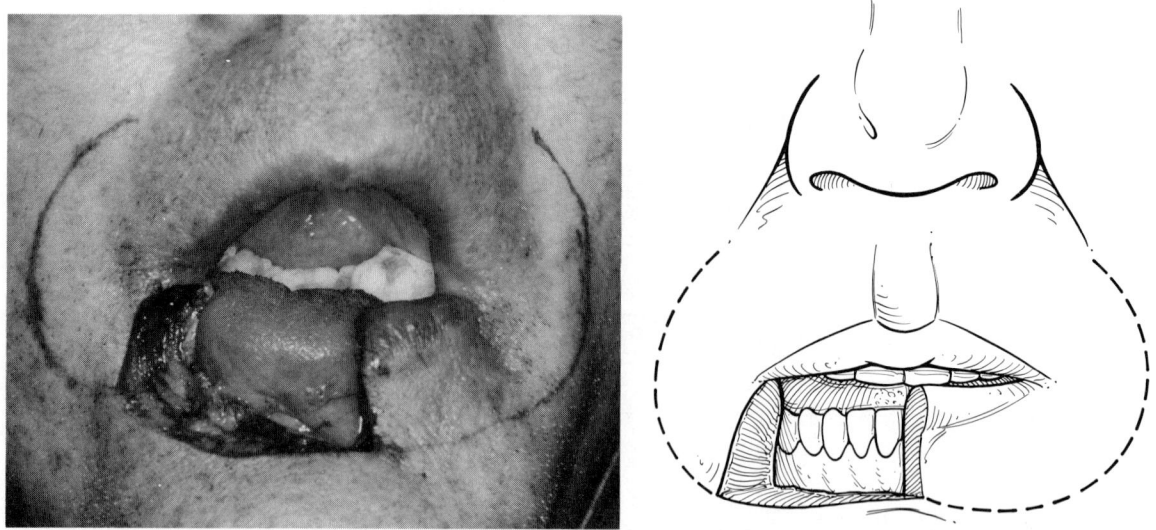

The resection is completed, and the position of the vessels is noted.

CHAPTER 8
LIP
RECONSTRUCTION

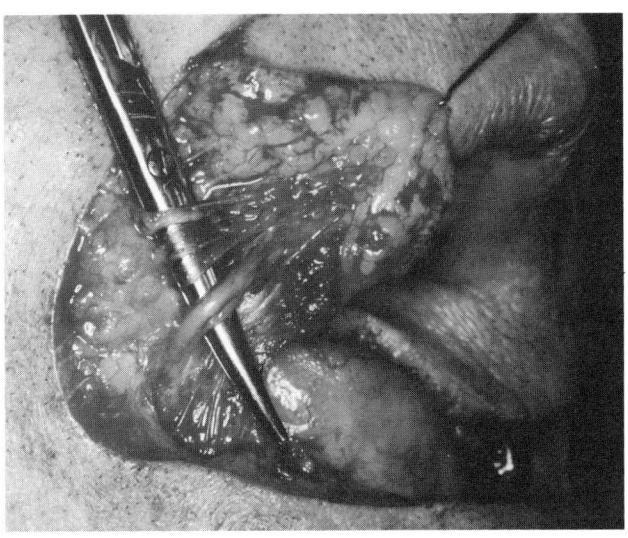
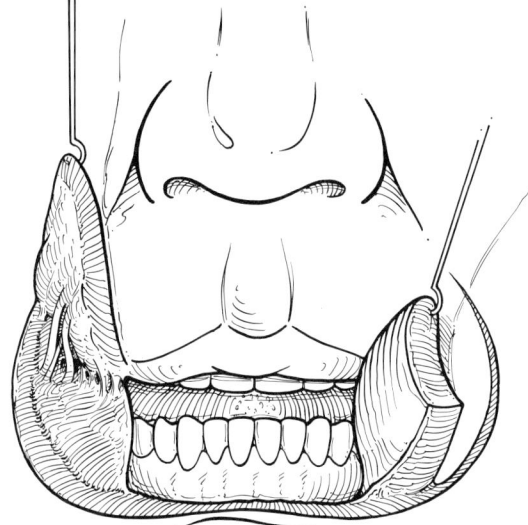

Incisions are made transversely from the base of the postexcisional defect on both sides. These extend around the commissures into the upper lip; with the use of scissors they are maintained equidistant from the free lip margin. The orbicularis muscle fibers are spread apart longitudinally, in the line of the skin incision, down to the submucosal layer. The nerves and vessels are maintained intact. The mucosa is incised for 1 to 2 cm from the edge of the defect.

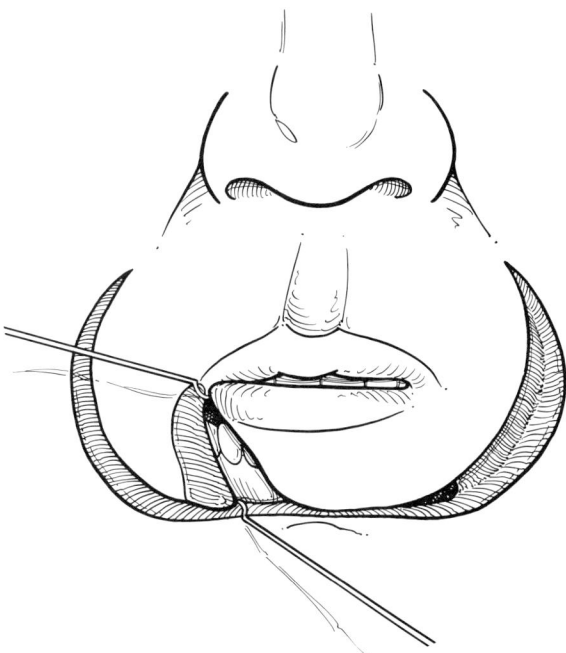

After this maneuver the edges of the defect can be approximated without tension.

381

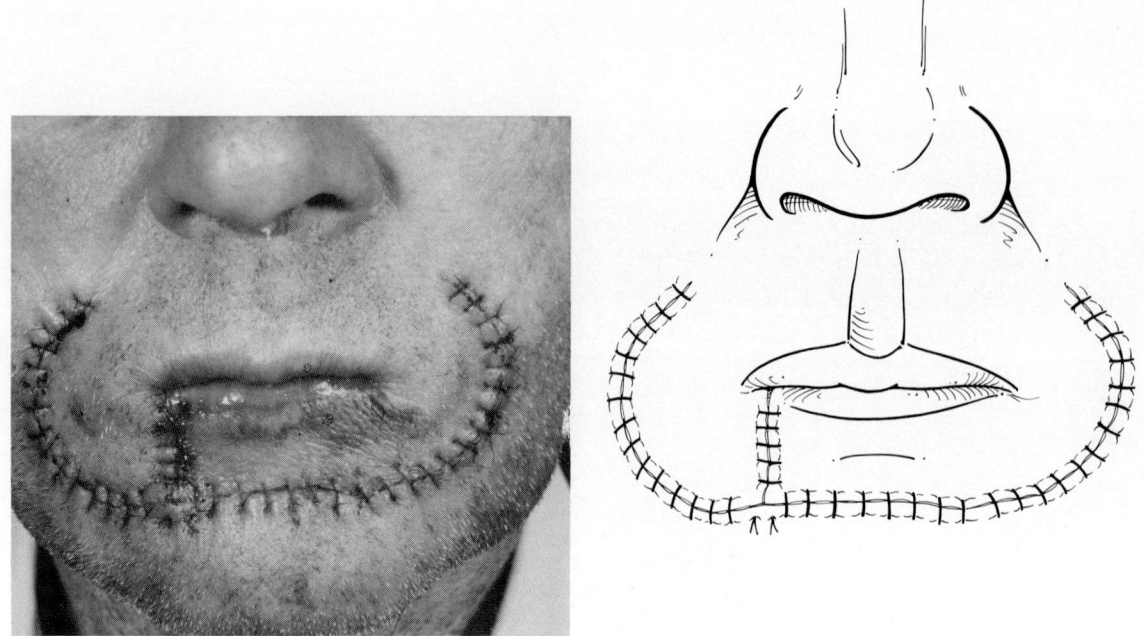

The lip reconstruction is sutured in layers.

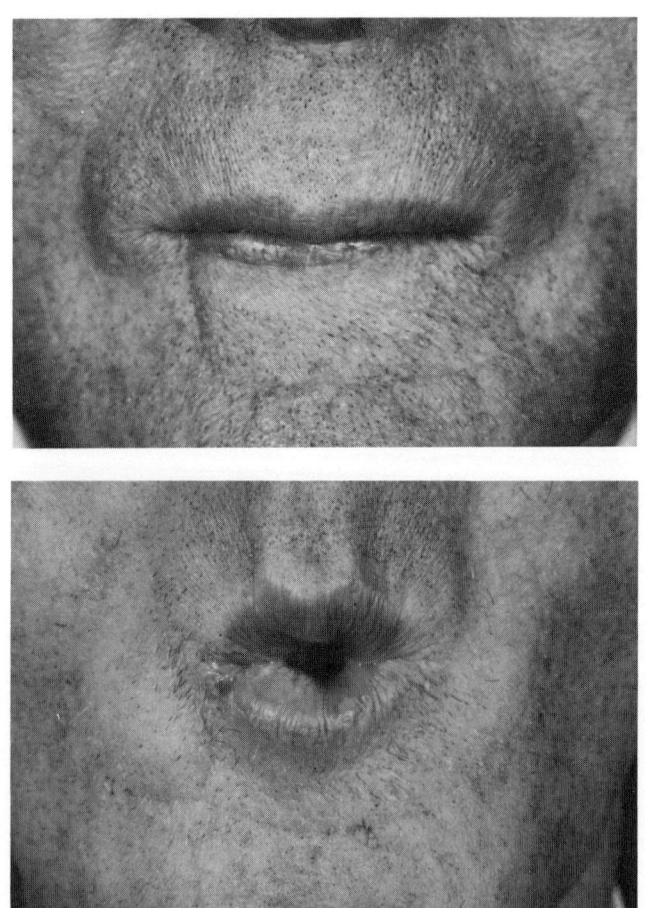

The result is a competent, sensate, fully functional lower lip with a slightly smaller oral stoma.

LOWER LIP AND CHEEK RECONSTRUCTION

When the lower lip is involved laterally and the defect extends onto the cheek, the postexcisional defect is considerable, consisting of lip and cheek. A more complex reconstruction is required. A single Karapandzic flap will close most of the lip defect, but a cheek and commissure reconstruction still needs to be done.

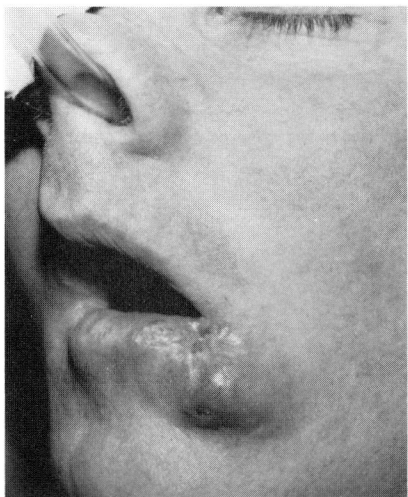

The figure above shows a patient with a recurrent squamous cell carcinoma of lip commissure and cheek.

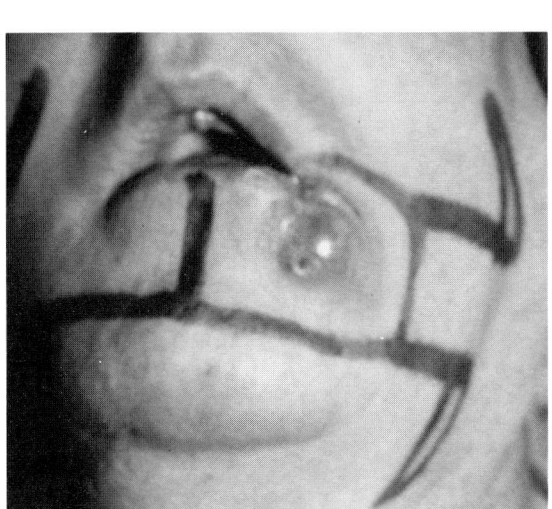
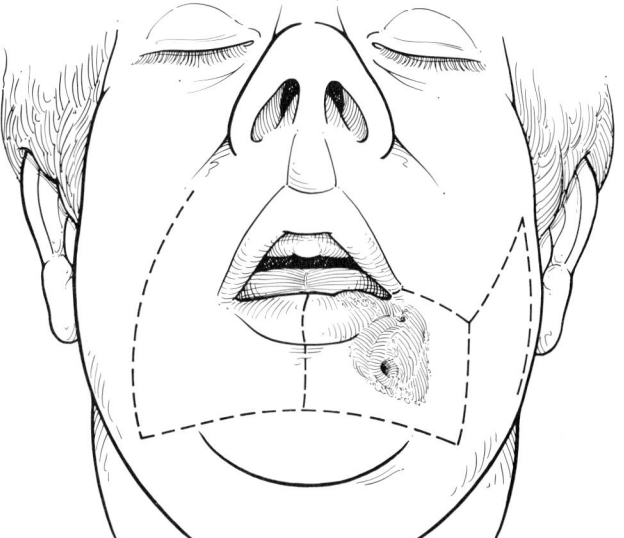

Initially, a Karapandzic flap and a Webster cheek advancement flap reconstruction was planned; the latter was changed to a rhomboid flap.

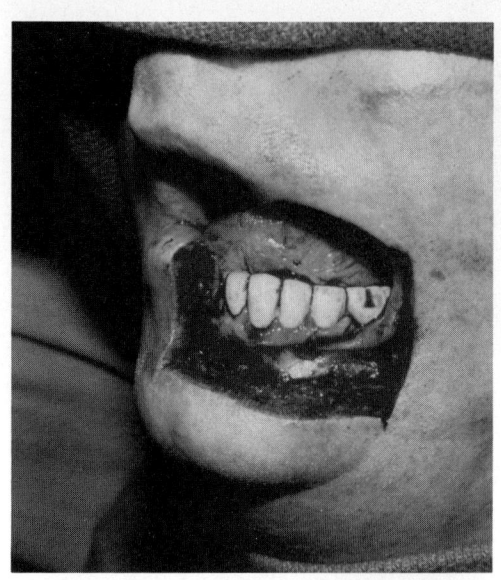

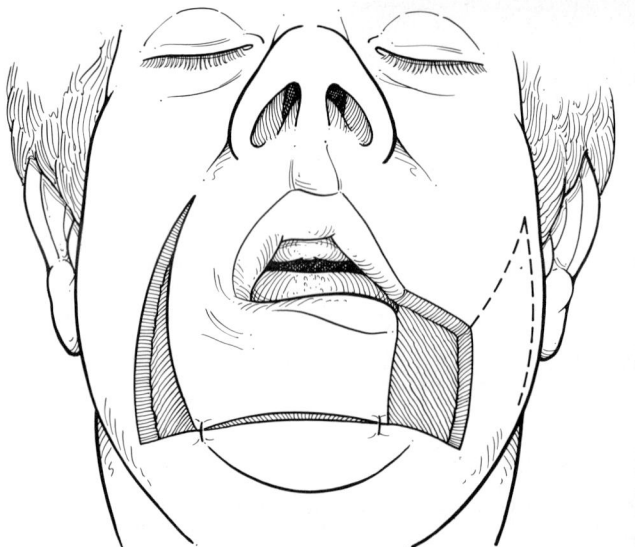
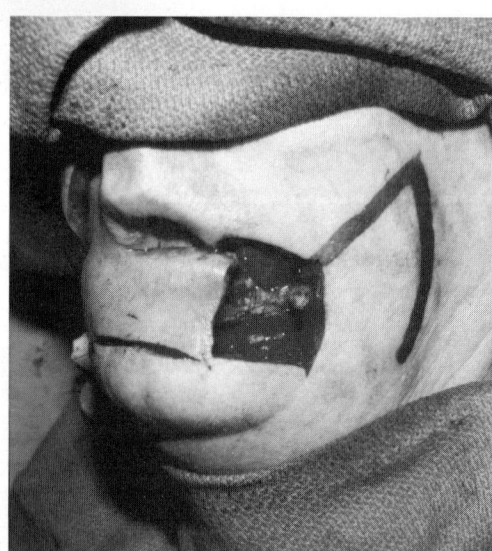

After excision of the lesion, the single Karapandzic flap can be used to reconstruct the whole lower lip.

CHAPTER 8
LIP RECONSTRUCTION

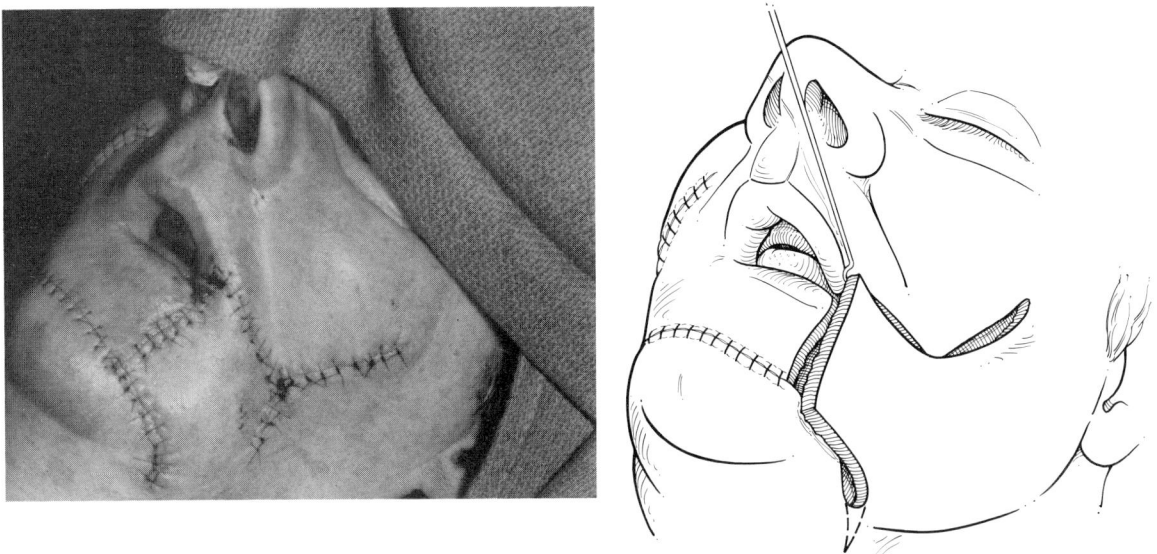

Intraoral mucosa in the cheek area could be reconstructed directly, and the skin defect was repaired with the rhomboid flap.

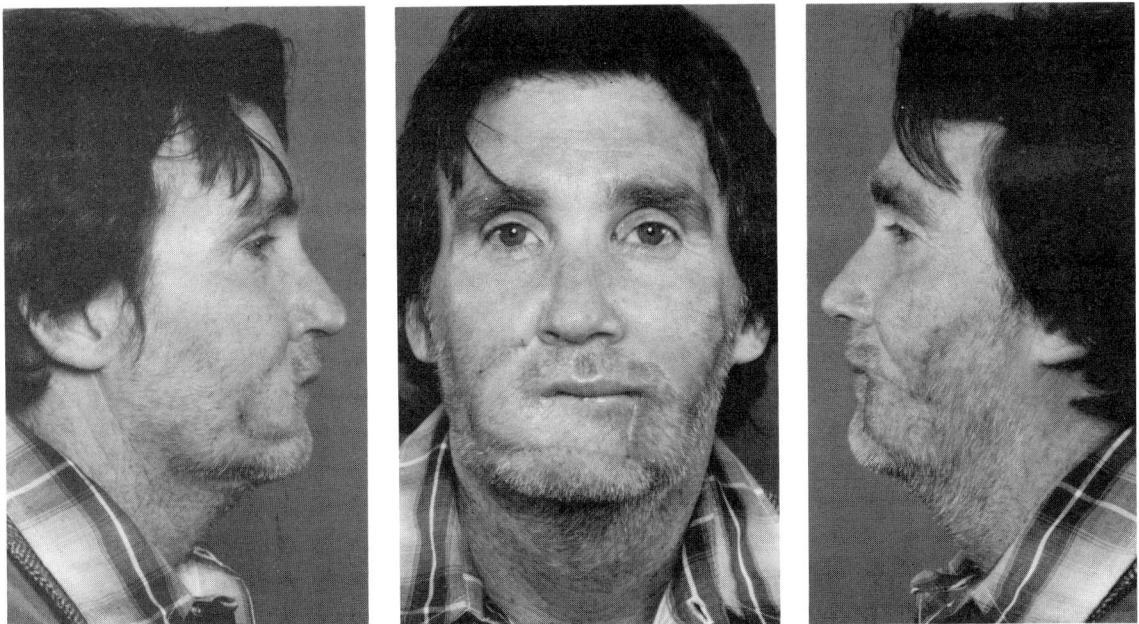

The result illustrated is early, but it is satisfactory and will improve with time, especially in relation to symmetry. Lip function is good.

385

PROBLEMS

If a single Karapandzic flap is used, asymmetry of the commissure results. Therefore this method is not recommended. However, as can be seen from the patient shown here, when one flap is used to close a defect resulting from excision of a squamous cell carcinoma, the situation improves with time.

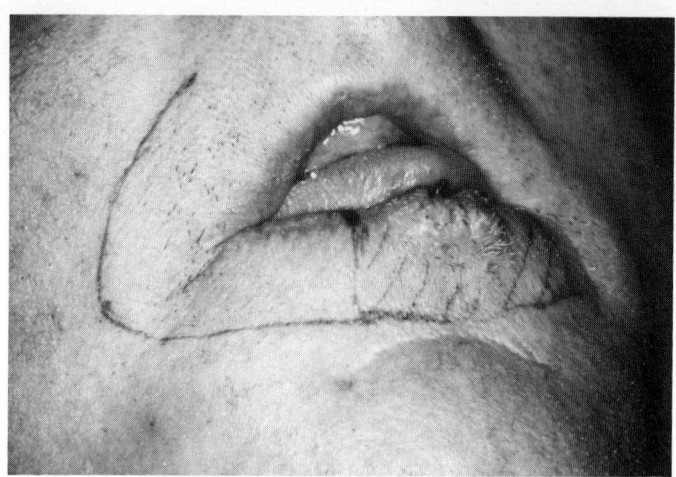

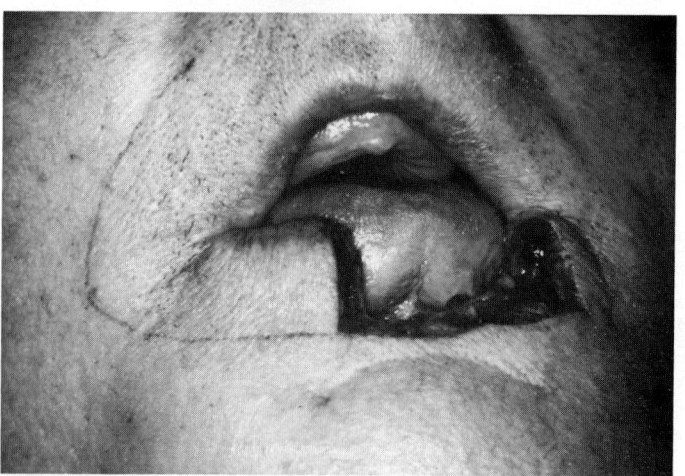

CHAPTER 8
LIP RECONSTRUCTION

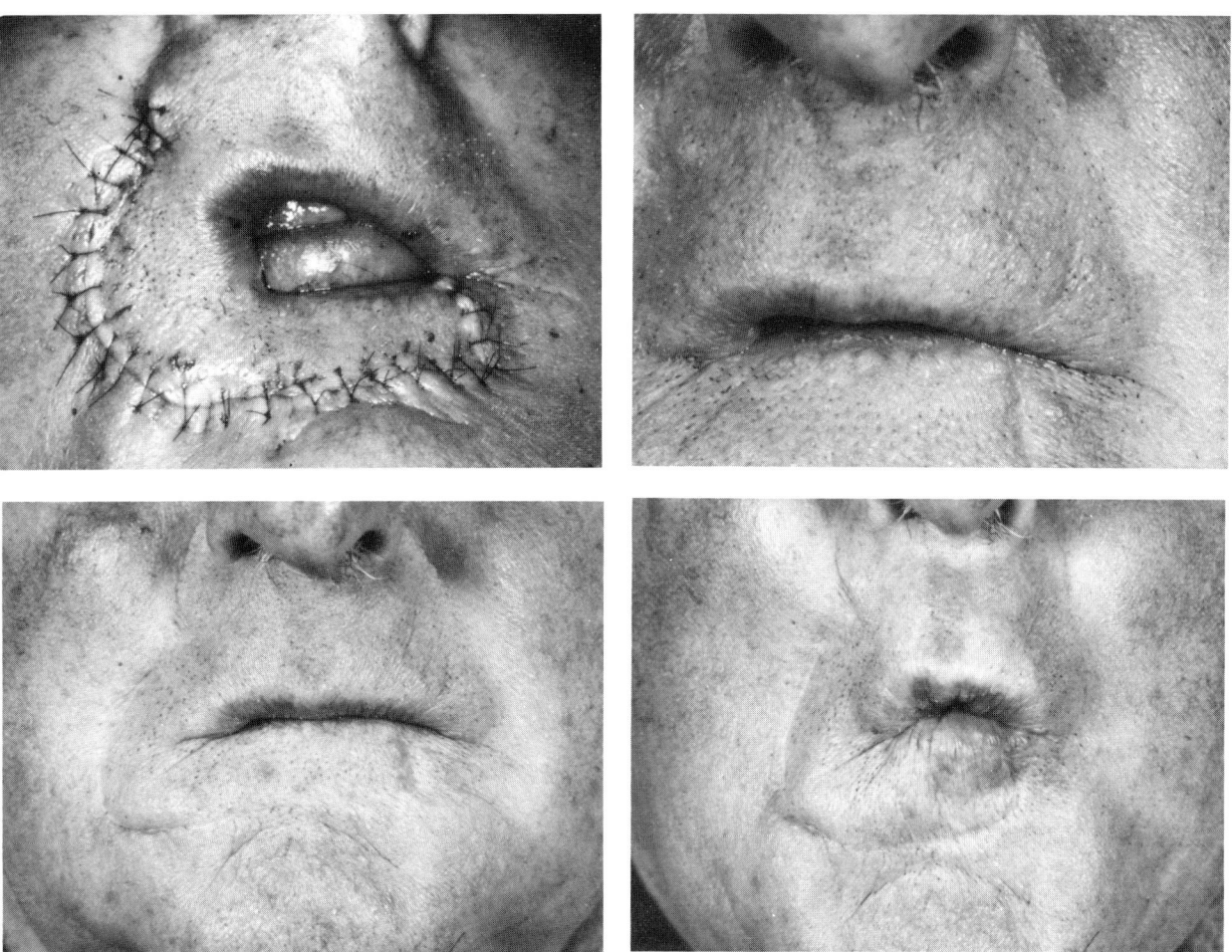

If the defect is more than three quarters of the lip length, this is not the method to use, since it results in a lower lip that is too tight, with an overhanging upper lip. Even in ideal circumstances there is some reduction in the size of the oral stoma. Patients with dentures must be instructed in how to remove and insert these appliances so that the least amount of strain is put on the lip.

Fan Flap

In 1920 Gillies[11] described a method of transposing nasolabial skin and mucosa into the lower lip by means of what he termed a fan flap. The flap base is superior, and the lateral flap is rotated to close the defect. This method has been modified in such a way that the flap is rectangular (as is the lip defect) and the pedicle is very small, containing only the labial vessels, some skin and subcutaneous tissues.

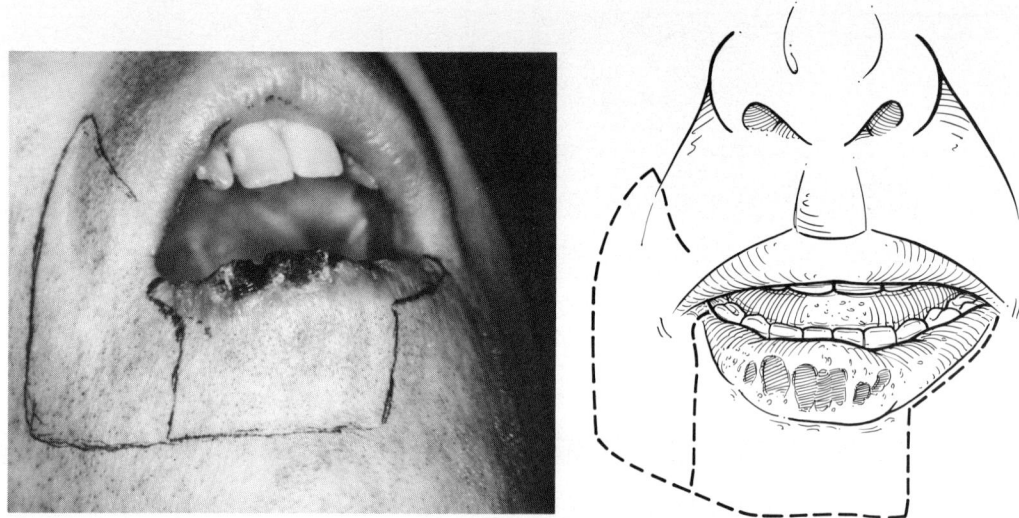

The patient presented here has a squamous cell carcinoma of the lower lip with premalignant change in the mucosa over the whole length of the lip.

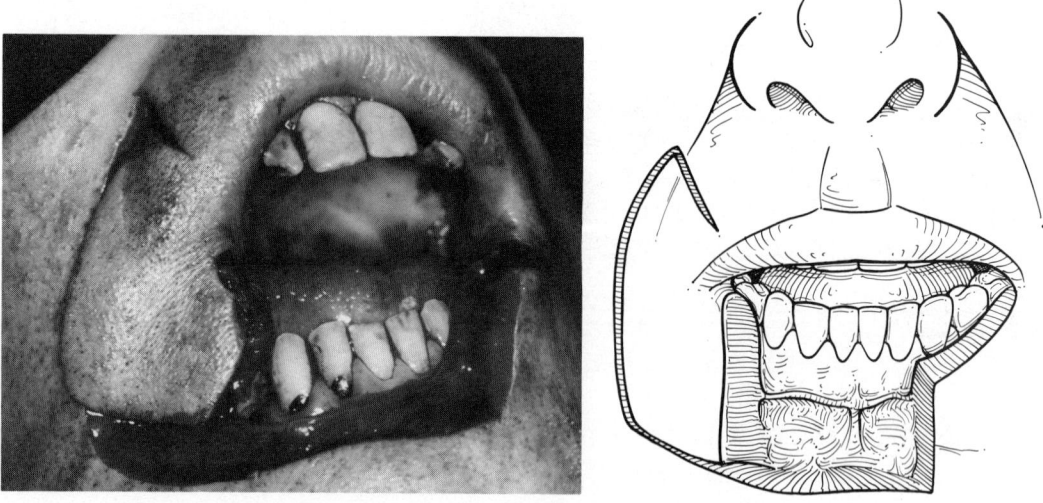

Three quarters of the lower lip is excised, and the modified fan flap is constructed.

CHAPTER 8
LIP RECONSTRUCTION

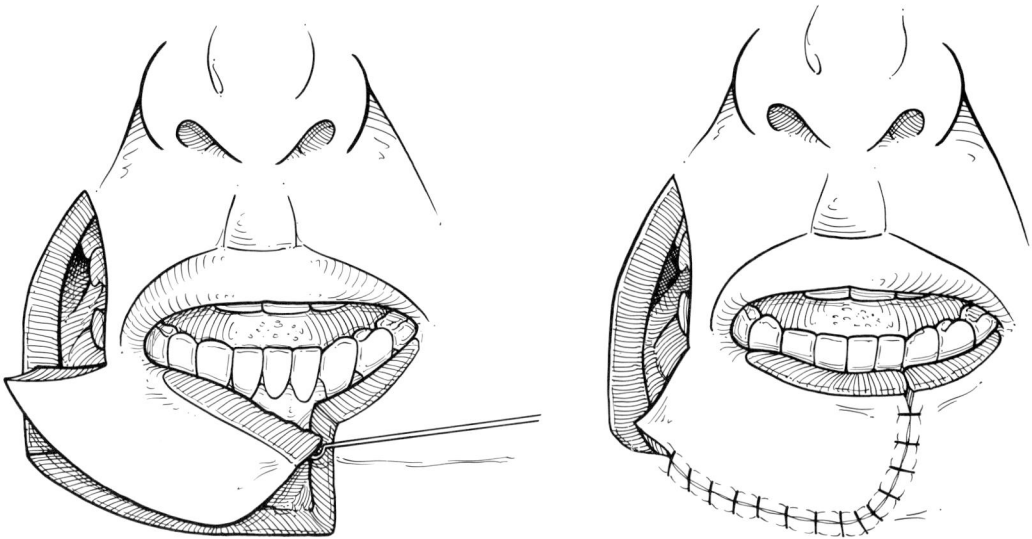

The narrow pedicle should be noted; it makes rotation easier. The lip can be reconstructed in one stage with minimal distortion of the oral commissure.

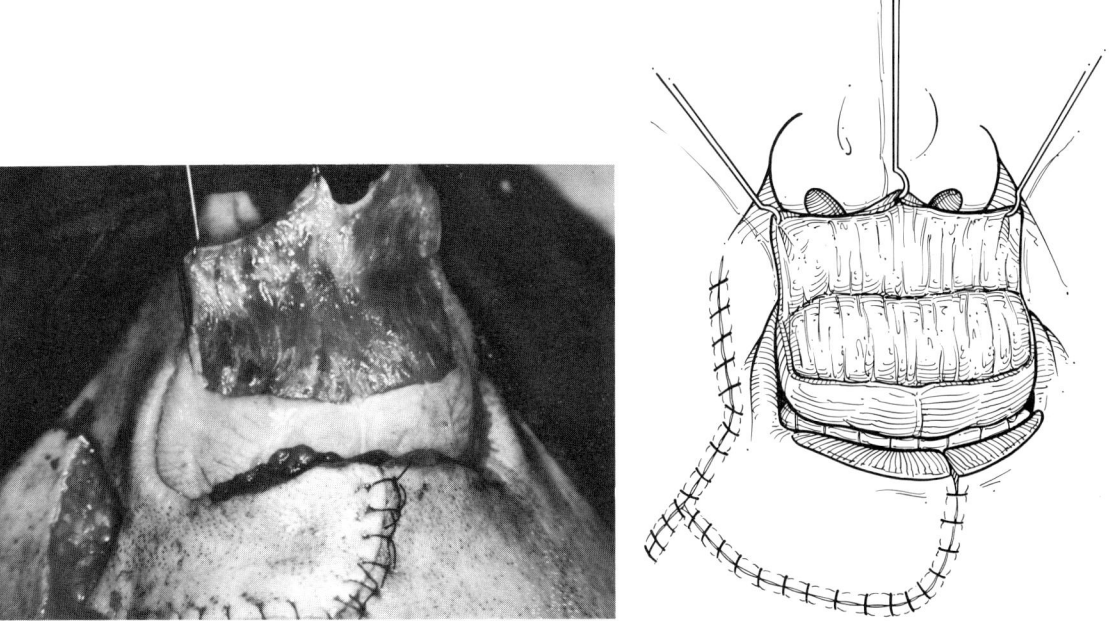

The great advantage of this method is that it does bring more tissue into the lip area. Thus there is little or no decrease in the size of the stoma. The donor defect closes directly. In the past the red margin of the newly reconstructed lip was somewhat deficient. This resulted from using mucosal advancement for red margin reconstruction. Now the inferior surface tongue flap is used to add bulk and mucosa to the new lip margin.

389

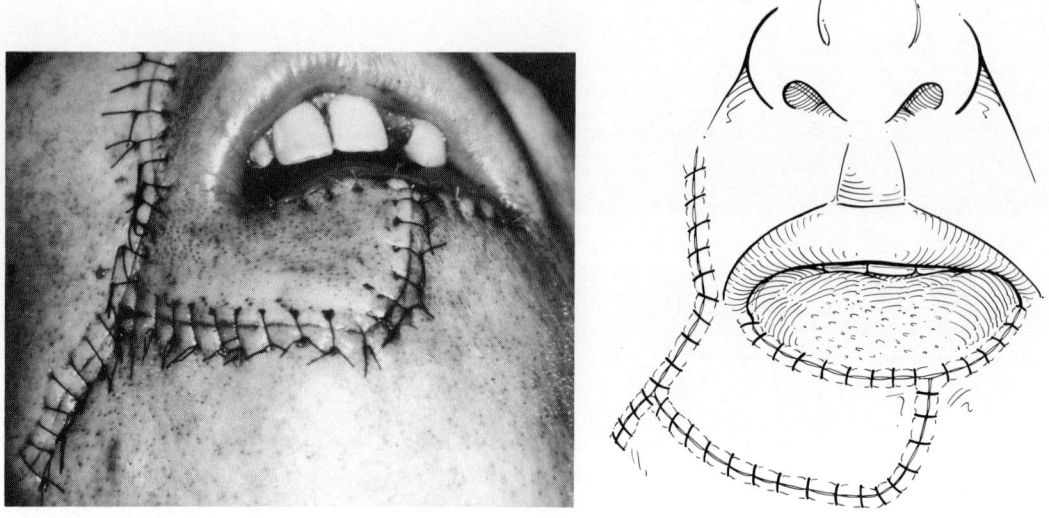

It is advisable to resurface the whole lip, since all of the mucosa is at risk.

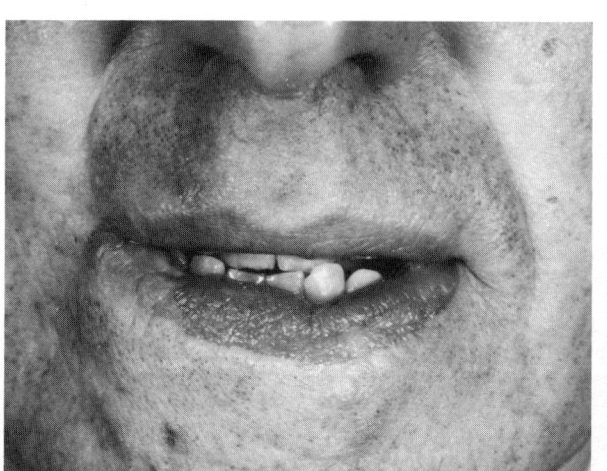
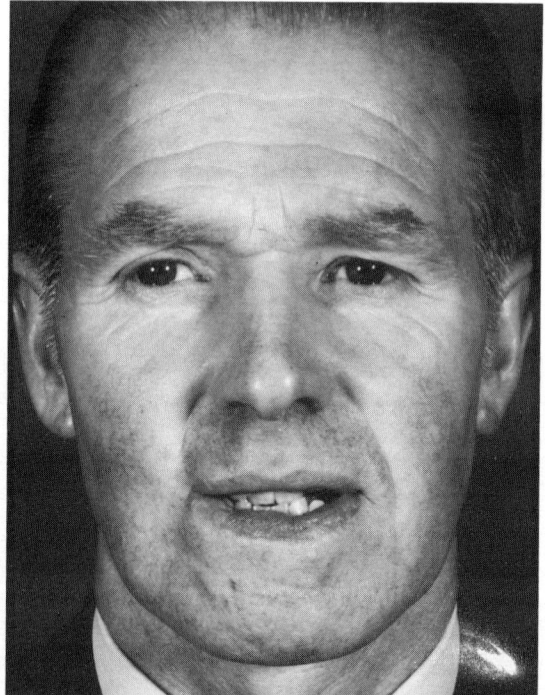

Improved aesthetic and functional results have been noted in comparison with older types of reconstruction for this problem.

PROBLEMS

With the fan flap the lip may have a degree of sensation, but little or no muscular function is present. In all but a few cases this lack of muscle function does not improve, and thus there are problems with oral competence. The flap often looks bulky and requires further procedures to deal with this. Some blunting or obliteration of the nasolabial fold almost always occurs, but this is a small price to pay for a good lip reconstruction.

Surgical Technique of Choice

Undoubtedly, the best choice in this group is the Karapandzic method. This technique is easy to perform and provides excellent results—a lip that has sensation and orbicularis function from the first postoperative day. Although the oral stoma is reduced, this rarely, if ever, causes significant problems. The cosmetic result is excellent in that the scars are good, the mouth is symmetric, and the nasolabial folds are unchanged. There is no evidence of pincushioning of the flaps. The vermilion area is normal because it has been undisturbed. In fact, the long-term results for many of the patients reveal little evidence of surgical intervention. This is the strength of the procedure, followed closely by the ease with which it can be performed.

TOTAL LOWER LIP RECONSTRUCTION

Total lower lip reconstruction varies only in degree from partial reconstruction, but the degree is significant. Since the Karapandzic method cannot be used, there is little possibility of having a truly functional and sensate lower lip. As with the upper lip, total lower lip reconstruction presents a considerable problem. In some ways it is more significant because oral competence depends greatly on a functional lower lip of an adequate height, having good muscular function and adequate sensation.

Webster Cheek Advancement Technique

The original description of the Webster cheek advancement technique[21] implies that it fulfills the criteria stated above, and on first encounter it seems ideal for total lower lip reconstruction. The problems of the tight lower lip and the overhanging upper lip, which were so ugly and characteristic of the earlier cheek advancement procedures such as the one described by Bernard,[2] appear to have been solved with this method. However, as will be seen later, it flatters to deceive.

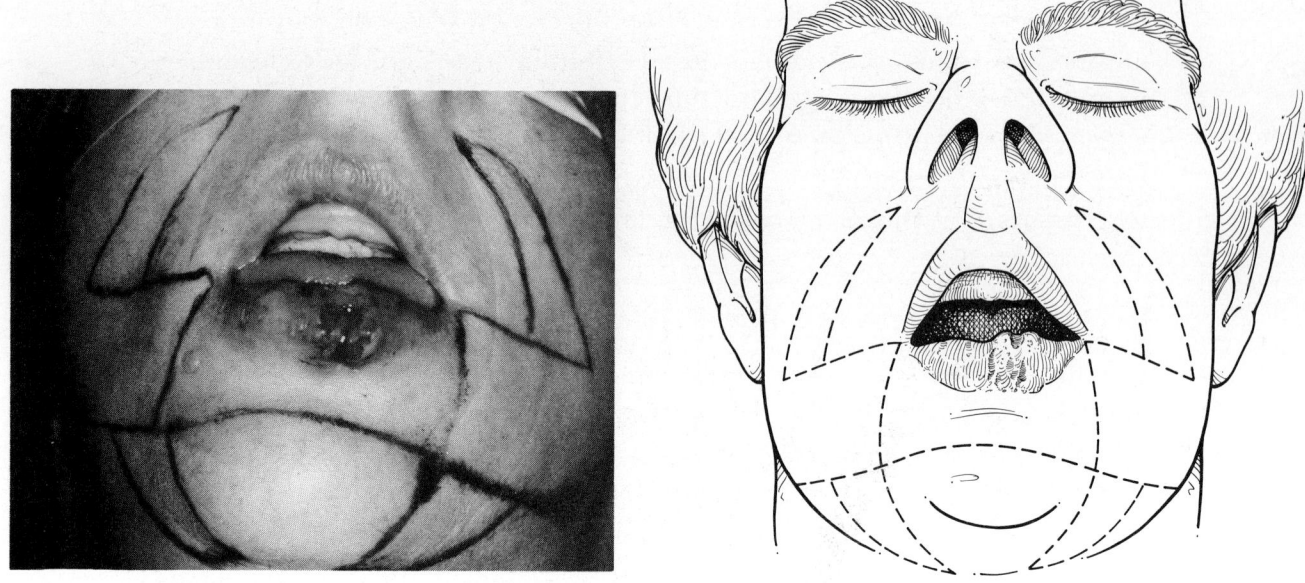

The patient shown here has an extensive lower lip squamous cell carcinoma, which requires a total lower lip resection. The Webster method of reconstruction is planned.

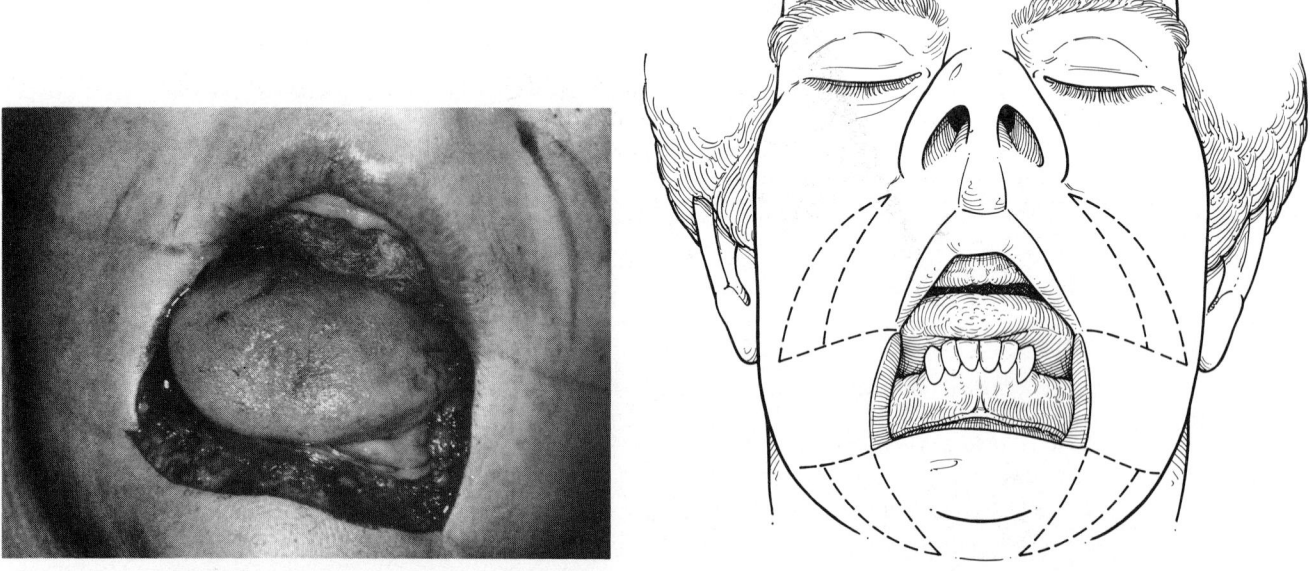

The total lower lip is resected from commissure to commissure along the lower limit of the buccal sulcus.

CHAPTER 8
LIP RECONSTRUCTION

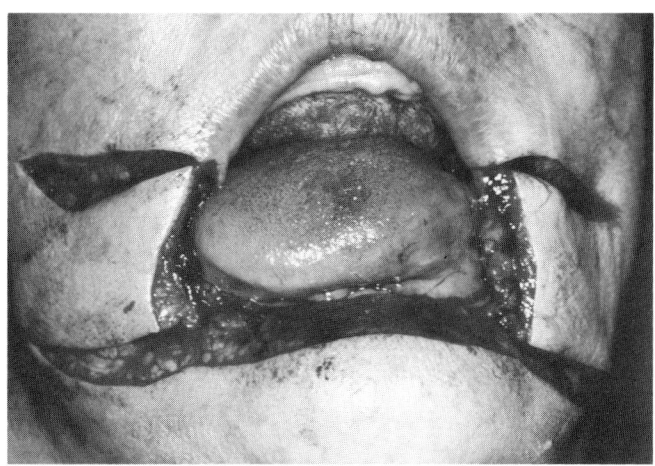

Horizontal incisions extend laterally from the commissure and from the base of the lower lip defect; they divide the orbicularis but maintain continuity of the buccinator and its nerve supply. If the flaps formed by these incisions were simply pulled together, the typical tight lower lip and excess upper lip, which has spoiled so many lower lip reconstructions, would result.

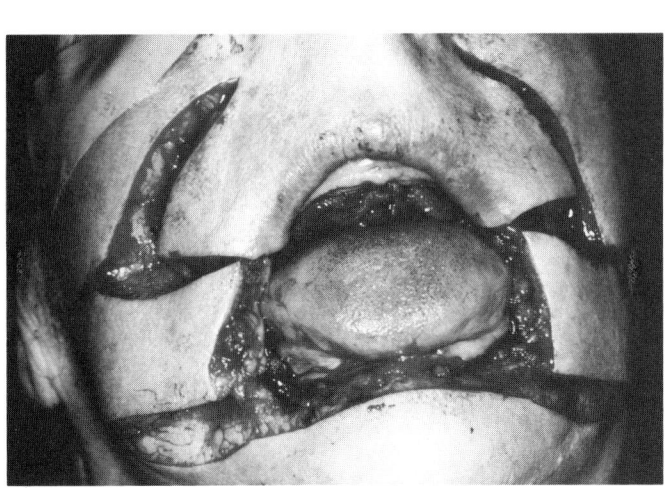

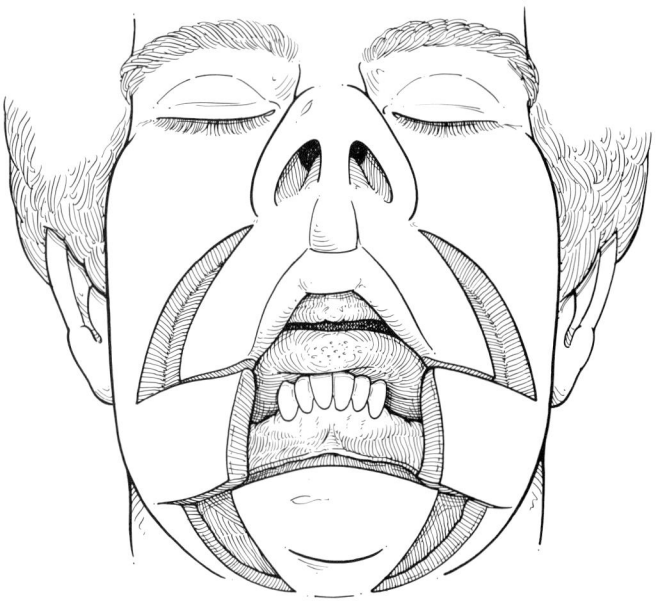

To prevent this situation from occurring and to advance the lower lip while stretching the upper lip laterally with resultant flattening of the upper lip, four Burow's triangles are excised. These are situated above and below the lateral end of the flaps and allow medial advancement to take place as the triangles are closed. The triangles are as wide as they can be to still allow closure without tension. Care is taken not to damage facial nerve branches. The mucosal incision is less extensive than the skin incision.

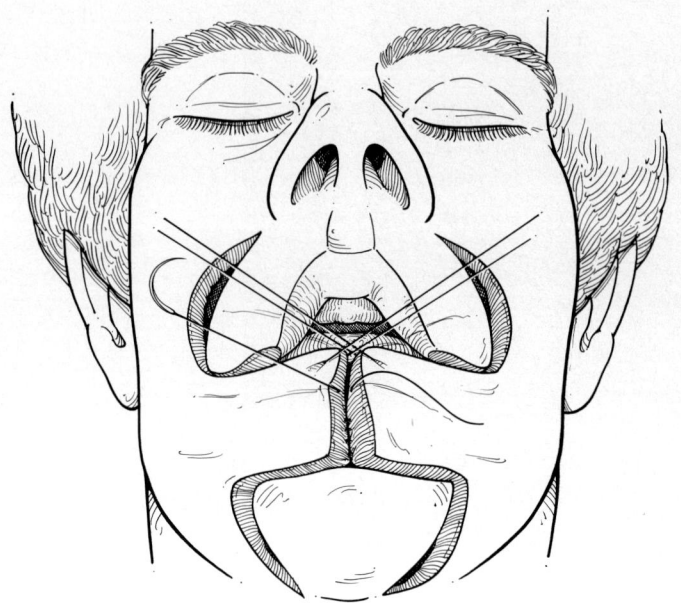

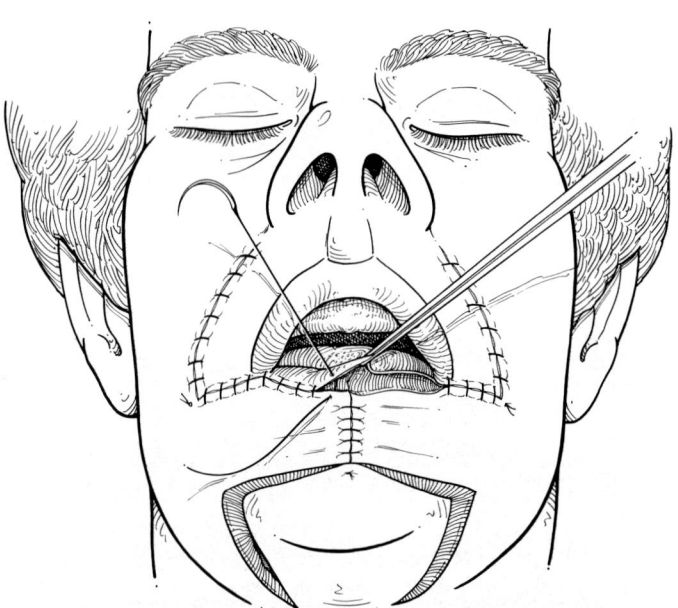

It is now possible to advance the bilateral flaps and suture them end to end in layers.

CHAPTER 8
LIP RECONSTRUCTION

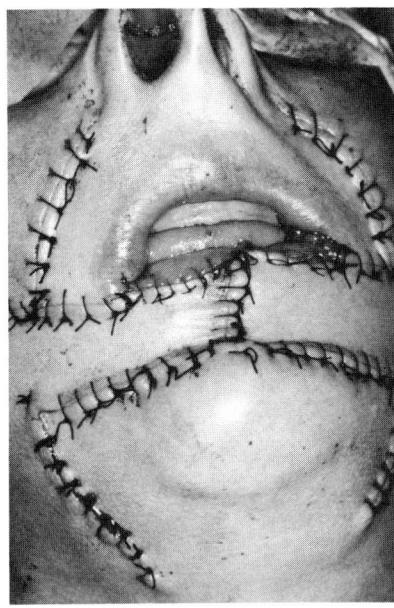 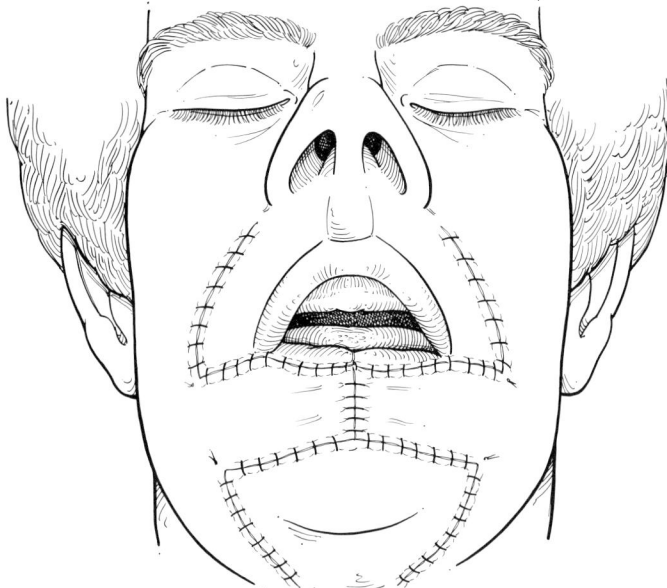

Some degree of tension in this suture line always exists. The superior and inferior triangles close as a result of the advancement and are sutured in layers. The vermilion border is recreated by mucosal advancement or, preferably, with a large tongue flap that is divided in 10 to 14 days. A tongue flap is used to provide continuity of mucosal cover and good vascularized tissue for the central flap junction area.

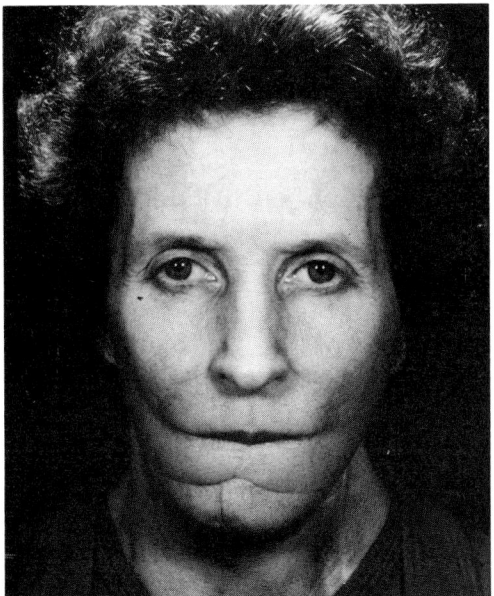 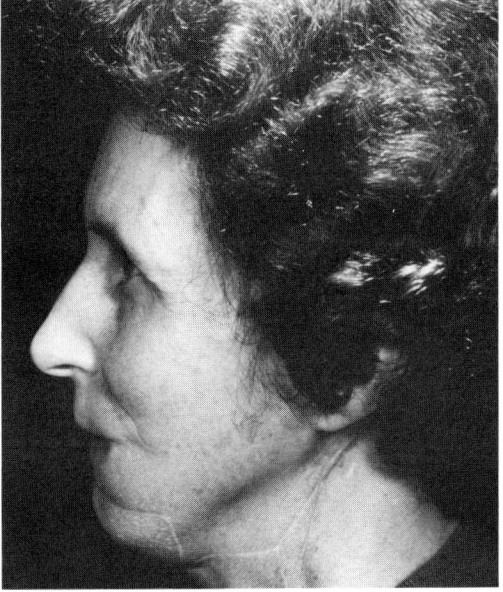

As shown here, the lower lip is somewhat tight, with reversal of lip relationships.

PROBLEMS

The Webster cheek advancement flap results in a tight lower lip and a bulky upper lip. Lower lip function is poor, resulting in less competence than is desirable. No procedure can adequately improve this situation; however, the tongue flap has overcome the mucosal deficiency so characteristic of this type of reconstruction. After initial enthusiasm for the Webster method, as with the Bernard method, it is now seldom used because of the problems outlined above. It does not meet the ideal criteria for lower lip reconstruction.

Bilateral Fan Flaps

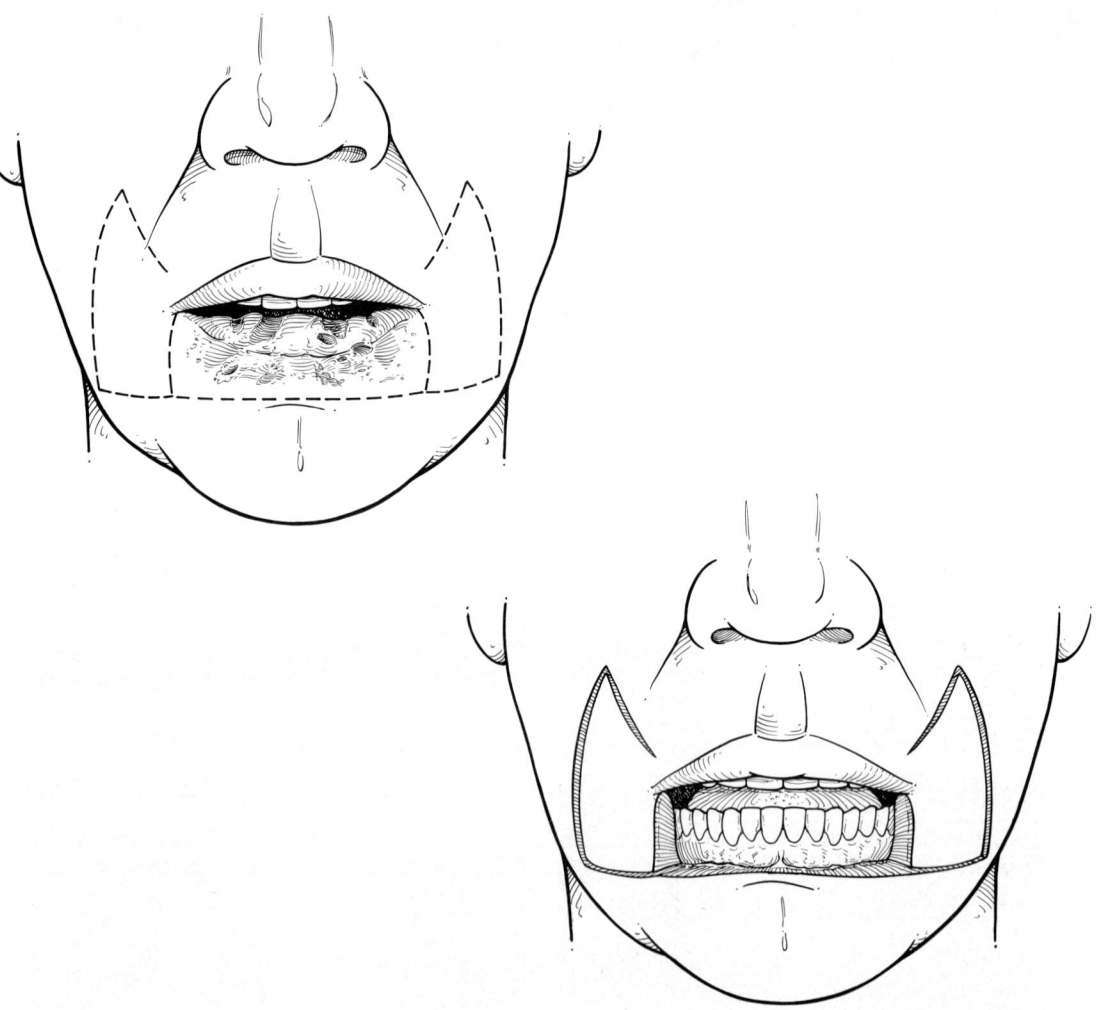

These fan flaps are constructed bilaterally, as illustrated for the unilateral fan flap.

CHAPTER 8
LIP RECONSTRUCTION

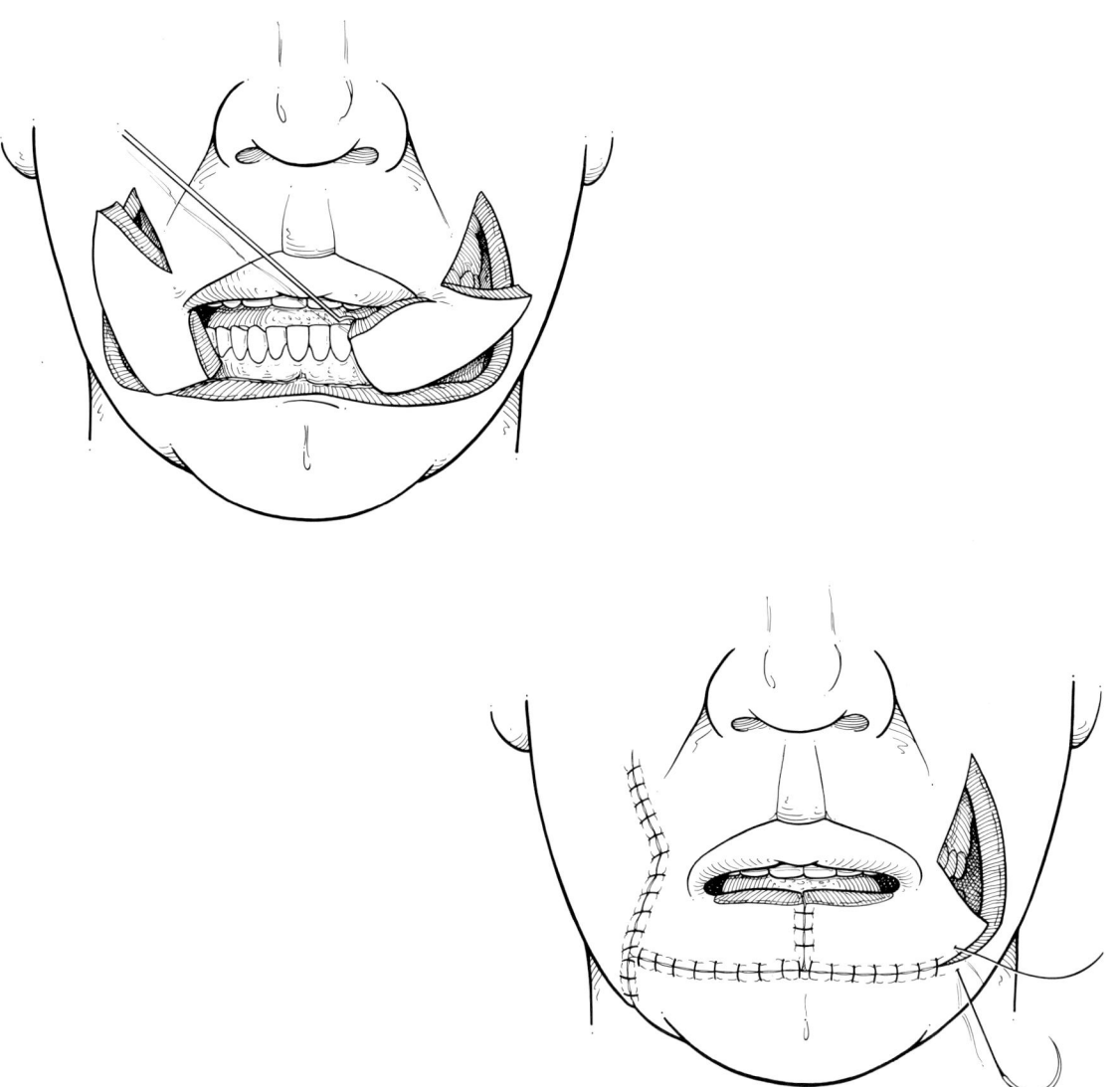

They are rotated on their pedicles and sutured end to end without tension.

397

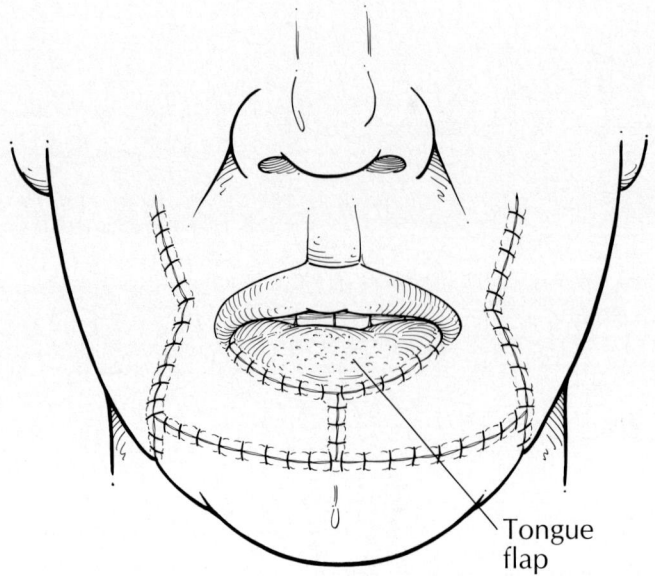

Bilateral fan flaps provide a lip of adequate bulk; the vermilion is supplied by a tongue flap, which is divided in 14 days. The donor defect can be closed directly without difficulty.

PROBLEMS

The lip created from fan flaps has little muscular function and poor sensation. It also tends to be pincushioned bilaterally. Even in the best reconstruction, there is always a degree of tightness with an excess of upper lip. In the past, when the vermilion was reconstructed by simple mucosal advancement, there was a problem with ischemia and delayed healing, with eventual notching where the four suture lines met in the midpoint of the reconstructed lip. This problem has been obviated by the use of the tongue flap, which, in addition to adding bulk for the vermilion, increases the vascularity of that area. Since the tongue flap has been used, ischemia and necrosis in this region has not been a problem. There is bilateral ablation of the nasolabial folds.

Surgical Technique of Choice

Undoubtedly, the bilateral fan flap and tongue flap reconstruction gives the best lower lip. This method brings in new tissue for lip reconstruction. The result is a lip that is bulkier and less tight than with other methods. Unfortunately, however, there is no ideal method for producing a sensate mobile lower lip to give normal competence to the mouth.

☐ Commissure Defects

Commissure defects often result from division of an old electrical burn or posttraumatic contractures. Reconstruction of the commissure is complex, both aesthetically and functionally. The normal contralateral commissure remains for comparison with the reconstruction; unfortunately asymmetry is common. Poor muscle reconstruction results in drooling and excoriation of the corner of the mouth.

MUCOSAL DEFECTS

Rhomboid Flaps

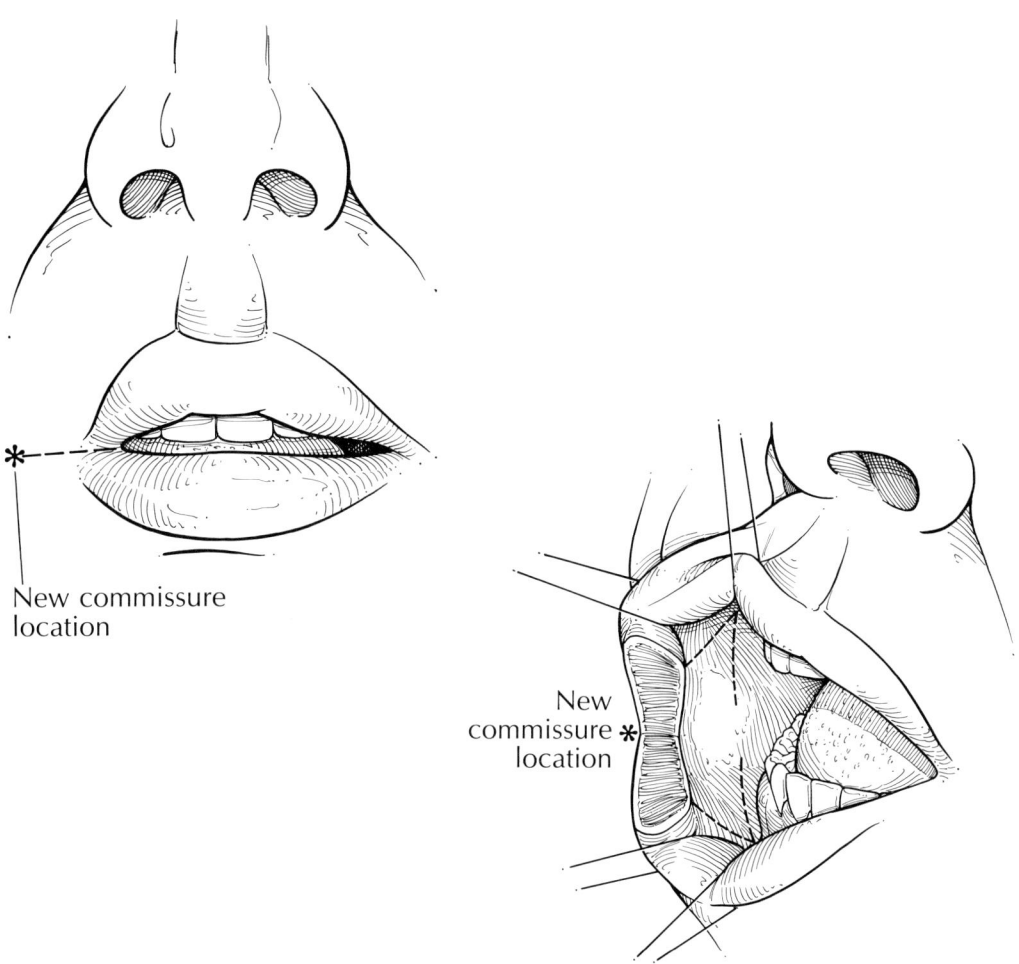

The position of the new commissure is marked in order to allow for some overcorrection. Division of the contracture forms two raw areas that are approximately two rhomboids, making the mucosal rhomboid flap the obvious choice for reconstruction.

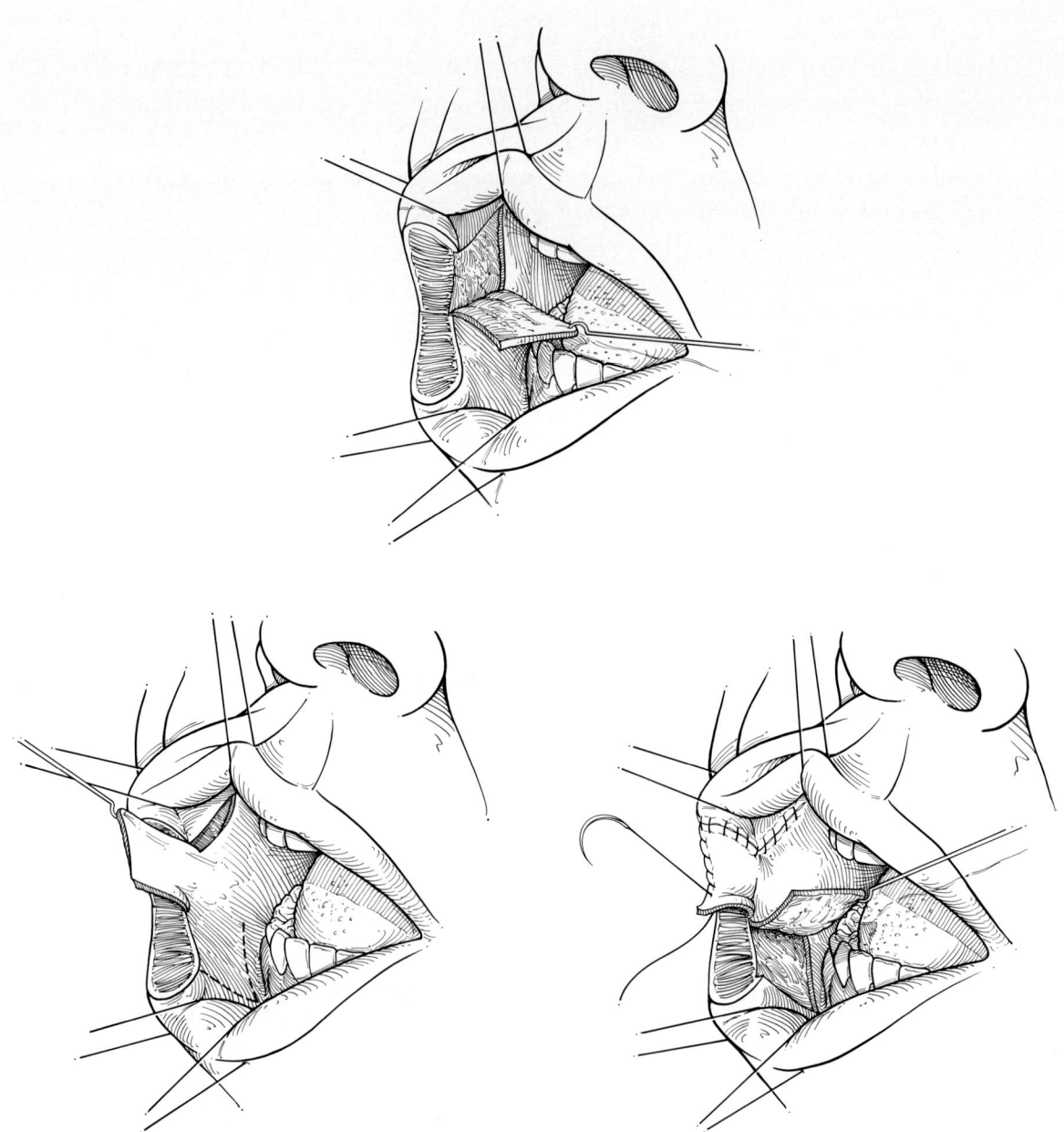

These flaps are constructed on a 120-degree angle (as described in Chapter 1). The flaps are rotated laterally to reconstruct the angle.

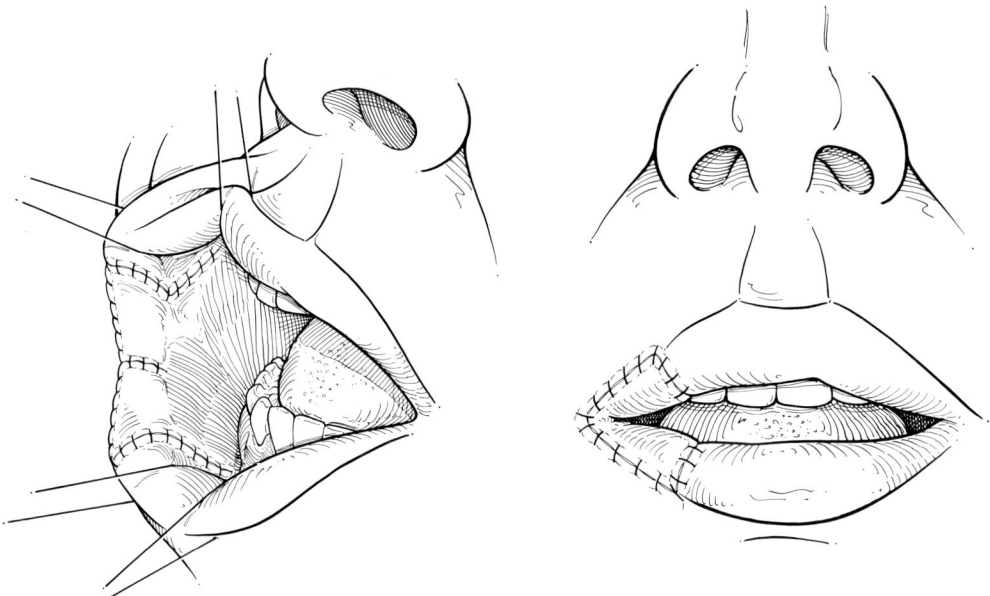

The donor sites are easily closed by direct suture.

Recently some aggressive splinting techniques have been introduced that may reduce the necessity for surgical correction of commissure contraction.

PROBLEMS

By and large, the results are satisfactory. Some contracture may take place because of the multiple suture lines, resulting in pincushioning and a partial recurrence of the deformity. Irregularity of the mucocutaneous junction also may occur, and this problem may be difficult to correct.

Tongue Flaps

If the mucosal defect is thick in the region of the commissure (for example, resection with skin flap reconstruction), tongue flaps can supply an adequate reconstruction. A flap based anteriorly on the side of the tongue can be raised and split to be inserted into the anterior portion of the commissural defect. In 10 days the flap is divided and inset into the apex of the commissure.

Another method is to raise two long posteriorly based flaps from the side of the tongue. These are rotated and sutured into the raw areas on the lips. Again, these flaps are divided in 10 days.

PROBLEMS

Tongue flaps are bulky; the color and texture are different from the normal lip mucosa. The method is technically difficult and should be used only in very unusual circumstances, as described below.

FULL-THICKNESS DEFECT OF COMMISSURE

Double Skin and Mucosal Rhomboid Flaps

The results of this technique have been consistently satisfactory as compared to other techniques. Commissural lesions can be excised in such a manner as to create rhomboid defects on the upper and lower lips.

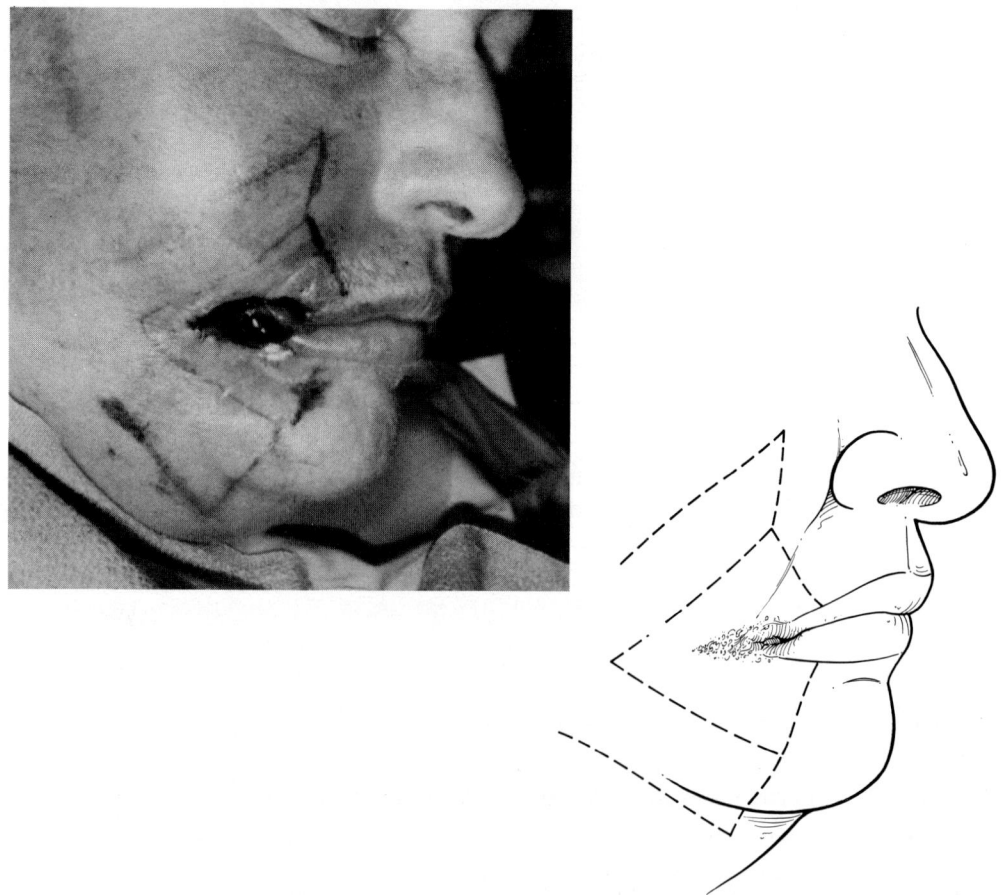

The patient shown here has a basal cell carcinoma of the oral commissure. From the 120-degree angles, rhomboid flaps are constructed.

CHAPTER 8
LIP RECONSTRUCTION

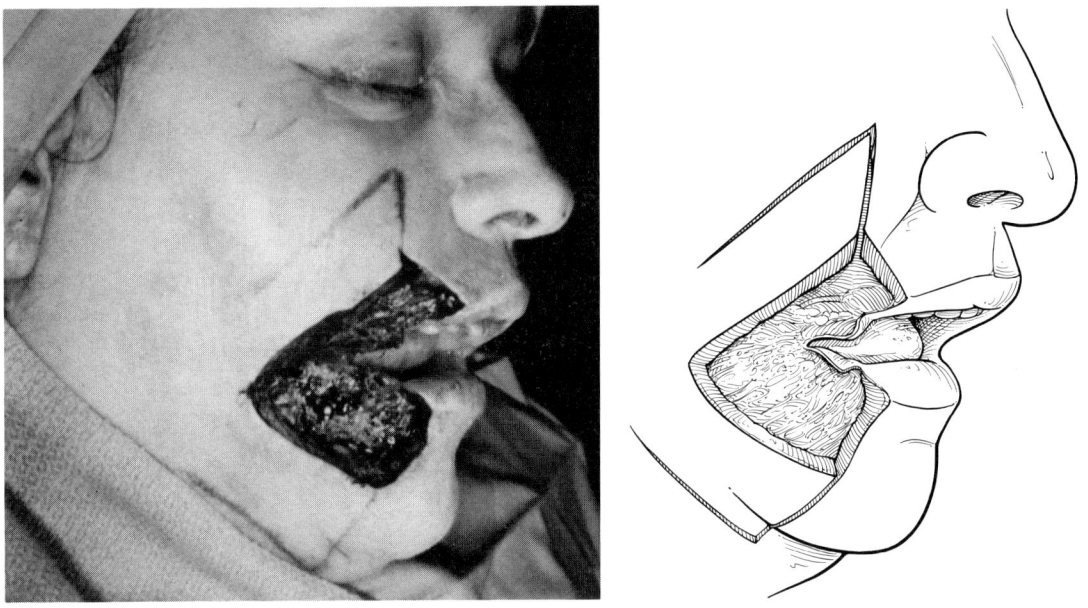

The defect is created and the rhomboid flaps are raised. These flaps may consist of skin only or skin and mucosa if necessary.

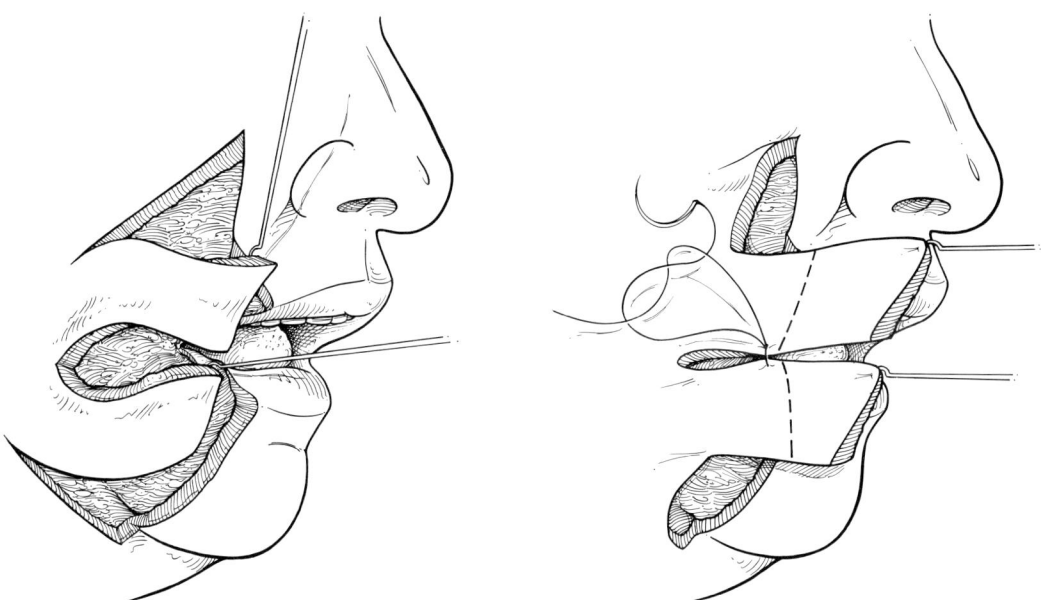

The 120-degree angles are moved together and sutured to form the commissure. Some adjustment may be necessary to place the commissure in the desired position.

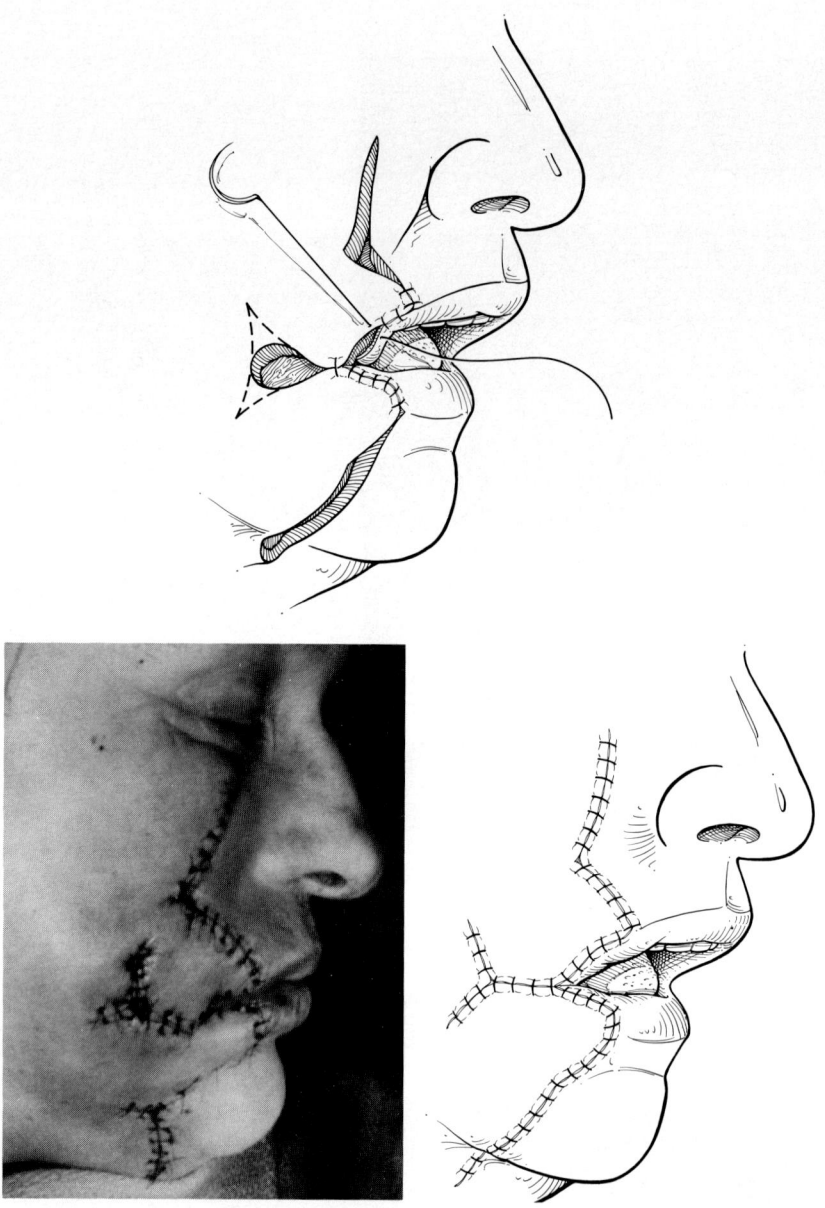

The defects on the lip and the cheek are closed directly after the commissure is formed. Raw edges remain on the reconstructed upper and lower lips; these raw areas are closed with mucosal advancement or mucosa rhomboids, as described earlier.

CHAPTER 8
LIP RECONSTRUCTION

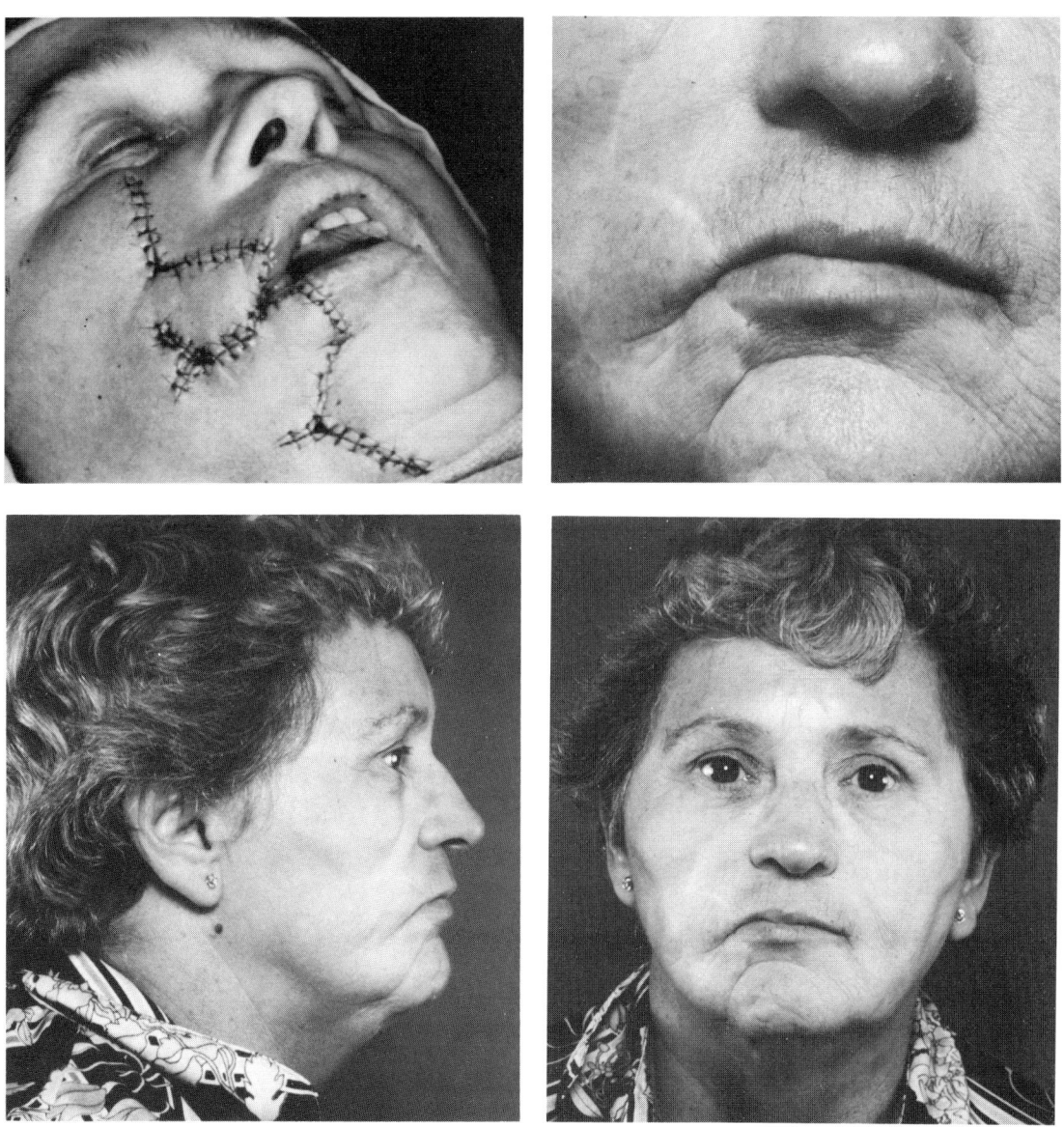

Although slight pincushioning occurs, symmetry and function are both good.

405

Double Skin Rhomboid Flaps and Tongue Flaps

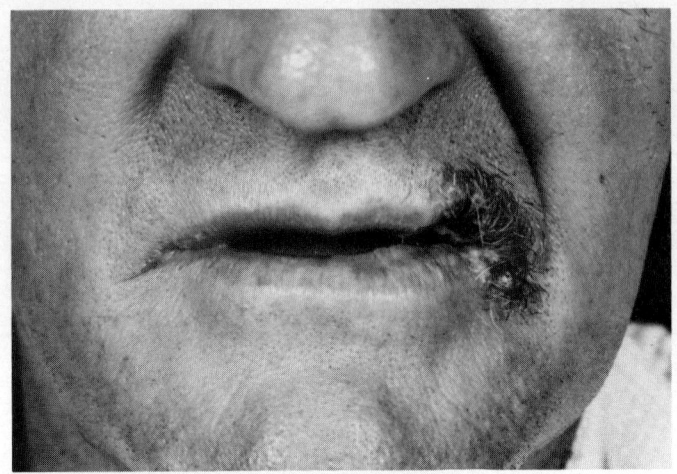

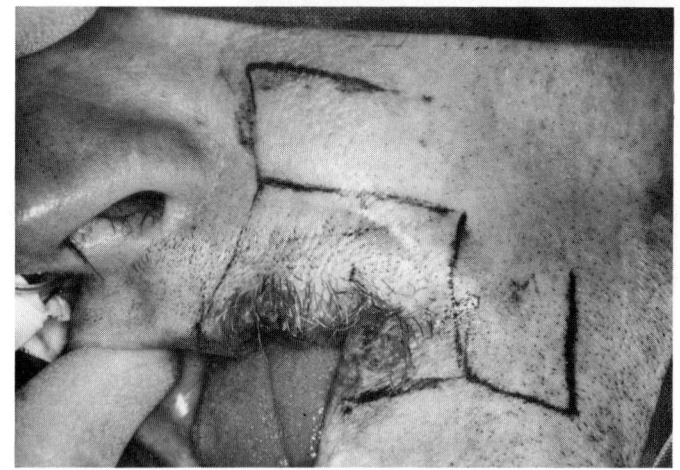

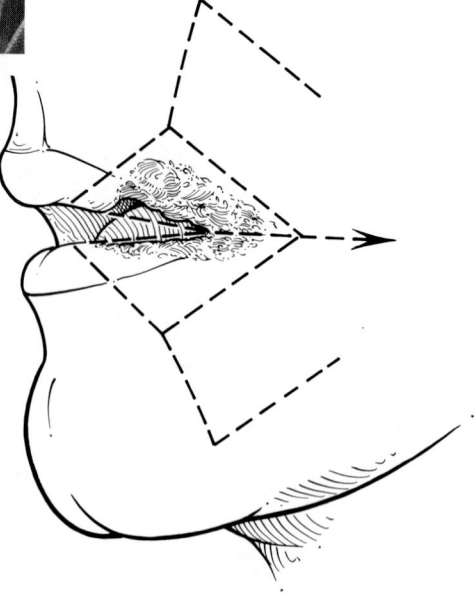

A double rhomboid defect is created by excision of a recurrent squamous cell carcinoma of the commissure.

CHAPTER 8
LIP
RECONSTRUCTION

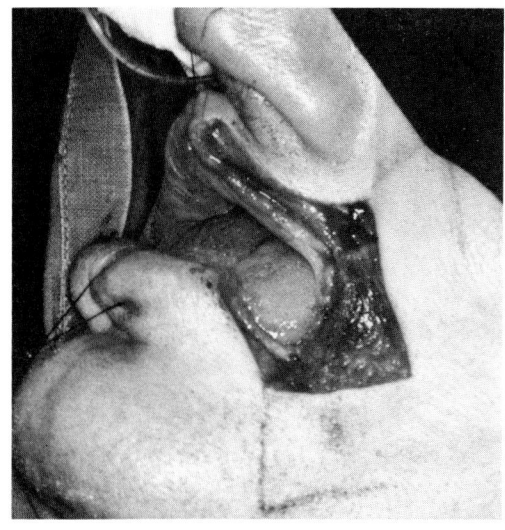

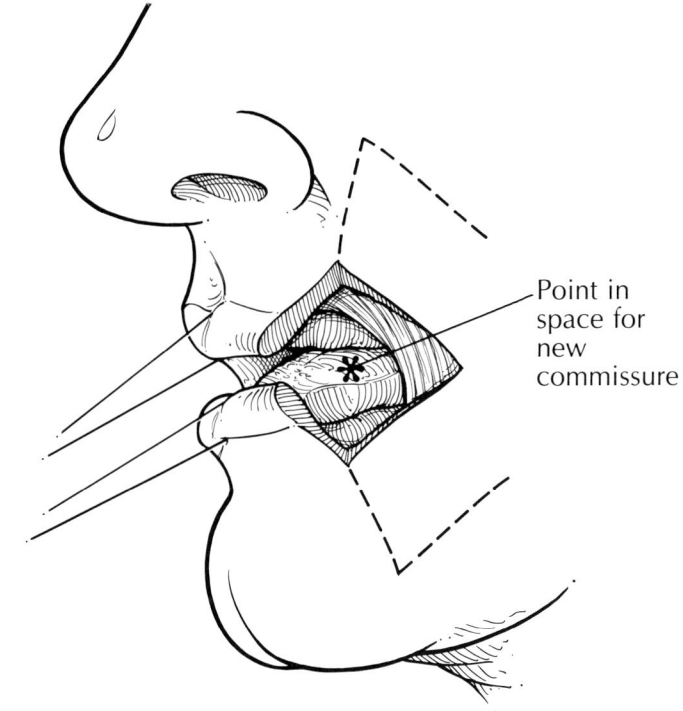

Point in space for new commissure

After excision, a full-thickness commissure defect is created. Rhomboid flaps are raised and rotated to close the defect and form the commissure.

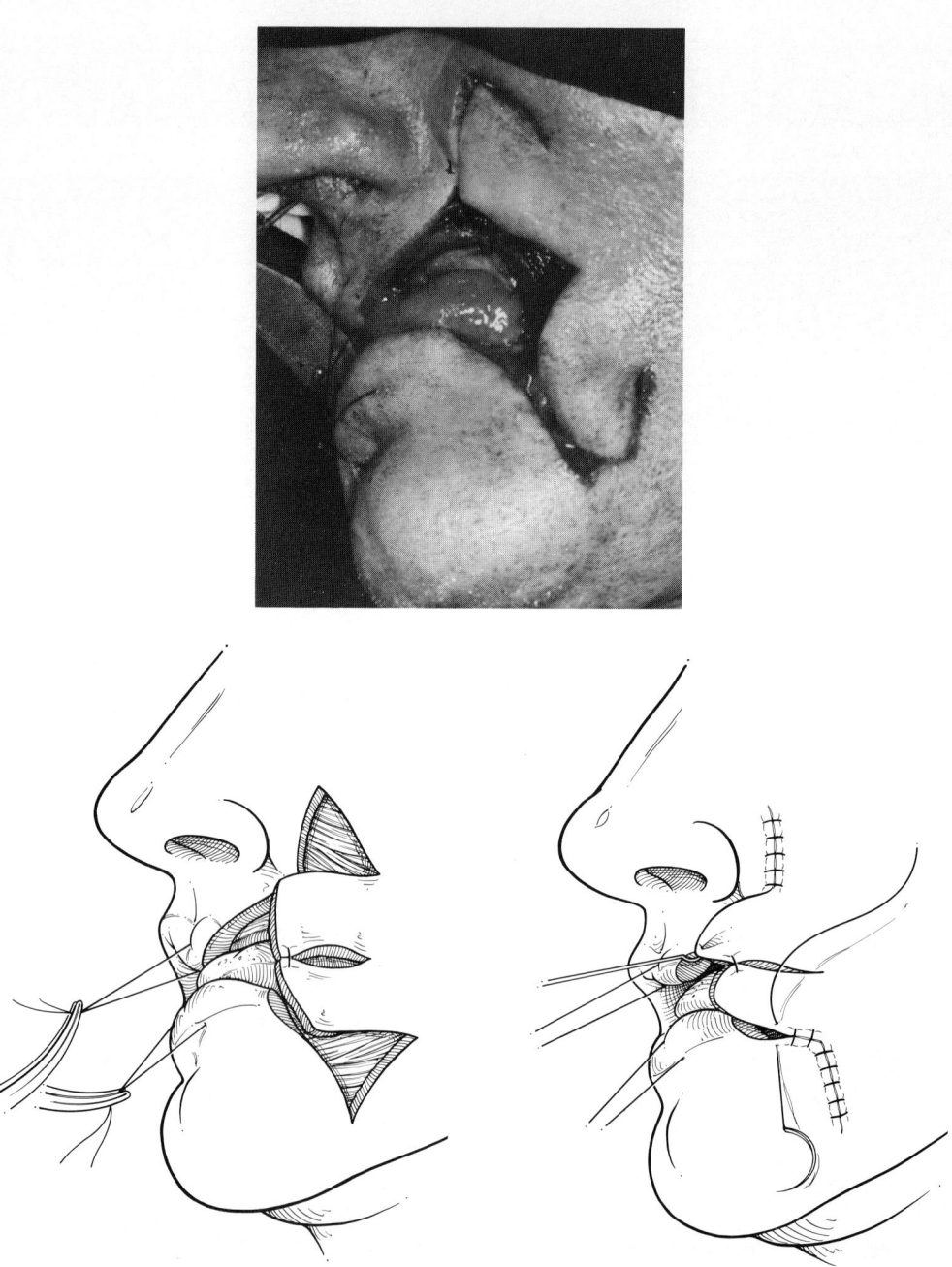

The flap is trimmed to obtain the ideal shape and position.

CHAPTER 8
LIP RECONSTRUCTION

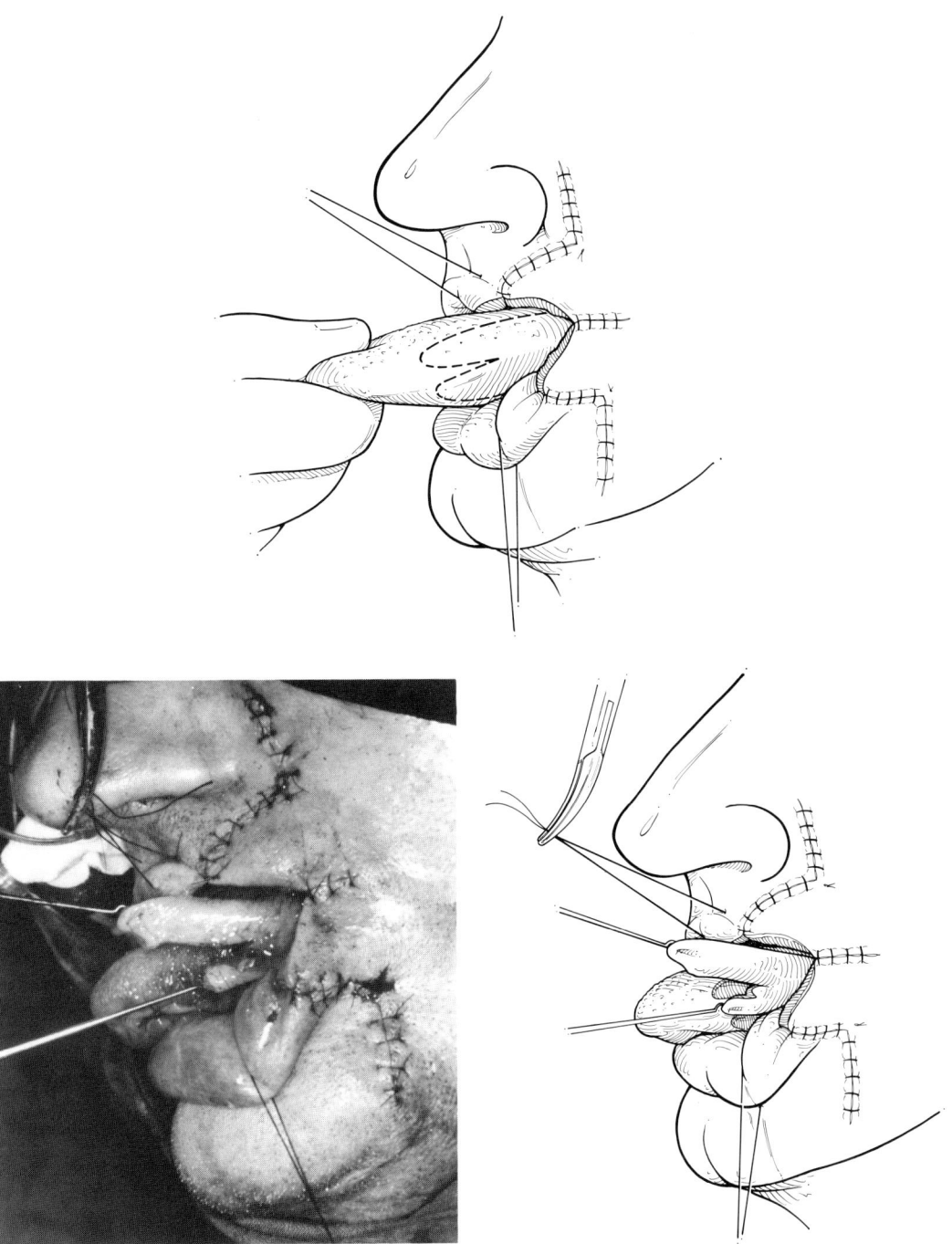

From the lateral side of the tongue, a flap is elevated, split in the midline, rotated, and used for the mucosa of the lips and commissure.

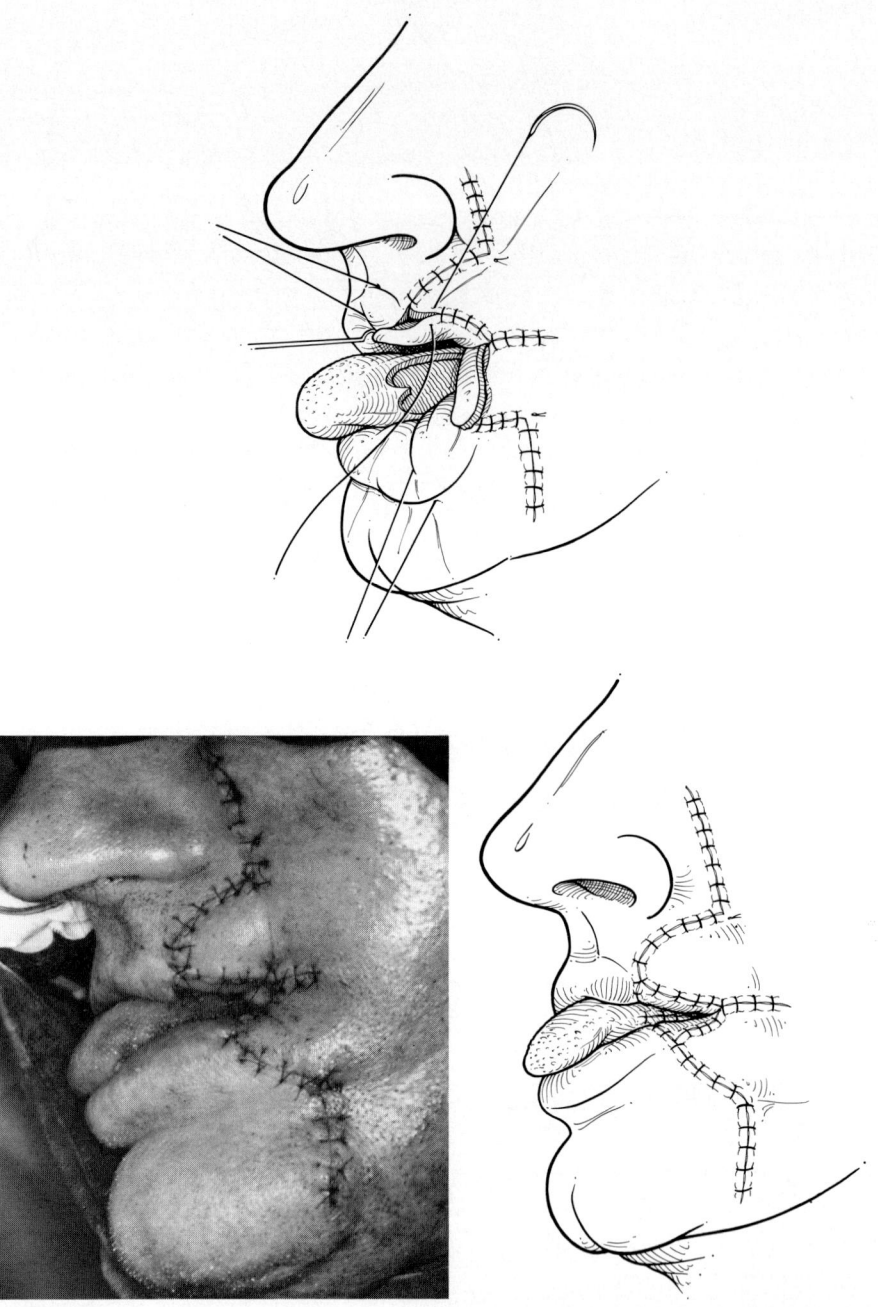

Ten days later the pedicle is divided, with the patient under local anesthesia.

PROBLEMS

Generally, the results of this technique are satisfactory. However, it is sometimes difficult to achieve a satisfactory skin-vermilion junction. In addition, a slight blunting of the commissure often occurs. These problems can be partially corrected later by a secondary procedure.

Apart from loss of definition of the commissure, pincushioning of the flaps, and occasional loss of competence at the oral angle, this has been a good method of reconstruction.

SURGICAL TECHNIQUE OF CHOICE

If buccal mucosal flaps can be used, these are preferable to tongue flaps because the latter involves a two-stage procedure that is technically more difficult. Only where significant bulk is required should tongue flaps be considered.

REFERENCES

1. Abbe, R.: A new plastic operation for the relief of deformity due to double harelip, Med. Rec. **53:**477, 1898.
2. Bernard, C.: Cancer de la levre inferieure; restauration à l' aide de deux lambeaux-lateraux quadrilataires, guerison. Bull. Mem. Soc. Chir., Paris, 1853.
3. Briedis, J., and Jackson, I.T.: The anatomy of the philtrum: observations made on dissection in the normal lip, Br. J. Plast. Surg. **34:**128, 1980.
4. Buck, G.: History of a case in which a series of plastic operations was successfully performed for the restoration of the right half of the upper lip and adjacent portions of the cheek and nose. Trans. Med. Soc. N.Y. State, p. 173, 1864.
5. Estlander, J.A.: En ny operationsmetod att atersralla en forstord lapp ellekkind, Finsak Lak-Sall SK Handl. **14:**1, 1872.
6. Fara, M.: Anatomy and arteriography of cleft lips in stillborn children, Plast. Recontr. Surg. **42:**29, 1968.
7. Fara, M.: The anatomy of cleft lip, Clin. Plast. Surg. **2:**205, 1975.
8. Fara, M.: The musculature of cleft lip and palate. In Converse, J.M., editor: Reconstructive plastic surgery, Philadelphia, 1977, W.B. Saunders Co.
9. Fara, M.: Functional anatomy of lip and palate and its application to cleft lip and palate surgery. In Jackson, I.T., editor: Recent advances in plastic surgery, ed. 2, Edinburgh, 1981, Churchill Livingstone.
10. Fara, M., Chlumsk, A., and Hrivnakova, J.: Musculis orbicularis oris in incomplete harelip, Acta. Chir. Plast. **7:**125, 1965.
11. Gillies, H.D.: Plastic surgery of the face, London, 1920, Frowde. Hodder & Stoughton, Oxford University Press.
12. Guerrero-Santos, J., Vasquez-Pallares, R., Vera-Strathmann, A., Machain, P., and Castaneda, A.: Tongue flap in reconstruction of the lip, Trans. Third Int. Congress Plastic Surgeons, Amsterdam, 1964, Excerpta Medica Foundation.
13. Jackson, I.T.: The use of tongue flaps to resurface lip defects and close palatal fistulae in children, Plast. Reconstr. Surg. **49:**537, 1972.
14. Jackson, I.T., and Sieber, H.: Closure of large anterior palatal fistulae using a tongue flap, Chir. Plastica **1:**313, 1973.

15. Kapetansky, D.I.: Double pendulum flaps for whistling deformities in bilateral cleft lips, Plast. Reconstr. Surg. **47:**321, 1971.
16. Karapandzic, M.: Reconstruction of lip defects by local arterial flaps, Br. J. Plast. Surg. **27:**93, 1974.
17. Nicolau, P.J.: The orbicularis oris muscle: a functional approach to its repair in the cleft lip, Br. J. Plast. Surg. **36:**141, 1983.
18. Sabattini, P.: Cenno storico dell'origine e progresso della rinoplastica e cheiloplastica seguito della descrizione de queste operazione sopra un solo individuo, Bologna, 1838, Belle Arti.
19. Stein, S.A.W.: Laebedannelse (Chelioplastik) udfort paa en ny methode, Hospitals-Middelelser (Copenhagen) **1:**212, 1848.
20. Webster, J.P.: Crescentic peri-alar cheek excision for upper lip flap advancement with a short history of upper lip repair, Plast. Reconstr. Surg. **16:**434, 1955.
21. Webster, R.C., Coffey, R.J., and Kelleher, R.E.: Total and partial reconstruction of lower lip with innervated muscle-bearing flaps, Plast. Reconstr. Surg. **25:**360, 1960.

BIBLIOGRAPHY

SURGICAL REPAIR AND RECONSTRUCTION

Barsky, A.J.: Principles and practice of plastic surgery, Baltimore, 1950, Williams & Wilkins.
Belbke, H.: Wiederherstellende und plastische chirurgie, vol. 3, Stuttgart, 1964, George Thieme Verlag.
Burian, F.: The plastic surgery atlas, London, 1967, Butterworth & Co., Ltd.
Conley, J.: Concepts in head and neck surgery, Stuttgart, 1970, George Thieme Verlag KG.
Denecke, H.J., and Meyer, R.: Plastische operationen an Kopf und Hals, vol. 1, Berlin, 1964, Springer-Verlag.
Doberl, A.: Illustrated handbook on local anesthesia, Copenhagen, 1969, Munksgaard.
Emmett, A.J.J., and O'Rourke, M.G.E.: Malignant skin tumors, New York, 1982, Churchill Livingstone, Inc.
Gillies, H.D., and Millard, D.R.: The principles and art of plastic surgery, Boston, 1957, Little, Brown & Co.
Gohrbandt, E., Gabka, J., and Berndorfer, A.: Handbuch der plastischen chirurgie, vol. 2, Berlin, 1967, Walter de Gruyter & Co.
Grabb, W.C., and Myers, M.B.: Skin flaps, Boston, 1975, Little, Brown & Co.
Haas, E.: Plastische chirurgie im Gesichts-Hals-Bereich, Stuttgart, 1976, George Thieme Verlag.
Jenkner, F.L.: Peripheral nerve block, Berlin, 1975, Springer-Verlag.
Kazanjian, V.H., and Converse, J.M.: Surgical treatment of facial injuries, ed. 3, Baltimore, 1974, Williams & Wilkins.
Limberg, A.A.: The planning of local plastic operations on the body surface: theory and practice, Lexington, Mass., 1984, The Collamore Press. [Originally published Leningrad, U.S.S.R., 1963, Government Publishing House for Medical Literature (Medgiz).]
McGregor, I.A.: Fundamental techniques of plastic surgery and their surgical applications, New York, 1980, Churchill Livingstone, Inc.
Mustarde, J.C.: Repair and reconstruction in the orbital region, Edinburgh, 1980, Churchill Livingstone, Inc.
Naumann, H.H.: Kopf-und Hals-Chirurgie, vol. 2, Stuttgart, 1974, George Thieme Verlag.
Petres, J., and Hundeiker, M.: Korrektive dermatologie, Berlin, 1975, Springer-Verlag.
Tanzer, R.C., and Edgerton, M.T.: Symposium on reconstruction of the auricle, St. Louis, 1974, The C.V. Mosby.
Zoltan, J.: Atlas of skin repair, Basel, 1984, S. Karger.

LOCAL FLAPS

Almasowa, N.W.: Skin repair of facial defects [Thesis, in Russian], 1935, University of Saratow.

Argamaso, R.V.: V-Y plasty for closure of a round defect, Plast. Reconstr. Surg. **53:**99, 1974.

Aubry, M., and Freidel, C.: Chirurgie de la face et de la region maxillofaciale, Paris, 1952, Masson & Cie.

Aufricht, G.: Evaluation of pedicle flaps versus skin grafts in reconstruction of surface defects and scar contractures of the chin, cheeks and necks, Surgery **15:**75, 1944.

Bethmann, W., and Zoltan, J.: Operations method en der plastischen chirurgie, Jena, German Democratic Republic, 1968, Gustav Fischer Verlag.

Borges, A.F.: Cirurgia plastica de una herida cutanea, Rev. Confed. Med. Panama **5:**1, 1958.

Borges, A.F.: La W-plastia en el tratamiento de la cicatrices, Rev. Latin Amer. Chir. Plast. **4:**10, 1959.

Borges, A.F.: Elective incisions and scar revision, Boston, Little, Brown & Co., 1973.

Breach, N.M.: Preauricular full-thickness skin grafts, Br. J. Plast. Surg. **31:**124, 1978.

Conley, J.J.: The use of regional flaps in head and neck surgery, Ann. Otolaryngol. **69:**1223, 1960.

Conley, J.J.: Regional flaps of the head and neck, Stuttgart, 1976, George Thieme Verlag.

Crickelair, G.F.: Surgical approach to facial scarring, JAMA **172:**160, 1960.

Deneck, H.M., and Meyer, R.: Plastische Operationen an Kopf und Hals, Berlin, 1964, Springer-Verlag.

Dufourmentel, C.: Les deplacements tegumenaires par lambeaux à deux pedicules, Restauration Maxillo-faciale **2:**44, 1918.

Emmett, A.J.J.: The closure of defects using adjacent triangular flaps with subcutaneous pedicles, Plast. Reconstr. Surg. **59:**45, 1977.

Escoffier, J.B.: La chirurgie plastique en cancerologie faciale, Ann. Chir. Plast. **32:**45, 1956.

Escoffier, J.B.: Chirurgie et rehabilitation en cancerologie faciale, Ann. Chir. Plast. **11:**21, 1966.

Farkas, L.G., and Krauss, M.: Surgical treatment of skin cancer (in Czech), Universitas Carolina Medika **1:**319, 1955.

Garrett, W.S., Giblin, T.R., and Hoffman, G.W.: Closure of skin defects of the face and neck by rotation and advancement of cervicopectoral flaps, Plast. Reconstr. Surg. **38:**342, 1966.

Gibson, T., and Kenedi, R.M.: Biomechanical properties of skin, Surg. Clin. North Am. **47:**279, 1967.

Gillies, H.D.: Plastic surgery of the face, London, 1920, Frowde, Hoddert, Stoughton.

Gillies, H.D., and Millard, D.R.: Principles and art of plastic surgery, Toronto, 1957, Little, Brown & Co.

Ginestet, G., Frezieres, H., DuPuis, A., and Pons, J.: Chirgurie plastique et reconstructure de la face, Paris, 1967, Flammarion.

Girardi, G.: Principles of local skin flaps, Facial Plast. Surg. **1:**31, 1983.

Goumain, A.J.M., and Fevrier, J.C.: Les autoplasties cutanees par lambeaux, J. Med. Bordeaux **2:**179, 1964.

Gunter, J.P.: Revision of scars of the head and neck, Otolaryngol. Clin. North Am. **7:**119, 1974.

Harashina, T., Maruyama, Y., and Kitamura, K.: The trilobed flap, Plast. Reconstr. Surg. **60:**623, 1977.

Kenedi, R.M., Gibson, T., and Daly, C.H.: Bioengineering studies of the human skin. In Jackson, S.F., Harkness, R., Partridge, S., and Tristam, G., editors: Structure and function of connective and skeletal tissue, London, 1965. Butterworth & Co., Ltd.

Kernahan, D.A., and Littlewood, A.H.: Experience on the use of arterial flaps about the face, Plast. Reconstr. Surg. **28:**207, 1961.

Koss, N.: The mathematics of flaps. In Krizek, T.J., and Hoopes, J.E., editors: Symposium on Basic science in plastic surgery, St. Louis, 1976, C.V. Mosby Co.

Kraissl, C.J.: The selection of appropriate lines for elective surgical incision, Plast. Reconstr. Surg. **8:**1, 1951.

Kraissl, C.J., and Conway, H.: Excision of small tumors of the skin of the face with special reference to the wrinkle lines, Surgery **23:**592, 1949.

Krupp, S., Daverio, P., and Brupbacher, J.P.: Island flaps for face and neck repair, Facial Plast. Surg. **1:**37, 1983.

Letenneur, G.P.: Quel-ques cas d'autoplastie faciale, Gazette des Hopitaux **28:**398, 1855.

Limberg, A.A.: Design of local flaps. In Gibson, T., editor: Modern trends in plastic surgery, ed. 2, London, 1966, Butterworth & Co., Ltd.

Limberg, A.A.: The planning of local plastic operations on the body surface: theory and practice, Lexington, MA, 1984, The Collamore Press. [Originally published Leningrad, U.S.S.R., 1963, Government Publishing House for Medical Literature (Medgiz).]

McGregor, I.A.: Local skin flaps in facial reconstruction, Otolaryngol. Clin. North Am. **15:**77, 1982.

Meyer, R.: Chirurgie reconstructive de la face et du cou apres l'ablation des tumeurs, Medicine et Hygiene **26:**542, 1968.

New, G.B., and Erich, J.B.: The use of pedicle flaps of skin in plastic surgery of the head and neck, Springfield, 1950, Charles C Thomas, Publisher.

Ohtsuka, H., Miki, Y., and Shioya, N.: Trilobed flap in facial reconstruction, Br. J. Plast. Surg. **35:**493, 1983.

Patterson, T.J.S.: The effects of tension on the survival of skin flaps. In Hueston, J., editor: Transactions of the Fifth International Congress of Plastic and Reconstructive Surgeons (Sydney), London, 1971, Butterworth & Co., Ltd.

Spira, M., Gerow, F.J., and Hardy, S.B.: Subcutaneous pedical flaps on the face, Br. J. Plast. Surg. **27:**258, 1974.

Trevaskis, A.E., Rempee, J., Okunski, W., and Rea, M.: Sliding subcutaneous-pedicle flaps to close a circular defect, Plast. Reconstr. Surg. **46:**155, 1970.

Webster, R.C., and Smith, R.C.: Cosmetic principles in surgery on the face, J. Dermatol. Surg. **4:**397, 1978.

Webster, R.C., Davidson, T.M., and Smith, R.C.: Broken line scar revision, Clin. Plast. Surg. **4:**263, 1977.

Webster, R.C., Smith, R.C., Smith, K.F., Barrera, A., and Hamdan, U.S.: Local flaps for the middle third of the face, Facial Plast. Surg. **1:**1, 1983.

Zoltan, J.: Our experiences and views in the reconstruction of the face, Acta Chir. Plast. **1:**16, 1959.

SKIN TENSION LINES

Borges, A.F.: Improvement of antitension line scars by the "W plastic" operation, Br. J. Plast. Surg. **12:**29, 1959.

Cox, H.T.: The cleavage lines of the skin, Br. J. Surg. **29:**234, 1941.

Gibson, T., Stark, H., and Evans, J.H.: Directional variations in extensibility of human skin in vivo, J. Biomech. **2:**20, 1969.

Gibson, T., Stark, H., and Kenedi, R.M.: The significance of Langer's lines, Transactions of the Fifth International Congress of Plastic and Reconstructive Surgeons, (Sydney), London, 1971, Butterworth & Co., Ltd.

Kraissl, C.J., and Conway, H.: Excision of small tumors of the skin of the face with special references to the wrinkle lines, Surgery **23:**592, 1949.

Kraissl, C.J.: The selection of appropriate lines for elective surgical incision, Plast. Reconstr. Surg. **8:**1, 1951.

Langer, K.: Zur Anatomie und Physiologie der Haut. Uber die spaltbarkeit der cutis. S.B. Akad. Wiss, Wien, **44:**19, 1861.

Rubin, L.R.: Langers lines and facial scars, Plast. Reconstr. Surg. **3:**47, 1948.

W-PLASTY

Borges, A.F.: Improvement of antitension skin lines by the "W plastic" operation, Br. J. Plast. Surg. **12:**29, 1959.

Borges, A.F.: La plastie en W dans le traitement des cicatrices, Rev. Latinoam. Chir. Plast. (Mexico) **4:**10, 1959.

Borges, A.F., and Alexander, J.E.: Relaxed skin tension lines, Z plasties on scars and fusiform excision of lesions, Br. J. Plast. Surg. **15:**242, 1962.

Borges, A.F.: The W plastic versus the Z plastic scar revision, Plast. Reconstr. Surg. **44:**58, 1969.

Borges, A.F.: Historical review of the Z and W plasty revision of linear scars, Int. Surg. **56:**182, 1971.

Borges, A.F.: Scar analysis and objectives of revision procedures, Clin. Plast. Surg. **4:**223, 1977.

Z-PLASTY

Berger, P.: Autoplastie par de doublement de la palmure et echange de lambeaux. In Berger, P., and Banzet, S., editors: Chirurgie orthopedique, Paris, 1904, Steinfeil.

Borges, A.F., and Alexander, S.E.: Relaxed skin tension lines, Z-plasties on scars and fusiform excision of lesions, Br. J. Plast. Surg. **15:**242, 1962.

Borges, A.F., Alexander, J.E., and Block, L.I.: Z-plasty treatment of unesthetic scars, Eye, Ear, Nose, Throat, Mon. **44:**39, 1965.

Borges, A.F., and Gibson, T.: The original Z-plasty, Br. J. Plast. Surg. **26:**237, 1973.

Cazelles, E.G.: Du traitement de l'ectropion cictriciel, Theses pour le doctorat en Medicine, 1980, Faculte de Medicine de Paris. Paris, Rognoux.

Cuono, C.B.: Double Z-plasty repair of large and small thrombic defects: the double-Z rhomboid, Plast. Reconstr. Surg. **71:**658, 1983.

Davis, J.C., and Kitlowski, E.A.: The theory and practical use of the Z-plasty incision for the relief of scar contractures, Ann. Surg. **109:**1001, 1939.

Davis, J.S.: Plastic Surgery, Philadelphia, 1919, P. Blakiston' Son & Co.

Davis, J.S.: Contracted scars. Section on Plastic Surgery, Practice of Surgery, vol. 5, Dean Lewis, 1930.

Davis, J.S.: The relaxation of scar contractures by means of the Z or revised Z-type incision, Ann. Surg. **94:**871, 1931.

Davis, J.S.: Present evaluation of the merits of the Z-plastic operation, Plast. Reconstr. Surg. **1:**26, 1946.

Denonvilliers, C.P.: Presentation de malades, Bulletin de la Societe de Chirurgie de Paris **5:**35, 1854.

Denonvilliers, CP.: Blepharoplastie, Bulletin de la Societe de Chirurgie de Paris **7:**243, 1856.

Denonvilliers, C.P.: De la methode autoplastique par pivotment appliquée, à la restauration des paupieres. Bulletin General de la Therapie, Medicale et Chirurgicale **65:**110, 1863.

Dingman, R.O.: Some applications of the Z-plastic procedure, Plast. Reconst. Surg. **16:**246, 1955.

Furnas, D.W.: The tetrahedral Z-plasty, Plast. Reconstr. Surg. **35:**291, 1965.

Furnas, D.W.: The four fundamental functions of the Z-plasty, Arch. Surg. **96:**458, 1968.

Furnas, D.W., and Fischer, G.W.: The Z-plasty: biomechanics and mathematics, Br. J. Plast. Surg. **24:**144, 1971.

Golomb, F.M.: Closure of circular defects with double rotation flaps and Z-plasties, Plast. Reconstr. Surg. **74:**813, 1985.

Hazratl, E.: Compound right-angle Z-plasty, Plast. Reconstr. Surg. **10:**133, 1952.

Horner, W.: Clinical report on the surgical department of the Philadelphia Hospital, Blockley for the months of May, June, July 1837, Am. J. Med. Sci. **21:**105, 1837.

Iselin, M.: La plastie en Z rectifies, Ann. Chir. Plast. **7:**295, 1962.

Iselin, M., and Iselin, F.: Types of Z-plasty and their technical determination, J. Int. Coll. Surg. **43:**276, 1965.

Ivy, R.H.: Who originated the Z-plasty? Plast. Reconstr. Surg. **47:**67, 1971.

Katoh, H., Nakajima, T., and Yoshimura, Y.: The double-Z rhomboid plasty: an improvement in design, Plast. Reconstr. Surg. **74:**817, 1985.

Letenneur, G.P.: Quelques cas d'autoplastie faciale, Gazette des Hopitaux **28:**398, 1855.

Limberg, A.A.: Skin plastic with shifting triangle flaps, Leningrad Trauma Inst. **8:**62, 1919.

Limberg, A.A.: Design of local flaps. In Gibson, T., editor: Modern trends in plastic surgery, vol. 2, London, 1966, Butterworth & Co., Ltd.

Marino, H.: The levelling effect of Z-plasties on lineal scars of the face, Br. J. Plast. Surg. **12:**34, 1959.

McCurdy, S.L.: Manual of orthopaedic surgery, Pittsburgh, 1898, Nicholson Press.

McCurdy, S.L.: Plastic operations to elongate cicatricial contractions across joints, Cleveland Med. J. **3:**123, 1904.

McCurdy, S.L.: Z-plastic surgery: plastic operation to elongate cicatricial contraction of the neck, lips, and eyelids and across joints, Surg. Gynecol. Obstet. **16:**209, 1913.

McCurdy, S.L.: Z-plastic surgery, Int. J. Surg. **30:**389, 1917.

McCurdy, S.L.: Correction of burn scar deformity by the Z plastic method, J. Bone Joint Surg. **6:**683, 1924.

McGregor, I.A.: The theoretical basis of the Z-plasty, Br. J. Plast. Surg. **9:**256, 1957.

McGregor, I.A.: The Z plasty, Br. J. Plast. Surg. **19:**82, 1966.

Mir, Y., and Mir, L.: The six flap Z-plasty, Plast. Reconstr. Surg. **52:**625, 1973.

Morel-Fatio, D.: La plastie en Z, J. Chir. Paris **65:**747, 1949.

Morestin, H.: De la correction des flexions permanentes des doigts, Revue de Chir. **50:**1, 1914.

Piechaud, T.: Deux observations de symphyse des membres à la suite de brulures etendues, Rev. d'Orthop. **7:**81, 1896.

Pieri, G.: Ricostruzione del pollice dal moncone della folange basale, La Chir. degli organi de movimento **3:**325, 1919.

Rahm, H.: Die morestin scheplastik bei fingerkontrakturen, Beitrg z Klin. Chir. **127:**214, 1922.

Smith, F.: Multiple excisions and Z-plasties in surface reconstruction, Plast. Reconstr. Surg. **1:**170, 1946.

Steindler, A.: Reconstructive surgery of the upper extremity, New York, 1923, D. Appleton & Co.

Webster, R.C.: Cosmetic concepts in scar camouflaging-serial excisional and broken line techniques, Trans. Amer. Acad. Ophthal. Otolaryng. **73:**256, 1969.

Webster, R.C., Davidson, T.M., and Smith, R.C.: Broken line scar revision, Clin. Plast. Surg. **4:**263, 1977.

Woolf, R.M., and Broadbent, T.R.: The four-flap Z-plasty, Plast. Reconstr. Surg. **49:**48, 1972.

BUROW'S TRIANGLES

Burow, C.A.: Beschreibung einer neuen Transplantatiosmethode zum Widerersatz verloren gegangener, Theile des Gesichts, Berlin, Nauck, 1855.

Burow, C.A.: Schmidt's Jahrbucher der in-und auslandischen Gesammten Medicin, pp. 140-145, 1856. (Abstract.)

Saemann O.: Die transplantations-methode des Prof. Dr. Burow Deutsche Klilnik 20. In: Schmidt's Jahrbucher der in-und auslandischen Gesammten Medicin, pp. 348-349, 1853.

ROTATION FLAPS

Crow, M.L., and Crow, F.J.: Resurfacing large cheek defects with rotation flaps from the cheek, Plast. Reconstr. Surg. **58:**196, 1976.

Golomb, F.M.: Closure of circular defects with double rotation flaps and Z-plasties, Plast. Reconstr. Surg. **74:**813, 1985.

Hardaway, R.M.: The useful rotation flaps, Am. J. Surg. **90:**1013, 1955.

Imre, J.: Lidplastik und Plastische Operationen an den Weichteilen des Gesichts, Budapest, 1924, Studium.

Imre, J.: Blepharoplasty and operation of other soft parts of the face (in Hungarian), Budapest, 1928, Studium.

Imre, J.: Plastic operations of the eyelids, Ophthalmol. Congr. part 2, 1936. Trans. Ophthalmol. Soc. U.K. **57:**494, 1938.

Loeb, R.: Temporo-mastoid flap for reconstruction of the cheek, Rev. Latin-Am. Chir. Plast. **6:**2, 1962.

Imre, J.: Operationen an den Liden, Ophthalmologische Operations Lehre, Stuttgart, 1942, George Thieme.

Imre, J.: Atlas d'autoplasties de la face, Paris, 1943, Dion.

Marchac, D.: Lambeaux de rotation fronto-nasal, Ann. Chir. Plast. **15:**44, 1970.

Saad, M.N., and Maisels, D.O.: Further applications of the rotation advancement technique, Br. J. Plast. Surg. **25:**116, 1972.

Stark, R.B., and Kaplan, J.M.: Rotation flaps, neck to cheek, Plast. Reconstr. Surg. **50:**230, 1972.

ISLAND FLAPS

Andrews, E.B.: Island flaps in facial reconstruction, Plast. Reconstr. Surg. **44:**49, 1969.

Barron, J.N., and Emmett, A.J.J.: Subcutaneous pedicle flaps, Br. J. Plast. Surg. **18:**51, 1965.

Biesenberger, H.: Deformitaten und kosmetische Operationen der Weiblichen Brust. Vienna, 1931, Wilhelm Maudrich.

Dufourmentel, C.: Le lambeau cerf-volant, lambeau insulalre de glissement avec plastie en VY, Ann. Chir. Plast. **15:**344, 1970.

Dufourmentel, C., and Talaat, S.M.: The kite flap. In Hueston, J., editor: Transactions of the Fifth International Congress of Plastic and Reconstructive Surgeons (Sydney), London, 1971, Butterworth and Co., Ltd.

Emmett, A.J.J.: The closure of defects by using adjacent triangular flaps with subcutaneous pedicles, Plast. Reconstr. Surg. **59:**45, 1977.

Esser, J.F.S.: Island flap, NY Med. J. **106:**264, 1917.

Fischl, R.A.: A flap for nasolabial defects—or "Save the dog ear," Br. J. Plast. Surg. **22:**351, 1969.

Goumain, A.J.M., and Fevrier, J.C.: Les transplants cutanes "en clot" ou "island flaps" en chirgurie plastique de la face, Ann. Chir. Plast. **10:**174, 1965.

Holevich, J., and Paneva-Holevich, E.: Bipedicled island flap, Acta Chir. Plast. **16:**106, 1971.

Jurkiewicz, M.J., and Walton, B.E.: Use of island flaps to restore facial loss, Ann. Surg. **31:**73, 1965.

Kubacek, V.: Transposition of flaps on the face on a subcutaneous pedicle, Acta Chir. Plast. **2:**108, 1960.

Milton, S.H.: Experimental studies on island flaps: ischemia and delay, Plast. Reconstr. Surg. **49:**444, 1972.

Rosic, A., and Platz, H.: Uber Gefassgestielte Lappen zur Defekdeckung im Gesichtsbereich, Fortschr. Kiefer. Gesichtschir. **23:**85, 1978.

Strahan, R.W., Sorosky, R., and Williams, D.: Vascular pedicled island flaps, Arch. Otolaryng. **92:**588, 1970.

Titova, A.T.: Local plasty with opposing triangular flaps in the treatment of scar contracture of the skin after burns, Acta Chir. Plast. **4:**156, 1962.

Trevaskis, A.E., Rempel, J., Okunski, W., and Rea, M.: Sliding subcutaneous pedicle flaps to close a circular defect, Plast. Reconstr. Surg. **46:**155, 1970.

Zaki, M.S., and Talaat, S.M.: The single pedicled kite flap: a new modified subcutaneous pedicle flap, Egypt. J. Plast. Reconstr. Surg. **1:**129, 1977.

BILOBED FLAPS

Babin, R.W., and Krause, C.: The nasal dorsum flap, Arch. Otolaryng. **104:**82, 1978.

Crowley, R.T., and Nickel, W.O.: Definitive treatment of decubitus ulcers in paraplegic patients by coverage with transposition bilobed flap grafts, Surg. Gynecol. Obstet. **100:**465, 1955.

Dean, R.K., Kelleher, J.C., Sullivan, J.G., and Baibak, G.: Bilobed flaps. In Grabb, W.C., and Myers, M.B., editors: Skin flaps, Boston, 1975, Little, Brown & Co.

Elliot, R.A.: Rotation flaps of the nose, Plast. Reconstr. Surg. **44:**147, 1969.

Esser, J.F.S.: Gestielte Plastiken, Bruns Beitr. Klin. Chir. **108:**514, 1915.

Esser, J.F.S.: Gestielte lokale Nasenplastik mit zweizipfeligem Lappen, Deckung des sekundären Defektes vom ersten Zipfel durch den zweiten. Deutsche Zeitschrift fur Chirurgie **143:**385, 1918.

Golomb, F.M., and Neumann, C.G.: An experimental method for comparing primary closures of skin defects, Plast. Reconstr. Surg. **22:**194, 1958.

Gunter, J.P.: Facial reconstruction using local skin flaps, J. Otolaryngol. **7:**171, 1978.

Harashina T., Maruyama, Y., and Kitamura, K.: The trilobed flap, Plast. Reconstr. Surg. **60:**623, 1977.

Hass, E.: Basic techniques of plastic surgical repair in defects of the skull and face, Arch. Otorhinolaryngol. **216:**1, 1977.

Kastenbauer, E.R.: Special methods of reconstructive surgery in the facial region, Arch. Otorhinolaryngol. **216:**123, 1977.

McGregor, J.C., and Soutar, D.S.: A critical assessment of the bilobed flap, Br. J. Plast. Surg. **34:**197, 1981.

Morgan, B.L., and Samian, M.R.: Advantages of the bilobed flap for closure of small defects on the face, Plast. Reconstr. Surg. **52:**35, 1973.

Narayanan, M.: Immediate reconstruction with bipolar scalp flap after excision of huge cheek cancers, Plast. Reconstr. Surg. **46:**548, 1970.

Ohtsuka, H., Miki, Y., and Shioya, N.: Trilobed flap in facial reconstruction, Br. J. Plast. Surg. **35:**493, 1983.

Tardy, M.E., Tenta, L.T., and Azem, K.: The bilobed flap in nasal repair, Arch. of Otorhinolaryngol. **95:**1, 1972.

Vilar-Sancho, B., Bermudez, M., and de la Fuente, A.: The extended use of bilobed flaps from the shoulder and thoracic wall in severe burn scarring of the face, Chirurgia Plastica (Berlin) **3:**49, 1975.

Weerda, H.: Die defektdekung mit Nahlappen nach Exstirpation von Tumoren in der Ohrregion, Laryngol. Rhinol. Otol. (Stuttgart) **57:**93, 1978.

Weerda, H.: The principles of the "bilobed flap" and its use for reconstruction of "multiple flaps" [in German] Arch. Otorhinolaryngol. **220:**133, 1978.

Weerda, H.: Multiple cheek rotation flaps in the reconstruction of face defects [in German], HNO **27:**358, 1979.

Weerda, H.: Trauma of the auricle [in German], HNO **28:**208, 1980.

Weerda, H.: One-stage reconstruction of wide defects [in German], Laryngol. Rhinol. Otol. **60:**312, 1981.

Weerda, H., and Munker, G.: Simultaneous multiple flaps in head and neck surgery [in German], HNO **26:**272, 1978.

Weerda, H.: Bilobed and trilobed flaps in head and neck repair, Facial Plast. Surg. **1:**51, 1984.

Zimany, A.: The bilobed flap, Plast. Reconstr. Surg. **11:**424, 1953.

CRESCENTIC ADVANCEMENT

Churchill, F.: Face and foot deformities, London, 1885, Churchill Livingstone.

Dieffenbach, J.F.: Die operative chirurgie, Liepzig, 1845, Brockhaus Verlag.

Lindemann, A., Lange, G., and Frenzel, H.: Die chirurgie des Gesichts der Mundhohle und der Luftweg, Berlin, 1941, Urban & Schwarzenberg.

Prince, D.: Report upon plastic surgery. Transactions of the Seventh Anniversary Meeting of the Illinois State Medical Society, Springfield, June 4-5, 1867, Chicago, Fergus.

Stone, J.S.: Plastic surgery. In Bryant, J.D., and Buck, A.H., editors: American Practice of Surgery, vol. 4, New York, 1908, Wood.

Webster, J.P.: Crescentic perialar cheek excision for upper lip flap advancement with a short history of upper lip repair, Plast. Reconstr. Surg. **16:**434, 1955.

TRANSPOSITION FLAPS

Hadjistamoff, B.: A plastic operative procedure for the repair of large circular or elliptical body surface defects, Plast. Reconstr. Surg. **2:**362, 1947.

Webster, R.C., Davidson, T.M., and Smith, R.C.: The thirty degree transposition flap, Laryngoscope **88:**85, 1978.

RHOMBOID FLAPS

Aubry, M., and Freidel, C.: Chirurgie de la face et de la region maxillo faciale, Paris, 1952, Masson & Cie.

Borges, A.F.: Elective incisions and scar revision, Boston, Little, Brown & Co., 1973.

Borges, A.F.: Choosing the correct Limberg flap, Plast. Reconstr. Surg. **62:**542, 1978.

Brobyn, T.J., Cramer, L.M., Hulnick, S.J., and Kodsi, M.S.: Facial resurfacing with the Limberg flap, Clin. Plast. Surg. **3:**481, 1976.

Bullock, J.D., and Hamdi, B.: Double rhomboid flap in ophthalmic plastic surgery, Ophthalmic Surg. **11:**431, 1980.

Bullock, J.D., Koss, N., and Flagg, S.V.: Rhomboid flap in ophthalmic plastic surgery, Arch. Ophthalmol. **90:**203, 1973.

Cuono, C.B.: Double Z-plasty repair of large and small rhombic defects: the double-Z rhomboid, Plast. Reconstr. Surg. **71:**658, 1983.

Friede, L., Girardi, G., and Martini, Z.: Utilizzazione clinica dei. lembi di Limberg e Dufourmentel, Rev. Ital. Chir. Plast. **5:**195, 1973.

Gunter, J.P.: Rhombic flaps, Facial Plast. Surg. **1:**69, 1983.

Gunter, J.P., Carder, H.M., and Fee, W.E.: Rhomboid flap, Arch. Otolaryngol. **103:**206, 1977.

Jervis, W., Salyer, K.E., Vargas-Busquets, M.A., and Atkins, R.W.: Further applications of the Limberg and Dufourmentel flaps, Plast. Reconstr. Surg. **54:**335, 1974.

Katoh, H., Nakajima, T., and Yoshimura, Y.: The double-Z rhomboid plasty: an improvement in design, Plast. Reconstr. Surg. **74:**817, 1985.

Koss, N., and Bullock, J.D.: A mathematical analysis of the rhomboid flap, Surg. Gynecol. Obstet. **141:**439, 1975.

Limberg, A.A.: Mathematical principles of local plastic procedures on the surface of the human body [in Russian], Leningrad, 1946, Medgiz.

Limberg, A.A.: The planning of local plastic operations on the body surface: theory and practice, Lexington, Mass., 1963, The Collamore Press. [Originally published Leningrad, USSR, 1894, Government Publishing House for Medical Literature (Medgiz).]

Limberg, A.A.: Design of local flaps. In Gibson, T., editor: Modern trends of plastic surgery, ed. 2, London, 1966, Butterworth & Co., Ltd.

Limberg, A.A.: Planimetrie und Stereometrie der Haut-plastik, Jena, 1967, Gustav Fischer, Verlag.

Lister, G.D., and Gibson, T.: Closure of rhomboid skin defects: the flaps of Limberg and Dufourmentel, Br. J. Plast. Surg. **25:**300, 1972.

Ombredanne, L.: Chirurgie reparatrice, Paris, 1920, Masson & Cie.

Roggendorf, E.: The oblong parallelogram-shaped "Schwenklappen"-plasty, Plast. Reconstr. Surg. **65:**635, 1980.

DUFOURMENTEL FLAPS

Dufourmentel, C.: Le fermeture des pertes de substance cutanée limitées, "Le lambeau de rotation en L pour Losange", dit "LLL", Ann. Chir. Plast. **7:**61, 1962.

Dufourmentel, C.: An L-shaped flap for lozenge-shaped defects, Transactions of Third International Congress Plastic Surgeons, Amsterdam, 1963, Excerpta Medical Foundation.

Jervis, W., Salyer, K.E., Vargas-Busquets, M.A., and Atkins, R.W.: Further applications of the Limberg and Dufourmentel flaps, Plast. Reconstr. Surg. **54:**335, 1974.

Lister, G.D., and Gibson, T.: Closure of rhomboid skin defects: the flaps of Limberg and Dufourmentel, Br. J. Plast. Surg. **25:**300, 1972.

RETROAURICULAR FLAPS

Maillard, G.F., and Montandon, D.: The Washio tempororetroauricular flap: its use in 20 patients, Plast. Reconstr. Surg. **70:**550, 1982.

Montandon, D., and Maillard, G.F.: Place du lambeau retroauriculaire dans les reconstruction du nez, Ann. Chir. Plast. **22:**189, 1977.

Orticochea, M.: A postauricular flap to reconstruct facial defects, Br. J. Plast. Surg. **29:**325, 1976.

Washio, H.: Retroauricular temporal flap, Plast. Reconstr. Surg. **43:**162, 1969.

Washio, H.: Further experiences with the retroauricular flaps, Plast. Reconstr. Surg. **50:**160, 1972.

Washio, H.: The retroauricular temporal flap. In Grabb, W.C., and Myers, B.M., editors: Skin flaps, Boston, 1975, Little, Brown & Co.

NASOLABIAL FLAPS

Cameron, R.R., Lotham, W.D., and Dawling, J.A.: Reconstruction of the nose and upper lip with nasolabial flaps, Plast. Reconstr. Surg. **52:**145, 1973.

Cameron, R.R.: Nasal reconstruction with nasolabial cheek flaps. In Grabb, W.C., and Myers, M.B., editors: Skin flaps, Boston, 1975, Little, Brown & Co.

Champion, R.: Reconstruction of the columella, Br. J. Plast. Surg. **12:**353, 1960.

Climo, M.S.: Nasolabial flap for alar defect, Plast. Reconstr. Surg. **44:**303, 1969.

Da Silva, G.: A new method of reconstruction of the columella with a nasolabial flap, Plast. Reconstr. Surg. **34:**63, 1964.

De Cholnoky, T.: Partial and total reconstruction of nostrils by pedicle nasolabial flaps, Proceedings of Fifth International Congress of Otorhinolaryngology, 1953.

Esser, J.F.S.: Mund-Lippenplastik aus der Nasolabialgegend, Beitr. Klin. Chir. **105:**545, 1916.

Georgiade, N.G., Mladick, R.A., and Thorne, F.L.: The nasolabial tunnel flap, Plast. Reconstr. Surg. **43:**463, 1969.

Guerrero-Satos, J., and Dicksheet, S.: Nasolabial flap with simultaneous cartilage graft in nasal alar reconstruction, Clin. Plast. Surg. **8:**599, 1981.

Hagerty, R.F., and Smith, W.: The nasolabial cheek flap, Ann. Surg. **24:**506, 1958.

Harii, K.: Reconstruction of traumatic short nose with iliac bone graft and nasolabial flaps, Plast. Reconstr. Surg. **69:**863, 1982.

Haybrock, G.: Some applications of the nasolabial flap in reconstruction of the nose and lips, Br. J. Plast. Surg. **23:**26, 1970.

Herbert, D.C., and Harrison, R.G.: Nasolabial subcutaneous pedicle flaps. I. Observations on their blood supply, Br. J. Plast. Surg. **28:**85, 1975.

Herbert, D.C., and De Geus, J.: Nasolabial subcutaneous pedicle flaps. II. Clinical experience, Br. J. Plast. Surg. **28:**90, 1975.

Jackson, I.T., and Reid, C.D.: Nasal reconstruction and lengthening with local flaps, Br. J. Plast. Surg. **31:**343, 1978.

McLaren, L.R.: Nasolabial flap repair for alar margin defects, Br. J. Plast. Surg. **16:**234, 1963.

Pers, M.: Cheek flaps in partial rhinoplasty, Scand. J. Plast. Reconstr. Surg. **1:**37, 1967.

Reginato, L.E., and Belda, W.: Correction of scaphoid facies and restoration of nasal foundations with bilateral nasolabial flaps, Rev. Paul. Med. **72:**130, 1968.

Walker, A.W., and Schewe, J.E.: Nasolabial flap reconstruction for carcinoma of the lower lip, Am. J. Surg. **113:**783, 1967.

Wesser, D.R., and Burt, G.B.: Nasolabial flap for losses of the nasal ala and columella, Plast. Reconstr. Surg. **44:**300, 1969.

Wynn, S.K.: Primary plastic repair of nasal defects with the nasal labial flap, Trans. Am. Acad. Ophthalmol. Otolaryng. **61:**614, 1957.

Wynn, S.K., and Wiviott, W.: Resurfacing of the nose with bilateral cheek flaps. In Transactions Fourth International Congress Plastic and Reconstructive Surgery, Amsterdam, 1968, Excerpta Medica.

FOREHEAD RECONSTRUCTION

Dufourmentel, C., and Mouly, R.: Chirurgie plastique du cuir chevelu, du crane et du front Paris, 1959, Flammarion & Cie.

Hamilton, R., and Royster, H.P.: Reconstruction of extensive forehead defects, Plast. Reconstr. Surg. **47:**421, 1971.

New, G.B., Figi, F.A., and Havens, F.Z.: Replacement of tissues of the forehead and scalp, Surg. Clin. North Am. **14:**607, 1934.

Orticochea, M.: Application de la technique des quatre lambeaux danss la reconstruction du front et des regions parietales, Ann. Chir. Plast. **14:**153, 1969.

Texier, M., and Preaux, J.: Le Lambeau frontal a pedicule scalpant pour la reparation des pertes de substance cutanee d'un hemi front, Ann. Chir. Plast. **11:**131, 1966.

Worthen, E.F.: Repair of forehead defects by rotation of local flap, Plast. Reconstr. Surg. **57:**204, 1976.

NOSE RECONSTRUCTION

Avahoff, J.C.: The dorsal nasal flap, Plast. Reconstr. Surg. **53:**671, 1974.

Bethea, H.: Closure of large nasal defects with double rotated pedicle flaps, Am. J. Surg. **95:**299, 1958.

Babin, R.W., and Krause, C.: The nasal dorsum flap, Arch. Otolaryngol. **104:**82, 1978.

Blair, V.P.: Total and subtotal reconstruction of the nose, JAMA **85:**1925, 1931.

Blair, V.P., and Byars, L.T.: Hits and strike-outs in the use of pedicle flaps for nasal restoration, Surg. Gynecol. Obstet. **82:**367, 1946.

Cameron, R.R., Lotham, W.D., and Dawling, J.A.: Reconstruction of the nose and upper lip with nasolabial flaps, Plast. Reconstr. Surg. **52:**145, 1973.

Cameron, R.R.: Nasal reconstruction with nasolabial flaps. In Grabb, W.C., and Myers, M.B.: Skin flaps, Boston, 1975, Little, Brown & Co.

Cardoso, A.D.: Loss of columella after leishmaniasis. Reconstruction with subcutaneous tissue pedicle flap, Plast. Reconstr. Surg. **21:**117, 1958.

Carpue, J.C.: An account of two successful operations for restoring a lost nose from the integument of the forehead, The Gentleman's Magazine, London, 1816, Longman.

Carson, W.E., Cameron, R.R., and Lotham, W.D.: Naso-orbital reconstruction in war casualties, Plast. Reconstr. Surg. **45:**536, 1970.

Champion, R.: Reconstruction of the columella, Br. J. Plast. Surg. **12:**353, 1960.

Chardot, C., and Carolus, J.M.: Le lambeau frontal a pedicule median en chirurgie cancerologique, Ann. Chir. Plast. **10:**106, 1965.

Climo, M.S.: Nasolabial flap for alar defect, Plast. Reconstr. Surg. **44:**303, 1969.

Converse, J.M.: New forehead flap for reconstruction of the nose, Proc. R. Soc. Med. **35:**811, 1942.

Converse, J.M.: Reconstruction of the nose by scalping flap technique, Surg. Clin. North Am. **49:**2, 1959.

Converse, J.M., and Wood-Smith, D.: Experiences with the forehead island flap with a subcutaneous pedicle, Plast. Reconstr. Surg. **31:**521, 1963.

Converse, J.M.: Reconstructive plastic surgery, Philadelphia, 1964, W.B. Saunders Co.

Converse, J.M.: Clinical application of the scalping flap in reconstruction of the nose, Plast. Reconstr. Surg. **43:**247, 1969.

Cort, D.F.: Nasal tip replantation, Plast. Reconstr. Surg. **52:**194, 1973.

Cronin, T.D.: V-Y rotational flap for nasal tip defect, Ann. Plast. Surg. **11:**282, 1983.

Da Silva, G.: A new method of reconstruction of the columella with a nasolabial flap, Plast. Reconstr. Surg. **34:**63, 1964.

Dawan, I.K., Aggarwal, S.B., and Hariharan, S.: Use of an off-midline forehead flap for repair of small nasal defects, Plast. Reconstr. Surg. **53:**537, 1974.

Denecke, H.J.: Plastische Operationen an Kopf und Hals, 1. Bd. Nasenplastik, Berlin, 1964, Springer-Verlag.

Edgerton, M.T., Lewis, C.M., and McKelly, L.: Lengthening of the short nasal columella by skin flaps from the nasal tip, Plast. Reconstr. Surg. **40:**343, 1967.

Elsahy, N.I.: The hocky stick nasal flap and its use in reconstruction around the nose, Acta Chir. Plast. **20:**24, 1978.

Erich, J.B.: A survey of skin grafts and pedicle flaps for repair of nasal defects, Ann. Otolaryngol. **72:**808, 1963.

Escoffier, J.B.: The forehead flap in nasal repair, Plast. Reconstr. Surg. **21:**94, 1958.

Farina, R.: Total rhinoplasty for deformities following leprosy, Plast. Reconstr. Surg. **20:**78, 1957.

Farrior, R.T.: Korrigierende und rekonstruktive plastische Chirurgie an der ausseren. In Naumann, H.H., editor: Kopf-und Halschirurgie, vol. 2, Stuttgart, 1974, George Thieme Verlag.

Figi, F.A., and Moorman, W.L.: The median forehead flap-indications and limitations, Plast. Reconstr. Surg. **24:**163, 1959.

Gaze, N.T.: Reconstructing the nasal tip with a midline forehead flap, Br. J. Plast. Surg. **33:**122, 1980.

Georgiade, N.G., Mladick, R.A., and Thorne, F.L.: The nasolabial tunnel flap, Plast. Reconstr. Surg. **43:**463, 1969.

Gillies, H.D.: Deformities of the syphilitic nose, Br. J. Med. **2:**977, 1923.

Gillies, H.D.: The columella, Br. J. Plast. Surg. **2:**192, 1949.

Gliosci, A., Sabbagh, E., and Hipps, C.J.: Reconstruction of the nose by local pedicle flap, Plast. Reconstr. Surg. **41:**149, 1968.

Guerrero-Santos, J., and Dicksheet, S.: Nasolabial flap with simultaneous cartilage graft in nasal alar reconstruction, Clin. Plast. Surg. **8:**599, 1981.

Haas, E., and Meyer, R.: Konstruktive und rekonstruktive Chirurgie der Nase. In Gohrbandt, E., Gabka, J., Berndorfer, A., editors: Handbuch der Plastischen Chirurgie, vol. 2, Berlin, 1968, W. de Gruyter.

Haas, E.: Zur Rekonstruktion von Nasendefekten, Z. Laryngol. Rhinol. **47:**251, 1968.

Haas, E.: Rekonstruktionen von Defekten in Stirn-Hals-Bereich. Plastische Chirurgie in Gesichts-Hals-Bereich, Stuttgart, 1976, George Thieme Verlag.

Hagerty, R.F., and Smith, W.: The nasolabial cheek flap, Ann. Surg. **24:**506, 1958.

Harii, K.: Reconstruction of traumatic short nose with iliac bone graft and nasolabial flaps, Plast. Reconstr. Surg. **69:**863, 1982.

Heanley, C.: The subcutaneous tissue pedicle flap in columella and outer basal reconstruction, Br. J. Plast. Surg. **8:**60, 1955.

Ivy, R.H.: Repair of acquired defects of the face, JAMA **84:**181, 1925.

Jackson, I.T., and Reid, C.D.: Nasal reconstruction and lengthening with local flaps, Br. J. Plast. Surg. **31:**343, 1978.

Jost, G., Walker, C., Bull, T., Lattole, P., and Vergnon, L.: Nasal defect repair, Facial Plast. Surg. **1:**75, 1983.

Jost G., Danon, J., Hadjean, E., Mahe, E., Vertu, J.: Preparations plastiques des pertes de substances cutanees de la face, Paris, 1977, Libraire Arnette.

Kaplan, J.: Reconstruction of the columella, Br. J. Plast. Surg. **25:**37, 1972.

Kazanjian, V.H.: The repair of nasal defects with the median forehead flap: primary closure of the forehead wound, Surg. Gynecol. Obstet. **83:**37, 1946.

Kazanjian, V.H.: Nasal deformities of syphilitic origin, Plast. Reconstr. Surg. **3:**517, 1948.

Kernahan, D.A.: Reconstruction of the nose. In Grabb, W.C., and Smith, J.W., editors: Plastic surgery, Boston, 1973, Little, Brown & Co.

König, F.: Zur Deckung von Defekten der Nasen flügel. Berl. Klin. Wschr. **39:**137, 1902.

König, F.: Über Nasenplastik, Bruns Beitrag Klin. Chir. **94:**515, 1914.

Labat, L.: De la rhinoplastie, Ann. de la Med. Physiologique **25:**56, 1834.

Lagrot, F.G., and Greco, J.M.: "Drawbridge" reconstructive rhinoplasty, Plast. Reconstr. Surg. **42:**37, 1968.

Langenbeck, B.: Über eine neue Methode der totalen Rhinoplastik. Berl. Klin. Wochenschr. **13,** 1864.

Lejour, M.: One-stage reconstruction of nasal skin defects with local flaps, Chir. Plast. **1:**254, 1972.

Leuders, H.W.: Regional nasal flap. In Conley, J.J., and Dickinson, J., editors: Plastic and reconstructive surgery of the face and neck, Proceedings of the First International Symposium, vol. 2, Stuttgart, 1972, George Thieme Verlag.

Loeb, R.: Backward insertion of median forehead flap in nasal deformities, Br. J. Surg. **12:**349, 1960.

Loeb, R.: Principles in reconstruction of the nose. In Conley, J.J., and Dickinson, J., editors: Plastic and reconstructive surgery of the face and neck, Proceedings of the First International Symposium, vol. 2, Stuttgart, 1972, George Thieme Verlag.

Macomber, W.B., and Berkeley, W.T.: Use of neck-tubed pedicles in reconstruction of defects of the face, Plast. Reconstr. Surg. **2:**585, 1967.

Maillard, G.F., and Montandon, D.: The Washio tempororetroauricular flap: its use in 20 patients, Plast. Reconstr. Surg. **70:**550, 1982.

Malbec, E.F., and Beaux, A.R.: Reconstruction of columella, Br. J. Plast. Surg. **9:**142, 1958.

Marchac, D.: Lambeau de rotation frontonasal, Ann. Chir. Plast. **15:**48, 1970.

Masson, J.K., and Mendelson, B.C.: The Banner flap, Am. J. Surg. **134:**419, 1977.

Mazzola, R., and Marcus, S.: History of total nasal reconstruction with particular emphasis on the folded forehead flap technique, Plast. Reconstr. Surg. **72:**408, 1983.

McFee, W.F.: Surgical treatment of cancer of the nose with emphasis on methods of repair, Ann. Surg. **140:**475, 1954.

Mendelson, B.C., Masson, J.K., Arnold, P.G., and Erich, J.B.: Flaps used for nasal reconstruction: a perspective based on 180 cases, Mayo Clin. Proc. **54:**91, 1979.

Meyer, R.: Rhinoplastica parziale au lembofrontale e frontotemporal, Minerva Chir. **15:**1, 1960.

Meyer, R.: Die partielle Ersatzplastik der Nase, Helv. Chir. Acta **31:**304, 1964.

Meyer, R.: Plastische Operationen an Kopf und. Hals, vol. 1, Nasenplastik (H.J. Denecke and R. Meyer, editors), Berlin, 1964, Springer Verlag.

Meyer, R.: Total nasal reconstruction. In Conley, J., and Dickinson, J., editors: Plastic and reconstructive surgery of the face and neck, Proceedings of First Int. Symp., Stuttgart, 1972, George Thieme Verlag.

Millard, D.R.: Total reconstructive rhinoplasty, Plast. Reconstr. Surg. **37:**167, 1966.

Millard, D.R.: Hemirhinoplasty, Plast. Reconstr. Surg. **40:**440, 1967.

Millard, D.R.: Reconstructive rhinoplasty for the lower half of the nose, Plast. Reconstr. Surg. **53:**133, 1974.

Nelaton, C., and Ombredanne, L.: La rhinoplastie, Paris, 1904, Steinheil.

New, G.B.: Sickle flap for nasal reconstruction, Surg. Gynecol. Obstet. **80:**497, 1945.

New, G.B.: Further uses of the sickle flap in plastic surgery, Plast. Reconstr. Surg. **8:**415, 1951.

Orticochea, M.: A new method for total reconstruction of the nose. The ear as a donor site, Clin. Plast. Surg. **8:**481, 1981.

Paletta, F.X., and Van Norman, R.T.: Total reconstruction of the columella, Plast. Reconstr. Surg. **30:**322, 1962.

Penn, J.: The pattern of the forehead flap in rhinoplasty, S. Afr. Med. J. **24:**937, 1950.

Pers, M.: Cheek flaps in partial rhinoplasty, Scand. J. Plast. Reconstr. Surg. **1:**37, 1967.

Pierce, G.W., and O'Connor, G.B.: Reconstructive surgery of the nose, Ann. Otorhinolaryngol. **47:**437, 1938.

Ploner, L.: Reconstruction of columella, Plast. Reconstr. Surg. **5:**212, 1968.

Reginato, L.E., and Belda, W.: Correction of scaphoid facies and restoration of nasal foundation with bilateral nasolabial flaps, Rev. Paul Med. **72:**130, 1968.

Reiger, R.A.: A local flap for repair of the nasal tip, Plast. Reconstr. Surg. **40:**147, 1957.

Richardson, G.S., Hanna, D.C., and Gaisford, J.C.: Midline forehead flap nasal reconstruction in a patient with a low brow line, Plast. Reconstr. Surg. **49:**130, 1972.

Rigg, B.M.: The dorsal nasal flap, Plast. Reconstr. Surg. **52:**361, 1973.

Rintala, A.E., and Asko-Seljavaara, S.: Reconstruction of midline skin defects of the nose, Scand. J. Plast. Reconstr. Surg. **3:**105, 1969.

Rogers, B.O.: Nasal reconstruction 150 years ago: aesthetic and other problems, Aesthetic Plast. Surg. **5:**283, 1981.

Rybka, F.J.: Reconstruction of nasal tip using nasalis myocutaneous sliding flaps, Plast. Reconstr. Surg. **40,** 1983.

Saad, M.N., and Barron J.N.: Reconstruction of the columella with alar margin flaps, Br. J. Plast. Surg. **33:**427, 1980.

Sanvanero-Rosselli, G.: Chirurgia plastica del naso, Rome, 1931, Pozzi.

Sawhney, C.P.: A longer angular midline forehead flap for the reconstruction of nasal defects, Plast. Reconstr. Surg. **58:**721, 1976.

Sawhney, C.P.: Reconstruction of partial loss of nose, Clin. Plast. Surg. **8:**511, 1981.

Schaupp, H.: Rekonstruktion des Nasenflügels unter Verwendung des frontotemporalen Lappens. Hals-Nas.-Oto. **21:**187, 1973.

Schimmelbusch, C.: Zit aus Joseph J. Nasenplastik und sanstige Geischtsplastik, vol. 3, **5:**643. Leipzig, 1931, C. Kabitzch Verlag.

Schmid, E.: Über neue Wege in der plastischen Chirurgie der nase, Beitr. Klin. Chir. **184:**385, 1952.

Schmid, E.: Partielle und totale Nasenplastik, Fortschr, Kiefer und Gesichtschirurgie **7:**80, 1961.

Schmid, E.: Nasal reconstruction. In Gibson, T., editor: Modern trends in plastic surgery, London, 1964, Butterworth & Co., Ltd.

Smith, F.: Total rhinoplasty, Warthin Ann. 601, 1927.

Snow, J.W., and Harris, H.W.: One stage columellar reconstruction, Plast. Reconstr. Surg. **42:**83, 1968.

Sung, R.Y.: Total nasal reconstruction, Chinese Med. J. (Eng.) **66:**243, 1948.

Sung, R.Y.: Total nose reconstruction: an infraclavicular tube method, Chinese Med. J. 74:223, 1956.

Sung, R.Y.: Total nose reconstruction: a single stage method, Chinese Med. J. **92:**75, 1979.

Taglilacozzi, G., and Joseph, J.: Nasanplastic, vol. 2, Leipzig, 1931, C. Kabitzsch Verlag.

Tagliacozzi, G.: De curtorum chirurgia per insitionem, Venice, 1957, Gasper-Bindoni.

Tardy, M., Tental, L., and Azem, K.: The bilobed flaps in nasal repair, Arch. Otolaryngol. **95:**1, 1972.

Walter, C.: Nasal reconstruction, Laryng. **7:**1227, 1975.

Warren, J.M.: Rhinoplastic operations, with some remarks on the autoplastic methods usually adapted for the restoration of parts lost by accident or disease, Boston, 1840, Clapp.

Wesser, D.R., and Burt, G.B.: Nasolabial flap for losses of the nasal ala and columella, Plast. Reconstr. Surg. **44:**300, 1969.

Wynn, S.K., and Wiviott, W.: Resurfacing of the nose with bilateral cheek flaps. In Transactions of Fourth International Congress of Plastic and Reconstructive Surgeons, Amsterdam, 1968, Excerpta Medica.

Young, F.: The repair of nasal losses, Surgery **20:**670, 1946.

Vecchione, T.R.: Columella reconstruction using internal nasal vestibular flaps, Br. J. Plast. Surg. **33:**399, 1980.

Wilkinson, T.S.: Alar hinge flap in heminasal reconstruction, Ann. Plast. Surg. **1:**481, 1978.

Zoltan, J.: La correction des brêches pénétrantes et circonscrites de l'arête nasale, Ann. Chir. Plast. **2:**217, 1957.

CHEEK RECONSTRUCTION

Becker, D.W.: A cervicopectoral rotation flap for cheek coverage, Plast. Reconstr. Surg. **61:**868, 1978.

Bergonzelli, V.: Il lembo cutaneo sottomandibolare nella riparazione dei tegumenti dei deu terzi inferiori della faccia, Minerva Chir. **10:**1, 1955.

Crow, M.L., and Crow, F.J.: Resurfacing large cheek defects with rotation flaps from the cheek, Plast. Reconstr. Surg. **58:**196, 1976.

De Cholnoky, T.: The repair of extensive soft tissue losses of the cheek, Plast. Reconstr. Surg. **16:**288, 1955.

Erich, J.P.: Traumatic defects of nose and cheeks, Surg. Clin. North Am. **29:**1, 1949.

Garrett, W.S., Giblin, T.R., and Hoffman, G.W.: Closure of skin defects of the face and neck by rotation and advancement of cervicopectoral flaps, Plast. Reconstr. Surg. **38:**342, 1966.

Hadjistamoff, B.: Restoration of the cheek by using the skin of the jaw-neck region, Plast. Reconstr. Surg. **62:**127, 1947.

Kaplan, I., and Goldwyn, R.M.: The versatility of the laterally based cervicofacial flap for cheek repairs, Plast. Reconstr. Surg. **61:**390, 1978.

Kruger, E.: Reconstruction of full thickness defects of the cheek and the lips with special reference to the replacement of oral mucosa. Transactions Fourth International Congress Plastic and Reconstructive Surgeons, Amsterdam, 1967, Excerpta Medica Foundation.

Lejour, M.: The cheek sliding flap, Chir. Plast. **2:**347, 1974.

Loeb, R.: Tempero-mastoid flap for reconstruction of the cheek, Rev. Lat. Amer. Chirurg. Plast. **6:**2, 1962.

Meyer, R.: La chirurgie reconstructive de la face et du cou apres l'ablation de tumeurs, Medicine and Hygiene **26:**542, 1968.

New, G.B., and Figi, F.A.: The repair of postoperative defects involving the lips and cheeks secondary to removal of malignant tumors, Surg. Gynecol. Obstet. **62:**182, 1936.

Stark, R.B., and Kaplan, J.M.: Rotation flaps, neck to cheek, Plast. Reconstr. Surg. **50:**230, 1972.

Sung, R., Yang, P., and Liu, J.: Reconstruction of the cheek and lips, Clin. Plast. Surg. **9:**71, 1982.

Weerda, H.: Multiple cheek-rotation flap in the reconstruction of face defects [in German], HNO **27:**358, 1979.

EAR RECONSTRUCTION

Alexandrov, N.M.: A method of plastic repair with the aid of Filatov's tubed flap in the formation of the external ear, Vestn. Otorhinolaryngol. **25:**23, 1963.

Alexandrov, N.M.: Traumatic defects of the auricle and methods of their repair, Acta Chir. Plast. (Prague) **6:**302, 1964.

Antia, N.H.: Repair of segmental defects of the auricle in mechanical trauma. Symposium on reconstruction of the auricle (R.C. Tanzer, and M.T. Edgerton, editors), vol. 10, St. Louis, 1974, The C.V. Mosby Co.

Antia, N.H., and Buch, V.I.: Chondrocutaneous advancement flap for the marginal defect of the ear, Plast. Reconstr. Surg. **39:**472, 1967.

Blake, G.B.: Malignant tumours of the ear and their treatment, Br. J. Plast. Surg. **27:**67, 1974.

Brent, B.: Reconstruction of ear, eyebrow and sideburn in the burned patient, Plast. Reconstr. Surg. **55:**312, 1975.

Brent, B., and Byrd, H.S.: Secondary ear reconstruction with cartilage grafts covered by axial, random, and free flaps of temporoparietal fascia, Plast. Reconstr. Surg. **72:**141, 1983.

Byars, L.T., and De Mere, M.: Restoration of missing ear, Plast. Reconstr. Surg. **5:**66, 1950.

Converse, J.M.: Reconstruction of the auricle. II. Plast. Reconstr. Surg. **22:**230, 1958.

Crikelair, G.F.: A method of partial ear reconstruction for avulsion of the upper portion of the ear, Plast. Reconstr. Surg. **17:**438, 1956.

Cronin, T.D.: One-stage reconstruction of the helix: two improved methods, Plast. Reconstr. Surg. **9:**547, 1952.

Dufourmental, C., and Vaillant, J.M.: Les possibilities de reconstruction du pavillon de l'oreille, Presse Med. **72:**1971, 1964.

Evans, A.J., and Gilles, H.: Reconstruction of the external ear, Trans. Int. Soc. Plast. Surg., Second Cong., Edinburgh, 1959, Churchill Livingstone.

Lewin, M.F.: Formation of the helix with a postauricular flap, Plast. Reconstr. Surg. **5:**432, 1950.

Lewin, M.L., and Argamaso, R.V.: Repair of major defects of the auricle in mechanical trauma. In Tanzer, R.C., and Edgerton, M.T., editors: Symposium on reconstruction of the auricle, St. Louis, 1974, The C.V. Mosby Co.

Lockwood, C.D.: Plastic surgery of the ear, Surg. Gynecol. Obstet. **49:**392, 1929.

Luna, C.: Partial auricular plastic surgery, Rev. Lat. Am. Chirurg. Plast. **5:**28, 1961.

Maliniac, J.W.: Reconstruction for partial loss of the ear, Plast. Reconstr. Surg. **2:**124, 1946.

Masson, J.K.: A simple island flap for reconstruction of concha-helix defects, Br. J. Plast. Surg. **25:**398, 1972.

McNichol, J.W.: Total helix reconstruction with tubed pedicles following loss by burns, Plast. Reconstr. Surg. **6:**373, 1950.

Millard, D.R.: The chondrocutaneous flap in partial auricular repair, Plast. Reconstr. Surg. **37:**523, 1966.

Nagel, F.: The reconstruction of partial auricular loss, Plast. Reconstr. Surg. **49:**340, 1972.

Navbi, A.: One-stage reconstruction of partial defect of the auricle, Plast. Reconstr. Surg. **33:**77, 1964.

Nelaton, C., and Ombredonne, L.: Les otoplasties, Paris, 1907, G. Steinheil.

Pegram, N., and Peterson, R.: Repair of partial defects of the ear, Plast. Reconstr. Surg. **18:**305, 1956.

Pennisi, V.R., Klabunde, E.H., and Pierce, G.W.: The preauricular flap, Plast. Reconstr. Surg. **35:**552, 1965.

Pierce, G.W.: Reconstruction of the external ear, Surg. Gynecol. Obstet. **50:**601, 1930.

Pigossi, N.: Repair of partial losses of the external ear, Rev. Lat. Am. Cir. Plast. **9:**35, 1965.

Spina, V.: A simpler method of partial reconstruction of the external ear, Plast. Reconstr. Surg. **13:**488, 1984.

Steffanoff, D.N.: Auriculo-mastoid tube pedicle for otoplasty, Plast. Reconstr. Surg. **3:**352, 1948.

Steffensen, W.H.: A method of total ear reconstruction, Plast. Reconstr. Surg. **36:**97, 1965.

Tanzer, R.C.: Total reconstruction of the external ear, Plast. Reconstr. Surg. **23:**1, 1959.

Tanzer, R.C.: Total reconstruction of the auricle. In Wallace, A.B., editor: Trans. Int. Soc. Plast. Reconstr. Surg., Baltimore, 1960, Williams & Wilkins.

Tanzer, R.C.: Congenital deformities of the auricle. In Converse, J.M., editor: Reconstructive plastics surgery, Philadelphia, 1964, W. B. Saunders Co.

Walter, C.: Reconstruction procedures on the auricle, Trans. Amer. Acad. Ophthalmol. Otolaryngol. **73:**266, 1969.

Weerda, H.: Trauma of the auricle [in German], HNO **28:**208, 1980.

Weerda, H.: One-stage reconstruction of auricle defects [in German], Laryngol. Rhinol. Otol. **60:**312, 1981.

EYELID RECONSTRUCTION

Cutler, N.L., and Beard, C.: Method for partial and total upper lid reconstruction, Am. J. Ophthalmol. **39:**1, 1955.

Dieffenbach, J.F.: Die operative chirurgie, Leipzig, 1845, F.A., Brockhaus.

Figi, F.A.: Plastic surgery of the eyelids, Plast. Reconstr. Surg. **4:**403, 1950.

Fricke, J.C.G.: Die Bildung never Augenlider (Blepheroplastik) nach Zerstörungen und dadurch hervorgebrachten Auswartswendungen derselben, Hamburg, 1829, Perthes & Besser.

Gorney, M., Falces, E., Jones, H., and Manis, J.R.: One stage reconstruction of substantial eyelid margin defects, Plast. Reconstr. Surg. **44:**592, 1969.

Hagerty, R.F., and Smoak, R.D.: Reconstruction of the lower eyelid, Plast. Reconstr. Surg. **38:**52, 1966.

Hay, D.: Reconstruction of both eyelids following traumatic loss, Br. J. Plast. Surg. **24:**361, 1971.

Hollwich, F., and Junemann, G.: Defektdekung nach Entfernung von Lidtumoren, Plast. Reconstr. Surg. **3:**200, 1967.

Holmstrom, H., Bartholdson, L., and Johanson, B.: Surgical treatment of eyelid cancer with special reference to tarsoconjunctival flaps, Scand. J. Plast. Reconstr. Surg. **9:**107, 1975.

Imre, J.: Lidplastik und plastiche Operationen anderer Weichteile des Gesichts. Budapest, 1928, Studium-Verlag.

Jackson, I.T., Laws, E.R., Jr., and Martin, R.D.: A craniofacial approach to advanced recurrent cancer of the central face, Head Neck **5:**474, 1983.

Kreibig, G.: Vereinfachte Operationsmethoden zum Ersatz der Augenlider, Klin. Mbl. Augenheilkunde, Stuttgart, 1940.

Lentrodt, J.: Ersatz der Lidhaut nach Verbrennungen, Klin. Monastsbl. fur Augenheilkunde 158, 770, 1971, Stuttgart.

Lentrodt, J.: Die Bedeutung des Knorpeltransplantates in der rekonstruktiven Lidchirurgie nach Tumoroperationen, Vortr. Jahrestag. Dtsch Ges f. Plast. u Widerherst. Chir. Stuttgart, 1975, George Thieme Verlag.

Lipschutz, H.: Experiences with upper lateral cartilage in reconstruction of the lower eyelid, Ann. Ophthalmol. **73:**592, 1973.

Manchester, W.M.: A simple method for the repair of full thickness defects of the lower eyelid with special reference to the treatment of neoplasms, Br. J. Plast. Surg. **3:**252, 1951.

McCoy, F.J., and Crow, M.L.: Adaptation of the "switch flap" to eyelid reconstruction, Plast. Reconstr. Surg. **35:**633, 1965.

McGregor, I.A.: Eyelid reconstruction following subtotal resection of upper or lower lid, Br. J. Plast. Surg. **26:**346, 1973.

McLaren, L.R., and Beard, C.H.: Repair of the lower eyelid after full thickness excision for cancer. In Bohmert, H., editor: Plast. Chir. des Kopf-und HalsBereiches und der weiblichen, Stuttgart, 1975, George Thieme Verlag.

Meyer, R.: Reconstruction orbito-palpebrales par lambeau frontotemporal. Ophthalmologica **154:**328, 1967.

Meyer, R.: Plastische Chirurgie bei Verstummelungen an Kopf und Hals, Helv. Chir. Acta **37:**296, 1970.

Meyer, R.: Reconstruction of the eyelids. In Conley, J., and Dickinson, J.T., editors: Plastic and reconstructive surgery of the face and neck, Vol. 2, Stuttgart, 1972, George Thieme Verlag.

Millard, R.: Eyelid repairs with chondromucosal graft, Plast. Reconstr. Surg. **30:**267, 1962.

Monks, G.H.: Reconstruction of a new eyelid with a flap from the temporal region, Boston Med. Surg. J. 139:385, 1898.

Monks, G.H.: The restoration of the lower eyelid by a new method, Boston Med. Surg. J. **139:**385, 1898.

Morax, J.: Une greffe avec pedicule vasculaire en deux cas d'epitheliome ulcere de l'angle nasal des paupieres et de la face, Annls. Oculist., 1926.

Mustarde, J.C.: The use of flaps in the orbital region, Plast. Reconstr. Surg. **45:**146, 1970.

Mustarde, J.C.: Reconstruction of the eyelids and eyebrows. In Grabb, W., and Smith, J.W., editors: Plastic surgery, Boston, 1973, Little, Brown & Co.

Mustarde, J.C.: Repair and reconstruction in the orbital region, Edinburgh, 1980, Churchill Livingstone, Inc.

Mustarde, J.C., Jones, L.T., and Callahan, A.: Ophthalmic plastic surgery, up-to-date, Birmingham, 1970, Aesculpaius Publishing Co.

Pollock, W.J., Gustavo, A.C., and Ryan, R.F.: Reconstruction of the lower eyelid by a different lid-splitting operation, Plast. Reconstr. Surg. **50:**184, 1972.

Schmid, E.: Reconstruction of the orbit and lids, Trans. Int. Soc. Plast. Surg. London, Edinburgh, 1960, E & S Livingstone, Ltd.

Schmid, E.: Grundlagen der Lidrekonstruktion, Klin. Mbl. Augenheilkunde **162:**296, 1973.

Schuchardt, K.: Ausgenwahlte Kapitel aus der Weiderherstellungschirurgie des Gesichtes unter besonderer Beruckischitigung der Augenlider und der Orbita. In Thiel, R.: Ophthalmologische Operationslehre, vol. 4, Leipzig, 1950, J.A. Barth.

Smith, B., and Cherubim, T.D.: Oculoplastic surgery, St. Louis, 1970, The C.V. Mosby Co.

Smith, B., and Obear, M.: Bridge flap technique for large upper lid defects, Plast. Reconstr. Surg. **38:**1, 1966.

Tripier, L.: Du lambeau musculocutane en forme de pont. appliqué à la restauration des paupières, Rev. Chir. **4,** 1890.

Walser, E.: Forschritte auf dem Gebiet der Lid und Orbitachirurgie, Med. Klin. **69:**1720, 1974.

TONGUE FLAPS

Bakamjian, V.: Use of tongue flaps in lower lip reconstruction, Br. J. Plast. Surg. **17:**76, 1964.

Cadenat, H., Combelles, R., and Fabie, M.: Lambeaux de langue vascularisation, morphlogie et utilisation, Ann. Chir. Plast. **18:**223, 1973.

Carvalhal Franca, J.G.: Lip reconstruction employing a lingual flap, Assoc. Med. Brasil **17:**123, 1971.

Gosserez, M., and Stricker, M.: La langue, materiau de choix dans la reparation des pertes de substance labiale. In Transactions of the Fourth International Congress of Plastic Surgery, Amsterdam, 1969, Excerpta Medica Foundation.

Guerrero-Santos, J., Vasquez-Pallares, R., Vera-Strathmann, A., Machain, P., and Castaneda, A.: Tongue flap in reconstruction of the lip. In Broadbent, R.T., editor: Transactions of the Third International Congress of Plastic Surgeons, Amsterdam, 1964, Excerpta Medica Foundation.

Guerrero-Santos, J., and Alta Mirano, J.T.: The use of lingual flaps in repair of fistulae of the hard palate, Plast. Reconstr. Surg. **38:**123, 1966.

Guerrero-Santos, J., Casteneda, A., and Barba, A.: Surgery for labial angioma, Arch. Surg. **94:**728, 1967.

Guerrero-Santos, J.: Use of a tongue flap in secondary correction of cleft lips, Plast. Reconstr. Surg. **44:**368, 1969.

Jackson, I.T.: Use of tongue flaps to resurface lip defects and close palatal fistulae in children, Plast. Reconstr. Surg. **49:**537, 1972.

Jackson, I.T., and Sieber, H.: Closure of large anterior palatal fistulae using a tongue flap, Chir. Plastica **1:**313, 1973.

Zarem, H., and Greer, D.M.: Tongue flap for reconstruction of the lips after electrical burns, Plast. Reconstr. Surg. **53:**310, 1974.

LIP RECONSTRUCTION

Abbe, R.: A new operation for the relief of deformity due to double harelip, Med. Rec. N.Y. **53:**477, 1898.

Alexandrov, N.M.: Repair of defects in the lower lip by two symmetrical flaps from the upper lip, Acta Chir. Plast. **8:**269, 1966.

Alquie, A.: Cheiloplastie de la levre inferieure, Bull. Soc. Paris **5:**137, 1854-1855.

Anderson, R., and Kurtay, M.: Reconstruction of the corner of the mouth, Plast. Reconstr. Surg. **47:**463, 1972.

Andrews, E.: Repair of lower lip defects by Hagendorn rectangular flap method, Plast. Reconstr. Surg. **34:**27, 1964.

Ashley, F.L.: Reconstruction of the lower lip, Plast. Reconstr. Surg. **15:**313, 1955.

Audoucet, J.: Autoplastie de la levre inferieure, Essai sur un nouveau procede. Thesis, Paris, 1895, Sorbonne.

Axhausen, G.: Technik und Ergebnisse der Spaltplastiken, München, 1952, Carl Hanser Verlag.

Bakamjian, V.Y.: Use of tongue flaps in lower lip reconstruction, Br. J. Plast. Surg. **17:**76, 1964.

Baker, S.R.: Lip reconstruction. In Holt G.R., Gates, G.A., and Mattox, D.E., editors: Decision making in otolaryngology, New York, 1983, B.C. Decker, Inc.

Baker, S.R., and Krause, C.J.: Cancer of the lip. In Suen, J.Y., and Myers, E.N., editors: Cancer of the head and neck, New York, 1981, Churchill Livingstone.

Baker, S.R., and Krause, C.J.: Pedical flaps in reconstruction of the lip, Facial Plast. Surg. **1:**61-68, 1983.

Barton, M., Spira, M., and Hardy, B.: An improved method for "V" excision of the lip combined with vermilionectomy, Plast. Reconstr. Surg. **33:**471, 1964.

Bennett, J., Lynch, J. Lewis, S., and Blocker, T.: The operative treatment of cancer of the lip, Amer. Surgeon **28:**537, 1962.

Berger, P.: Cheiloplastie Methode italienne, Bull. Mem. Soc. Chir. Paris **16:**679, 1890.

Bernard, C.: Cancer de la levre inferieure opere par un procede nouveau, Gazette des Hopitaux **44,** 1853.

Bernard C.: Cancer de la levre inferieur: restauration a l'aide de lambeaux quadrilataires-lateraux querison. Scalpel Liege 1851-1853, **5:**162,

Bowers, D., and Lolonel, U.: Double cross lip flaps for lower lip reconstruction, Plast. Reconstr. Surg. **47:**209, 1971.

Bradley, C., and Leake, J.E.: Compensatory reconstruction of the lips and mouth after major tissue loss, Clin. Plast. Surg. :637, 1984.

Bretteville-Jensen, G.: Reconstruction of the lower lip after central excisions, Br. J. Plast. Surg. **26:**247, 1973.

Briedis, J., and Jackson, I.T.: The anatomy of the philtrum: observations made on dissection in the normal lip, Br. J. Plast. Surg. **34:**128, 1980.

Brusati, R.: Reconstruction of the labial commissure by sliding V-shaped cheek flap, J. Max. Facial Surg. **7:**11, 1979.

Buchanan, A.: On a method of restoring the lower lip after complete or partial excision in cases of extensive cancerous disease, London Med. Gaz. **29:**79, 1841.

Buck, G.: History of a case in which a series of plastic operations were successfully performed for the restoration of the right half of the upper lip and adjacent portions of the cheek and nose, Trans. Med. Soc. State of N.Y., 1864.

Burow, C.A.: Beschreibung einer neuen Transplantations-Methode (Methode der seitlichen Dreiecke) zum Wiederersatz verloren gegangener Teile des Gesichts, Berlin, 1855, Nauck.

Campbell, Reid, D.A.: A mucosal cross-lip flap, Br. J. Plast. Surg. **9:**106, 1956.

Cannon, B.: The use of the vermilion bordered flaps in surgery about the mouth, Surg. Gynecol. Obstet. **74:**458, 1942.

Chardot, C., Carolus, J.M., and Fieve, G.: La cheiloplastie en un temps, apres, exerese canceriologique: Resultats pour 51 observations dont 47 reparations immediates, Ann. Chir. Plast. **12:**287, 1967.

Clodius L: Reconstruction of upper lip by means of composite innervated neck-flap. Transactions of Fourth International Congress on Plastic Surgery, 1967. Amsterdam, Excerpta Medica, 1969 (International Congress Series No. 174).

Cohney, C.: Reconstruction de la levre inferieure apres excision chirurgicale pour cancer, Ann. Chir. Plast. **8:**105, 1963.

Converse, J.M.: The "over and out" flap for restoration of the corner of the mouth, Plast. Reconstr. Surg. **56:**575, 1975.

Cubey, R.B.: Lip-plug carcinoma and its management by modified Abbe flap, Br. J. Plast. Surg. **28:**80, 1975.

Demjen, S., Simun, L., and Dolezal, B.: Operation of Sabattini, Acta Chir. Plast. **1:**34, 1959.

Dieffenbach, J.F.: Die operative chirurgie Leipzig, 1845, Brockhaus.

Dieu-Lafoy, B.: Cited in Rigaud, P.H. "L'Anaplastie des levres, de Joues, et des paupieres, Thèse de Concours, Paris, 1841, Rorevier et Cie.

Eberle, R.C.: Chirurgische Versorgung von Hautdefekten im Bereich von Kopfhaut, Stirn, Wange und Lippen. In H.H. Naumann, editor: Kopf-und Hals-Chirurgie, vol. 2 Stuttgart, George Thieme Verlag, 1974.

Erikson, E., and Johanson, B.: Reconstruction of the oral commissure with Z-plasty, Scand. J. Plast. Reconstr. Surg. **16:**305, 1982.

Estlander, J.A.: En ny operationsmetod att atersralla en forstord lapp ellekkind, Finsak. Lak-Sall SK Handl. **14:**1, 1872.

Estlander, J.A.: En method. att fran den ena lappen fylla. substansforluster i den andra och i kinder. Noral. Med. Arkiv. **4:**1, 1872.

Estlander, J.A.: Eine methode, aus der einen Lippe Substanzverluste der anderen zu ersetzen. Langenbeck's Arch. Klin. Chir. **14:**622, 1872.

Estlander, J.A.: Methode d'autoplastic de la joue d'une levre par un lambeau emprente a l'autre, Rev. Meds. et Chir. 1. 1877.

Estlander, J.A.: A method of reconstructing loss of substance in one lip from the other, Plast. Reconstr. Surg. **42:**361, 1968.

Fernandez Villoria, J.M.: Reconstruction of the lip in the surgical treatment of cancer. In Chambers, R.G., Janssen de Limpens, A.M.P., Jaques, D.A., and Routledge, R.T., editors: Cancer of the head and neck, Amsterdam, 1975, Excerpta Medica Foundation.

Flanigan, W.S.: Reconstructive surgery of the lip region, Am. Surg. **17:**735, 1951.

Flanigan, W.S.: Free composite grafts from lower to upper lip, Plast. Reconstr. Surg. **17:**376, 1956.

Freeman, B.S.: Myoplastic modifications of the Bernard cheiloplasty, Plast. Reconstr. Surg. **21:**453, 1958.

Freidel, M., Schweizer, F., and Beziat, J.L.: A propos de la reparation de la levre superieure, Ann. Chir. Plast. **26:**144, 1981.

Fries, R.: The merits of Bernards operation as a universal procedure for lower lip reconstruction after resection of carcinoma, Chir. Plast. **1:**45-52, 1971.

Fries, R.: Advantages of a basic concept in lip reconstruction after tumor resection, J. Maxillofac. Surg. **1:**13, 1973.

Fujimori, R.: "Gate flap" for the total reconstruction of the lower lip, Br. J. Plast. Surg. **33:**340, 1980.

Gelbke, H.: An unusual application of the Estlander Abbe plastic operation of the lip, Plast. Reconstr. Surg. **14:**68, 1954.

Gilles, H.D., and Millard, D.R.: The principles and art of plastic surgery, Boston, 1957, Little, Brown & Co.

Ginestet, G.: Reconstruction de toute la levre inferieure par les lambeaux naso-geniens totaux, Rev. Odont. Stomat. **8:**28, 1946.

Ginestet, G., Dupois, A., and Merville, L.: Le lambeau unipedicule de cuir chevalu dans les reconstructions de la region genienne et de la levre superieure, Ann. Chir. Plast. **2:**183, 1957.

Goleman, B., Friedhofer, H., Anger, M., and Glina, S.: Reconstrucciones parciales del labio inferior con la technica de Camille Bernard, Cir. Plast. Ibero-Latinio-Am. **4:**75, 1978.

Goleman, B., Friedhofer, H., Anger, M., and Glina, S.: Von Bruns' technique for lower lip reconstruction, Rev. Col. Bras. Cir. **7:**5, 1980.

Gosserez, M., and Stricker, M.: Apropos de la reparation des levres, Ann. Chir. Plast. **13:**7, 1968.

Goto, K., Suzuki, E., and Marumo, E.: Analysis of the results of the lip switch operations, Jpn. J. Plast. & Reconstr. Surg. **18:**302, 1975.

Grimm, G.: Eine neue Methode der Nahlappenplastik zum Ersatz tumorbedingter totaler Underlippendefekte. Zentralbl. Chir. **91:**1621, 1966.

Guerrero-Santos, J., Vasquez-Pallares, R., Veram, A., Vera-Strathman, A., Machain, P., and Castaneda, A.: The tongue flap in reconstruction of the lip. In Broadbent, R.T., editor: Transactions of Third International Congress Plastic and Reconstructive Surgeons (Washington, 1963), Amsterdam, 1964, Excerpta Medica Foundation.

Günther, H.: Die chirurgische Behandlung des unterlippencarcinomas. Fortschr. Kiefer-u. Gesichtschir. **13:**118, 1968.

Günther, H., and Spiessl, B.: Rekonstruktion der Unterlippe nach Carcinomentfernung und gleichzeitiger Ausräumung regionärer Lymphknoten. Chir. Plast. Reconstr. **3:**230, 1967.

Hendrick, J.W., and Ward, G.E.: Treatment of cancer of the lip, J. Int. Coll. Surg. **15:**7, 1951.

Hollmann, K.: Bipedicled VY flap technique for primary repair of lower lip defects, Acta Chir. Plast. **12:**223, 1970.

Huffstadt, A.J.C.: Fan flaps in cheiloplasty, Acta Chir. Neerl. **16:**103, 1964.

Huffstadt, A.J.C.: Lip reconstruction by means of local tissue transposition, Ned. Tijdschr. Geneeskd. **3:**346, 1967.

Hughes, A., Maree, D., and Salis, R.J.L.: Technique de cheiloplastie pour les cancers etendus des levres, Presse Med. **79:**1690, 1971.

Imbert, G.: Etude sur la Restauration de la levre inferieure suivie de la description d'vu nouveau procede pour refaire le bord libre au moyeu d'un lambeau muqueux en forme de pont. Thesis, Lyon, 1883, University of Lyon.

Imes, R.: Advantages of a basic concept in lip reconstruction after tumor resection, J. Max. Fac. Surg. **1:**13, 1973.

Isaksson, I., and Johanson, B.: Partial reconstruction of the lower lip, Panminerva Med. **9:**420, 1967.

Jabaley, M.E., Clement, R.L., and Orcutt, T.W.: Myocutaneous flaps in lip reconstruction, Plast. Reconstr. Surg. **59:**680, 1977.

Jabaley, M.E., Orcutt, T.W., and Clement, R.L.: Applications of the Karapandzic principle of lip reconstruction after excision of lip cancer, Am. J. Surg. **132:**529, 1976.

Jesse, R.H.: Extensive cancer of the lip, Arch. Surg. **94:**509, 1967.

Johanson, B., Aspelund, E., Breine, U., and Holmstrom, H.: Surgical treatment of nontraumatic lower lip lesions with special reference to the step technique, Scand. J. Plast. Reconstr. Surg. **8:**232, 1974.

Juraha, Z.L.: Reconstruction of the lower lip with two flaps from the upper lip hinged on the superior labial vessels. Br. J. Plast. Surg. **33:**87, 1980.

Kapetansky, D.I.: Double pendulum flaps for whistling deformities in bilateral cleft lips, Plast. Reconstr. Surg. **47:**321, 1971.

Karapandzic, M.: Reconstruction of lip defects by local arterial flaps, Br. J. Plast. Surg. **27:**93, 1974.

Kawamoto, H.: Correction of major defects of vermilion with a cross-lip vermilion flap, Plast. Reconstr. Surg. **64:**315, 1979.

Koechlin, H.: Restauration de la moitie de la levre superieure, Praxis **48/49:**1142, 1959.

Kruger, E.: Reconstruction of full thickness defects of the cheek and the lips with special reference to the replacement of oral mucosa, Transactions of Fourth International Congress Plastic and Reconstructive Surgeons, Amsterdam, 1967, Excerpta Medica.

Langenbeck, B.: Carcinoma Labii inferioris cheiloplastik, Gosch. D. Klin. 278, 1854.

Lee, E.S., and Wilson, J.S.P.: Cancer of the lip, Proc. R. Soc. Med. **63:**685, 1970.

Le Fort, L.: Cheiloplastie de la levre superieure. In Malgaigne, J.F., and Le Fort, L.: Manual de Medicine Operatoire, ed. 9, Paris, 1889, Alcen.

Lentrodt, J.: Zur lippenrekonstruktion nach Tumoroperationen, Dtsch. Zahnarztl. Z. **25:**670, 1970.

Lentrodt, J., and Luhr, H.: Reconstruction of the lower lip after tumor resection combined with radical neck dissection, Plast. Reconstr. Surg. **48:**579, 1971.

Lupo, G., and Mazzola, R.F.: Our experience with lip reconstruction—a lesson from history, Clin. Plast. Surg. **11:**619, 1984.

MacFee, W.F.: A method of reconstructing the lower lip following excision for cancer, Ann. Surg. **149:**903, 1959.

Madden, J.J., Erhardt, W.L., Franklin, J.D., Withers, E.H., and Lynch, J.B.: Reconstruction of the upper and lower lip using a modified Bernard-Burow technique, Ann. Plast. Surg. **5:**100, 1980.

Marino, H., Gandolfo, E.A., and Rizzo, M.: Reconstructive surgery in cancer of the lower lip, Prensa. Med. Argent. **52:**973, 1965.

Martin, H.E.: Cheiloplasty for advanced carcinoma of the lip, SGO **54:**914, 1932.

May, H.: One-stage operation for closure of large defects of the lower lip and chin, Surg. Gynecol. Obstet. **73:**236, 1941.

May, H.: The modified Dieffenbach operation for closure of large defects of lower lip and chin, Plast. Reconstr. Surg. **1:**196, 1946.

May, H.: Surgical treatment of cancer of the lip, Plast. Reconstr. Surg. **9:**424, 1952.

Mazzola, R.F., and Lupo, G.: Evolving concepts in lip reconstruction, Clin. Plast. Surg. **11:**583, 1984.

McGregor, I.A.: Reconstruction of the lower lip, Br. J. Plast. Surg. **36:**40, 1983.

McHugh, M.: Reconstruction of the lower lip using a neurovascular island flap, Br. J. Plast. Surg. **30:**316, 1977.

McLaren, L.R.: Reconstructive surgery in the treatment of malignant disease of the mouth, Br. J. Plast. Surg. **16:**305, 1963.

Mentre, C.: Les levres, Etude anatomique, Ann. Chir. Plast. **26:**112, 1981.

Meyer, R.: A technique for the immediate reconstruction of the lower lip after ablation of tumour, Chir. Plastica (Berlin) **2:**1, 1973.

Meyer, R., and Failat, A.: New concepts in lower lip reconstruction, Head Neck Surg. **4:**240, 1982.

Millard, D.R.: A lip "fleur-de-lys" flap, Plast. Reconstru. Surg. **34:**34, 1964.

Moller, G.: Reparative surgery in cancer of the lower lip, Cir. Plast. Uruguaya **8:**101, 1967.

Morestin, H.: Technique de l'ablation des cancers de la levre inferieure, Bull. Mem. Soc. Anat. **77:**697, 1902.

Morgan, N.C.: Operation for new lip, Lancet **9:**394, 1825.

Morgan, N.C.: Operation for new under lip, Lancet **12:**537, 1828.

Morgan, N.C.: Operation for new upper lip, Lancet **13:**357, 1829.

Murphy, A.L.: An operation for cancer of the lip, Surg. Gynecol. Obstet. **111:**786, 1960.

Murray, J.F.: Total reconstruction of a lower lip with bilateral Estlander flaps, Plast. Reconstr. Surg. **49:**658, 1972.

Nelaton, C., Ombredanne, L.: Les autoplasties levres, joues, oreilles, tronc, membres, Paris, 1907, Steinheil.

New, G.B., and Figi, F.A.: The repair of postoperative defects involving the lips and cheeks secondary to the removal of malignant tumors, Surg. Gynecol. Obstet. **62:**182, 1936.

New, G.B., and Erich, J.B.: Repair of postoperative defects of the lips, Am. J. Surg. **43:**237, 1939.

Nicolau, P.J.: The orbicularis oris muscle: a functional approach to its repair in the cleft lip, Br. J. Plast. Surg. **36:**141, 1983.

O'Brien, B.: A muscle skin pedicle for total reconstruction of the lower lip, Plast. Reconstr. Surg. **45:**395, 1970.

O'Connor, C.M.: Carcinoma of the lips, reparative plasties, Bull. Acad. Argent. Cir. **54:**542, 1970.

Olivari, N.: One-stage reconstruction of the whole lower lip, Br. J. Plast. Surg. **26:**66, 1973.

Padgett, E.C.: Cheiloplasty for cancer of the lip, Int. J. Orthod. Oral Surg. **22:**939, 1936.

Page, R.E., and Stranc, M.F.: Normal lip function in adults, Ann. Plast. Surg. **9:**502, 1982.

Parsons, R.W.: Reconstruction of the lower face and lip, Clin. Plast. Surg. **2:**551, 1975.

Pelley, A.D., and Tan, E.P.: Lower lip reconstruction, Br. J. Plast. Surg. **34:**83, 1981.

Perko, M.: An interesting case of lower lip reconstruction, Br. J. Plast. Surg. **18:**285, 1965.

Perras, C.: The cancer of the lip, Am. J. Surg. **104:**746, 1962.

Pierce, G.W., Klabunde, E.H., and Brobst, H.T.: Surgical reconstruction of large lip losses. Collective review, Plast. Reconstr. Surg. **9:**68, 1952.

Pierre, M., and Jouglard, J.P.: Destruction complete de la levre inferieure chez un enfant de cinq ans. Reconstruction. Resultat eloigne. Am. Chir. Plast. **13:**119, 1968.

Platz, H., and Wepner, F.: Results of standardized lip repair after tumor resection, J. Maxillofac. Surg. **5:**108, 1977.

Reid, F.: In Wegner, E.A., editor: De Chiliplastice Labii inferioris, Jena, E. Germany, 1853, Schreiber et Fil.

Reynaud, J., and Diop, L.: Lambeaux de rotation ou lambeaux migrateurs dans les plasties labiales et labiocommissurales des nomas, Ann. Chir. Plast. **13:**128, 1968.

Romieu, C., Pujol, H., Solassol, C., and Meiss, L.: Place des reparations plastiques dans le traitment du cancer des levres, Ann. Chir. Plast. **13:**115, 1968.

Roux, J.N.: Memoire sur le cancer des levres er sur une nouvelle methode operatoire, Rev. Med. Fr. Etrang. **1:**30, 1828.

Sabattini, P.: Cenno storico dell'origine e progresso della rhinoplastica e cheiloplastica seguito della descrizione de queste operazione sopra un solo individuo, Bologna, 1838, Belle. Arti.

Sanvenero-Rosselli, G.: Plastic surgery in cancer of the face and neck. In Plastic surgery of head and neck tumors, Proceedings of First Annual Meeting of Swiss Society of Plastic and Reconstructive Surgeons (Locarno), Amsterdam, 1965, Excerpta Medica.

Sainte-Martin, L.: De la restauration de la levre inferieure apres l'ablation du cancroide, Thesis, 1873, Paris, Sorbonne.

Sawhney, C.P.: Restoration of function to a lower lip reconstructed by flaps, Plast. Reconstr. Surg. **60:**77, 1977.

Schewe, E.J.: A technique for reconstruction of the lower lip following extensive excision for cancer, Ann. Surg. **146:**285, 1957.

Schmid, E.: Plastic operations for partial or total losses of the lip, Plast. Reconstr. Surg. **14:**138, 1954.

Schmid, E.: Uber neue Moglichkeiten zur WiederHerstellung eines fehlenden Philtrums, Langenbecks Arch. f. Klin. Chir. **309:**96, 1965.

Schroder, F.: Zur Rekonstruktion von Unterlippen und Wangendefekten vach Tumorresektion, Therapiewoche **25:**44, 6618, 1975.

Schuchardt, K.: Operationen im Gesicht und im Kieferbereich, Operationen an den lippen. In Bier Braun and Kummel, eds.: Chirurgische Operationslehre, Leipzig, 1954, J.A. Barth.

Schuchardt, K.: Grundsätzliches zur primären und sekundären Defektdeckung nach der Operation von gutartigen und bösartigen Gesichtstumoren. Chir. plast. reconstr., **3:**180, 1967.

Schuchardt, K., and Luhr, H.G.: Operationen an den Lippen. In *Chirurgische Operationslehre*, Edited by Bier, Braun, Kümmell. J.A. Barth, Leipzig, 1972.

Schulten, M.W.: En method att erstta en defekt af ena lappen medelst en bryggformad lamba fran den andra, Finska Lak-Sallsk-Hande **35:**859, 1894.

Sedillot, C.: Nouveau procede de cheiloplastie procede a double lambeau, Gaz. Med. Paris, **3:**8, 1848.

Sedillot, C.: Nouveau procede de cheiloplastie par transport du bord libre de la levre saine sur la levre restauree, Compt. Rend. Ac. Sci. **42:**189, 1856.

Shimizu, H.J.: A simple method of reconstruction for extensive lower lip loss. In Marchac, D., editor: Transactions Sixth International Congress Plastic Surgeons, Paris, 1976, Masson & Cie.

Smith, F.: Some refinement in reconstructive surgery of the face, JAMA **120:**352, 1942.

Smith, J.W.: The anatomical and physiological acclimatisation of tissue transplanted by lip switch techniques, Plast. Reconstr. Surg. **26:**40, 1960.

Soussaline, M., and Kauer, C.: Reconstruction of the lower lip after radical resection for cancer, Plast. Reconstr. Surg. **60:**172, 1977.

Spiessl, B.: Möglichkeiten der Schnittführung zur en-bloc-Resektion von fortgeschrittenen regionär metastasierenden Tumoren der Mundhöhle und des Gesichtes. Dtsch. Zahn-, Mundund Kieferheilk., **43:**190, 1964.

Stein, S.A.W.: Laebedannelse (Cheiloplastik) udfort paa en ny methode, Hospitalsmiddelelser (Copenhagen) **1:**212, 1848.

Stranc, M.F., and Page, R.E.: Functional aspects of the reconstructed lip, Ann. Plast. Surg. **10:**103, 1983.

Stranc, M.F., and Robertson, G.A.: Steeple flap reconstruction of the lower lip, Ann. Plast. Surg. **10:**4, 1983.

Stricker, M.: La commissure buccale, Structure mouvent a geometrie variable, Ann. Chir. Plast. **26:**131, 1981.

Sullivan, D.E.: "Staircase" closure of lower lip defects, Ann. Plast. Surg. **1:**392, 1978.

Sung, R., Yang, P., and Liu, J.: Reconstruction of the cheek and lips, Clin. Plast. Surg. **9:**71, 1982.

Szlazak, J.: The application of a Burow's triangular flap in reconstruction of the lower lip, Br. J. Plast. Surg. **11:**128, 1958.

Szymanowski, J.: Zur plastichen chirurgie, Vierteljahr. Zeitschr. f.d. Prakt. Heilk **60:**152, 1870.

Tagliacozzi, G.: De curtorum chirurgia per insitionem, Venice, 1597, Gasper Bindoni.

Tange, I., and Takano, Y.: The lip-switch flap for the acquired defect of the lip: report on four cases, Japan, J. Plast. Reconstr. Surg. **9:**263, 1966.

Teale, T.P.: On plastic operations for the restoration of the lower lip and for the relief of several deformities of the face and neck, London, 1857, Churchill.

Thompson, N., and Pollard, A.C.: Motor function in Abbe flap, Br. J. Plast. Surg. **14:**66, 1961.

Timosca, G., Pasnicu, M., and Streba, P.: Cheiloplasty after surgical excision of the lower lip for cancer, Rev. Med. Chir. Soc. Med. Nat. Iasi. **75:**909, 1971.

Tschopp, H.M.: Reconstructive surgery after severe animal bite injuries of the head and neck area, Chir. Plast. **7:**88, 1983.

Tsur, H., Shafir, R., and Orenstein, A.: Hairbearing neck flap for upper lip reconstruction in the male, Plast. Reconstr. Surg. **71:**262, 1983.

Van Dorpe, E.J.: Simultaneous repair of the upper lip and nostril floor after tumor excisions, Plast. Reconstr. Surg. **60:**381, 1977.

Volpato, B., and Leidi, P.: Lo "staircase advancement flap" nella ricostruzione del labbro inferiore: indicazioni e risultati, Riv. It. Chir. Plast. **14:**587, 1982.

Von Bruns, V.: Chirurgischer Atlas. Bildliche Darstellung der chirurgischen Krankheiten und der zu ihrer Heilung erforderlichen Instrumente, Bandagen und Operationen, Tubingen, 1857/1860, H. Laupp'sche Buchhandlung.

Walker, A.W., and Schewe, J.E.: Nasolabial flap reconstruction for carcinoma of the lower lip, Am. J. Surg. **113:**783, 1967.

Webster, J.P.: Crescentic peri-alar cheek excision for upper lip flap advancement with a short history of upper lip repair, Plast. Reconstr. Surg. **16:**434, 1955.

Webster, R.C., Coffey, R.J., and Kelleher, R.E.: Total and partial reconstruction of the lower lip with innervated muscle-bearing flaps, Plast. Reconstr. Surg. **25:**360, 1960.

Wegner, E.A.: De chiliplastice labii inferioris, Jena, E. Germany, 1853, Schreiber et Fil.

Wexler, M.R., and Dingman, R.O.: Reconstruction of the lower lip, Chir. Plast. **3:**23, 1975.

Wilson, J.S.P., Walker, E., and Walker, E.P.: Reconstruction of the lower lip, Head Neck Surg. **4:**29, 1981.

Wustrack, K.O., and Silsby, J.J.: Reconstruction of the incompetent oral commissures with dermal muscle flaps from the face, Plast. Reconstr. Surg. **62:**118, 1978.

Yarington, C.T., and Larrabee, W.F.: Reconstruction following lip resection, Otolaryngol. Clin. North Am. **16:**407, 1983.

Zisser, G.: A contribution to the primary reconstruction of the upper lip and labial commissure, J. Maxillofac. Surg. **3:**211, 1975.

ACKNOWLEDGMENTS

I would like to thank *The British Journal of Plastic Surgery* and Churchill Livingstone for permission to reproduce photographs that appear on the following pages:

Pages 150 to 154 from Jackson, I.T., and Reid, C.D.: Nasal reconstruction and lengthening with local flaps, Br. J. Plast. Surg. **31:**343, 1978.

Pages 303 to 306 from Mustarde, J.C.: Repair and reconstruction in the orbital region, ed. 2, Edinburgh, 1980, Churchill Livingstone.

INDEX

A

Abbe flap
 for full-thickness upper lip defects, 357-360
 reversed, for small full-thickness lower lip defects, 376-379
 problems with, 379
Abbe-Estlander flap for full-thickness upper lip defects, 360-361
 problems with, 361
Advancement flap, 12-13
 crescentic, 23
  perialar
   for alar base–nasolabial region reconstruction, 245-247, 248
    problems with, 247
   for full-thickness upper lip skin defect, 362-364
    bilateral, 365-368
   for upper lip skin defects, 344-347, 355
    modification of, 348-351
 direct, 13
 horizontal, for supramedial cheek reconstruction, 232-233
  problems with, 233
 inferior, for lateral to alar base reconstruction, 248-249
  problems with, 249
 nasolabial triangular, for alar base–nasolabial region reconstruction, 242-244, 248
  problems with, 244

Advancement flap—cont'd
 for supramedial cheek reconstruction, 229-231, 241
  problems with, 231
 transverse triangular, for supramedial cheek reconstruction, 239-241
  problems with, 241
 triangular island, for lip mucosa reconstruction, 331-333
  problems with, 333
  transverse, 333-334
   problems with, 334
 vertical triangular, for supramedial cheek reconstruction, 234-236, 241
  problems with, 236
 V-Y, 12
  for lip mucosa reconstruction, 330
   problems with, 330
Aesthetics
 of cheek reconstruction, 192
 of ear reconstruction, 254
 of eyelid and canthal region reconstruction, 275
 of forehead reconstruction, 46
 of lip reconstruction, 329
 of nose reconstruction, 89
Alar base, lateral to, reconstruction, 248-249
 inferior advancement flap for, 248-249
  problems with, 249
Alar base–nasolabial region reconstruction, 242–248
 nasolabial triangular advancement flap for, 242–244, 248
  problems with, 244

441

Alar base–nasolabial region reconstruction—cont'd
  perialar crescentic advancement flap for, 245-247, 248
    problems with, 247
    surgical technique of choice for, 248
Alar rim flaps for reconstruction of columella, 139-140
Anatomy
  of cheek, 190-192
  of ear, 252-254
  of eyelid, 274
  of forehead, 44-45
  of lip, 328
  of nose, 88-89
Anesthesia
  eye, 40
  intranasal, 40
Anesthetic infiltration
  direct, 40
  local, 37
Anesthetics, administration of, 37-40

B

Back cut, 7, 29
Banner flap for lateral aspect of nose, 101-102, 127
  problems with, 102
Bilobed flap, 21-22
  for lateral reconstruction of cheek, 199-201
    problems with, 201
  for malar region reconstruction, 214-215, 223
    problems with, 215
  for nasal tip reconstruction, 134-135, 137
  for nose reconstruction, lateral aspect of, 109-117, 127
    problems with, 117
Biomechanics, skin, 4
Blood supply
  of cheek, 192
  of ear, 254
  of eyelid, 274
  of forehead, 45
  of lip, 328
  of nose, 89
Burow's triangles, 13

C

Cancer, skin, treatment of, 2
Canthal region, 275
  and lid reconstruction, 273-326
    aesthetics of, 275
    areas of, 276-325
    incisions for, placement of, 276
    tissue availability for, areas of, 276
Canthus, 275
  lateral, 275
    reconstruction of, with forehead flap, 323-325
      problems with, 325
      surgical technique of choice for, 325
  medial, 275
    reconstruction of, 90-99, 312-316
      complex, 316-322
      finger flap for, 94-95, 99
        problems with, 95
      with full-thickness lid reconstruction, 316-322
        forehead and cheek rotation flaps for, 317-322
        problems with, 322
      glabellar flaps for, 90-99
        classic, 91-94
        problems with, 94
      glabellar island flap for, 96-99
        problems with, 99
      split finger flap for, 313-316
        problems with, 316
      surgical technique of choice for, 99
Cheek
  aesthetics of, 192
  anatomy of, 190-192
  blood supply of, 192
  incisions in, placement of, 192
  and lower lip reconstruction, 383-387
  lymphatic system of, 192
  malar region of; *see* Malar region reconstruction
  musculature of, 190
  nerve supply of, 190-191
    motor, 190
    sensory, 191
  reconstruction of, 189-249
    areas of, 193-249
      lateral, 193-204
        bilobed flap for, 199-201

Cheek—cont'd
  reconstruction of—cont'd
    lateral—cont'd
      bilobed flap for—cont'd
        problems with, 201
      preauricular transposition flap for, 194-195, 204
        problems with, 195
      rhomboid flap for, 202-203
        problems with, 203
      rotation flap for, 196-198, 204
        problems with, 198
      surgical technique of choice for, 204
    lower, 204-210
      rhomboid flap for, 205-206, 210
        problems with, 206
      rotation flap for, 209-210
        problems with, 210
      surgical technique of choice for, 210
      transposition flap for, 207-208, 210
        problems with, 208
    supramedial; see Supramedial cheek reconstruction
  skin of, 190
  tissue availability for, areas of, 193
Cheek advancement technique, Webster, for total lower lip reconstruction, 391-396
  problems with, 396
Cheek axial flap for reconstruction of nasal lining, 155-157
Cheek rotation flap; see Rotation flap, cheek
Chondromucosal graft and cheek rotation flap for total lower lid reconstruction, 289-293
  problems with, 293
Cocaine for intranasal anesthesia, 40
Columella, reconstruction of, 137-140
  alar rim flaps for, 139-140
  fork flaps for, 139
  nasolabial flap for, 138
Commissure defects, 399-411
  full-thickness, reconstruction of, 402-411
    double skin and mucosal rhomboid flaps for, 402-405, 411
    double skin rhomboid flaps and tongue flaps for, 406-411
      problems with, 411

Commissure defects—cont'd
  mucosal, reconstruction of, 399-402
    rhomboid flaps for, 399-401
      problems with, 401
    tongue flaps for, 401-402
      problems with, 402
Complications of forehead reconstruction, management of, 84
Creep and stress relaxation of skin, 5
Crescentic advancement flap, 23
  perialar
    for alar base–nasolabial region reconstruction, 245-247, 248
      problems with, 247
    for full-thickness upper lip skin defect, 362-364
      bilateral, 365-368
        problems with, 368
    for upper lip skin defect, 344-347, 356
      modification of, 348-351
        problems with, 351

D

Defect and donor area, examination of, 6
Direct closure of small full-thickness lip defects, 376
  problems with, 376
Direct local infiltration, 40
Direct transverse closure of nasal tip, 136-137
"Dog ear," 8, 30-31
Donor and defect area, examination of, 6
Dufourmentel flap, 20-21
  for temporal skin defects, 70-76
    problems with, 76

E

Ear
  anatomy of, 252-254
  blood supply of, 254
  conchal defect of, anterior, 257-261
    postauricular "revolving door" island flap for reconstruction of, 257-261
      problems with, 261
  lobule of, reconstruction of, 271
  lymphatic drainage of, 254
  musculature of, 253
    extrinsic, 253
    intrinsic, 253

Ear—cont'd
  nerve supply of, 253
    motor, 253
    sensory, 253
  partial defect of, 261-266
    postauricular flap for, 262-266
      problems with, 266
  reconstruction of, 251-271
    aesthetics of, 254
    areas of, 255-261
    incisions for, placement of, 254
    tissue availability for, areas of, 255
  rim defects of, 255-257
    neck tube pedicles for, 271
    rim advancement for, 256-257
      problems with, 257
  total resurfacing of, 267-271
    temporalis fascia flap for, 267-271
      problems with, 271
Epinephrine for anesthesia, 37
Examination and evaluation of patient, 35
Extension curve, in vitro, of skin, 4
Eye anesthesia, 40
Eyelid
  anatomy of, 274
    blood supply of, 274
  and canthal region reconstruction, 273-326
    aesthetics of, 275
    areas of, 276-325
    complex, 316-322
    incisions for, placement of, 276
    tissue availability for, areas of, 276
  function of, 276
  lower, reconstruction of, 277-293
    partial, 280-286
      cheek rotation flap for, 280-286
        problems with, 286
      for skin defect, 277-280
        bilateral Tripier flap for, 279-280
          problems with, 280
      unilateral Tripier flap for, 277-278
      surgical technique of choice for, 293
    total, 286-293
      cheek rotation flap and chondromucosal graft for, 289-293
        problems with, 293
      forehead flap for, 286-289
        problems with, 288-289
  lymphatic drainage of, 275
  musculature of, 274

Eyelid—cont'd
  nerve supply of, 274
  skin of, 274
  upper, reconstruction of, 294-312
    partial, 294-302
      lid rotation flap for, 298-302
        problems with, 302
      lid switch flap for, 294-297
        problems with, 297
      surgical technique of choice for, 302
    total, 303-312
      cheek rotation and lower lid switch flap for, 303-307
        problems with, 307
      surgical technique of choice for, 312
      two-stage lower lid switch and cheek rotation flap for, 307-311, 312
        problems with, 311
Eyelid switch flap
  for partial upper lid reconstruction, 294-297
    problems with, 297
  total lower, and cheek rotation flap for upper lid reconstruction, 303-307
    problems with, 307
  two-stage lower, and cheek rotation flap for upper lid reconstruction, 307-311, 312

F

Fan flap for reconstruction of lower lip, 388-391
  bilateral, 396-398
    problems with, 398
  problems with, 391
Finger flap
  for reconstruction of medial canthus, 94-95, 99
    problems with, 95
  split, for reconstruction of medial canthus, 313-316
    problems with, 316
Flap
  Abbe, 257-360
    reversed, 376-379
      problems with, 379
  Abbe-Estlander, 360-361
    problems with, 361
  advancement; *see* Advancement flap
  alar rim, 139-140

Flap—cont'd
  Banner, 101-102, 127
    problems with, 102
  bilobed; *see* Bilobed flap
  cheek axial, 155-157
  cheek rotation; *see* Rotation flap, cheek
  disadvantages of, 3
  Dufourmentel; *see* Dufourmentel flap
  effectiveness of, compared to graft, 2
  eyelid, upper, rotation, 298-302
    problems with, 302
  eyelid switch; *see* Eyelid switch flap
  failure of, 32
  fan, 388-391
    bilateral, 396-398
      problems with, 398
    problems with, 391
  finger; *see* Finger flap
  forehead; *see* Forehead flap
  fork, 139
  Fricke; *see* Forehead flap
  galeal frontalis, 165-168
  Gillies, 371-372
  glabellar; *see* Glabellar flap
  glabellar island, 96-99
    problems with, 99
  hatchet, 63-65
    problems with, 65
  in head and neck reconstruction
    general considerations in, 1-34
    general principles in, 3-6
  island; *see* Island advancement flap; Island flap
  Karapandzic; *see* Karapandzic flap; Karapandzic technique
  Lambeau en L pour losange "LLL"; *see* Dufourmentel flap
  Limberg; *see* Rhomboid flap
  local; *see* Local flap
  movement of, procedures to facilitate, 24-31
  nasolabial; *see* Nasolabial flap
  necrosis of, 32
  postauricular, 262-266
    problems with, 266
    "revolving door" island, 257-261
  preauricular transposition, 194-195
    problems with, 195
  rhomboid; *see* Rhomboid flap
  Rintala, 132-133, 137
    problems with, 133

Flap—cont'd
  rotation; *see* Rotation flap
  Schmid, 172-177
    problems with, 177
  temporalis fascia, 267-271
    problems with, 271
  tongue; *see* Tongue flap
  transposition; *see* Transposition flap
  triangular island advancement; *see* Advancement flap, triangular island
  triangular kite, 136
  Tripier
    bilateral, 279-280
      problems with, 280
    unilateral, 277-278
  Washio, 178-184, 187
    problems with, 184
  Webster cheek advancement, 391-396
    problems with, 396
Forehead
  anatomy of, 44-45
  blood supply of, 45
  lymphatics of, 45
  musculature of, 44
  nerve supply of, 45
  reconstruction of, 43-85
    aesthetics of, 46
    areas of, 47
    complications from, management of, 84
    main, 48-59
      bilateral rotation flap for, 58-59
        problems with, 59
      factors to consider in, 48
      scalp rotation for, 48
      surgical techniques of choice for, 84
      unilateral rotation flap for, 49-53
        problems with, 52-53
      Worthen rotation flap for, 54-57
        problems with, 57
    surgical options for, 47
    tissue availability for, areas of, 47
  skin of, 44
    appearance of, 44
    color of, 44
    texture of, 44
Forehead flap
  and cheek rotation flap for complex reconstruction of medial canthus, 317-322
    problems with, 322

Forehead flap—cont'd
  for reconstruction of lateral canthus, 323-325
    problems with, 325
  for subtotal reconstruction of nose, 169-172, 187
  for total lower lid reconstruction, 286-293
  for total nose reconstruction, 158-162, 168
    and local in-turned flap, 163-165
Fork flaps for reconstruction of columella, 139
Fricke flap; *see* Forehead flap

G

Galeal frontalis flap for total reconstruction of nose, 165-168
Gillies flap for total upper lip reconstruction, 371-372
Glabellar flap
  classic, for medial canthus reconstruction, 91-94
    problems with, 94
  extended, for reconstruction of lateral aspect of nose, 107-109
    problems with, 109
  for medial canthus reconstruction, 90-99
    problems with, 94
Glabellar island flap for reconstruction of medial canthus, 96-99
  problems with, 99
Glabellar reconstruction, 77-83
  rhomboid flaps for, 77-79
    problems with, 83
  transposition flaps for, multiple, 80-83
    problems with, 83
Graft
  chondromucosal, and cheek rotation flap for total lower eyelid reconstruction, 289-293
    problems with, 293
  effectiveness of, compared to flap, 2
  for nasal lining, 141
    problems with, 141
  nasolabial, 2

H

Hatchet flaps for supraeyebrow reconstruction, 63-65
  problems with, 65
Head and neck reconstruction, flaps in, general considerations, 1-34

History, medical, 35
Hyaluronidase for anesthesia, 37

I

Incisions, placement of
  for cheek reconstruction, 192
  for ear reconstruction, 254
  for eyelid and canthal region reconstruction, 276
  for forehead reconstruction, 46-47
  for lip reconstruction, 329
  for nose reconstruction, 89
Intranasal anesthesia, 40
Intraoperative care, 41
Island advancement flap, triangular, for reconstruction of lip mucosa, 331-333
  problems with, 333
  transverse, 333-334
    problems with, 334
Island flap, 14-15
  for supraeyebrow reconstruction, 60-69
    problems with, 62

K

Karapandzic flap
  for large full-thickness defects of lower lip, 380-382
  for lower lip and cheek reconstruction, 383-387
    problems with, 386-387
  reversed, for full-thickness defects of upper lip, 369-370
    problems with, 370
Karapandzic technique, 380-381

L

Lambeau en L pour losange "LLL" flap; *see* Dufourmentel flap
Lateral canthus; *see* Canthus, lateral
Lid; *see* Eyelid
Lidocaine hydrochloride and epinephrine for anesthesia, 37
Limberg flap; *see* Rhomboid flap
Lines of minimal relaxed tension, 6
Lip
  anatomy of, 328
  blood supply of, 328

INDEX

Lip—cont'd
  commissure defects of, reconstruction of, 399-411
    full-thickness, 402-411
      double skin and mucosal rhomboid flaps for, 402-405
      double skin rhomboid flaps and tongue flaps for, 406-411
      problems with, 411
    mucosal, 399-402
      rhomboid flaps for, 399-401
        problems with, 401
      tongue flap for, 401-402
        problems with, 402
  defects of, full-thickness
    large, reconstruction of, 376-391
      Abbe flap, reversed, for, 376-379
      fan flap for, 388-391
        problems with, 391
      Karapandzic technique for, 380-382, 391
      surgical technique of choice for, 391
    small, direct closure of, 376
      problems with, 376
  lower, reconstruction of, 373-398
    and cheek, 383-387
      Karapandzic flap for, 383-387
        problems with, 386-387
    mucosal defect of, extensive, 335-340
      factors to consider in, 335
      mucosal advancement for, 335
        problems with, 335
      tongue flap for, 335-340
        problems with, 339-340
    skin defects of, 373-375
      inferiorly based nasolabial flap for, 373-374
      problems with, 374
    total, 391-398
      fan flaps, bilateral, for, 396-398
        problems with, 398
      surgical technique of choice for, 398
      Webster cheek advancement technique for, 391-396
        problems with, 396
  lymphatic drainage of, 329
  mucosa of, reconstruction of, 330-343
    rotation flap for, 330
      problems with, 330
    surgical technique of choice for, 334

Lip—cont'd
  mucosa of, reconstruction of—cont'd
    triangular island advancement flap for, 331-333
      problems with, 333
    transverse, 333-334
      problems with, 334
    V-Y advancement flap for, 330
      problems with, 330
  musculature of, 328
  nerve supply of, 328
  reconstruction of, 327-412
    aesthetics of, 329
    areas of, 329-411
    commissure defect of, 399-411
    incisions for, placement of, 329
    tissue availability for, areas of, 329
  upper, reconstruction of, 344-370
    full-thickness defects of, 357-370
      Abbe flap for, 357-360, 370
      Abbe-Estlander flap for, 360-361
        problems with, 361
      perialar crescentic advancement flap for, 362-364
        bilateral, 365-368
        problems with, 368
      reversed Karapandzic flap for, 369-370
        problems with, 370
    mucosal defect of, extensive, 341-343
      tongue flap for, 341-343
        problems with, 343
    skin defects of, 344-356
      perialar crescentic advancement flap for, 344-347, 355
        modification of, 348-351
      surgical technique of choice for, 355-356
      two-stage nasolabial flap for, 352-354, 355-356
        problems with, 354
    total, 371-372
      Gillies flap for, 371
      nasolabial flap for, 371-372
LLL flap; *see* Dufourmentel flap
Local anesthetic infiltration, 37
  direct, 40
Local flap
  advantages of, 2
  complications of, 32-33

Local flap—cont'd
  in-turned
    and forehead flap for total reconstruction of nose, 163-165
    for reconstruction of nasal lining, 142-146
      problems with, 146
  types of, 16-23
Lymphatic drainage
  of ear, 254
  of eyelid, 275
  of lip, 329
  of nose, 89
Lymphatic system of cheek, 192
Lymphatics of forehead, 45

M

Malar region reconstruction
  bilobed flap for, 214-215
    problems with, 215
  lateral cheek rotation flap for, 218-223
    problems with, 223
  rhomboid flap for, 210-213
    problems with, 213
  surgical technique of choice for, 223
  transposition flap for, 216-217
    problems with, 217
Medial canthus; see Canthus, medial
Medical history, 35
Mental nerve block, 39
Musculature
  of cheek, 190
  of ear, 253
  of eyelid, 274
  of forehead, 44
  of lip, 328
  of nose, 88

N

Nasal lining, reconstruction of, 141
  cheek axial flap for, 155-157
  local in-turned flap for, 142-146
    problems with, 146
  nasolabial flap for, 147-149
    bilateral, 150-154
    problems with, 154
  skin graft for, 141
    problems with, 141
  surgical technique of choice for, 158
Nasal reconstruction; see Nose, reconstruction of

Nasal skin reconstruction, 158
Nasal tip, reconstruction of, 128-136
  bilobed flap for, 134-135, 137
  direct transverse closure of, 136-137
  nasolabial flap for, 128-131, 137
    problems with, 131
  Rintala flap for, 132-133, 137
    problems with, 133
  surgical technique of choice for, 137
  triangular kite flap for, 136
Nasolabial flap
  for columella reconstruction, 138
  inferiorly based, for skin defects of lower lip, 373-375
    problems with, 375
  island, for reconstruction of lateral aspect of nose, 124-127
    problems with, 126-127
  for lip reconstruction, upper, 371-372
  for nasal lining reconstruction, 147-149
    bilateral, 150-154
    problems with, 154
  for nasal tip reconstruction, 128-131, 137
    problems with, 131
  for nose reconstruction, lateral aspect of, 118-123
  transposition, for supramedial cheek reconstruction, 237-238
    problems with, 238
  triangular advancement, for alar base–nasolabial reconstruction, 242-244
    problems with, 244
  two-stage, for skin defects of upper lip, 352-354, 355-356
    problems with, 354
Nasolabial region–alar base; see Alar base–nasolabial region reconstruction
Nasolabial skin graft, 2
Neck skin for subtotal reconstruction of nose, 185-187
  problems with, 187
Neck tube pedicles for reconstruction of rim of ear, 271
Necrosis, flap, 32
Nerve block
  infraorbital, 39
  mental, 39
  supraorbital, 38
  technique for, 38-39

Nerve supply
    of cheek, 190-191
    of ear, 253
    of eyelid, 274
    of forehead, 45
    of lip, 328
    of nose, 88
Nose
    anatomy of, 88-89
    blood supply of, 89
    lateral aspect of, reconstruction of, 100-127
        Banner flap for, 101-102, 127
            problems with, 102
        bilobed flap for, 109-117, 127
            problems with, 117
        extended rhomboid flap for, 107-109
            problems with, 109
        nasolabial flap for, 118-123
        nasolabial island flap for, 124-127
        rhomboid flap for, 103-106
            problems with, 106
        surgical procedure of choice for, 127
    lining of; see Nasal lining
    lymphatic drainage of, 89
    medial canthus of; see Canthus, medial
    musculature of, 88
    nerve supply of, 88
    reconstruction of, 87-188
        aesthetics of, 89
        areas of, 90-140
        complex, 141-187
        complications of, 188
        incisions for, placement of, 89
        subtotal, 169-187
            forehead flap for, 169-172, 187
            neck skin for, 184-187
                problems with, 187
            Schmid flap for, 172-177
                problems with, 177
            surgical technique of choice for, 187
            Washio flap for, 178-184, 187
                problems with, 184
        total, 158-168
            forehead flap for, 158-162, 168
                and local in-turned flap, 163-165
            galeal frontalis flap for, 165-168
            surgical procedure of choice for, 168
        tissue availability for, areas of, 89

Nose—cont'd
    skin of, 88
        reconstruction of, 158
    tip of; see Nasal tip

O

Opthaine; see Proparcaine for topical anesthesia

P

Patient
    examination and evaluation of, 35
    intraoperative care of, 41
    management of, 35-41
    postoperative care of, 41
    preoperative care of, 36
Pincushioning, 19, 32-33
Postoperative care, 41
Preauricular transposition flap for lateral cheek reconstruction, 194-195, 204
    problems with, 195
Preoperative care, 36
Proparcaine for topical anesthesia, 40

R

Regional nerve block, 37-39
"Revolving door" island flap, postauricular, for reconstruction of anterior conchal defect, 257-261
    problems with, 261
Rhomboid flap, 16-19
    for commissure mucosal defect, 399-401
        problems with, 401
    double, 18
        and mucosal flap, for full-thickness commissure defect, 402-405
        and tongue flap, for full-thickness commissure defect, 406-411
            problems with, 411
    for glabellar reconstruction, 77-79
        problems with, 83
    for lateral reconstruction of cheek, 202-203
        problems with, 203
    for lower cheek reconstruction, 205-206, 210
        problems with, 210
    for malar region reconstruction, 210-213, 223
        problems with, 213
    for nose reconstruction, lateral aspect of, 103-106

449

Rhomboid flap—cont'd
  for nose reconstruction—cont'd
    problems with, 106
  for supraeyebrow reconstruction, 66-69
    problems with, 69
  for temporal skin defect, 70-76
  triple, 19
Rim defects of ear, 255-257
  rim advancement for, 256-257
    problems with, 257
Rintala flap for reconstruction of nasal tip, 132-133
Rotation flap, 7-10
  bilateral, for forehead reconstruction, 58-59
    problems with, 59
  cheek
    and chondromucosal graft, for total lower lid reconstruction, 289-293
      problems with, 293
    and forehead flap, for complex reconstruction of medial canthus, 316-322
      problems with, 322
    lateral, for malar region reconstruction, 218-223
      problems with, 223
    for partial lid reconstruction, 280-286
      problems with, 286
    and total lower lid switch flap for upper lid reconstruction, 303-307
      problems with, 307
    and two-stage lower lid switch flap for total upper lid reconstruction, 307-311, 312
      problems with, 311
    inferior, for supramedial cheek reconstruction, 226-228
      problems with, 228
    lateral, for supramedial cheek reconstruction, 223-225
    for lateral cheek reconstruction, 196-198, 204
      problems with, 198
  for lip mucosa reconstruction, 330
  for lower cheek reconstruction, 209-210
    problems with, 210
  unilateral, for forehead reconstruction, 49-53
    problems with, 52-53

Rotation flap—cont'd
  upper eyelid, for partial lid reconstruction, 298-302
    problems with, 302
  Worthen, for forehead reconstruction, 54-57
    problems with, 57

S

Scalp rotation for forehead reconstruction, 48
Schmid flap for subtotal reconstruction of nose, 172-177
  problems with, 177
Skin
  advancement of, 12-13
  biomechanics of, 4
  cheek, 190
  eyelid, 274
  forehead, 44
    appearance of, 44
    color of, 44
    texture of, 44
  neck, for subtotal reconstruction of nose, 185-187
    problems with, 187
  nose, 88
    reconstruction of, 158
  rotation of, 7-10
  stress relaxation and creep of, 5
  transposition of, 10-11
  viscoelastic properties of, 5
Skin cancer, treatment of, 2
Skin defects, temporal; *see* Temporal skin defects
Skin flap; *see* Flap
Skin graft; *see* Graft
Skin in vitro extension curve, 4
Skin movement, methods of, 7-15
Split finger flap for reconstruction of medial canthus, 312-316
  problems with, 316
Stress relaxation and creep of skin, 5
Supraeyebrow reconstruction
  hatchet flap for, 63-65
    problems with, 65
  island flap for, 60-62
    problems with, 62
  rhomboid flap for, 66-69
    problems with, 69
Supramedial cheek reconstruction, 223-241
  advancement flap for, 229-231, 241

Supramedial cheek reconstruction—cont'd
    advancement flap for—cont'd
        horizontal, 232-233
            problems with, 233
        nasolabial, 237-238
            problems with, 238
        problems with, 231
        transverse triangular, 239-241
            problems with, 241
        vertical triangular, 234-236, 241
            problems with, 236
    rotation flap for
        inferior, 226-228
            problems with, 228
        lateral, 223-225
            problems with, 225
    surgical technique of choice for, 241
Supraorbital nerve block, 38
Surgical approach, planning, 6-31

T

Temporal skin defects, reconstruction of, 70-76
    with double rhomboid flap, 73-76
        problems with, 76
    with rhomboid or Dufourmentel flap, 70-72
        problems with, 76
Temporalis fascia flap for total ear resurfacing, 267-271
Tension
    minimal relaxed, lines of, 6
    and vascularity, relationship between, 5
Tissue availability, areas of, 6
    for cheek reconstruction, 193
    for ear reconstruction, 255
    for eyelid and canthal region reconstruction, 276
    for forehead reconstruction, 47
    for lip reconstruction, 329
    for nose reconstruction, 89
Tissue expanders, 5
Tongue flap
    for commissure mucosal defects, 401-402
        problems with, 402
    and double skin rhomboid flaps for full-thickness commissure defects, 406-411
        problems with, 411
    for lower lip mucosal defects, 335-340
        problems with, 339-349

Tongue flap—cont'd
    for upper lip mucosal defects, 341-343
        problems with, 343
Transposition flap, 10-11
    for lower cheek reconstruction, 207-208, 210
        problems with, 208
    for malar region reconstruction, 216-217
        problems with, 217
    multiple, for glabellar reconstruction, 80-83
        problems with, 83
    nasolabial, for supramedial cheek reconstruction, 237-238
        problems with, 238
    preauricular, for lateral cheek reconstruction, 194-195, 204
        problems with, 195
"Trap-dooring," 19
Triangular advancement flap
    nasolabial, for alar base–nasolabial region reconstruction, 242-244, 248
        problems with, 244
    transverse, for supramedial cheek reconstruction, 239-241
        problems with, 241
    vertical, for supramedial cheek reconstruction, 234-236, 241
        problems with, 236
Triangular island advancement flap for lip mucosa defects, 331-333
    problems with, 333
    transverse, 333-334
        problems with, 334
Triangular kite flap for reconstruction of nasal tip, 136
Tripier flap for lower lid skin defect
    bilateral, 279-280
        problems with, 280
    unilateral, 277-278
Tumor recurrence, 32

V

Valium for sedation, 35
Vascularity and tension, relationship between, 5
Viscoelastic properties of skin, 5
V-Y advancement flap, 12
    for lip mucosa reconstruction, 330
        problems with, 330

W

Washio flap for subtotal reconstruction of nose, 178-184, 187
  problems with, 184
Webster cheek advancement technique for total lower lip reconstruction, 391-396
  problems with, 396
Worthen rotation flap for forehead reconstruction, 54-57

X

Xylocaine; *see* Lidocaine hydrochloride and epinephrine for anesthesia

Z

Z-plasty, 24-26
  four-flap, 27